HIV/AIDS
in South Africa

THIS DEFINITIVE TEXT covers all aspects of HIV/AIDS in South Africa, from basic science to medicine, sociology, economics and politics. It has been written by a highly respected team of South African HIV/AIDS experts and provides a thoroughly researched account of the epidemic in the region.

The book comprises seven sections, the first of which describes the evolving epidemic, presents the numbers behind the epidemic, and captures its nature in one of the worst affected parts of the world. This is followed by a section on the science of the virus, covering its structure, and its diagnosis. HIV risk factors and prevention strategies, focal population groups and the impact of HIV/AIDS in all aspects of South African life are discussed in the next four sections. The final sections look at the treatment of HIV/AIDS, the politics of HIV/AIDS treatment, mathematical modelling to extrapolate the potential impact of treatment and finally a discussion of the future of HIV/AIDS in South Africa.

This text has been written at an accessible level for the general reader, undergraduate and postgraduate students, health care providers, researchers and policymakers in this field as well as international scholars studying HIV/AIDS in Africa.

"... taken altogether this wealth of information illuminates the path of this dark disease ... As you, the reader, page through this book, I hope and trust that you will hear the call to action."
– Nelson Mandela

"South Africa possesses the capacity to both curb the epidemic and to minimise its impact – dedicated efforts by its government and civil society are already underway. A wealth of essential evidence is available in this book, making it a valuable contribution to the effort against AIDS in South Africa."
– Peter Piot

D1451990

HIV/AIDS
in South Africa

Edited by S. S. Abdool Karim and Q. Abdool Karim

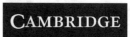

CAMBRIDGE UNIVERSITY PRESS
Cambridge, New York, Melbourne, Madrid, Cape Town, Singapore, São Paulo

Cambridge University Press
The Water Club, Beach Road, Granger Bay, Cape Town 8005, South Africa

Published in the United States of America by Cambridge University Press, New York

www.cambridge.org
Information on this title: www.cambridge.org/9780521616294
© Cambridge University Press 2005, 2008

First published 2005

Editor: Dr Bridget Farham
Indexer: Jeane Cope
Proof reader: Ethné Clark
Illustrators: James Whitelaw, Vanessa Wilson, Adele Wilson
Design: The Nimble Mouse, Cape Town
Cover design: Karen Ahshläger
Typesetting: Vanessa Wilson (Serengeti Media)
Typeset in 9.5 pt Swift-Regular

Printed in South Africa by Creda Communications

ISBN-13 978-0-521-61629-4 paperback
ISBN-10 0-521-61629-8 paperback

. . . .

This book is dedicated to
    all those infected and affected by HIV,
    those who valiantly protect the rights and dignity of those
        infected,
    those in the frontline of service provision for prevention and
        care, and
    those who persevere in finding new prevention and treatment
        options to enhance our response to impact on this pandemic

Special tribute to Zubada Bibi Abdool Karim – mother, carer and humanitarian.

Contents

Section 1 **The evolving HIV epidemic**

1 Introduction..31
   Salim S. Abdool Karim and Cheryl Baxter
2 Overview of the book...37
   Salim S. Abdool Karim, Quarraisha Abdool Karim and Cheryl Baxter
3 HIV infection in South Africa: the evolving epidemic.............48
   Eleanor Gouws and Quarraisha Abdool Karim
4 HIV incidence rates in South Africa...67
   Eleanor Gouws

Section 2 **The virus, the human host and their interactions**

5 Viral structure, replication, tropism, pathogenesis and
   natural history...79
   Lynn Morris and Tonie Cilliers
6 HIV diagnostics...89
   Adrian Puren
7 Origin, diversity and spread of HIV-1.....................................109
   Carolyn Williamson and Darren P. Martin
8 Cellular immunity in HIV: a sythesis of responses to
   preserve self..119
   Clive Gray

Section 3 **HIV risk factors and prevention strategies**

9 Reducing sexual risk behaviours: Theory and research,
   successes and challenges..143
   Catherine Mathews
10 Barrier methods...166
   Landon Myer
11 Mother-to-child transmission (MTCT) of HIV-1.....................183
   Hoosen 'Jerry' Coovadia
12 Sexually transmitted infections...193
   David Coetzee and Leigh Johnson
13 Safe blood supplies..203
   Anton Heyns and Johanna P. Swanevelder
14 Intravenous drug use in South Africa......................................217
   Ted Leggett

15 New prevention strategies under development and
    investigation..226
    Salim S. Abdool Karim and Cheryl Baxter

Section 4 Focal groups for understanding the HIV epidemic

16 Heterosexual transmission of HIV – the importance of
    a gendered perspective in HIV prevention.................................243
    Quarraisha Abdool Karim
17 Young people and HIV/AIDS in South Africa: Prevalence
    of infection, risk factors and social context...........................262
    Abigail Harrison
18 Female sex workers...285
    Gita Ramjee
19 Population movement and the spread of HIV in
    southern Africa..298
    Mark Lurie
20 Young men..313
    Gethwana Makahye

Section 5 The impact of AIDS

21 Shattering the silence – an auto-biographic, reflective
    narrative on living with HIV/AIDS...321
    Lilian Benita Mboyi
22 Impact of AIDS – the health care burden...................................336
    Mark Colvin
23 The impact of AIDS on the community..351
    Janet Frohlich
24 The achilles heel? The impact of HIV/AIDS on democracy
    in South Africa...371
    Mark Heywood
25 The impact on ethics...384
    Jerome Singh
26 The economic impact of AIDS...405
    Alan Whiteside
27 AIDS-related mortality in South Africa.......................................419
    Debbie Bradshaw and Rob Dorrington

Section 6 Treating HIV

28 TB and HIV...433
       Gavin Churchyard and Elizabeth Corbet
29 Prevention of opportunistic infections in adults 454
       Gary Maartens
30 Nutritional prophylaxis 463
       Marianne Visser
31 Challenges in managing AIDS in South Africa 477
       Douglas Wilson and Lara Fairall
32 Antiretroviral therapy 504
       Robin Wood
33 The challenges of implementing antiretroviral treatment
       in South Africa...524
       Andrew Gray
34 The political history of AIDS treatment................................538
       Nawaal Deane

Section 7 What does the future hold?

35 Models and trends 551
       Brian Williams
36 The future of the HIV epidemic in South Africa...................567
       Salim S. Abdool Karim and Quarraisha Abdool Karim

Contributors

Cheryl Baxter, MSc is an associate researcher for the Centre for the AIDS Programme of Research in South Africa (CAPRISA). She assists with writing of research grants and contributes to the scientific output of the Centre through publications and annual reports. Her current research interests include prevention of HIV infection, particularly women-controlled methods. She also assists the corresponding editor of the *International Journal of Infectious Diseases* to source and select reviewers.

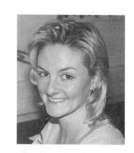

Debbie Bradshaw, MSc, DPhil (Oxon) is an established researcher in mortality and epidemiology in South Africa. She heads the Medical Research Council Burden of Disease Research Unit and is an honorary associate Professor in the University of Cape Town Department of Public Health and Family Medicine. Her main research interests are mortality profiles and health transition. She was part of the team that developed methods to assess the impact of AIDS on adult mortality and led the team that conducted the first South African National Burden of Disease Study. She has published many papers and serves on several advisory committees in the health and health research arena.

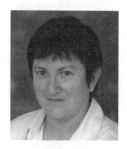

Gavin Churchyard, MBChB, MMED (Internal Medicine), FCP (SA), PhD is a specialist physician, internationally-renowned for his contributions in tuberculosis (TB). He is the Chief Executive Officer of Aurum Health Research, an independent industry-based health research unit and a honorary associate Professor, Department of Medicine, School of Clinical Sciences in the Faculty of Health Sciences, University of KwaZulu-Natal, Honorary Associate Professor at the University of Cape Town, School of Public Health and Family Medicine and Honorary Senior Lecturer at the London School of Hygiene and Tropical medicine. Churchyard is the principal investigator on a number of industry-based studies focusing on TB, HIV and occupational lung disease. He is a member of the executive committee of the International Consortium to Respond Effectively to the AIDS/TB Epidemic (CREATE), funded by the Bill and Melinda Gates Foundation. He serves on the executive committee of the NIH funded Centre for the AIDS Programme of Research in South Africa (CAPRISA) and on the South African AIDS Vaccine Initiative senior investigators committee. He is a member of the South African Tuberculosis Trials Consortium and has consulted for the World Health Organisation and UNAIDS on TB and cotrimoxazole preventive therapy for HIV infected individuals. He has contributed to industry, national and international guidelines for TB preventive therapy.

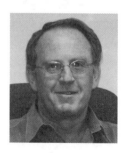

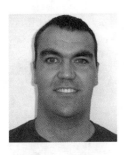

Tonie Cilliers, MSc has submitted his PhD at the University of the Witwatersrand and is based at the National Institute for Communicable Diseases. He has worked on HIV-1 coreceptors and has isolated and characterised over 200 HIV-1 subtype C viruses. His main project was to determine the sensitivity of HIV-1 subtype C isolates to entry inhibitors that target different stages of the viral entry process. In November 2000, he received a Fogarty International AIDS Fellowship to visit Dr John Moore's laboratory where he acquired the skills to perform entry inhibitor studies. As a follow-up he received training in Dr Alexandra Trkola's laboratory sponsored by a WHO African AIDS Vaccine Program training fellowship. He has ten publications in peer-reviewed journals. A large portion of his work has been presented at international conferences. He received a grant from Bristol-Meyers Squibb 'Secure-the-Future' to perform pre-cinical studies on the effectiveness of a new class of antiretroviral drugs targeting the coreceptor or binding regions of HIV-1 subtype C viruses.

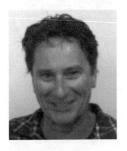

David Coetzee, BA, MBBCh, FFCH, MS is a clinical infectious diseases epidemiologist whose main research interests are in the prevention and management of HIV infection including the implementation of antiretroviral therapy in resource-constrained settings. He is a Senior Specialist and Head of the Infectious Disease and Epidemiology Unit at the School of Public Health and Family Medicine at the University of Cape Town. The Unit has worked with Médecins Sans Frontières to develop the HIV services in Khayelitsha where antiretrovirals are provided. His unit is currently conducting a microbicide trial and a trial to measure the efficacy of twice daily acyclovir suppressive therapy in preventing HIV transmission among heterosexual HIV-discordant couples.

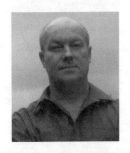

Mark Colvin, BSc, MBChB, DOH, MS is a senior research associate at CADRE, South Africa and an honorary lecturer in the School of Public Health, Nelson R. Mandela School of Medicine, University of KwaZulu-Natal, Durban. He an infectious diseases epidemiologist. Dr Colvin's research interests centre around the epidemiology of STIs and HIV in southern Africa with a focus on surveillance studies. He has conducted HIV surveillance and behavioural studies on the general population, in prisons, health services and in numerous workplaces. Other related research activities include STI intervention trials, research into preventing mother-to-child transmission of HIV and investigating how traditional healers may be incorporated into community-based TB DOTS programmes. Currently Dr Colvin has active collaborations with several other national research organisations including the Health Systems Trust and the Human Sciences

Research Council and he has been a principal investigator or collaborator on grants received from the NIH, Wellcome Trust, the World Health Organisation, DFID, the European Union and the World Bank.

Hoosen (Jerry) Coovadia, MBBS, MD is a paediatrician and expert in perinatal HIV transmission. Dr Coovadia was the Head of the Department of Paediatrics at the University of Natal until 2000, and is now the Victor Daitz Professor for HIV/AIDS research at the University of KwaZulu-Natal. He has made substantial contributions in paediatric diseases, including the definitive work on nephrosis in South African black children, malnutrition and immunity, measles, particularly the effect of Vitamin A supplementation on children with measles and other infections. He is internationally recognised for his ground-breaking research in HIV/AIDS transmission from mother to child, especially through breastfeeding and is the Protocol Chair for HIVNET 023 and HPTN 046. He is particularly committed to developing research capacity, having supervised over 40 postgraduate students and taught in the medical, nursing and allied health professions for more than 20 years. He is also a Fellow of the University of KwaZulu-Natal and was awarded the Star of South Africa by President Nelson Mandela for his contribution to democracy in South Africa. In 1999, he was awarded the Silver Medal by the Medical Research Council for his achievements in medical research.

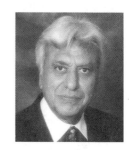

Elizabeth Corbett, MBBCh, PhD is a clinical epidemiologist and a Senior Lecturer in the Clinical Research Unit, London School of Hygiene and Tropical Medicine. She has extensive research experience in the field of HIV and TB in Africa, and has been a close collaborator of Dr Churchyard since 1996. She has published widely on mycobacterial diseases, and is a regular reviewer for journals including the *Lancet* and *International Journal of Tuberculosis and Lung Disease*. She is a member of the TB Expert Committee that advises the Ministry of Health and Child Welfare, Zimbabwe. She has collaborated with the Stop TB Department of the World Health Organisation in estimating the burden of HIV-associated TB and direction of trends. Dr Corbett is engaged in full-time epidemiological research, based in the Biomedical Research and Training Institute, Harare, Zimbabwe. Her ongoing research projects are centred on TB epidemiology and control in high HIV prevalence areas.

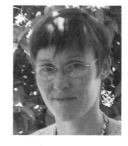

Nawaal Deane, BA has been a reporter for the *Mail & Guardian* since 2000 and has been their HIV/AIDS correspondent since 2002. Ms Deane has written extensively on the HIV/AIDS epidemic and two of her articles have been published in the MG Bedside Book. She is a

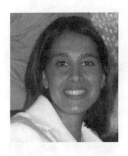

regular contributor to BBC focus on Africa, International Press Services, and Dutch magazine, *'Zuidelike Afrika'*. Ms Deane studied journalism and communication at Rand Afrikaans University, including visual studies, Internet journalism, and media law. She also holds an International Relations degree from the University of the Witwatersrand. Ms Deane has completed several other journalism courses including an Internet Economic and Financial Journalism, the Idasa Budget Information Service Journalist course, and the Standard Bank Economic Journalist course. Ms Deane assists with the annual Newspaper School Camp.

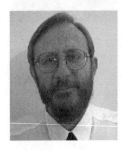

Rob Dorrington, BCom (UND), BSc (Hons) (UCT), BA (UNISA), MPhil (UCT), FIA, ASA, FASSA is an actuary and a demographer, Professor of Actuarial Science and Director of the Centre for Actuarial Research at the University of Cape Town. He is convener of the AIDS Committee of the Actuarial Society of South Africa, and as such has worked extensively on the ASSA2000 suite of AIDS and demographic projection models. He currently serves on the South African Statistics Council, the Research Monitoring and Evaluation Task Team of the South African National AIDS Council, and on a national reference group to assist Statistics South Africa with producing official mortality tables and population projections. He has served on the Council of the Actuarial Society of South Africa and as Vice-President of the Demographic Association of Southern Africa, and is a past winner of the President's award of the Actuarial Society of South Africa. He has consulted for a number of large organisations including the Cape Metropolitan Council, the Western Cape Provincial Administration and the national Road Accident Fund. Over the past year he has participated in numerous seminars and workshops and authored or co-authored several papers and posters at national and international conferences.

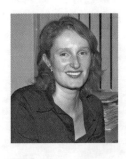

Lara Fairall, MBChB is a research fellow at the University of Cape Town Lung Institute. Her main research interests are the implementation of clinical practice guidelines in primary care and prospective multi-method evaluation of complex health interventions using pragmatic cluster randomised controlled trials. She is a member of the team adapting and testing the Practical Approach to Lung Health (PAL) guidelines of the WHO for use in South Africa. Recently these guidelines were expanded to HIV/AIDS care including antiretroviral treatment (PALSA PLUS). Dr Fairall is the principal investigator of a trial to assess their impact on the quality of HIV/AIDS care provided by primary care nurses, currently underway in the Free State Province.

Janet Frohlich, DipMGC, BCur (Ed et Ad), D Cur is the Community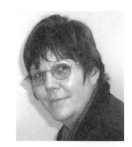
Programmes Manager and Operations Manager for the Centre for the
AIDS Programme of Research in South Africa's (CAPRISA) rural
research site in Vulindlela. She coordinated the first South African
National STI/HIV/AIDS Review in 1997. She has served as the project
leader of the HASA Nurse Educators Forum that designed and imple-
mented the first South African short course in Palliative Nursing
Care; a member of the UNAIDS International task team to develop
Best Practices for Community Mobilization; Director of the Hospice
Association of Southern Africa; a member of the Independent Study
Group into an Enabling environment for NGOs; a member of the
Executive Committee of the National AIDS Convention for southern
Africa; consultant to the National Department of Health and Gauteng
Provincial Health Department for the Development of AIDS Palliative
Care Guidelines and Guidelines. She was the Project Leader of the
SAMRC Hlabisa HIV Vaccine Preparedness Study and Site Manager of
the SAMRC rural research site in Hlabisa. She was awarded a post-
doctoral fellowship from the Southern Africa Fogarty Aids Training
Programme in 2002. She is currently the International co-chair of the
Community Working Group for the NIH HIV Prevention Trials
Network.

Eleanor Gouws, MSc, MPH is a biostatistician with several years of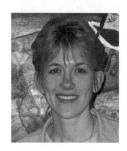
experience in analysing HIV and AIDS-related data. She worked as
statistical consultant and scientist at the Medical Research Council in
Durban, South Africa, between 1990 and 2001, before joining the
World Health Organisation to work on the Multi-Country
Evaluation of the Integrated Management of Childhood Illness
strategy. She is currently employed as adviser in statistics, modelling and estimations by the Joint United Nations Programme on
HIV/AIDS in Geneva. Research areas of particular interest include
studying the dynamics of HIV infection and estimating HIV prevalence and incidence. She has published widely in the medical
research field, with several scientific publications on HIV and AIDS.

Andrew Gray, MSc (Pharm) has research interests that include the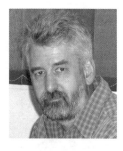
development of quality management tools for pharmaceutical
services at district level, the implementation of District Health
Systems, policy analysis, rational medicines use and the application
of highly active antiretroviral therapy in resource-constrained
settings. He is a senior lecturer in the Department of Experimental
and Clinical Pharmacology, Nelson R Mandela School of Medicine,
University of KwaZulu-Natal, Durban. He is also the study pharmacist
for the Centre for the AIDS Programme of Research in South Africa

(CAPRISA). He has been appointed to the Scheduling Committee of the South African Medicines Control Council.

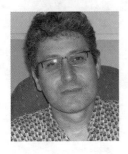

Clive Gray, PhD is an immunologist and Head of the CTL laboratory at the National Institute for Communicable Diseases in Johannesburg. He is co-chair of HIVNET 028 – a five-country study on immune responses in acute HIV infection. His initial research was in transplantation immunology and understanding allo-recognition and innate immunity. He later moved into HIV/AIDS research. He was awarded the prestigious James Gear Fellowship in 1995, which allowed him to work at the Center for AIDS Research at Stanford University as a Postdoctoral Fellow. From 1996 to 1998, he was involved in investigating specific cellular immunity to HIV in individuals receiving antiretroviral drug therapy. Since 1997, he has been actively involved in the scientific agenda of vaccine development in South Africa. At present, he directs a laboratory within the AIDS Unit at the National Institute for Virology specifically addressing cellular immunity in southern African HIV-1 infected individuals.

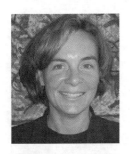

Abigail Harrison, PhD is a social scientist focusing on the interdisciplinary application of medical anthropology, demography and epidemiology in public health. She is an Instructor in the Department of Medicine, Division of Infectious Diseases, Brown University Medical School/The Miriam Hospital, Providence Rhode Island, USA, where she is also an associate of the Population Studies and Training Centre. Her current research is concerned with the patterns and social causes of HIV infection in young people, with an emphasis on sexual risk behaviours. She has been Principal Investigator for three studies related to young people and the social aspects of sexual risk throughout the adolescent lifecourse, with funding from the Wellcome Trust, National Institutes of Health, and the World Health Organisation. She has a strong interest in HIV prevention research, and has just completed a study to evaluate a school-based intervention aimed at sexual risk reduction among teens in rural KwaZulu-Natal. She serves as a consultant to the South African Medical Research Council in Durban, where she worked from 1996–2000 as a Senior Scientist directing fieldbased research on HIV/AIDS in rural Kwa-Zulu-Natal province.

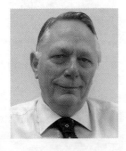

Anthon du P Heyns MB ChB, DTM&H, FCPath, MD, DSc is a haematologist whose main current interests are blood safety and estimating and minimising the risk of the impact of the HIV/AIDS pandemic on the safety of the blood supply. He is chief executive officer of the South African National Blood Service. He is also Honorary Professor in the Department of Haematology and Molecular Medicine of the

University of the Witwatersrand, and Extraordinary Professor in the Department of Haematology and Molecular Biology of the Medical Faculty at University of the Free State. He is on the editorial board of the *Cardiovascular Journal* of South Africa. He has published widely in the fields of haematology, blood platelets, blood transfusion and blood safety.

Mark Heywood, MA is a Senior Researcher and Head of the AIDS Law Project (ALP) at the Centre for Applied Legal Studies (CALS), University of the Witwatersrand. He is also National Treasurer of the Treatment Action Campaign (TAC). At the ALP he has been involved in successful public impact litigation around the rights of people living with HIV, including South Africa's first Constitutional Court judgement dealing with HIV (Hoffmann v SAA, where the ALP was amicus curiae); the Pharmaceutical Manufacturers' Association v SA Government case where the TAC was admitted as an amicus curiae; and the case brought by the TAC against the SA government on mother-to-child HIV transmission, which also led to a groundbreaking judgement in South Africa's Constitutional Court. He has undertaken consultancy work on AIDS, the law and human rights for orginisations such as UNAIDS, the UNDP, the ILO and the Office of the High Commission on Human Rights (OHCHR). He assisted drafting the Southern African Development Community (SADC) Code on AIDS and Employment (1996) and WHO/UNAIDS Guidance on Disclosure, Partner Notification and AIDS Reporting (1999). He was involved in consultative processes that drew up the United Nations International Guidelines on HIV and Human Rights (1996) and the UNAIDS manual on HIV/AIDS and Human Rights for Members of Parliament (1999). He is one of the editors of the *HIV/AIDS and the Law: Resource Manual* and has published more than 100 articles on legal, ethical and human rights questions linked to HIV/AIDS.

Leigh Johnson, BBusSc, PGDipActSc is a researcher at the Centre for Actuarial Research, at the University of Cape Town. His research interests are in the modelling of HIV/AIDS and other sexually transmitted diseases, and in the modelling of prevention and treatment strategies for these diseases. He is a member of the AIDS Committee of the Actuarial Society of South Africa (ASSA), and he has been closely involved in the development of the ASSA AIDS models. He has also been closely involved in the development of a national antiretroviral treatment plan for South Africa.

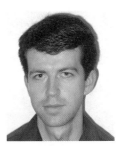

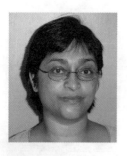

Quarraisha Abdool Karim, PhD is an infectious diseases epidemiologist whose main research interests are in understanding the evolving HIV epidemic in South Africa; factors influencing acquisition of HIV infection in adolescent girls; and sustainable strategies to introduce HAART in resource-constrained settings. She is an Adjunct Associate Professor in Epidemiology at the Mailman School of Public Health at Columbia University. In addition she co-ordinates the Columbia-University Southern African Fogarty AIDS International Training and Research Programme in Durban, South Africa. She is also an Adjunct Associate Professor in Public Health and Family Medicine at the Nelson R Mandela School of Medicine, University of KwaZulu-Natal, South Africa. She is Head of the Women and AIDS Programme and an Executive Committee member of CAPRISA (Centre for the AIDS Programme of Research in South Africa) – a large multi-institutional AIDS Research Centre and of the HPTN (HIV Prevention Trials Network) Leadership Group – a NIH funded network for HIV prevention science with US and international sites.

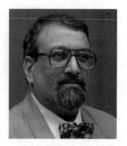

Salim S. Abdool Karim, MBChB, PhD is a clinical infectious diseases epidemiologist whose main current research interests are in microbicides and vaccines to prevent HIV infection and implementing antiretroviral therapy in resource-constrained settings. He is Deputy Vice-Chancellor (Research and Development) at the University of Natal in Durban, South Africa. He is also Professor in Clinical Epidemiology at the Mailman School of Public Health at Columbia University and Adjunct Professor in Medicine at the Weill Medical College of Cornell University. He is Director of the Centre for the AIDS Programme of Research in South Africa (CAPRISA) – a large multi-institutional AIDS Research Centre. Within CAPRISA, he is the protocol chair of a randomised controlled trial to assess the effect of integrated tuberculosis and HIV care.

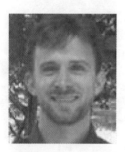

Ted Leggett, MSocSci, JD was formerly a senior researcher in the Crime and Justice Programme at the Institute for Security Studies in Pretoria, and a senior researcher at the School of Development Studies at the University of KwaZulu-Natal in Durban. He has written extensively on crime and justice issues in South Africa, including work on crime statistics, criminal justice policy, policing, and crime prevention. He has also done ethnographic research on drugs and sex work, and is the author of a book on the topic 'Rainbow Vice: The drugs and sex industries in the new South Africa' (Zed Books: London).

Mark Lurie, PhD is a social epidemiologist and an Assistant Professor of Community Health (Research) at Brown University Medical School/The Miriam Hospital in Providence, Rhode Island USA. As a Senior Scientist with the South African Medical Research Council between 1996 and 2000, Dr Lurie conducted research on the concurrent HIV/AIDS, STI, and TB epidemics in sub-Saharan Africa. His primary research has been on the role of population movement, or migration, on the spread of HIV in South Africa. He was the PI of a 3-year cohort study, with behavioural and biological outcomes, among migrant and non-migrant men and their rural partners in South Africa. Dr Lurie's current research is on the public health impact of antiretroviral therapy.

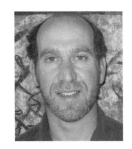

Gary Maartens, FCP(SA), MMed (Int Med), DTM&H is Head of the Division of Pharmacology, Department of Medicine, University of Cape Town and former Head of the Division of Infectious Diseases. He is a contributor to national treatment guidelines for antiretroviral therapy, management of HIV-associated opportunistic infections, adult vaccinations, community acquired pneumonia and tuberculosis in HIV infection. He is an editorial board member of *Lancet Infectious Diseases*, the *Southern African Journal of Epidemiology and Infection* and the *Southern African Journal of HIV Medicine*. Current research projects include: host immune response to tuberculosis, clinical epidemiology and prevention of tuberculosis in HIV infection, the natural history of HIV infection in resource poor settings and the healthcare costs of HIV.

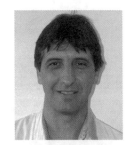

Lilian Benita Mboyi, BA Gen (Psychology, Linguistics) is a 38-year old single mother of two boys aged 16 and 9. Born and raised in Zimbabwe, she graduated from the University of Zimbabwe in 1989. She worked in corporate South Africa for thirteen years and specialised in Corporate Internal Communications. She read for a Masters in Philosophy in HIV/AIDS and Society at the University of Cape Town in 2002–2003 and is currently a CAPRISA pre-doctoral research fellow. Academic interests are pursuing a deeper understanding of the role played by stigma and discrimination in the spread of HIV/AIDS. Social interests are reading, watching movies, dancing, dining out and taking scenic walks. Her greatest ambition is to write an international best seller by the age of 40.

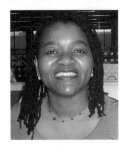

Gethwana Makhaye, B Soc Sci (Hons) is a nurse who specialised in family planning, STI management and primary health care. She is the founder and Director of the Targeted AIDS Interventions (TAI) Organisation and has worked extensively with women's groups since 1996. Her research interests include disclosure of HIV status and its

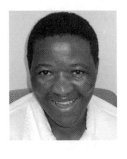

impacts on people living with HIV/AIDS and the role that young men play in the HIV/AIDS epidemic. She founded the 'Shosholoza' project in 1998 and the 'Inkunzi Isematholeni' project in 2001 which focuses on young soccer players. She has also piloted work with churches and traditional healers in the province of KwaZulu-Natal. Her effort in these projects has resulted in her being voted as one of the top 10 innovative women in South Africa. She was awarded a Fogarty Fellowship in 2002 and is currently completing her Masters degree in Medical Science.

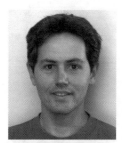

Darren Marten, PhD is a post-doctoral fellow at the Institute for Infectious Diseases and Molecular Medicine, Division of Medical Virology at the University of Cape Town. He is developing computer software for the detection and analysis of recombination among nucleic acid sequences. His main focus is the development of computational and experimental techniques for studying viral recombination within infected host organisms.

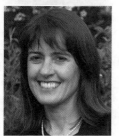

Catherine Mathews, PhD is a social scientist and epidemiologist in the Health Systems Research Unit at the South African Medical Research Council. She is an honorary lecturer in the Women's Health Research Unit, School of Public Health and Family Medicine, University of Cape Town. She is also a member of the Adolescent Health Research Institute at the University of Cape Town. She has an interest in adolescent reproductive health and HIV/AIDS prevention. She is currently involved in school-based and clinic-based research to develop and evaluate reproductive health interventions. In the past, she has led quantitative and qualitative research projects to evaluate and improve the management of STIs in public health services.

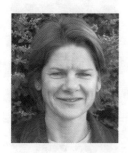

Lynn Morris, DPhil is a Chief Specialist Scientist at the National Institute for Communicable Disease in Johannesburg where she heads the AIDS Unit. She is also a Professor at the University of Witwatersrand where she holds a joint appointment. Dr Morris received her undergraduate degrees from the University of the Witwatersrand and her DPhil at the University of Oxford. She studied macrophage biology while at Oxford, examining aspects such as developmental biology, hematopoiesis and surface receptors on macrophages. This was followed by a three-year Royal Society post-doctoral fellowship at the Walter and Eliza Hall Institute in Melbourne, Australia where she examined cellular immunity, particularly the role of cytokines in the response to the human parasite *Leishmania major*. She has been at the NICD for the past 12 years and has been instrumental in studying the genetic and biologic characterisation of HIV-1 subtype C strains and the humoral immune responses of subtype C-infected individuals. Her current research focus is on the envelope glycoproteins of HIV-1 subtype C viruses and how they interact with cellular receptors on host cells, with a view to ultimately developing agents, including antibodies that can inhibit this interaction. She also has an active programme studying HIV drug resistance. She currently holds a Wellcome Trust International Senior Research Fellowship in Biomedical Sciences.

Landon Myer, PhD is a Senior Lecturer in the School of Public Health and Family Medicine at the University of Cape Town. His interests are in infectious disease epidemiology including HIV, other sexually transmitted infections, and tuberculosis. With a background in social anthropology, he was the principal investigator of a countrywide study of condom use sponsored by the National Department of Health and directed a randomised controlled trial of on-site syphilis testing in antenatal care in KwaZulu-Natal. More recently, he worked with the MTCT-Plus Initiative at the Mailman School of Public Health, Columbia University, a multi-country programme to delivery comprehensive HIV care including antiretroviral therapy to women and families. His current work focuses on the delivery of health services for HIV infected individuals and the social and economic determinants of population health.

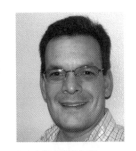

Adrian Puren, MBBCh, PhD heads the Specialised Molecular Diagnostics Unit at the National Institute of Communicable Diseases (NICD). Dr Puren's interests include HIV-1 and other viral diagnostics, epidemiology and immunology. Projects he is involved in include: the HIV-1 long-term non-progressor clinic; a collaborative project with INSERM on the relationship between HIV-1 infection and HIV-1 and HSV-2 transmission; diagnostic support of the PMTCT nevirapine resistance project in collaboration with Lynn Morris (NICD) and PRHU; the immunogenetics in HIV-1 infection in acute seroconverters in collaboration with CIPRA; the role of HLA in HIV-1 vaccine development, a SAAVI-supported programme and a PHASE 1 ACIDFORM microbicide trial in collaboration with the RHRU. Dr Puren's research is sponsored by the Poliomyelitis Foundation, SAAVI, INSERM, CONRAD and the CIPRA initiative through the NIH. He publishes regularly and his teaching responsibilities include undergraduate and postgraduate students in aspects of Virology and Immunology.

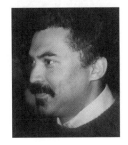

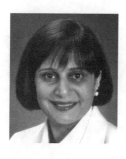

Gita Ramjee, PhD is the Director of the HIV Prevention Research Unit of the South African Medical Research Council. As a Chief Specialist Scientist, she is involved in numerous international research programmes and clinical trials in HIV prevention. Dr Ramjee is the Director of the HIV Prevention Trials Unit (HPTU) in South Africa which forms part of the global HIV Prevention Trials Network (HPTN). Her expertise in the clinical testing of vaginal microbicides has earned her international acclaim and brought the HIV Prevention Research Unit to the forefront in its field. Dr Ramjee is currently the Principle Investigator on three Phase III trials, and one Phase II/IIb trial, and her Unit is the only centre globally involved in testing of all microbicides that have reached this advanced stage of development. Dr Ramjee pioneered the South African Microbicide Research Initiative that works in collaboration with microbicide and barrier method advocacy groups to accelerate the testing of microbicides and other HIV prevention technologies.

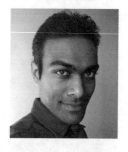

Jerome Amir Singh, BA, LLB, LLM, PhD (Natal), MHSc (Toronto), is Head of the Bioethics and Health Law Programme at the Centre for the AIDS Programme of Research in South Africa (CAPRISA), Nelson R. Mandela School of Medicine, University of KwaZulu-Natal, Durban, South Africa; Adjunct Professor in the Department of Public Health Sciences and Joint Centre for Bioethics at the University of Toronto, Canada; and Course Director for Bioethics and the Law at Howard College School of Law, University of KwaZulu-Natal, Durban, South Africa. He serves on the International Research Ethics Board of Médecins Sans Frontières, the United States National Institutes of Health International Therapeutic Data Safety Monitoring Board, the Research Ethics Committee of the South African Human Sciences Research Council, the Scientific Advisory Board of Aurum Health Research, the Ethics Committee of Docline Medical Aid Scheme, and the Executive Committe of CAPRISA.

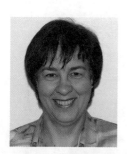

Johanna Petronella Swanevelder, MSC (Quantitative Health Sciences) is the National Data Analyst for the South African National Blood Service. Ms Swanevelder has been responsible for development of a model to manage the transfusion risk in blood services. This model forms the basis for continuous evaluation of the risk profile of donors/donations enabling the targeting of safe blood procurement to ensure a safe blood supply is available to all South African patients. Prior to joining the South African National Blood Service in 1997, she was employed by the Department of Health in the Epidemiology Directorate where she started and conducted the annual national surveys in attenders of antenatal clinics from 1990 to 1996.

Marianne Visser, BNutr, MPhil (Epidemiology) is a registered dietician who has a research interest in the epidemiology of micronutrient deficiencies in HIV-infection and tuberculosis. She is currently involved in a systematic review examining the role of micronutrient supplementation in HIV-infected children and adults. She is an honorary lecturer at the Nutrition and Dietetics unit, School of Health and Rehabilitation Sciences at the University of Cape Town.

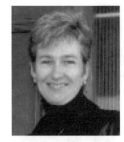

Alan Whiteside, MA, DEcon is a development economist who has been working on HIV/AIDS and health issues for the past 20 years. His main research interests are around the interactions of health and development and the impact of HIV/AIDS and its consequences for societies and economies. He is a professor at the University of KwaZulu-Natal and is the Director of the Health Economics and HIV/AIDS Research Division at the university, which he established in 1998. He also holds associate posts with the Liverpool School of Tropical Medicine and the School of Development Studies at the University of East Anglia.

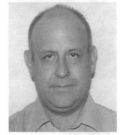

Brian Williams, PhD studied physics at the Universities of Natal, South Africa and Cambridge, England. He has extensive experience of the mathematical modelling of the epidemiology of infectious diseases. In 1994 he became the Director of the Epidemiology Research Unit where he worked on diseases of mine workers focusing on tuberculosis, silicosis and HIV and in 1998 moved to the Council for Scientific and Industrial Research. During this time he set up and ran the Carletonville Mothusimpilo ('Working-together-for health') project, a community-based intervention for the control of HIV. In 2001 he moved to the World Health Organisation in Geneva where he works on tuberculosis and HIV/AIDS. His interests are in public health, especially TB and HIV, and in modelling disease processes and dynamics. He has published widely on a range of diseases, including measles, trypanosomiasis, leishmaniasis, silicosis, malaria, tuberculosis and HIV.

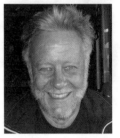

Carolyn Williamson, PhD is a virologist and Associate Professor in the Institute for Infectious Diseases and Molecular Medicine, University of Cape Town. She currently directs a molecular HIV research programme on HIV diversity, pathogenesis and vaccine development. Her group was central to the initial elucidation of HIV-1 diversity in South Africa and has collaborated nationally and internationally in programmes involved in vaccine design, developement and testing. She is currently chair of the Biomedicaal and Clinical Sciences Working Group of the WHO/African AIDS Vaccine Programme, is a

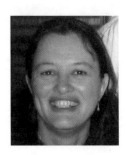

principal investigator in the SAAVI funded project to develop DNA subtype C vaccine for clinical trials and is Protocol Chair of Study based at the Centre for the AIDS Programme of Research in South Africa (CAPRISA) which is investigating clinical, immunological and virological characteristics in acute HIV-1 subtype C infection.

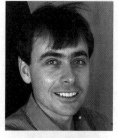

Douglas Wilson, MBChB, FCP (SA) is a specialist physician and Head of the Department of Medicine at Edendale Hospital. He provides a specialist antiretroviral service in Pietermaritzburg and is presently doing research in the diagnosis of smear negative tuberculosis. Dr Wilson is a Lecturer in the Department of Medicine at the University of KwaZulu-Natal.

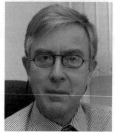

Robin Wood, BSc (Lond), BM (Oxon), DTM&H (Liv), MMed (UCT), FCP (SA) is Professor of Medicine, Groote Schuur Hospital and Director of the Desmond Tutu HIV Centre, Institute of Infectious Disease and Molecular Medicine, University of Cape Town, South Africa. He completed his undergraduate training at Oxford and London University, and carried out post-graduate training in Internal Medicine at the University of Cape Town, and Infectious Diseases training at Stanford Medical School, California. Since 1993 he has supervised the first dedicated HIV clinic in the Western Cape at Somerset Hospital (Cape Town, South Africa). Dr Wood's major research interests are in the fields of infectious diseases and HIV. He has published widely in the areas of HIV management, tuberculosis interaction with HIV and new drug development.

Foreword

There is no question that the AIDS epidemic has had a devastating impact on Africa, and particularly in South Africa. A tragedy of unprecedented proportions is unfolding. So far, the AIDS epidemic in Africa has created 14 million orphans. Today, AIDS in Africa is claiming more lives than the sum total of all wars, famines and floods, and the ravages of such deadly diseases as malaria. It is devastating families and communities, overwhelming and depleting health care services; and robbing schools of both students and teachers. Business has suffered, or will suffer, losses of personnel, productivity and profits; economic growth is being undermined and scarce development resources have to be diverted to deal with the consequences of the pandemic. Decades have been chopped from life expectancy and young child mortality is expected to more than double in the most severely affected countries of Africa. AIDS is clearly a disaster, effectively wiping out the development gains of the past decades and threatens the future.

South Africa has been especially hard hit. Every day in South Africa, an estimated 1700 people are newly infected with HIV. In the face of the grave threat posed by HIV/AIDS, we have to rise above our differences and combine our efforts to save our people. History will judge us harshly if we fail to do so now, and right now.

The experience in a number of countries has taught that HIV infection can be prevented through investing in information and life skills development for young people. Promoting abstinence, safe sex and the use of condoms and ensuring the early treatment of sexually transmitted diseases are some of the steps needed. Ensuring that people, especially the young, have access to voluntary and confidential HIV counselling and testing services and introducing measures to reduce mother-to-child transmission have been proven to be essential in the fight against AIDS. Just as we will not succeed until we appreciate the gender dimension of vulnerability to HIV, we will also not succeed until we have addressed the stigmatisation and discrimination, and provide safe and supportive environments for people affected by HIV/AIDS. We need to break the silence, banish stigma and discrimination, and ensure inclusiveness within the struggle against AIDS; those who are infected with this terrible disease do not want stigma, they want love.

We need bold initiatives to prevent new infections among young people, and large-scale actions to prevent mother-to-child transmission, and at the same time we need to continue the international effort of searching for an effective microbicide and vaccine; and we need to aggressively treat opportunistic infections; to work with families and communities to care for children and young people to protect them from violence and abuse, and to ensure that they grow up in a safe and supportive environment. For this there is need for us to be focused, to be strategic, and to mobilise all of our resources and alliances, and to sustain the effort until this war is won.

It is not as if all sectors of South Africa have not moved significantly on many of these areas; the government, private sector, non-governmental organisations, and civil society have made great strides in the struggle against AIDS but much more remains to be done. The challenge is to move from rhetoric to action, and action at an unprecedented intensity and scale. There is a need for us to focus on what we know works based on evidence.

For this we all need to be well informed and I am pleased to see such a large group of South Africa's leading AIDS researchers come together to produce this book on HIV/AIDS in South Africa. The comprehensive picture of the epidemic in our country provided by this book is a carefully woven tapestry of information of AIDS – while each thread of information is important; taken altogether this wealth of information illuminates the path of this dark disease. This text, edited by the Abdool Karims and written for and by South Africans, comes at a time when the country's AIDS treatment rollout is gathering momentum and the thirst for information is rapidly growing. As you, the reader, page through this book, I hope and trust that you will hear the call to action. It is imperative that we respond with all the energy and resources that we can bring to bear in the fight against AIDS.

Nelson Mandela

Acknowledgements

This book would not have been possible without the contributions of a wide number of people. The editors would like to acknowledge the efforts of each of the contributors in preparing this comprehensive account of the HIV/AIDS epidemic in southern Africa. In particular, the editors would like to point out that the book would not have been possible without the dedication, time and effort put in by Cheryl Baxter, associate researcher for the Centre for the AIDS Programme of Research in South Africa (CAPRISA). David Newmarch provided invaluable assistance with the early drafts of the book.

The publisher gratefully acknowledges permission from the following sources:
Chapter 5: p 87. Fig 5.6 from *Oxford Handbook of* HIV *Medicine*, Fig 6.2, p 52 Chapter 9: p 160. Poster from Soul City, Johannesburg. Chapter 18: p 292. Tables 18.2, p 293. 18.3 and 18.4 from *Sexually Transmitted Diseases* 2002; 29(1): 44–49: 721–724. Chapter 27 Figs 27.2 and 27.3 from Dorrington RE, Bourne D, Bradshaw D, Laubscher R, Timeaus IM. 2001. The impact of HIV/AIDS on adult mortality in South Africa. MRC Technical Report. MRC Cape Town. (ISBN 1-919809-14-7). Chapter 30: p 466. Fig 30.1 from *Oxford Handbook of* HIV *Medicine*, Fig 47.1, p 413; p 469 Fig 30.2 from *British Journal of Nutrition* 1999; 81: 181–189. Chapter 31: p 482. Fig 31.2 from AIDS 2004; Apr 9; 18(6): 887–95. Chapter 36 p 571. Fig 36.2 from *The Lancet* 2004: Vol 363: pp 1394; general source material from *The Lancet* 2003; 362: pp 1499.

Every effort has been made to trace copyright holders. Should infringements have occurred, please inform the publishers who will correct these in the event of a reprint.

SECTION 1
Birth of a rapidly growing epidemic

CHAPTER 1
Introduction

Salim S. Abdool Karim

THE NUMBER OF PEOPLE infected with HIV worldwide has increased exponentially from just a handful of cases in the early 1980s to about 40 million by the end of 2003 and more than 20 million people have already died of AIDS. Catastrophically, the extent of its impact turned out to be far worse than ever predicted.

In South Africa, the early phase of the epidemic was restricted to just a few hundred cases among men who have sex with men and persons receiving unsafe blood transfusions. However, by the early 1990s, heterosexual transmission came to dominate as the mode of spread of HIV infection, and with it, the concomitant HIV epidemic in newborns and young children through perinatal transmission. South Africa now is the country estimated to have the largest number of people (5.3 million HIV positive people as at December 2002) living with HIV/AIDS. Despite this, the South African response to the HIV epidemic has been characterised by a unique form of denialism in the highest echelons of political power. However, with the announcement in 2003 by the South African government to adopt a national antiretroviral roll-out plan, there is renewed optimism that South Africa can turn the tide of the epidemic.

More than two decades have passed since the first case of AIDS was described. In this relatively short period the number of people infected with HIV has increased exponentially from just a handful of cases in the early 1980s to about 40 million worldwide by the end of 2003. Already, more than 20 million have died of AIDS. Undoubtedly, AIDS is the world's most devastating epidemic, the deadliest in the history of humankind, its impact already far worse than could first have been predicted.

AIDS epidemic first identified in USA

The report published by the Atlanta-based Centers for Disease Control and Prevention (CDC) in June of 1981 was the first to take note of the disease and marked the beginning of awareness of the epidemic potential of AIDS in the USA. This report described the occurrence, without identifiable cause, of *Pneumocystis carinii* pneumonia (PCP) in five gay men in Los Angeles. (Note: The specific name of *Pneumocystis carinii* is in the process of being changed to *jiroveci*. Both specific names will be used in this book.)

Very little was known about the epidemiology and transmission of what seemed to be a new disease, and initially it was thought that only homosexuals were affected. However, it soon became evident that the disease affected other groups when the first cases of PCP were reported in injecting drug users in December 1981. At this time, reports emerged that the disease was also occurring in haemophiliacs and Haitian immigrants in the USA.

In 1982 the disease was named Acquired ImmunoDeficiency Syndrome (AIDS). The mode of transmission of AIDS became clearer after a 20-month-old child who had received multiple blood transfusions died from infections related to AIDS. This caused worldwide concerns about the safety of the blood supply. At about this time, the first cases of possible mother-to-child transmission of AIDS were reported by the CDC.

The realisation then became all too inescapable that the number of people who could become infected might continue to grow when it was then reported that the disease could be transmitted heterosexually as well.

Discovery of HIV

In 1983, Dr Luc Montagnier, Dr Francois Barre-Sinoussi and colleagues at the Institute Pasteur in France reported that they had isolated a new virus which they believed was the cause of AIDS. This virus was named lymphadenopathy-associated virus (LAV). Soon thereafter, Dr Robert Gallo from the National Cancer Institute in the USA also announced that he had isolated the virus which caused AIDS, and he named it human T-lymphotropic virus type III (HTLV-III). Following the publication of a number of more detailed reports concerning LAV and HTLV-III, it became apparent that the viruses were actually the same and that the electron-micrographs published by Dr Gallo and his research team of HTLV-III were actually pictures of LAV obtained from Dr Montagnier. After an ensuing investigation, a compromise was reached and both Dr Gallo and Dr Montagnier were credited as co-discoverers of HIV. The isolation of the virus provided the essential material for the first blood test for detecting HIV.

AIDS in South Africa

AIDS was first reported in South Africa in 1983. A report in the *South African Medical Journal* described two cases of AIDS in male homosexuals. In the early part of the epidemic in South Africa (1982–1987), AIDS was associated mainly with homosexuals, blood transfusion recipients and haemophiliacs. The first peak in the AIDS epidemic in the mid-1980s occurred in male homosexuals, who were being diagnosed with AIDS-related opportunistic diseases.

Prior to this in the early 1980s, before the cause of AIDS was recognised and blood donations routinely screened for the presence of HIV-antibodies, several haemophiliacs acquired HIV through transfusions of factor VIII, a component of blood. Each transfusion of factor VIII was derived from hundreds of blood donations, thereby increasing the risk of HIV transmission. By 1985, a safe blood supply was secured throughout South Africa when all blood transfusion services introduced self-exclusion questionnaires for their donors and, more importantly, routine HIV screening of all donated blood.

Currently, in South Africa all blood donations are routinely screened for the presence of HIV-antibody and a marker of early HIV infection known as the P24 antigen by sensitive and specific third-generation Enzyme ImmunoAssay (EIA) test systems. Since the introduction of the Blood Safety Policy in South Africa in 1999, which actively selects low-risk donors, the HIV prevalence rate in blood collections has decreased significantly and in 2002 was at the same level as 1991 (0.06%). The 1999 Blood Safety Policy included racial profiling and was revised in 2004 to remove race as a criterion for excluding donations.

The number of male homosexuals admitted to HIV clinics had reached a plateau in 1989 while the visits from the general population started to rise. By the end of 1989, a number of surveillance studies confirmed the entry of HIV into the heterosexual population in South Africa. Between 1990 and 1994 it became increasingly apparent that the heterosexual epidemic was rapidly exceeding the homosexual epidemic.

As in most of Africa, AIDS first became apparent as an urban phenomenon in South Africa but it spread rapidly into rural areas. An important feature of the HIV epidemic in the heterosexual population was the age difference of those infected with HIV; predominantly these are young women and older men, and overall a disproportionate number of people between the ages of 15 and 40.

Since the mid-1990s the AIDS epidemic has risen steadily (FIGURE 1.1) in South Africa and by the end of 2002 an estimated 5.3 million South Africans were HIV positive. Approximately 2.95 million women and 2.3 million men between the ages of 15 to 49 years were infected with HIV in 2002.

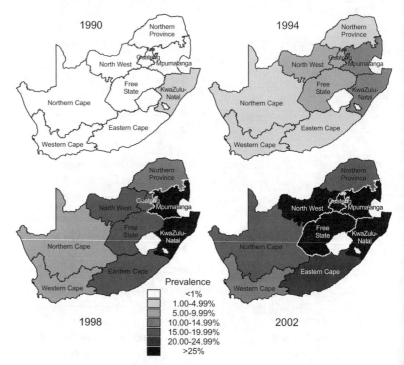

FIGURE 1.1 Rapidly growing HIV epidemic in South Africa
Source: Department of Health antenatal HIV surveys

South Africa's response to the AIDS epidemic

The response to the AIDS epidemic in South Africa developed slowly at first. In the 1990s it suffered huge crises of credibility, faltering seriously in the late 1990s despite some initial momentum in the period just after the dawn of democracy in 1994, but in the present decade it has been gathering momentum once again with the announcement by the government in 2003 that it would make free antiretroviral treatment available in the public health service.

In the mid-1980s, HIV/AIDS was seen in South Africa as a gay epidemic confined to select high-risk sub-groups within the larger urban centres of the country. As a result it evoked minimal response from the government. In contrast, various non-governmental initiatives responded by initiating localised preventive, care and support programmes for those infected and affected.

During this period in the mid-1980s, the state Department of National Health and Population Development focused on the need for information dissemination, counselling and HIV testing by establishing a number of AIDS Training and Information Centres (ATICs). Subsequently, the recognition of the need for a more specific response from central government led to the establishment of a dedicated AIDS Unit within the National Health Department. Among other responsibilities, this unit was given the task of drawing up a national AIDS strategy, as well as co-ordinating all AIDS-related activities in the country. The government's response was, however, seen as tainted and its judgemental approach (by attacking African culture) undermined its credibility. At about this time, an independent body, the AIDS Programme of the National Progressive Primary Health Care Network (NPPHCN) was established to offer an unprejudiced alternative to AIDS prevention, more in tune with community needs.

From a political perspective, South Africa's response to the epidemic has been characterised by a unique form of denialism in the highest echelons of political power. The first post-apartheid government of President Mandela was faced with the urgent need for reconciliation and nation building which took precedence over the need to accord AIDS the necessary priority and commitment. The subsequent government, under the leadership of President Thabo Mbeki, is probably best characterised by its litany of errors in AIDS policy and for its failure to rise to the challenge that AIDS posed for South Africa. The creation of the Mbeki presidential panel, comprising AIDS denialists on the one hand and AIDS researchers and doctors on the other, marked the lowest point of the degeneration of the government's response into confusion and obtuseness. However, 2003 saw a change of heart – in recognition of the extent of devastation caused by AIDS, the South African government made a far-reaching decision to provide free antiretroviral drugs in the state health care service. The spirit of hope this has engendered has been an incentive for this book in its aim of providing a comprehensive picture of AIDS as it besets one of the world's youngest but most vibrant democracies: a country emerging from the oppression of apartheid only to encounter the devastation of AIDS just when it expected to be enjoying the hard-earned fruits of freedom.

Bibliography

ALTMAN, L.K. Rare cancer seen in 41 Homosexuals. *The New York Times*, 1981.

ALTMAN L.K. New U.S. Report Names Virus that May Cause AIDS. *The New York Times*, 1984.

BARRE-SINOUSSI F, CHERMANN J-C, REY F, NUGEYRE MT, CHAMARET S, GRUEST J, DAUGUET C, AXLER-BLIN C, BRUN-VEZINET F, ROUZIOUX C, ROZENBAUM W, MONTAGNIER L. 'Isolation of a T-Lymphotropic Retrovirus from a Patient at Risk for Acquired Immune Deficiency Syndrome (AIDS)'. *Science* 1983; 220: 868–871.

CENTERS FOR DISEASE CONTROL. PNEUMOCYSTIS PNEUMONIA – LOS ANGELES. *Mobidity and Mortality Weekly Report* 1981; 30: 1–3.

CENTERS FOR DISEASE CONTROL. OPPORTUNISTIC INFECTIONS AND KAPOSI'S SARCOMA AMONG HAITIANS IN THE UNITED STATES. *Mobidity and Mortality Weekly Report* 1982; 31: 353–354, 360–361.

COHN RJ, MACPHAIL AP, HARTMAN E, SCHWYZER R, SHER R. 'Transfusion-related human immunodeficiency virus in patients with haemophilia in Johannesburg'. *South African Medical Journal* 1990; 78: 653–656.

EPIDEMIOLOGIC NOTES AND REPORTS. PNEUMOCYSTIS CARINII PNEUMONIA AMONG PERSONS WITH HEMOPHILIA A. *Morbidity and Mortality Weekly Report* 1982; 31: 365–367.

EPIDEMIOLOGIC NOTES AND REPORTS. POSSIBLE TRANSFUSION-ASSOCIATED ACQUIRED IMMUNE DEFICIENCY SYNDROME, (AIDS) – CALIFORNIA. *Morbidity and Mortality Weekly Report* 1982; 31: 652–654.

EPIDEMIOLOGIC NOTES AND REPORTS. IMMUNODEFICIENCY AMONG FEMALE SEXUAL PARTNERS OF MALES WITH ACQUIRED IMMUNE DEFICIENCY SYNDROME (AIDS) – NEW YORK. *Morbidity and Mortality Weekly Report* 1982; 31: 697–698.

RAS GJ, SIMSON IW, ANDERSON R, PROZESKY OW, HAMERSMA T. 'Acquired immuno-deficiency syndrome. A report of 2 South African cases'. *South African Medical Journal* 1983; 64: 140–142.

DEPARTMENT OF HEALTH, SOUTH AFRICA. '*Summary report: National HIV and syphilis antenatal sero-prevalence survey in South Africa, 2002*'. Pretoria, South Africa.

THE AIDS EPIDEMIC IN SAN FRANCISCO: THE MEDICAL RESPONSE, 1981–1984. VOLUME I, AN ORAL HISTORY CONDUCTED IN 1992–1993. Regional Oral History Office 1995, The Bancroft Library, University of California, Berkeley.

UNEXPLAINED IMMUNODEFICIENCY AND OPPORTUNISTIC INFECTIONS IN INFANTS – NEW YORK, NEW JERSEY, CALIFORNIA. *Morbidity and Mortality Weekly Report* 1982; 31: 665–667.

UNAIDS/WHO. *Report on the global HIV/AIDS epidemic. 2002*. Geneva, Switzerland.

CHAPTER 2
Overview of the book

Salim S. Abdool Karim, Quarraisha Abdool Karim and Cheryl Baxter

AT PRESENT, AFRICA BEARS the brunt of the HIV epidemic. And it is southern Africa that has the highest burden of disease on the continent. In South Africa alone, by the end of 2003 around five million adults were living with HIV. That figure is growing. Every day another 1700 people are estimated to become infected with the virus. The disease has rightly been likened to a whirlwind, sweeping everything before it as millions become infected, fall ill and die. HIV is a particularly fascinating virus. As a retrovirus it insinuates itself into the DNA of its host, becoming a Trojan horse in the immune system and systematically weakening the host until the body can no longer efficiently fight infection. What is particularly devious is the way in which the body's initial response to the infection is incorporated into HIV's attack strategy. The very immune cells produced in defence allow the virus to penetrate further and further into the host's tissues, ensuring a lifetime of infection. It is probably the infinitely fascinating science of the virus that initially stimulated researchers around the world to spend so much time elucidating the cause of the mysterious syndrome that first appeared in the medical literature in 1981.

Since then it has become clear that HIV affects all aspects of our lives – even those who are not infected with the virus; from the molecular level, to the level of the immune system, to the way in which the virus causes disease – to the community level. And it is at the community level that an understanding of HIV is perhaps most important. HIV is more than a simple infection. Its nature means that society is inextricably entwined with this disease. The impact on those infected, the stigma attached to infection and the social and economic effects of that infection cause HIV to have an enormously broad impact; on the economy, on the practice of ethics, on politics at a national level. There is no aspect of people's lives in South Africa that is not affected by the levels of infection seen in this country. It is the single most important challenge facing us in the twenty-first century and we have not yet turned the corner, although the rate of growth of the epidemic is mercifully slowing. Prevention efforts are being scaled up and treatment programmes are being planned and, in some areas, already rolled out.

We have come a long way in our understanding of the molecular biology, epidemiology, medicine and sociology of HIV since 1981. But where, in fact, are we going and how can the devastation that is being wrought across Africa in particular and the developing world in general be brought to an end? It is these questions that stimulated the authors of this book to put pen to paper. Without knowledge we can fight nothing and South Africa arguably has among the highest level of understanding in the world of all aspects of HIV. In these pages the country's leading experts have put together a detailed account of the epidemic – one that will illustrate their commitment to ending the carnage.

Birth of a rapidly growing epidemic

It is always difficult to know where to start in any book that attempts to provide comprehensive cover of a diverse subject. However, before plunging into the science of the virus itself, the book's editors have given an overview of the epidemiology of the disease – unique to the region. Detailed epidemiological information is the foundation for understanding the epidemic and this is provided by Eleanor Gouws and Quarraisha Abdool Karim who outline the distinct phases of the epidemic. In South Africa there have been five distinct phases, marking key milestones in the regional spread of the virus from the first reported cases of AIDS in the early 1980s to the current gener-alised major epidemic with a prevalence that may start to decline soon, but may also simply appear to decline as incidence and mortal-ity converge. At first, the disease was, as elsewhere, confined to homosexuals and those who had received infected blood products. However, the trajectory of the epidemic changed as heterosexual transmission became predominant. This change was important to the demographics of the disease. Young, economically active people and young women in particular became particularly vulnerable. Taking analysis of the patterns of the epidemic further Eleanor Gouws provides an overview of temporal trends in the geographical distribu-tion of HIV in South Africa using mathematical modelling techniques to derive incidence estimates from HIV prevalence surveys. The epidemic at present seems to be close to a steady state. But the ques-tion of how it will continue to unfold remains.

Part of the mystery of HIV lies in the molecular, virological and immunological features of the virus. Some of the most significant advances in the field of HIV research have been at these levels and Lynn Morris and Tonie Cilliers has been involved in the genetic and biological characterisation of HIV-1 subtype C strains. They have also looked at the immune responses of subtype C infected individuals. The importance of this work lies in its potential application in developing novel antibodies that may inhibit the interaction of the envelope glycoproteins of HIV and cellular receptors on host cells. In this book, they describe the structure of the virus, its replication cycle and pathogenesis and provide an overview of the natural history of the clade C HIV subtype.

The technologies for detecting HIV are varied. The latest generation of HIV tests are fast, accurate and practical in both the clinic and at home. The identification of individuals with primary HIV infection (also referred to as acute infection) is critical from an epidemiological perspective and possibly from a therapeutic intervention and counselling perspective. Adrian Puren gives an account of diagnostic tests for HIV infection, emphasising how the tests have been adapted for subtype C viruses. The importance of acute infection is highlighted in this chapter. This is particularly relevant in South Africa where the incidence of HIV is so high, with large numbers of people in the acute phase of infection. During the acute phase, the actual numbers of virus in the blood, the viral load, is high – several times higher than set point levels during established infection. High viral load is associated with a greater risk of HIV transmission; hence the importance of acute infection and being able to recognise and detect it. Not only this, but the early cellular responses, thought to be HLA dependent may be important in determining the set point viral load level. The practical importance of this lies in the studies that are currently underway to assess the potential of prevention and anti-retroviral treatment during acute infection to reduce this set point. At this stage we have no idea how effective this will be, but the importance of accurate diagnosis remains clear.

HIV's ability to evolve rapidly in response to environmental pressures gives it its capacity for continual adaptation and escape from selective forces such as immune responses and antiretroviral drugs. Carolyn Williamson and Darren Martin present molecular data to describe the origin and growth of the epidemic in South Africa, explaining mechanisms of HIV diversification, the clade distribution, and the implications of HIV's extreme diversity. It is this extreme diversity and the ability of the virus to continue to diversify that concern Willamson and Martin. Can the global HIV population be controlled at its current level and will we be able to maintain this control in the face of HIV's inevitable future diversification?

The immune response is the body's first line of defence against infection. HIV attacks a class of T-helper cells and has the ability, over time, to cripple the immune system, inevitably making AIDS fatal. The cellular immune responses to HIV are complex and Clive Gray not only provides an overview of these, but presents additional data on a rare number of individuals who appear to have natural resistance to HIV-1 infection. These individuals could provide important clues about protective immune responses and could influence HIV vaccine development.

Risk factors and prevention strategies

A continuing rise in the number of HIV infected people in Africa is not inevitable. Success is being achieved in some prevention interventions, leading to a reduction in sexual risk behaviour. Catherine Mathews reviews the prevalence of sexual risk behaviours in South Africa and provides examples of the personal, interpersonal, social, structural and environmental forces that shape these behaviours. She also analyses specific risk reduction interventions that have been demonstrated to be effective locally and internationally and considers some of the particular challenges of implementing and evaluating HIV prevention programmes in South Africa.

Despite recent advances in other areas of HIV prevention, including behavioural interventions, microbicides, and vaccines, barrier methods remain a pivotal part of the fight against HIV/AIDS. The successes in promoting condom uptake and utilisation are described by Landon Myer. However, there are still important barriers to condom use across the country. Myer shows how ongoing interventions to improve the accessibility of condoms, as well as make condoms more comfortable to use, have the potential to increase their use substantially.

AIDS is claiming more lives in Africa than the sum total of all wars, famines and floods to date, leaving many hundreds of thousands of orphaned children. Furthermore, sub-Saharan Africa is home to roughly 90% of the 800 000 infants who contract HIV from their mothers before or during birth or as a result of breastfeeding. In some African countries, around 25% of the pregnant women are infected with HIV. Jerry (Hoosen) Coovadia provides an overview of mother-to-child transmission in South Africa, dealing frankly with some of the controversial issues around nevirapine and how to reduce transmission during breastfeeding.

The association between sexually transmitted infections (STIs) and HIV transmission is well established – the presence of STIs enhances the acquisition of HIV. Hence, identifying and treating STIs remains an important prevention mechanism. David Coetzee and Leigh Johnson describe the interaction between HIV and other STIs and give an overview of the extent of STIs in South Africa. They explain that the challenge for South African researchers is to identify and test different combinations of interventions including improved STI services with syndromic management, mass STI treatment, and periodic presumptive STI treatment to define cost-effective programmes with the potential for containing the HIV epidemic in South Africa.

The HIV epidemic potentially compromises the safety and sufficiency of the blood supply in South Africa and in the early days of the epidemic instances of transmission did occur. Fortunately this has been significantly reduced over the years and contributes only fractionally to the number of new HIV cases in South Africa annually. Anthon Heyns and Johanna Swanevelder of the South African Blood Transfusion Service discuss strategies to ensure the safety of blood supply, governance of the blood service, the window period of infectivity and South Africa's Blood Safety Policy and its outcomes.

Since 1994 South Africa has opened up to drug dealers, who have connections to both the Far East and Central Asia. They have set up operations in inner Johannesburg, Pretoria, and Cape Town with a resultant rise in intravenous drug use, known to be a major risk factor for HIV transmission elsewhere in the world. Ted Leggett gives a brief history of injection drug use in South Africa and warns that while intravenous drug use is currently a minor part of HIV transmission in South Africa, the growing popularity of heroin is likely to make it an issue in the future.

Salim Abdool Karim and Cheryl Baxter conclude this section by discussing future prevention strategies. In particular, they touch on new approaches to the prevention of HIV transmission, namely microbicides, vaccines, antiretroviral prophylaxis and reducing herpes simplex Type 2 virus infection and its sequelae.

Focal groups for understanding the HIV epidemic

Although, worldwide, there are as many women as there are men with HIV infection, this averaged figure conceals marked geographical differences in the gender distribution of the disease. In South Africa the HIV epidemic is well established in the general heterosexual population, but a disproportionate burden of infection is borne by discrete high-risk groups in which there is a strong gender bias. This section of the book analyses the gender issues in the HIV epidemic and highlights the important risk groups of sex workers, adolescents, migrant workers and young women.

Not only do more women have HIV infection in South Africa compared to men but they also acquire infection with HIV at a younger age. As early as 1992, it was noted that young women in the early childbearing years (15–29 years) have the highest rates of HIV infection in South Africa. This trend has continued. Quarraisha Abdool Karim describes the factors that have contributed to increased HIV risk in women in South Africa, making it clear how crucial it is for men to take greater responsibility and be more actively involved, individually and at a community level, in efforts to reduce women's risk of acquiring infection with HIV.

Abigail Harrison expands on her work on HIV in rural Zulu adolescents by exploring the high risk of HIV infection in young South Africans. She examines HIV prevalence, sexual risk behaviours and the proximate determinants of HIV infection in young people. She discusses youth-focused prevention strategies and concludes with a discussion of the challenges inherent in preventing HIV infection among young South Africans.

Despite sex work being illegal in South Africa, desperate economic circumstances force many women to engage in commercial sex for survival. This places them at risk both of contracting and transmitting the virus. Gita Ramjee considers case studies on commercial sex work from three South African cities and highlights the need for the government to recognise and decriminalise the sex worker industry as a pre-condition for interventions to promote health-seeking behaviour among sex workers and their partners.

The spread of disease in societies is shaped, at least in part, by the political, social and economic environment in which people live. In South Africa, 'circular' migration between urban centres and mines for work and rural areas as home bases served as the fundamental building block for the apartheid society. Migration has been an important determinant of the spread of infectious diseases and was a critical factor responsible for the extraordinarily rapid spread of HIV in South Africa. Young women in both urban and rural areas are uniquely vulnerable to acquiring HIV and migration is an important factor contributing to the high prevalence of HIV among women. Mark Lurie's chapter discusses how population movement has contributed to the spread of HIV in South Africa, explaining the importance of conjugal instability and concomitant high STI incidence rates in the spread of HIV among migrants.

Men are, obviously, important in the spread of any sexually transmitted infection and their role in the spread of HIV in South Africa is examined in detail by Gethwana Makahye. Gender is a social construct and is about different roles and responsibilities in society. While much is written about the disempowered role that women have in many societies, few people understand that the male role – of strength, decision making and responsibility – can be equally disempowering under certain circumstances. It is this dichotomy that Makahye explores in her chapter on young men, explaining how the social constructs of men's role in society can be used to help men understand how they can be a part of preventing the further spread of the virus in South Africa.

Impact of AIDS

HIV/AIDS is a pandemic whose impact on societies is without precedent in recorded human history. There is no segment of society that can claim to have escaped its effects. It is devastating families and communities, overwhelming health care services and depleting schools of both students and teachers. Business has suffered and continues to suffer losses of personnel productivity and profits, economic growth is being undermined and scarce resources have to be diverted to deal with the consequences of the epidemic.

The greatest impact of HIV has obviously been on those living with the virus. Lilian Mboyi gives a searing account of her infection with HIV and the effects this has had on her and her family over the years. Now stable on antiretrovirals, her story takes the reader on a roundabout of emotions, from despair to hope and finally acceptance. This very human account of living with HIV is one of the most important chapters in the book.

AIDS has placed a huge added burden on an already strained health care system in South Africa. The epidemic is drastically changing the case mix and demographic pattern of those who seek care in the public health service: increasingly young adults whose health status would normally be good and for whom health care services have not previously had to provide. Not only can the current health system not cope with the numbers of AIDS patients but patients who don't have HIV/AIDS are being severely compromised because of a lack of capacity. Mark Colvin warns that the worst of the impact on the health care system is still to come. Health care costs in the public sector are likely to double by 2010 if current levels of care are maintained. Although the greatest burden of the disease will be borne by the public sector, the disease is likely to cause an escalation in medical aid and medical insurance scheme rates.

AIDS has an impact on all levels of the social fabric: individual, family and community. With sharply rising child mortality, life expectancy has contracted by decades rather than years. And though all are affected, it is the economically disadvantaged that have been the most vulnerable. Janet Frohlich describes the effects on family structure and discusses the complexity of the challenges created by the increasing number of orphans within poor communities.

AIDS and research into AIDS has raised many ethical challenges and has led to a rethink of the way research should be conducted and what is owed to research participants in the developing world. Jerome Singh provides a detailed analysis of the effects of the epidemic on the conduct of research and clinical practice and the ethical issues that this has raised, including an in-depth discussion of the issues posed by clinical trials in resource-poor areas.

Economic activity and social progress are under threat from HIV and AIDS in Africa. The disease has effectively wiped out the development gains of the past decade and is poised to sabotage future economic growth in the continent. UNAIDS estimates that AIDS is reducing per capita growth in more than half of the countries in sub-Saharan Africa by 0.5%–1.2% annually. Alan Whiteside describes the complex and interrelated nature of the economic impact of AIDS in South Africa, detailing the impacts at the macro- and micro-economic level. Although the data are far from clear cut, it would seem clear that HIV will have far-reaching effects on the economies of all the countries in sub-Saharan Africa with high burdens of disease.

The 1990s saw a rapid increase in young adult mortality in South Africa, caused largely by the effects of HIV. Debbie Bradshaw and Rob Dorrington provide a detailed analysis of the available statistics on mortality in South Africa, showing how these can be interpreted in a way that increases our understanding of the impact of HIV on the demographics of the country.

Mark Heywood examines the impact of HIV on the young democracy that is South Africa. Unfortunately, the political history of HIV in South Africa has been one of controversy and denial. Although the South African government has recognised the importance of the epidemic to the country, they have been slow to implement programmes that can mitigate its effects. Heywood traces this history and shows how, even now, it is possible that HIV has had a serious and negative effect on South Africa's journey to full democracy.

Treating AIDS

Even before the emergence of AIDS, South Africa was already experiencing a major TB epidemic. The AIDS epidemic has exacerbated this and TB is now a leading cause of mortality in South Africa, the two epidemics running in parallel. Drawing on studies in the mining sector Gavin Churchyard and Elizabeth Corbet give an overview of the epidemiology, pathogenesis, clinical features, treatment and control of HIV-associated TB.

Several opportunistic infections are associated with AIDS. The best way to prevent opportunistic diseases is to improve the level of immune function with highly active antiretroviral therapy (HAART). Yet even when HAART becomes widely accessible in South Africa, prevention of opportunistic disease will remain an essential component of care for the HIV-infected person. Gary Maartens details ways to minimise opportunistic infections through recommendations of environmental safety, and provision of chemoprophylaxis and vaccinations that are available in South Africa.

Chronic weight loss is common in patients with AIDS. AIDS dietician Marianne Visser reviews current data regarding the clinical significance of weight loss in HIV infection and the effect of antiretroviral therapy, as well as nutritional support, on body weight and body composition. She outlines the role of micronutrient deficiencies in the pathogenesis of HIV infection and the effects of supplementation of various micronutrients on nutritional, immunological and clinical outcomes in HIV disease and she reviews the implications of these for clinical practice.

Despite the substantial change that the health care system has undergone over the past ten years, it remains ill-equipped to comprehensively tackle the HIV epidemic. For the foreseeable future many HIV-infected individuals will be unable to access antiretrovirals and will need palliative care, which can be therapeutically challenging and emotionally demanding. Douglas Wilson and Lara Fairall, drawing on long clinical experience in managing AIDS patients, describe the current health care structures for AIDS care in the private and public sectors. There are many potential obstacles to effective care in South Africa. Among them are adherence to therapy and the lack of infrastructure in the health services generally. Wilson contributes a broad discussion of important clinical issues affecting AIDS patients in South Africa and underlines the importance of mobilising human resources in coordinated and well-focused primary-care programmes.

Treating and caring for the millions of South Africans living with HIV/AIDS poses an enormous challenge. Highly active antiretroviral therapy (HAART) can transform the course of HIV infection into a manageable disease, as has been observed in many industrialised countries. Robin Wood details the fiscal and operational challenges in implementing HAART in South Africa. He discusses the importance for patient outcome of issues involved in diagnosis, staging, clinical management, and therapeutic choices.

The challenge of treating the millions of South Africans with antiretroviral therapy is not limited to operational issues. Drug procurement, use of generics, and monitoring of drug resistance all pose equally daunting challenges. Andrew Gray outlines antiretroviral drug issues of particular importance to developing countries, including complexities such as the legal ramifications of using generic drugs and the challenge to notions of intellectual property rights in the face of an international catastrophe.

The political response to AIDS in the pre-1994 era was characterised by homophobia, denial, xenophobia, racial profiling and scare tactics. This changed post-1994 but the hope of a genuine and committed response was not immediately met, as successive government responses failed to meet the threat head on. An in-depth political analysis of the history of the response to HIV since 1994 is presented by Nawaal Deane, an investigative journalist from the *Weekly Mail and Guardian*. She presents the key political events that shaped the response to the AIDS epidemic in South Africa and argues that the errors and misunderstandings of the past have undermined even the country's positive attempts to deal with HIV/AIDS. The government's decision to adopt a comprehensive approach to HIV/AIDS in South Africa, including a national antiretroviral roll-out plan could be a turning point in the relationship between AIDS activists and government authorities.

However, at the time of writing, there does appear to be political will to continue with the planned roll-out of antiretrovirals across all provinces. At the same time, differences in infrastructure and capacity between provinces present a major challenge to government, both national and provincial.

What does the future hold?

To understand the complex HIV/AIDS epidemic patterns, dynamic, non-linear, mathematical models have been developed that can be used to make predictions about the future course of the epidemic and to explore the consequences of different scenarios. Brian Williams discusses some of the implications of modelling disease processes and dynamics, offers projections of the impact of HIV on TB and the likely impact of behavioural change programmes and programmes to manage curable and treatable STIs, predicts how many people will die if we continue only with current prevention programmes, and gives us a statistical perspective on how best to mount a serious response to the epidemic.

The book concludes by capturing the imperative of a national concerted response to the AIDS epidemic. The social movements that

characterised past changes in health-related behaviours need to be
emulated. Indeed, South Africa is well placed to achieve a remarkable
turnaround in the epidemic if it chooses the right future – a future
that integrates prevention and treatment to address stigma and
create a new level of openness on AIDS as the major challenge facing
the future South Africa.

CHAPTER 3

HIV Infection in South Africa: the evolving epidemic

Eleanor Gouws and Quarraisha Abdool Karim

CROSS-SECTIONAL DATA ON HIV prevalence in South Africa is widely available, the most extensive being based on the annual surveillance set up by the National Department of Health in 1990 to monitor the prevalence of HIV infection in women attending public antenatal clinics. Many additional surveys have been conducted in South Africa over the last 15 years and these provide crucial information on epidemic trends, patterns of infection, and factors that contribute to the spread of the epidemic.

South Africa has experienced one of the fastest growing HIV epidemics in the world and currently bears about 10% of the global burden of HIV infection. The epidemic is characterised by high HIV prevalence, fuelled by high rates of new infections in young women and is predominantly of subtype C. The prevalence varies by age, gender and geographic area.

Data collected over recent years indicates that the epidemic has started to level off, an effect that is unlikely to be due to interventions, but simply reflects the natural saturation of the epidemic. While the HIV prevalence is no longer increasing significantly, the incidence of new infections is balanced by rising mortality rates.

This chapter provides an introduction to factors that influence the transmission dynamics of epidemics and key epidemiological tools for measuring the burden of infection in a defined population at a given point in time as well as over a defined time period. Our understanding of the HIV epidemic in South Africa depends largely on a range of seroprevalence surveys that have been conducted in a variety of settings and populations; a brief description of these sources of HIV data is provided.

The evolving epidemic in South Africa is described in relation to times that mark key milestones in the spread of HIV in South Africa, from the first reported cases of AIDS in the early eighties as a localised subtype B epidemic among men having sex with men, haemophiliacs and recipients of unscreened blood products, to the current point of a generalised, mature, subtype C epidemic where the prevalence of infection appears to have stabilised although morbidity and mortality are still on the increase. Distinctive characteristics of the South African HIV epidemic are described, ranging from the rapid spread of HIV infection to differences in terms of gender, age and geographic area. The chapter concludes by considering the implications of current epidemic trends for prioritising and targeting interventions to alter the nature and the future course of the epidemic.

Transmission dynamics, prevalence and incidence rates

Sexual transmission of HIV depends upon direct contact between infected and susceptible individuals. The simplest model of the population dynamics of HIV is shown schematically in FIGURE 3.1. People are born susceptible, putting aside the issue of mother-to-child transmission, and the rate at which infections are acquired is proportional to the number of encounters between susceptible (S) and infected (I) cases. In the case of HIV, the rate at which infection spreads at a population level depends on: the number of infected people; the number of susceptible people who are available to be infected; the rate at which these two groups make contact; the probability that the infection is transmitted (per sexual contact); and the life expectancy of infected people.

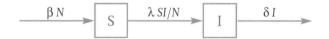

FIGURE 3.1 The population grows at a per capita rate β, susceptible people become infected at a rate λ times the current prevalence (I/N), and people die of AIDS at a rate δ. The population growth rate is the birth rate minus the background death rate.

Most epidemics are shaped by the interplay of these factors. Initially there is an exponential increase in the number of newly infected individuals. As the number of infected individuals increases, the susceptible pool decreases, and the prevalence levels off.

After a steady state has been reached and depending on behaviour change or other interventions that serve to reduce transmission, the prevalence may eventually start to fall, as shown in FIGURE 3.2 for Uganda and Zimbabwe.

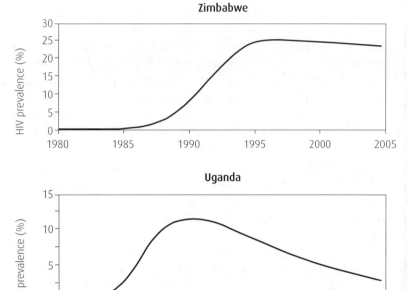

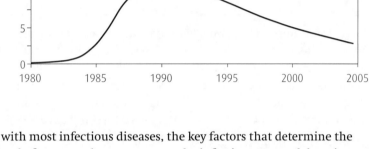

FIGURE 3.2 HIV epidemic trends showing stabilisation in Zimbabwe and a decline in Uganda. *Source: Curves fitted to UNAIDS/WHO data (UNAIDS/WHO Epidemiological Fact Sheets)*

As with most infectious diseases, the key factors that determine the spread of AIDS are the contact rate, the infectiousness and duration of infectiousness. In the case of AIDS these depend on demographic factors including age and gender; social factors including sexual networking patterns and sexual practices; biological variables such as the presence of other sexually transmitted infections and male circumcision; and medical factors including the provision of anti-retrovirals and the treatment of AIDS-related opportunistic infections.

As the epidemic of HIV infection threatens to overwhelm South Africa, it is important to understand the basic dynamics in order to deal with it. It is necessary to know not only how much disease there is in a population at any time but also how the burden of infection and disease is changing with time, The two most fundamental measurements for monitoring trends in an epidemic are prevalence and incidence rates. These measures enable one to determine how much infection there is in a population at a specific time as well as how the burden of infection is changing with time.

Prevalence is defined as the proportion of individuals in the population who are infected or who have the condition of interest or disease at a given point in time, while the incidence rate of infection or disease is the frequency of occurrence of *new* cases of infection or disease in a defined time period.

While the prevalence of infection provides a measure of the cumulative risk of infection, the incidence of infection gives the rate at which new infections are acquired (FIGURE 3.3). Prevalence data provide a snapshot view of the current number of people infected with HIV, which is essential for understanding the health impact of a disease within a community, for assessing the need for medical care and for targeting and evaluating interventions. In contrast, incidence data provide information on current infection rates by measuring rates of new infections in individuals who were previously uninfected. Incidence data are therefore more sensitive to the dynamics of disease transmission and exploring causal theories concerning the course of the diseases, as well as for measuring the immediate or short-term impact of interventions.

In this and the following chapters, measures of both prevalence and incidence will be used to describe trends and characteristics of the HIV epidemic in South Africa. This chapter primarily utilises prevalence data. The next chapter focuses on the HIV incidence rates in South Africa.

$$\text{Prevalence} = \frac{\textit{Number of individuals who are infected with HIV at a specific time}}{\textit{Number of individuals in the population at that point in time}}$$

$$\text{Incidence rates} = \frac{\textit{Number of new cases of HIV infection during a certain time period}}{\textit{Number of uninfected individuals in the population x time period of observation}}$$

FIGURE 3.3 Calculating prevalence and incidence rate

Sources of data on HIV infection in South Africa

Numerous HIV seroprevalence surveys have been undertaken in South Africa over the past 15 years that have enabled us to understand how the HIV epidemic in South Africa is evolving, identify factors that contribute to the spread of the epidemic and offer guidance for prioritising and targeting interventions.

Antenatal clinic surveys

National, annual, anonymous, antenatal clinic surveys

The rise in the number of HIV infections among heterosexual, voluntary blood donors during 1988 and 1989 prompted the then Department of National Health and Population Development to initiate a national HIV surveillance programme in 1990. This was based on anonymous, unlinked, cross-sectional surveys of pregnant women attending antenatal clinics in the public health sector throughout South Africa. Only women who were attending an antenatal clinic for their first visit for their current pregnancy were included in order to minimise the chance of the same woman being included in the study more than once.

Pregnant women were chosen as a proxy marker for monitoring the spread of HIV in the heterosexual population. All pregnant women attending antenatal clinics in the public health services routinely submit blood samples to be tested for syphilis, rhesus factor (RH) and ABO blood grouping in order to prevent haemolytic disease in the newborn. After removal of personal identifiers, these blood specimens are used for the annual HIV surveys.

Notwithstanding several biases inherent in this population, the national, annual antenatal HIV surveys conducted during October and November each year provide the most reliable estimates of temporal trends of HIV infection in the general population, as well as age-specific HIV prevalence and geographical distribution of HIV infection in South Africa.

Thus far, 14 such surveys have been completed. The large sample size in each survey, consistent methodology and the timing of these cross-sectional surveys have aimed to minimise several biases inherent in cross-sectional studies. Data from these surveys have been used to monitor the progress of the HIV epidemic in the heterosexually active population in South Africa.

Western Cape district-wide HIV surveillance

Since 2001, the Western Cape Department of Health has been conducting annual, anonymous district-wide HIV seroprevalence surveys among first visit antenatal clinic attendees using public sector health facilities in conjunction with the national antenatal surveys. These surveys, three completed to date, provide useful insights into the wide variation in the distribution of HIV infection within the Western Cape and have assisted the Western Cape Department of Health with prioritising and targeting their response at a provincial level.

The Hlabisa health district, situated in rural northern KwaZulu-Natal, is home to about 215 000 largely Zulu-speaking people. Hlabisa has a large male migrant population and a relatively stable female population. In addition to migrant labour, most people rely on subsistence farming and pension remittances.

Since 1992, repeat cross-sectional, anonymous, antenatal surveys have been undertaken in Hlabisa by the South African Medical Research Council in the same months as the national ANC surveys and provide comparative data from a rural area that is consistent with the temporal trends in HIV infection in KwaZulu-Natal observed through the national survey. Ten such surveys have been completed to date.

Prevention of mother-to-child transmission (PMTCT) studies
Additional seroprevalence data from pregnant women have been collected in KwaZulu-Natal and Gauteng as part of natural history studies of HIV infection from infected mother-to-child (MTCT), trials of interventions to reduce MTCT and more recently through pilot PMTCT sites.

With the recently established PMTCT programmes, additional linked HIV data are becoming available and will enable comparisons between linked and unlinked surveys.

Population-based surveys

Population-based surveys in KwaZulu-Natal
Three population based surveys were conducted in conjunction with the Malaria Control Programme between 1990–1992. These surveys provide data on temporal trends in HIV infection in a predominantly rural population in the early stages of the epidemic. In addition, these surveys provided data on age and gender differences in HIV infection. The HIV seroprevalence trends observed in these surveys were consistent with the provincial data from the national ANC surveys.

Mandela Foundation/HSRC population-based survey
In 2002 the Mandela Foundation, in conjunction with the Human Sciences Research Council (HSRC), undertook the first national community-based study on behavioural and socio-cultural determinants of vulnerability to HIV/AIDS and tested consenting people for HIV. The study provides data on HIV prevalence by geographic area, race, gender and age. The data on HIV distribution by race is consistent with data from the National Blood Transfusion Services; and the data on gender and age distribution of HIV infection is consistent

with the population-based studies described above. However, this survey differs significantly in terms of the magnitude of, and provincial distribution of, HIV infection in South Africa in comparison to the national ANC surveys and other *ad hoc* studies. It is anticipated that this survey will be repeated every two years.

Carletonville/urban population survey

The Carletonville project, conducted in one of the world's largest mining complexes, was designed as a community-based intervention with a strong social evaluation component to identify and explore the contextual factors that influence the course of the epidemic and which can be used as markers of the effectiveness of the intervention. Information was obtained on HIV and STI prevalence, as well as on a range of social and behavioural determinants. In addition to the approximately 56 000 people living in the township, there are about 70 000 migrant mine workers recruited from rural areas in South Africa and neighbouring countries. The majority of the mine workers live in single sex hostels around the mines without their wives and frequently visit sex workers who operate in informal settlements in townships around the mines. In addition to baseline assessments undertaken in 1998, follow-up surveys were conducted in 1999 and 2000.

Other studies

Sex workers and clients at truck-stops in KwaZulu-Natal

Since the early 1990s the South African Medical Research Council has been undertaking research with sex workers at truckstops in the KwaZulu-Natal Midlands. In addition to HIV prevalence data, HIV sero-incidence data is also available from this population through the women's participation in a Phase III microbicide trial.

In 1998 a cross-sectional HIV seroprevalence study was undertaken with clients of sex workers at these truck-stops, enabling comparison of HIV prevalence in sex workers and their clients.

National workplace survey

Additional data on HIV infection in men and women by age and race is available from several workplace-based, anonymous surveys undertaken in South Africa. However, these data cannot be easily accessed.

HIV infection in South Africa

As in many parts of North America, Europe, central and eastern Africa, the first cases of AIDS in South Africa were diagnosed in 1982.

From 1983 to 1987, the spread of HIV in South Africa was mainly among men who have sex with men, and prior to the introduction of universal screening of all blood products for HIV in 1985 there were about 100 medically acquired infections among haemophiliacs. Several surveys conducted between 1985 and 1987 in a diverse range of populations demonstrated that up to 1987, HIV infection in the heterosexual population was rare.

Prevalences of zero were observed in a rural community in 1985, among sex workers in Transvaal in 1986 and among antenatal clinic attendees and out-patients in KwaZulu-Natal in 1987. In a study conducted among 29 312 mine workers in South Africa in 1986, only three men tested positive for HIV infection.

Despite the relatively late introduction of HIV infection in the heterosexual population in South Africa compared to eastern and central Africa, it accounts for currently 10% of the global burden of infection. In a 10-year period from 1990 to 2000, HIV sero-prevalence among antenatal clinic attendees has increased 'explosively' from 0.8% to 24.5% (FIGURE 3.4).

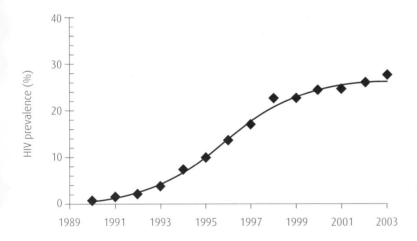

FIGURE 3.4 HIV prevalence among ANC attendees 1990–2002

The period 1988 to 1993 marks the beginning of the generalised or 'major' epidemic of subtype C HIV infection in South Africa. During the early stages of the epidemic, between 1990 and 1993 there was an exponential increase in HIV infection with a doubling time of a little over one year and by 1994 it had reached 10% among antenatal clinic attending women.

Between 1994 and 1998 the incidence of new infections reached a peak. Young women were at especially high risk (CHAPTER 16) and recombination of different genotypes was seen (CHAPTER 7). Fitted to a logistic curve, the epidemic reached half its peak value between 1995 and 1996 and has an expected maximum prevalence at the plateau of the epidemic of 26.5%. Despite the high rates of new HIV infections and increasing morbidity, mortality remained relatively low during this period. The high prevalence of HIV infection during this period is indicative of the demand for health care to be anticipated in the next period as individuals progress to AIDS.

The period 1999 to 2002 epitomises the maturation of the HIV epidemic in South Africa, characterised by the epidemic reaching saturation. The overall HIV prevalence data, as well as the provincial and age-specific data (TABLES 3.1) since 2000 indicate that the epidemic is reaching a plateau. While the HIV prevalence is no longer increasing, the mortality continues to rise (CHAPTER 25) and the incidence of new infections balances deaths (CHAPTER 4).

Anonymous HIV serosurveys were conducted among antenatal clinic attendees in the Hlabisa district between 1992 and 2001. As in KwaZulu-Natal generally, Hlabisa experienced a very dramatic increase in HIV and prevalences among prenatal clinic attendees have risen from 4.2% in 1992 to 14% in 1995 and 36% in 2001 (TABLE 3.2). The progression in rural KwaZulu-Natal is similar to that observed nationally.

The major epidemic as a result of heterosexual spread of HIV is associated with a concomitant epidemic in infants born to HIV-infected mothers. The epidemic of mother-to-child transmission of

PROVINCE										
Year	WC	EC	NC	FS	KZN	MP	NP	GT	NW	National
1990	0.1	0.4	0.2	0.6	1.6	0.4	0.3	0.7	1.1	0.7
1991	0.1	0.6	0.1	1.5	2.9	1.2	0.5	1.1	6.5	1.7
1992	0.3	1.0	0.7	2.9	4.5	2.2	1.1	2.5	0.9	2.2
1993	0.6	1.9	1.1	4.1	9.5	2.40	1.8	4.1	2.2	4.0
1994	1.2	4.5	1.8	9.2	14.4	12.2	3.0	6.4	6.7	7.6
1995	1.7	6.0	5.3	11.0	18.2	16.2	4.9	12.0	8.3	10.4
1996	3.1	8.1	6.5	17.5	19.9	15.8	8.0	15.5	25.1	14.2
1997	6.3	12.6	8.6	20.0	26.9	22.6	8.2	17.1	18.1	17.0
1998	5.2	15.9	9.9	22.8	32.5	30.0	11.5	22.5	21.3	22.8
1999	7.1	18.0	10.1	27.9	32.5	23.8	11.4	23.8	23.0	22.4
2000	8.7	20.2	11.2	27.9	36.2	29.7	13.2	29.4	22.9	24.5
2001	8.6	21.7	15.9	30.1	33.5	29.2	14.5	29.8	25.2	24.8
2002	12.4	23.6	15.1	28.8	36.5	28.6	15.6	31.6	26.2	26.5
2003	13.1	27.1	16.7	30.1	37.5	32.6	17.5	29.6	29.9	27.9

TABLE 3.1 HIV prevalence (%) in antenatal clinic attendees by province between 1990 and 2003

HIV is not discussed in this chapter as it is elaborated in great detail in CHAPTER 11.

Year	N	Prevalence of HIV (95% CI)	
1992	884	4.2%	(3.0–5.7)
1993	709	7.9%	(6.0–10.1)
1995	314	14.0%	(10.4–18.4)
1997	4731	27.2%	(25.9–28.5)
1998	3166	29.9%	(28.4–31.6)
1999	3001	34.0%	(32.5–35.7)
2001	906	36.1%	(32.9–39.2)

TABLE 3.2 Prevalence of HIV infection among antenatal clinic attendees, aged 15–49 in Hlabisa; 1992–2001

Geographical distribution

There is considerable geographical variation in the distribution of HIV infection in South Africa, with a gradient of infection that is highest in the east coast and lowest in the west coast of South Africa (TABLE 3.1). Antenatal HIV prevalence increased from 1.6% in 1990 to 37.5% in 2003 in KwaZulu-Natal compared to 0.06% to 13.1% in the Western Cape during the same period.

One explanation for the wide variation in the geographical distribution of HIV infection is the uneven population distribution. The distribution of people infected with HIV obtained by combining the provincial prevalence data with the population density is illustrated in FIGURE 3.5.

Although the Western Cape has low rates of infection, Cape Town has a large population and thus a high density of people infected with HIV. In contrast, while the overall infection rates in KwaZulu-Natal are high, the population is patchily distributed and infections do not occur evenly through the province. In the former Transkei, to the north-east of East London, infected people are more evenly spread over a large area. The mining centres at Carletonville, Klerksdorp and Welkom show high densities of infected people as do the port cities of Port Elizabeth, East London and Durban and the major industrial and commercial centre of Johannesburg.

While the overall doubling time at the start of the epidemic in South Africa was 13.8 months, the doubling time at a provincial level varied from 9.2 months in Northern province to 14.1 months in KwaZulu-Natal (TABLE 3.3).

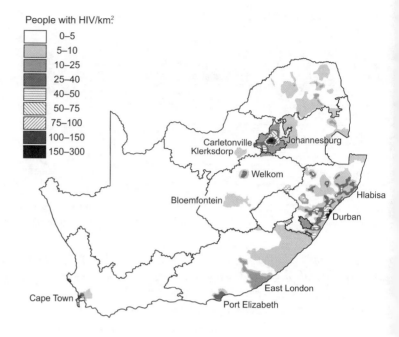

People with HIV/km²

- 0–5
- 5–10
- 10–25
- 25–40
- 40–50
- 50–75
- 75–100
- 100–150
- 150–300

FIGURE 3.5 The number of people living with HIV infection per square kilometre (adapted from Williams & Gouws, 2001 *Phil Trans R Soc Lond*)

TABLE 3.3 The 2002 HIV prevalence, the expected peak HIV prevalence, doubling times at the start of the epidemic (with 95% confidence interval) for data collected from antenatal clinic attendees by province

Province	Prevalence (%) (95% CI)		Doubling Time (months)
	2002	Asymptote	
Western Cape	12.4 (8.8–15.9)	11.1 (9.8–12.4)	12.3 (10.5–14.9)
Eastern Cape	23.6 (21.1–26.1)	23.5 (21.8–25.2)	13.5 (12.3–15.0)
Northern Cape	15.1 (11.7–18.6)	14.1 (12.1–16.1)	11.4 (9.3–14.6)
Free State	28.8 (26.3–31.2)	29.8 (28.0–31.6)	13.0 (11.7–14.7)
KwaZulu-Natal	36.5 (33.8–39.2)	36.1 (35.0–37.2)	14.1 (13.1–15.3)
Mpumalanga	28.6 (25.3–31.8)	28.8 (27.3–30.3)	10.5 (9.6–11.7)
Northern Province	15.6 (13.2–17.9)	14.7 (13.6–15.8)	9.2 (8.1–10.7)
Gauteng	31.6 (29.7–33.6)	31.1 (29.9–32.3)	13.2 (12.2–14.3)
North-West	26.2 (23.1–29.4)	25.9 (24.2–27.6)	12.2 (10.3–15.0)
National	26.5 (25.5–27.6)	26.5 (25.9–27.1)	13.8 (13.3–14.4)

Note: The expected peak prevalence is the point at which the HIV epidemic is expected to plateau in each province and is estimated by fitting a logistic curve with variable asymptote using a least squares fit.

TABLE 3.3 also shows that the HIV prevalence in 2002 is close to an asymptote in all provinces but at much higher rates in KwaZulu-Natal than elsewhere.

HIV prevalence by age estimated in 1998 for the national antenatal clinic attendees, two sentinel sites and selected risk groups in South Africa are summarised in TABLE 3.4. The prevalence of HIV infection among women in the general population in South Africa is increasing at the same rate among all age-groups and the shape of the age-distribution follows that of a log-normal distribution, as illustrated in FIGURE 3.6 using data from antenatal clinic attendees in Hlabisa. The prevalence is close to zero among girls younger than 15 years and then increases rapidly with age to a peak among 20- to 24-year old women and a slow decline with age among older women.

In 1998, the national ante-natal clinic surveillance data showed that 26% of women aged 20 to 24 years were infected with HIV, compared to a prevalence of 10% among women 40 years and older. Thirty nine percent of 20- to 24-year-old women in Hlabisa and an alarming 54% in Carletonville were infected in 1998, compared to 12% and 24%, respectively, of 40- to 44-year-old women (TABLE 3.4).

The age-specific HIV prevalence data nationally (TABLE 3.5) and from Hlabisa (TABLE 3.6) demonstrate the rapid progression of infection from 1990 to 2002 across all age groups and also highlight the alarmingly high increase in young women under the age of 30 years to unprecedented levels by 2001.

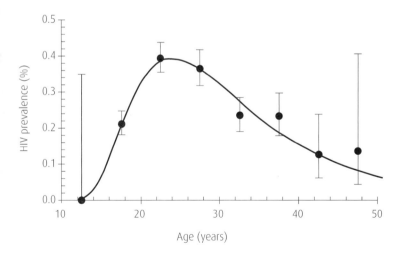

FIGURE 3.6 Age prevalence of HIV infection among women attending antenatal clinics in Hlabisa in 1998. The curve was fitted to the data recorded by one year age groups but is averaged in five yearly groups for clarity. Error bars are 95% confidence limits. The fitted curve is a log-normal function

In Hlabisa, the prevalence of HIV among 20- to 24-year-old women grew from 6.9% in 1992, to 21.1% in 1995, 39.3% in 1998 and 50.8% in 2001 (TABLE 3.6). The rapid increase in prevalence in the youngest group of women is a major cause for concern.

Age	WOMEN					MEN		
	Antenatal clinics: National survey	Hlabisa ANC	Carletonville	Sex workers at truckstops in KZN	Sex workers: Carletonville	Carletonville	Truck drivers in KZN	Mine workers: Carletonville
<15		7 0%	30 0.0%			31 0.0%		
15–19	874 21.0%	819 21.1%	101 20.8%	31 38.7%		99 2.0%		
20–24	1852 26.1%	994 39.3%	119 53.8%	56 58.9%		89 16.9%	23 47.8%	82 29.3%
25–29	1634 26.9%	608 36.4%	117 58.1%	41 68.3%	14 92.9%	59 42.4%	61 50.8%	167 28.1%
30–34	1484 19.1%	398 23.4%	105 46.7%	41 70.7%	34 67.6%	49 42.9%	56 57.1%	191 28.3%
35–39	921 13.4%	265 23.0%	93 33.3%	11 45.5%	26 69.2%	60 36.7%	58 50.0%	196 31.6%
40–44	271 10.5%	57 12.3%	68 23.5%	2 0.0%	25 52.0%	42 31.0%	43 60.5%	129 27.9%
45–49	37 10.2%	15 13.3%	30 20.0%	4 50.0%	11 81.8%	35 14.3%	44 65.9%	83 28.9%
50–54		3 33.3%	27 14.8%		5 60.0%	20 14.3%	22 59.1%	38 23.7%
55–59						15 13.3%		11 9.1%

TABLE 3.4 Age-specific prevalence of HIV in various groups studied in South Africa in 1998. Numbers and percentages are given

PREVALENCE (%) (95% CI)				
Age	1992	1995	1998	2001
15–19	2.4 (1.6–3.3)	10.3 (8.8–11.8)	21.0 (18.4–23.8)	15.4 (13.8–16.9)
20–24	3.5 (2.8–4.3)	14.3 (12.9–15.7)	26.1 (24.1–28.1)	28.4 (26.5–30.2)
25–29	1.8 (1.2–2.4)	12.1 (10.7–13.6)	26.9 (24.7–29.0)	31.4 (29.5–33.3)
30–34	1.8 (1.0–2.7)	9.1 (7.7–10.7)	19.1 (17.1–21.1)	25.6 (23.5–27.7)
35–39	1.6 (0.5–2.8)	6.7 (5.1–8.6)	13.4 (11.2–15.6)	19.3 (17.0–21.5)
40–44	0.1 (0–0.3)	4.5 (2.5–7.8)	10.5 (6.8–14.1)	9.1 (6.2–11.9)
45–49	0 (0–4.9)	2.5 (0.6–13.1)	10.2 (0.4–20.0)	17.8 (4.3–31.4)

TABLE 3.5 Temporal trends in the age-specific HIV prevalence among women attending antenatal clinics in the annual national survey 1992–2001. Prevalence is presented as percentage with 95% confidence intervals

Age group	1992	1995	1998	2001
20–24	6.9%	21.1%	39.3%	50.8%
25–29	2.7%	18.8%	36.4%	47.2%
30–34	1.4%	15.0%	23.4%	38.4%
35–39	0.0%	3.4%	23.0%	36.4%

TABLE 3.6 Temporal trends in the age-specific prevalence of HIV infection in antenatal clinic attendees in Hlabisa, northern KwaZulu-Natal

FIGURE 3.7 shows that, although prevalence increased dramatically over time, the shape of the antenatal HIV age prevalence curves, fitted to a log-normal function, has remained much the same over a period of nine years, with peak prevalences occurring at around 24 years. In 1992, prevalence peaked at 4% at age 24.4 years; in 1995 it peaked at 14% among women aged 23.7 years; in 1998 it peaked at 27.6% among women aged 23.4 years; and in 2001 it peaked at 30.5 among women aged 24.3-years-old.

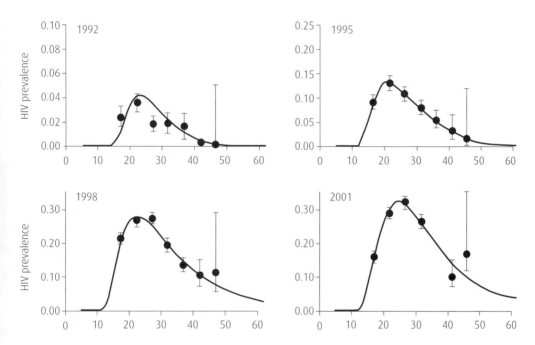

FIGURE 3.7 Age-prevalence curves showing temporal trends of the HIV epidemic among women attending national antenatal clinics

Age and gender differences

Population-based surveys undertaken in rural KwaZulu-Natal during 1990 to 1992 demonstrate that in addition to the rapid rise in HIV infection, there is a striking difference in age and gender distribution of HIV infection. FIGURE 3.8 illustrates the early rise of infection in young women between the ages of 15 to 19 years compared to a later rise of infection in men at about age 25 to 29 years of age in Kwazulu-Natal. The high incidence rate in young women is a key factor driving the spread of HIV in South Africa during this period and is discussed further in CHAPTER 16.

In Carletonville in 1998, the prevalence of infection is close to zero for both sexes before the age of 15 years but increases rapidly there-

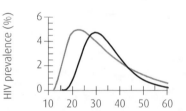

FIGURE 3.8 Age and gender distribution of HIV infection in rural Kwazulu-Natal

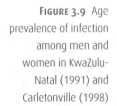

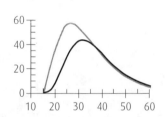

FIGURE 3.9 Age prevalence of infection among men and women in KwaZulu-Natal (1991) and Carletonville (1998)

after reaching 39% in 20-year-old women but only 8% in 20-year-old men (FIGURE 3.9). The peak prevalence is 58% at 24 years of age among women and 45% at 32 years of age among men. The median age at first sex was close to 16 years for both men and women in Carletonville and the prevalence of infection increases rapidly thereafter.

The age-specific prevalence of infection for rural men and women in KwaZulu-Natal in 1991 and for urban men and women in Carletonville in 1998, as illustrated in FIGURE 3.9, shows that while there are important gender differences between men and women, the shapes of the age-prevalence curves, reflecting the age-specific risk of infection, have not changed over time and are similar in urban and rural settings. Although the overall prevalence in the later urban survey is approximately ten times higher than in the earlier rural survey the shapes of the age-prevalence curves for men and women are statistically the same.

The more recently conducted HSRC survey is consistent with earlier observations on gender and age differences in HIV infection (FIGURE 3.10). Factors underlying these striking differences in HIV prevalence are covered in Section 4.

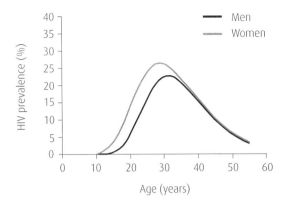

FIGURE 3.10 National 63

FIGURE 3.10 National prevalence of HIV by sex and age in 2002. Log-normal curves were fitted to data collected from the Nelson Mandela/HSRC study of HIV/AIDS

Racial differences in HIV prevalence

Marginalisation and discrimination on the basis of race and/or ethnicity is a key factor influencing vulnerability to HIV infection.

As in most countries collection of data by race is politically sensitive. The major users of public sector health facilities are Black Africans and therefore most data collected from public sector facilities are from Black African users. Data on racial distribution of HIV infection are available from voluntary blood donors through the National Blood Transfusion Services and the more recently conducted Mandela Foundation/HSRC national population-based survey. While HIV infection is found in all race groups, it is substantially more common in the Black African population (TABLE 3.7).

Race Group	Prevalence (%)	95% CI
African	12.9	11.2–14.5
White	6.2	3.1–9.2
Coloured	6.1	4.5–7.8
Indian	1.6	0–3.4

TABLE 3.7 HIV prevalence by race in South Africa 2002
Source: HSRC national survey

Migration and its effect on other sexually transmitted infections

Two key risk factors influencing the spread of HIV in South Africa are the migrant labour system and the high burden of other sexually transmitted infections. As both these issues are covered extensively in CHAPTER 19 and CHAPTER 12 respectively they are not covered in this chapter.

Morbidity and mortality

Given the long lag period between HIV infection and disease progression to illness and death, it is not surprising that it is only in the past three years that the disease burden has started to be felt at the health facilities level. The impact of advancing HIV disease is discussed in greater detail in CHAPTER 21.

As in other African countries, tuberculosis (TB) is the most common presenting opportunistic infection associated with advancing HIV disease. FIGURE 3.11 illustrates how the TB burden in one rural community has increased as the HIV prevalence has increased despite major advances and successes in TB control attained in the early 1990s. The interaction between HIV and TB is discussed more fully in CHAPTER 29.

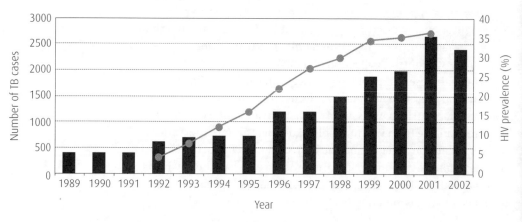

FIGURE 3.11
Tuberculosis caseload and antenatal HIV prevalence in Hlabisa
Source: Hlabisa Hospital records

While limited data are available on AIDS-related mortality, data on all cause mortality from the national demographic and health survey conducted by the South African Medical Research Council illustrate the substantial rise in mortality in both men and women in the age groups most affected by the HIV epidemic, and are discussed in more detail in CHAPTER 25. Similar to the age and gender patterns of HIV infection and AIDS-related morbidity patterns, there are stark age and gender differences in mortality, suggesting that the increase in deaths observed since 1998 is AIDS-related.

Conclusion

The HIV epidemic in South Africa can be considered in different stages: before 1987 the epidemic was concentrated among men who have sex with men and recipients of blood products and was predominantly of subtype B. Once introduced into the heterosexual population, the prevalence of HIV subtype C started to rise exponentially reaching 4%

in 1993. During the period 1994 to 1998 the prevalence of infection continued to increase rapidly among antenatal clinic attendees from 7.6% to 22.8%. Mathematical models show that the peak incidence of infection occurred during this period, although AIDS-related mortality was still relatively low. Since 1998 the rate of increase in the epidemic has slowed substantially and prevalence data suggest that the epidemic is reaching a plateau. Mortality rates, however, are still rising and the incidence of new infections is balanced by deaths. Post-2002, AIDS-related morality rates may exceed HIV incidence, resulting in a slow decline in HIV prevalence.

In the current stage of the HIV epidemic, South Africa has had to deal with continued large numbers of new HIV infections, ongoing high mother-to-child transmission rates, rising morbidity, rapidly rising deaths, and an increasing number of orphans.

Each of these factors demands effective and rapid interventions if the epidemic is to be brought under control. In particular, it is essential that comprehensive prevention programmes to reduce new HIV infections are in place; that PMTCT programmes to reduce the ongoing mother-to-child transmission of HIV are implemented; that care services are strengthened to ensure the provision of prophylaxis, treatment of opportunistic infections and antiretroviral treatment; that social services for families who are affected by AIDS deaths are strengthened; that programmes and social services to take care of and provide for orphans are established. Finally, the high rates of new infections in young women highlight the importance of targeting interventions at youth, addressing gender inequities, and the need for greater involvement of men in prevention programmes. Subsequent chapters in this book provide details and specifics relating to these interventions.

Bibliography

ABDOOL KARIM Q, ABDOOL KARIM SS, SINGH B, SHORT R, NGXONGO S. 'Seroprevalence of HIV infection in rural South Africa'. *AIDS* 1992; 6: 1535–1539.

DEPARTMENT OF HEALTH, SOUTH AFRICA 1998. National HIV sero-prevalence survey of women attending antenatal clinics in South Africa. Summary report. Pretoria: Health Systems Research and Epidemiology, DOH 1999.

DEPARTMENT OF HEALTH, RSA. *National HIV and syphillis antenatal sero-prevalence survey in South Africa 2003.* Summary report. Pretoria: Health Systems Research, Research Coordination and Epidemiology, DOH 2003.

DUSHEIKO GM, BRINK BA, CONRADIE JD, MARIMUTHU T, SHER R. Regional prevalence of hepatitis B, delta, and human immunodeficiency virus infection in Southern Africa: A large population survey. *American Journal of Epidemiology* 1989; 129: 138–45.

KUSTNER HGV, SWANEVELDER JP, VAN MIDDELKOOP A. 'National HIV surveillance – South Africa, 1990–1992'. *South African Medical Journal* 1994; 84: 195–200.

SHISANA O, BEZUIDENHOUT F, BROOKES HJ, CHAUVEAU J, COLVIN M, ET AL. *Nelson Mandela/ HSRC study of HIV/AIDS.* Human Sciences Research Council. Cape Town, South Africa, 2002.

RAMJEE G, GOUWS E. 'Prevalence of HIV among truck drivers visiting sex workers in Kwazulu Natal, South Africa'. *Sexually Transmitted Diseases* 2002; 29: 44–49.

SHER R. 'HIV infection in South Africa, 1982–1988 – a review'. *South African Medical Journal* 1989; 76: 314–318.

SCHOUB BD, SMITH AN, JOHNSON S, MARTIN DJ, LYONS SF, PADAYACHEE GN, HURWITZ HS. 'Considerations on the further expansion of the AIDS epidemic in South Africa – 1990'. *South African Medical Journal* 1988; 74: 153–157.

WILLIAMS BG, GOUWS E. 'The epidemiology of the human immunodeficiency virus in South AFrica'. *Philosophical Transactions of the Royal Society of London* 2001; 356: 1–10.

WILLIAMS BG, GOUWS E, COLVIN M, SITAS F, RAMJEE G, ABDOOL KARIM SS. 'Patterns of infection: Using age prevalence data to understand the epidemic of HIV in South Africa'. *South African Journal of Science* 2000; 96: 305–312.

WILLIAMS BG, MACPHAIL C, CAMPBELL C, TALJAARD D, GOUWS E, MOEMA S, MZAIDUME Z, RASEGO B. 'The Carletonville-Mothusimpilo Project: Limiting transmission of HIV through community-based interventions'. *South African Journal of Science* 2000; 96: 351–359.

CHAPTER 4
HIV incidence rates in South Africa

Eleanor Gouws

TO FULLY UNDERSTAND TEMPORAL changes in the epidemic of
HIV we need to know how incidence and mortality have changed over
time. Unfortunately, incidence is difficult to measure directly for logistical and ethical reasons, and mortality is difficult to measure directly
because of the stigma associated with AIDS. Prevalence provides a
measure of incidence and mortality averaged over the previous five to
ten years so that it is much more difficult to interpret immediate
changes in the dynamics of the epidemic using prevalence than it is
using incidence. Ideally, incidence rates should therefore be used to
measure changes in the HIV epidemic.

Several studies have shown very high rates of HIV incidence in
South Africa. The UNAIDS sponsored Col-1492 trial measuring HIV
incidence rates directly among a cohort of sex workers in KwaZulu-
Natal showed an incidence rate of 18% between 1996 and 1998.

Indirect methods applied to data collected from women attending
public antenatal clinics in South Africa showed a national incidence
rate of close to 6% in 2001 with provincial variation between 1.7%
(Western Cape) and 9.5% (KwaZulu-Natal). Incidence peaked for most
provinces between 1997 and 1999. In Hlabisa, a rural site in KwaZulu-
Natal, HIV incidence peaked among antenatal clinic attendees at
10.5% in 1998. Equally high incidence rates were shown for an urban
mining community in Carletonville, Gauteng, in 1998: 13.5% among
women and 9.6% among men aged 15–49 years.

Incidence estimates for South Africa

With the HIV epidemic in South Africa reaching maturity, incidence
is falling, prevalence is stabilising and mortality is still rising.
Although incidence provides a much better measure of the dynamics

of the epidemic than prevalence, incidence is more difficult to measure than prevalence. Ideally, a cohort of people needs to be followed for a year or more to determine the number who became infected with HIV during the course of the study. Very few cohort studies have been performed in South Africa because of the cost, logistics and the ethical problems involved in following negative individuals until they seroconvert. More recently, a number of Phase III HIV prevention trials have been initiated with HIV infection as the endpoint and it is likely that more incidence data will become available in the near future. To date, however, the only incidence data available are those collected from the UNAIDS sponsored Col-1492 Phase III microbicide trial among sex workers in KwaZulu-Natal.

Several indirect methods, including mathematical and statistical methods, many of which utilise cross-sectional age-prevalence data, have been developed to estimate the incidence of HIV infection. These include:

- Back-calculation methods, assuming that trends in new AIDS cases reflect existing and past trends in HIV incidence.
- Birth cohort methods, based on the assumption that HIV incidence rates in the population are stable over time and that prevalence in young people increases linearly with age.
- Statistical models for estimating incidence from age-specific disease prevalence, allowing for differential mortality between people with and without disease.
- Dynamic models, some of which use data on the age-specific prevalence of infection and data on the time-trends in the average prevalence of infection together with assumptions about the form, age dependence and survivorship function for people infected with HIV.
- Demographic models, the main purpose of which is often to investigate the demographic consequences of HIV for use in life insurance, health and pension applications.

Although models are extremely important for the understanding of the dynamics of the HIV epidemic, model estimates should be interpreted with care because there is always a degree of uncertainty around the estimates. The estimates depend both on the structure of the model and assumptions about the key parameters that cannot necessarily be determined directly from the raw data. A detailed description of mathematical models, with comparisons of various models and notes on the limitations of mathematical modelling, is given by Williams in CHAPTER 36.

Incidence rates can also be determined through laboratory techniques either by using a standardised algorithm for recent HIV

seroconversion (STARHS or 'detuned' ELISA) or by detecting the presence of p24 antigen, which indicates whether an infection has been
acquired recently. These laboratory methods are described in more
detail in CHAPTER 6.

CASE STUDY

Incidence rates estimated directly from the UNAIDS sponsored Phase III
Col-1492 microbicide trial A cohort of female sex workers operating at
truck-stops along the national road linking Durban to Johannesburg
was established in 1996, in preparation for a Phase III multi-centre
microbicide trial. Among the 477 sex workers screened for possible
participation in the trial, HIV prevalence was 51.3%. The demographic characteristics, risk behaviours and safer sex practices are
described in greater detail in CHAPTER 18.

A cohort of 198 HIV negative sex workers were then followed up as
part of the microbicide trial for a period of about three years between
1996 and 1998 and represents the only data set in South Africa
providing direct estimates of incidence from longitudinal data. The
overall incidence rate per annum in this cohort study of women of
mean age 25 years (range 15–48 years) was 18% (13%–23%), ranging
from 16.8% in 1996/1997 to 20% in 1999 (TABLE 4.1). This high incidence was not surprising given the sexual risk, in terms of number of
clients, low condom use and high incidence of other STIs, that this
cohort was exposed to.

Year	Number HIV +	Person-months of follow-up	HIV incidence rate (%) (per year); 95% CI
1996/1997	14	996	16.8 (8–26)
1998	25	1644	18.2 (11–25)
1999	13	780	20.0 (9–31)
1996–1999	52	3420	18.2 (13–23)

TABLE 4.1 HIV incidence rate in a cohort of sex workers participating in a microbicide trial in KwaZulu-Natal

Estimating incidence rates indirectly

The following section presents incidence rates estimated indirectly
using dynamic models developed by Williams and Gouws specifically
for South Africa. The models, here applied to data collected from the
National and Hlabisa ante-natal surveys and the Carletonville
surveys, use age-specific prevalence of infection and data on the time-
trends in the average prevalence of infection to estimate age-specific
incidence, and use Monte Carlo methods to estimate confidence
limits on the projections.

Incidence rates estimated for South Africa

National and provincial estimates of incidence rates for the period 1991 to 2001 are provided in TABLE 4.2 and FIGURE 4.1. Incidence for the national data appeared to have peaked in 1997 at 6.46% while rates vary substantially between provinces, reflecting the differences in the spread of HIV between provinces.

The peak incidence rate in most provinces seems to have occurred between 1997 and 1999. Similar to the prevalence data, the highest peak incidence was in KwaZulu-Natal in 1997 at 9.8% while the lowest occurred in the Western Cape in 1998 at 2.1%. In contrast, incidence in Gauteng peaked only in 2000 (FIGURE 4.1). Both national and provincial incidence data indicate that the HIV epidemic in South Africa may be reaching a steady state. Of note is that although the incidence rates have declined from their peak values they remain high.

Year	WC	EC	NC	FS	KZN	MP	NP	GT	NW	National
1990										
1991	0.10	0.36	0.31	0.86	1.62	0.81	0.34	0.83	0.41	0.71
1992	0.18	0.64	0.51	1.46	2.73	1.57	0.58	1.33	0.82	1.25
1993	0.34	1.09	0.80	2.40	4.34	2.88	0.94	2.09	1.60	2.11
1994	0.61	1.79	1.22	3.71	6.35	4.79	1.47	3.14	2.93	3.32
1995	1.03	2.77	1.75	5.29	8.38	6.85	2.12	4.46	4.72	4.73
1996	1.55	3.92	2.33	6.76	9.49	8.11	2.74	5.87	6.35	5.91
1997	1.98	4.95	2.84	7.69	9.76	8.07	3.16	7.08	6.92	6.46
1998	2.12	5.52	3.16	7.93	9.48	7.34	3.26	7.82	6.44	6.38
1999	1.99	5.57	3.25	7.75	9.19	6.74	3.15	8.09	5.70	6.04
2000	1.78	5.34	3.20	7.54	9.18	6.57	3.01	8.10	5.29	5.81
2001	1.65	5.14	3.13	7.52	9.47	6.77	2.93	8.09	5.27	5.81

TABLE 4.2 Incidence estimates (%) for antenatal clinic attendees by year and by province 1990–2001

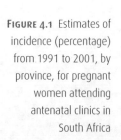

FIGURE 4.1 Estimates of incidence (percentage) from 1991 to 2001, by province, for pregnant women attending antenatal clinics in South Africa

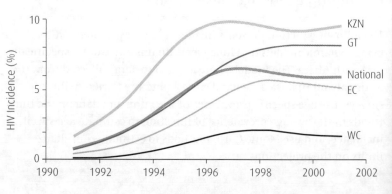

Model estimates based on data collected annually from antenatal clinic attendees in the rural district of Hlabisa between 1992 and 2001, where the HIV prevalence rose from 4.2% in 1992 to 14% in 1995 and 36% in 2001, show a peak incidence of 10.5% in 1998 (FIGURE 4.2). As observed with the HIV prevalence data, the estimated incidence rates for Hlabisa district are similar to that for KwaZulu-Natal province.

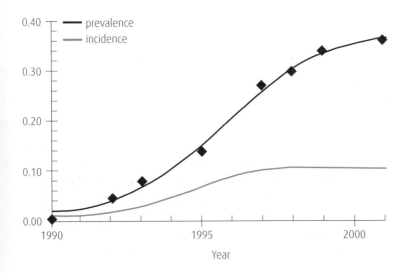

FIGURE 4.2 Temporal trends in prevalence and incidence among women attending antenatal clinics in Hlabisa

Estimates of annual incidence rates for Hlabisa, using two different models developed by Williams and Gouws, are presented in TABLE 4.3. Model 1 was fitted to antenatal clinic data collected from 1997 to 2001 and estimates were derived from age-specific prevalence and changes in overall prevalence with time. A method described by Podgor and Leske was used to estimate age-specific data for 1993 and 1995, because of the unavailability of age-specific data for these two years. Model 2 utilises time trends in prevalence. The two sets of estimates are similar and both indicate that the epidemic in rural KwaZulu-Natal has reached a steady state. Estimates of incidence using the Williams and Gouws models were standardised using the age distribution of the Hlabisa female population attending antenatal clinics.

The *age-specific* estimates of incidence for women attending antenatal clinics in Hlabisa from 1997 to 2001, using the Williams and Gouws model with a Weibull survival distribution function, are presented in TABLE 4.4 and FIGURE 4.3 together with the corresponding prevalence data for this period. While age-specific incidence estimates did not show dramatic changes between 1997 and 1999, estimates for 2001 were slightly lower. Similar to prevalence data, incidence peaked in the 20 to 24 year age groups at 13.1% in 1997, 14.6% in 1998, 14.6% in 1999, and 12.1% in 2001.

TABLE 4.3 Prevalence and estimated incidence of HIV infection (using two different models) among antenatal clinic attendees, aged 15–49 in Hlabisa: 1992–2001

Year	N	Prevalence of HIV (95% CI)	Estimated Annual Incidence	
			Model 1	Model 2
1992	884	4.2% (3.0–5.7)		2.0%
1993	709	7.9% (6.0–10.1)	2.3%	3.3%
1995	314	14.0% (10.4–18.4)	7.2%	7.1%
1997	4731	27.2% (25.9–28.5)	10.6%	10.2%
1998	3166	29.9% (28.4–31.6)	10.5%	10.5%
1999	3001	34.0% (32.5–35.7)	11.0%	10.3%
2001	906	36.1% (32.9–39.2)	9.9%	10.2%

TABLE 4.4 Prevalence and incidence with 95% confidence intervals for women attending antenatal clinic in Hlabisa, by age 1997–2001

Age (years)	1997	1998	1999	2001
Prevalence				
10–14		0 (0–34.8)	0 (0–45.1)	0 (0–52.7)
15–19	23.2 (20.5–26.3)	21.1 (18.1–24.5)	24.2 (20.6–28.2)	22.9 (17.0–29.8)
20–24	35.5 (32.6–38.7)	39.3 (35.5–43.4)	40.2 (36.0–44.8)	50.8 (43.4–58.2)
25–29	28.5 (25.3–32.0)	36.4 (31.7–41.5)	45.3 (39.9–51.3)	47.2 (36.5–58.1)
30–34	22.5 (18.9–26.5)	23.4 (18.9–28.6)	32.5 (26.9–38.9)	38.4 (27.3–50.5)
35–39	17.2 (13.2–22.1)	23.0 (17.6–29.6)	22.4 (16.4–29.9)	36.4 (22.4–52.3)
40–44	8.8 (4.3–15.7)	12.3 (5.1–23.7)	20.7 (11.2–33.4)	26.7 (7.8–55.1)
45–49	11.5 (2.4–30.2)	13.3 (1.7–40.5)	28.6 (3.7–71.0)	33.3 (0.8–90.5)
Incidence				
10–14		0.75 (0.4–1.4)	0.98 (0.53–1.76)	1.0 (0.35–2.89)
15–19	11.1 (9.9–12.3)	10.0 (8.7–11.3)	10.2 (8.9–11.6)	8.9 (7.0–11.0)
20–24	13.1 (11.8–14.4)	14.6 (13.0–16.2)	14.6 (13.1–16.3)	12.1 (9.5–15.7)
25–29	10.1 (9.0–11.1)	11.5 (10.3–12.9)	12.2 (10.9–13.8)	10.2 (7.8–12.9)
30–34	6.8 (5.7–8.0)	7.4 (6.3–8.9)	8.6 (7.1–10.3)	7.4 (5.0–10.5)
35–39	4.5 (3.4–5.8)	4.5 (3.3–6.14)	5.8 (4.3–7.5)	5.1 (2.7–8.1)
40–44	2.9 (1.9–4.2)	2.6 (1.7–4.2)	3.8 (2.4–5.7)	3.5 (1.4–6.8)
45–49	1.9 (1.1–3.0)	1.6 (0.9–2.8)	2.5 (1.4–4.3)	2.3 (0.8–5.7)

Estimated incidence rates by gender and age in an urban community in Gauteng

Using the Williams and Gouws model with a Weibull survival distribution function, incidence rates were estimated from age-prevalence data collected from an urban mining community in Carletonville in 1998. The overall incidence for men aged 15 to 49 years was 9.6% (assuming a flat age distribution) compared to 13.5% for women in the same age range. Age specific incidence rates for men and women are provided in FIGURE 4.4 and TABLE 4.5, and show a dramatic peak incidence of 22.8% among women aged 24 years and of 16.4% among men aged 30 years. Of note is that the incidence rate among young

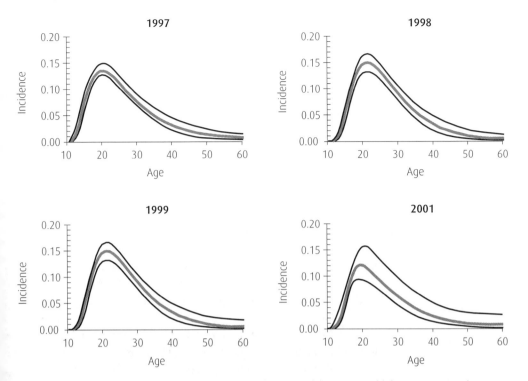

Figure 4.3 Age-specific estimates of HIV incidence (with 95% confidence intervals) for women attending antenatal clinics in Hlabisa in 1997, 1998, 1999 and 2001

women in this community in 1998 was higher than that reported for the truck-stop sex worker population described above and is of grave concern.

Age	Women		Men	
	Prevalence	Incidence	Prevalence	Incidence
10–14	0.5 (0.13–1.8)	0.52 (0.15–1.6)	0 (0–0.06)	0 (0–0.07)
15–19	18.7 (11.9–27.7)	10.7 (7.4–14.6)	1.73 (0.52–5.3)	1.3 (0.44–3.24)
20–24	48.7 (41.0–56.8)	21.5 (17.4–26.4)	17.1 (10.3–24.9)	8.5 (5.5–12.3)
25–29	55.6 (47.8–63.1)	21.3 (17.2–25.6)	37.6 (27.5–48.8)	15.3 (10.4–20.8)
30–34	49.4 (42.9–55.9)	16.6 (13.6–19.9)	44.1 (32.8–55.9)	15.7 (10.9–21.6)
35–39	38.5 (31.7–45.3)	11.6 (8.9–14.9)	39.1 (29.0–49.2)	12.4 (8.5–17.2)
40–44	27.7 (20.6–36.1)	7.9 (5.3–11.2)	29.6 (20.5–39.7)	8.5 (5.4–12.6)
45–49	18.9 (12.3–27.6)	5.2 (3.1–8.3)	20.0 (12.0–29.9)	5.5 (2.9–9.2)
50–54	12.6 (7.1–20.7)	3.5 (1.8–6.3)	12.5 (5.8–23.2)	3.4 (1.3–7.1)
55–59	8.1 (4.0–15.7)	2.3 (1.1–4.8)	7.4 (2.5–17.5)	2.0 (0.6–5.4)

Table 4.5 Age-specific HIV prevalence and incidence for men and women in Carletonville in 1998

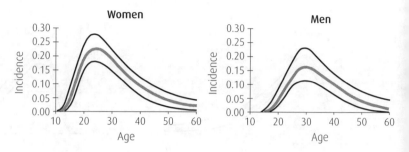

FIGURE 4.4 Age-specific incidence (with 95% confidence intervals) for women and men in the general population in Carletonville in 1998

Conclusion

South Africa has experienced one of the fastest growing HIV epidemics in the world and in 2002 more than 25% of women attending public antenatal clinics were infected with HIV. In order to understand the dynamics of HIV infection we need to know more about the current burden of disease, the rate of new infections and the rate of deaths, for which reliable estimates of prevalence and incidence are required. While prevalence data are widely available in South Africa, direct estimates of HIV incidence remain rare and only one cohort study to collect information on longitudinal incidence among a group of sex workers in KwaZulu-Natal has been conducted in South Africa. Incidence can be estimated indirectly from HIV prevalence data and in this chapter we report on incidence rates estimated using dynamic models developed specifically for South Africa.

The incidence estimates demonstrate extraordinarily high rates of HIV infection. Age-specific incidence curves, similar to age-specific prevalence curves, show peak incidences among young people with a decline among older age groups. Young women aged 20 to 24 years are at highest risk of being infected with HIV, while infection among men peaks at a later age (around 30 years). Shapes of age-specific incidence curves are similar between urban and rural populations.

Data in South Africa suggest that the epidemic is levelling off. Incidence estimated among national antenatal clinic attendees peaked in 1997 at around 6.5%. The slight decrease in incidence after 1997/1998 probably reflects the natural course of the epidemic as it reaches a steady state. If there is no change in behaviour in the coming years, the epidemic curve is likely to stay steady. However, should the HIV transmission rate fall significantly as a result of natural behaviour change or effective interventions, this will be seen first in falling incidence, as incidence rates respond to change much quicker than does prevalence. Prevalence reflects the average incidence over the past five to ten years and a change in the epidemic will take a longer time to manifest in estimates of prevalence.

The models described here can be used to obtain good fits to the prevalence of infection and reliable estimates of the incidence of infection. However, if we wish to explore the biological and social factors that influence the course of the epidemic or investigate the likely impact of different interventions we need dynamic models firmly based on what we know of the natural history of the epidemic. This is the subject of CHAPTER 36.

Bibliography

ABDOOL KARIM Q, ABDOOL KARIM SS, SINGH B, SHORT R, NGXONGO S. 'Seroprevalence of HIV infection in rural South Africa'. *AIDS* 1992; 6: 1535–1539.

BROOKMEYER R, QUINN TC. 'Estimation of current human immunodeficiency virus incidence rates from a cross-sectional survey using early diagnostic tests'. *American Journal of Epidemiology*1995; 141: 166–172.

DEPARTMENT OF HEALTH, RSA. 1998. *National HIV sero-prevalence survey of women attending antenatal clinics in South Africa. Summary report.* Pretoria: Health Systems Research and Epidemiology, DOH, 1999.

DEPARTMENT OF HEALTH, RSA. 2001. *National HIV and syphilis sero-prevalence survey of women attending public antenatal clinics in South Africa. Summary report.* Pretoria: Health Systems Research and Epidemiology, DOH 2001.

DORRINGTON R, BRADSHAW D, BUDLENDER D. *HIV/AIDS profile in the provinces of South Africa – indicators for 2002.* Centre for Actuarial Research, Medical Research Council and the Actuarial Society of South Africa. 2002. (The model and more detailed statistics can be accessed at www.assa.org/aidsmodel.asp)

DOYLE PR, MILLAR DB. 'A general description of an Actuarial Model application to the HIV epidemic in South Africa'. *Transactions of the Actuarial Society of South Africa* 1990; 8: 561–593.

GHYS PD, BROWN T, GRASSLY NC, GARNETT G, STANECKI K, STOVER J, WALKER N. The UNAIDS Estimation and Projection Package: A software package to estimate and project national HIV epidemics. *Sexually Transmitted Infections* 2004; 80 (Suppl 1): I5–I9

GOUWS E, WILLIAMS BG, SHEPPARD HW, ENGE B, ABDOOL KARIM SS. 'High incidence of HIV-1 in South Africa using a Standardized Algorithm for recent HIV sero-conversion'. *Journal of Acquired Immune Deficiency Syndrome* 2002; 29: 531–535.

GREGSON S, DONNELLY CA, PARKER CG, ANDERSON RM. 'Demographic approaches to the estimation of incidence of HIV-1 infection among adults from age-specific prevalence data in stable endemic conditions'. *AIDS* 1996; 10: 1689–1697.

JANSSENS RS, SATTEN GA, STRAMER SL, ET AL. 'New testing strategy to detect early HIV-1 infection for use in incidence estimates and for clinical and prevention purposes'. *Journal of the American Medical Association* 1998; 280: 42–48.

KUSTNER HGV, SWANEVELDER JP, VAN MIDDELKOOP A. 'National HIV surveillance – South Africa, 1990–1992'. *South African Medical Journal* 1994; 84: 195–200.

PODGOR MJ, LESKE MC. 'Estimating incidence from age-specific prevalence for irreversible diseases with differential mortality'. *Statistics in Medicine* 1986; 5: 573–578.

SAIDEL T, SOKAL D, RACE J, BUZINGO T, HASSIG S. 'Validation of a method to estimate age-specific Human Immunodeficiency Virus (HIV) incidence rates in developing countries using population-based seroprevalence data'. *American Journal of Epidemiology* 1996; 144: 214–223.

WILLIAMS BG, GOUWS E, COLVIN M, SITAS F, RAMJEE G, ABDOOL KARIM SS. 'Patterns of infection: Using age prevalence data to understand the epidemic of HIV in South Africa'. *South African Journal of Science* 2000; 96: 305–312.

WILLIAMS B, GOUWS E, WILKINSON D, ABDOOL KARIM S. 'Estimating HIV incidence rates from age prevalence data in epidemic situation'. *Statistics in Medicine* 2001; 20: 2003–2016

WILLIAMS BG, MACPHAIL C, CAMPBELL C, TALJAARD D, GOUWS E, MOEMA S, MZAIDUME Z, RASEGO B. 'The Carletonville-Mothusimpilo Project: Limiting transmission of HIV through community-based interventions'. *South African Journal of Science* 2000; 96: 351–359.

The virus, the human host and their interactions

CHAPTER 5

Viral structure, replication, tropism, pathogenesis and natural history

Lynn Morris and Tonie Cilliers

HIV IS A RETROVIRUS that infects and replicates primarily in human CD4+ T-cells and macrophages. The virus gains entry to the cell by attaching to the CD4 receptor and a coreceptor via its envelope glycoproteins. HIV is unusual in that it encodes the enzyme reverse transcriptase allowing a DNA copy to be made from viral RNA. This process is highly error prone and accounts for the enormous genetic variability that is characteristic of HIV. Once integrated into the cellular DNA, the provirus resides in the nucleus of infected cells and can remain quiescent for extended periods of time. These latent reservoirs pose the greatest challenge to continued treatment success and to the possibility of clearing HIV from the body.

The viral enzymes, reverse transcriptase and protease, have afforded the best target for interrupting the viral life cycle. Antiretroviral drugs targeting these two enzymes have proven highly effective in reducing the morbidity and mortality of AIDS. However, as a result of HIV's ability to mutate, resistance to these drugs has emerged and poses a threat to their continued success. Newer targets are being studied, the most advanced of which are the entry inhibitors. This class of drugs (many of which are still to be tested in humans) bind to either the viral envelope glycoprotein or the host receptors, preventing the interaction between the virus and host cell. Because of their mechanism of action these drugs may prove to be particularly useful as preventive agents and many are being considered in microbicide formulations.

An HIV vaccine is considered the best hope for controlling the HIV pandemic. However, developing a vaccine able to stimulate protective immune responses has proven to be extremely difficult. In particular, developing a vaccine able to stimulate antibodies that could serve as entry inhibitors (neutralising antibodies) has been elusive. Intensive efforts are underway to more fully understand the HIV envelope protein and to design vaccines able to expose the neutralization-sensitive regions of the viral envelope glycoprotein. Antibodies that target these 'achilles heels' of the envelope may be able to block viral entry and provide sterilising immunity against HIV.

Viral structure

HIV is a retrovirus, so named because it encodes the enzyme reverse transcriptase. This unique enzyme allows a DNA copy to be made from viral RNA, going against what is considered the normal flow of genetic information, hence retro 'to go backwards' (FIGURE 5.1). HIV genetic material exists both as genomic RNA inside viral particles and as proviral DNA in the nucleus of infected cells. Both forms are infectious and the latter allows HIV to persist in long-lived reservoirs, thwarting efforts to clear HIV from the body.

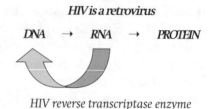

HIV is a retrovirus

DNA → *RNA* → *PROTEIN*

HIV reverse transcriptase enzyme

FIGURE 5.1 Schematic diagram of the genetic flow of HIV-1

Viral particles are spherical with a diameter of approximately 100 nm and as such can only be viewed under an electron microscope (FIGURE 5.2A). The outer lipid membrane is derived from the human host and contains the two major envelope glycoproteins, gp120 and gp41 ('gp' stands for glycoprotein and the number is the molecular weight in kilodaltons) (FIGURE 5.2B). These proteins are linked together and exist as trimers on the viral surface facilitating binding and entry to the host cell. The envelope protein can be referred to as 'Env'. Other major structural proteins are the group-associated antigens or *Gag* proteins. The matrix protein (p17), which lies just beneath the envelope, provides structure to the particle, while the capsid protein (p24) encloses the viral RNA. The capsid protein is clearly visible under the electron microscope as a dark conical structure in the centre of the particle (FIGURE 5.2A). HIV encodes three unique enzymes that are the major targets for antiretroviral therapies. These are reverse transcriptase, integrase and protease, collectively called polymerases or 'Pol' for short. All three enzymes are carried inside the viral particle where they remain active.

In addition to the major structural proteins, HIV also produces a number of regulatory and accessory proteins. In general these are

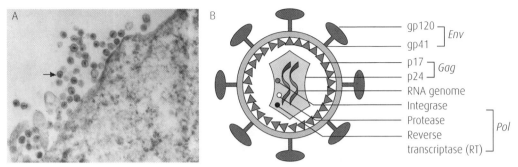

FIGURE 5.2 (A) Mature HIV particles with dense central core accumulate at the plasma membrane of infected cell (arrow). Cell lines expressing both CD4 and CCR5 receptors were infected with HIV for two days prior to harvesting. Ultra-thin sections were stained with lead citrate and uranyl acetate and viewed in the TEM Jeol 1200EX. Photograph courtesy of Nishi Prabdial-Sing. (B) Schematic representation of HIV-1 particle.

only produced once the virus infects cells and are not present inside viral particles. These include *Tat* and *Rev*, which enhance levels of gene expression and *Vif*, *Vpr*, *Vpu* and *Nef*, which function to increase viral production and infectivity.

Viral replication

HIV infects and replicates in human CD4+ T-cells and macrophages. Viral particles bind to surface CD4 and a coreceptor molecule via gp120. This interaction causes conformational changes allowing gp41 to insert itself into the host cell membrane, effecting fusion between the two membranes. The capsid is then injected into the cytoplasm where it releases the viral RNA with its bound reverse transcriptase enzymes. Once inside this enabling cellular environment, the RNA is reverse-transcribed to DNA. Reverse transcription is a highly error-prone process and is the major source of genetic variability that typifies HIV. The DNA molecule is then transported to the nucleus where, with the aid of the viral enzyme integrase, it is incorporated into human DNA. Proviral DNA can remain quiescent for extended periods of time or become transcriptionally active, particularly in cases where there is inflammation. At this stage the virus makes use of the host cell machinery to replicate itself. Viral RNA is either single-spliced or unspliced to make structural proteins, or they are multiple-spliced to make regulatory and accessory proteins. Full-length unspliced genomic RNA is transported to the plasma membrane to be included in new viral particles. The precursor *Gag-Pol* polyprotein (containing p17, p24 and all viral enzymes) is cleaved by viral protease to generate individual proteins that aggregate just beneath the plasma membrane surface for inclusion into the new virions. Envelope glycoproteins insert themselves into the cell membrane and mature viral particles

82

are formed when the virus buds through the membrane. The replication cycle is shown in FIGURE 5.3.

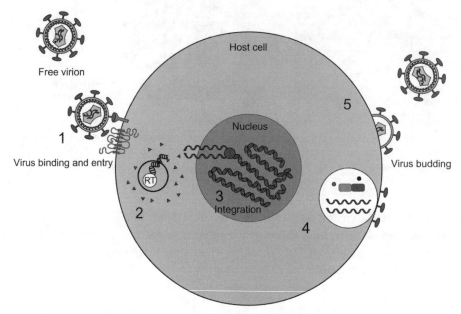

FIGURE 5.3 The replication cycle of HIV-1 is shown. (1) Virus attachment and entry via CD4 and a coreceptor. (2) Reverse transcription of the viral RNA to DNA. (3) Integration of viral DNA into the host DNA. (4) Production of provirus and assembly of proteins at the cell membrane ready for cleavage by the protease enzyme. (5) Virus budding from the cell membrane.

Viral targets

Viral enzymes, by virtue of the fact that they are essential in the virus replication cycle and are unique to the virus, have afforded the best target for antiretroviral therapies. Nucleoside reverse transcriptase inhibitors (NRTI), such as zidovudine, mimic the natural building blocks of DNA and act as chain terminators while non-nucleoside reverse transcriptase inhibitors (NNRTI), such as nevirapine, bind directly to the enzyme reverse transcriptase and inhibit its activity. Protease inhibitors prevent cleavage of viral proteins, resulting in the production of immature viral particles. Both reverse transcriptase and protease inhibitors are widely used in anti-HIV treatment and have had a dramatic impact on morbidity and mortality in HIV-infected patients. However, these drugs are not able to clear HIV infection because the virus can integrate into host DNA and remain quiescent in long-lived cellular reservoirs. Newer drugs that target integrase are in development. There is also considerable interest in a newer class of drugs that block HIV entry, opening up many possibilities for both therapeutic and preventive strategies.

In 1986, shortly after the discovery of HIV, the CD4 molecule was shown to serve as the primary receptor used by HIV to enter cells. However, it was soon realised that CD4 was not sufficient for entry. The discovery that chemokines secreted by CD8 cytotoxic T-cells inhibit HIV infection, as well as the existence of persons exposed to HIV who remained uninfected, provided clues to this second receptor. Subsequently fusin was discovered as the receptor for viruses that caused syncitia (SI) in T-cells and was later renamed CXCR4. A second coreceptor, termed CCR5 was shown to serve as the coreceptor for macrophage tropic or non-syncitium inducing (NSI) HIV isolates.

CCR5 and CXCR4 are used by most, if not all, HIV strains regardless of genetic subtype. These receptors are seven-transmembrane molecules of the G-protein-coupled receptor family. CCR5 is expressed on activated lymphocytes, macrophages, dendritic cells and brain cells while CXCR4 is expressed in resting T-cells and monocytes. Viruses isolated from recently infected individuals are almost exclusively CCR5-using, indicating that CCR5 viruses are selectively transmitted. It is thought that CCR5+ macrophages and dendritic cells, which are abundant in mucosal tissues, transport the virions to the lymphoid tissues and are responsible for dissemination of the virus throughout the body. Virus isolates from persons with late-stage disease can often use CXCR4 (referred to as X4), sometimes in addition to CCR5 (R5). The CXCR4 and the CCR5-CXCR4 (R5X4) phenotypes are considered to be more pathogenic, causing more rapid CD4+ T-cell depletion. However, many individuals develop terminal AIDS in the absence of a coreceptor switch (from R5 to X4 or R5X4), particularly those infected with HIV subtype C viruses, indicating that this is not a pre-requisite for developing AIDS.

HIV variants transmitted sexually are associated with CCR5 as the coreceptor of preference. This coreceptor was first discovered by analysing cells from people who engaged in high-risk sexual behaviour but remained HIV-uninfected. Subsequently a 32-base pair deletion (Δ32) in the CCR5 gene was discovered, which results in a frameshift and premature truncation of the protein. This truncated polypeptide is expressed, but does not appear on the cell surface and lacks coreceptor activity. Individuals who are homozygous for Δ32 CCR5 are highly resistant, but not immune, to HIV infection as they can be infected by viruses that use CXCR4. Individuals who are heterozygous for Δ32 CCR5 progress to disease more slowly and have a much lower viral load, probably as a result of reduced expression of CCR5. The allele frequency of Δ32 CCR5 in the Caucasian population is approximately 10%, with 1% being homozygous and approximately

18% being heterozygous. It is very rare among African populations, including those in South Africa.

Targeting viral entry

HIV entry occurs in three distinct phases offering multiple opportunities for intervention: the attachment of gp120 to CD4, the interaction of the gp120-CD4 complex with a coreceptor and the gp41 mediated membrane fusion process (FIGURE 5.4). Agents that target these three steps are broadly referred to as entry inhibitors and work by preventing the virus from gaining entry into the cell. The advent of entry inhibitors not only represents another target for therapeutic intervention, but also opens up exciting possibilities for these molecules to be used as preventive agents. By blocking HIV entry, the sequelae of viral integration and persistence is prevented. In particular, the use of entry inhibitors as topical, vaginal or rectal microbicides to prevent sexual transmission of HIV has received considerable attention.

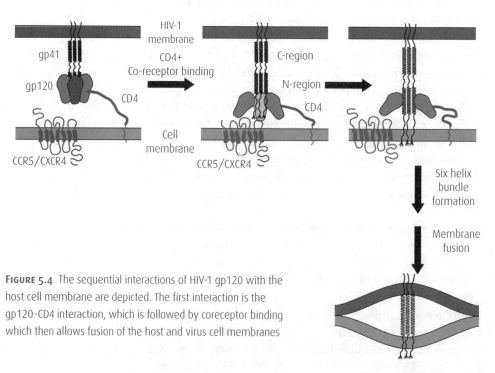

FIGURE 5.4 The sequential interactions of HIV-1 gp120 with the host cell membrane are depicted. The first interaction is the gp120-CD4 interaction, which is followed by coreceptor binding which then allows fusion of the host and virus cell membranes

Heterosexual transmission of HIV

HIV is present in vaginal fluids and semen as free virions and within infected cells. Infection takes place when the virus crosses the mucosal surface and binds to cells that express CD4 and CCR5 and/or

CXCR4. Sexual transmission of HIV is highly inefficient; the risks of acquiring infection after a single exposure are estimated to be less than 20 per 100 000 contacts and to 33 per 100 000 for occupational exposure contacts. However, various biological, social and virological factors play a role in influencing the rate of HIV transmission in different populations. The risks of HIV transmission are affected by the frequency of sexual contact, condom use, immunological status (including whether the infected partner has acute HIV infection or AIDS), male circumcision, and the presence of sexually transmitted diseases. Plasma levels of HIV are highly predictive of the risk of transmission; individuals with fewer than 1500 viral particles per ml rarely transmit the virus to a partner. Plasma levels of virus broadly correspond to viral loads in genital secretions – hence the risk of transmission is associated with viral load in semen and vaginal fluids.

Natural history and viral set-point

Within a few weeks of infection, there is a high level of HIV replication in the blood that can exceed ten million viral particles per microlitre of plasma. Concomitant with this is a decline in the numbers of CD4+ T lymphocytes. However, within a few weeks an immune response to HIV develops that curtails viral replication, resulting in a decline in the viral load and a return of CD4+ T-cell numbers to near normal levels (FIGURE 5.5). The control of viraemia has largely been attributed to the emergence of killer cells named cytotoxic T lymphocytes (CTL) (see CHAPTER 7 for more information on CTL) and to a lesser extent the development of a neutralising antibody response. As a result of these immune responses, individuals remain clinically well (asymptomatic) for many years. Kinetic studies have shown that during the asymptomatic period up to a billion HIV particles and two billion CD4+ T-cells are destroyed and produced each day. Thus while individuals may be clinically well, the virus continues to replicate, particularly in the lymph nodes, causing a gradual decline in CD4+ T-cell numbers. The drop in CD4+ T-cell numbers results in individuals becoming susceptible to various opportunistic infections, signaling the onset of AIDS. With this deterioration in immune function, the viral load increases and death ensues about eighteen months to two years after a diagnosis of AIDS.

In the absence of any antiretroviral therapy, the median time to AIDS from the point of HIV infection is eight to ten years, at least in the USA and Europe where there is generally good access to health care. There is accumulating evidence that the natural history of HIV disease in Africa may be about one to two years shorter than in the

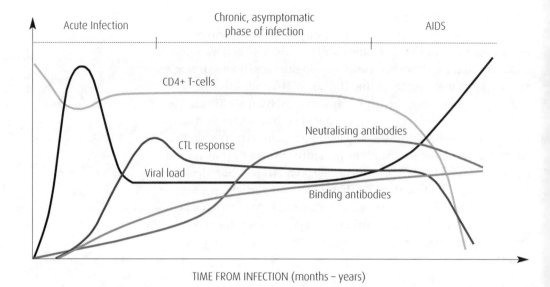

Acute Infection

Chronic, asymptomatic phase of infection

AIDS

CD4+ T-cells

Neutralising antibodies

CTL response

Viral load

Binding antibodies

TIME FROM INFECTION (months – years)

FIGURE 5.5 Schematic diagram showing the natural history of HIV-1 infection. During the acute stage the viral load increases dramatically and the number of CD4+ T-cells decline. After a few weeks CTL develop, which reduces the viral load and the CD4+ T-cell number returns to near normal levels. Neutralising antibodies take much longer to develop and are thought to play a role in controlling viral levels during chronic stages of infection. The onset of AIDS is associated with an increase in viral levels and collapse of the immune system. Drawing courtesy of Natasha Taylor.

developed world. Whether this is related to viral factors, such as differences in viral subtypes, or to socio-economic factors, such as poverty and poor access to health care, or to the generally higher burden of infectious diseases in Africa are all issues that need to be more fully explored.

The levels of HIV in the blood are highly predictive of the rate of disease progression: individuals with low viral set-points progress more slowly than those with higher levels of virus in their blood (FIGURE 5.6). For reasons that are not fully understood, some individuals never gain a temporary measure of control over viral replication and progress to AIDS within two to three years of infection (rapid progressors) while others have remained disease-free for up to 20 years with often undetectable viral loads (long-term non-progressors). At this stage very few long-term non-progressors have been identified in South Africa, but it would be important to identify and study such individuals, as they provide important clues as to the immune responses needed to control subtype C HIV replication.

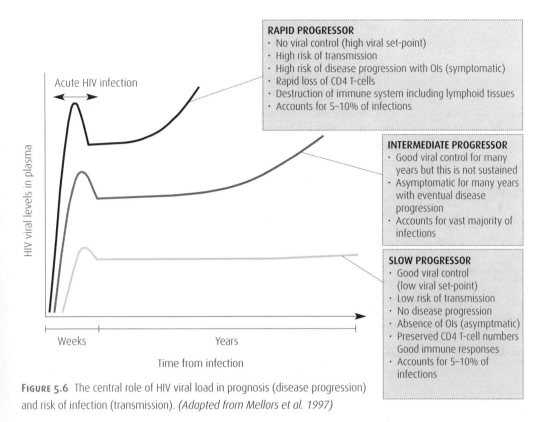

FIGURE 5.6 The central role of HIV viral load in prognosis (disease progression) and risk of infection (transmission). *(Adapted from Mellors et al. 1997)*

Humoral immunity to HIV

Antibodies to HIV proteins are made within a few weeks following infection and are often used in the diagnosis of infection (FIGURE 5.5). Although antibodies are made to all HIV proteins, only those to the envelope glycoproteins possess functional activity, ie can prevent or neutralise HIV infection. These neutralising antibodies take a considerably longer time to develop than binding antibodies, often months to years, and do not develop in all individuals. The ability of HIV to escape neutralising antibodies through a process of genetic change renders such antibodies ineffective. The targets of neutralising antibodies have been difficult to identify, largely because of their conformational and discontinuous nature. The neutralisation-sensitive face of gp120 comprises the functionally constrained domains of CD4 and coreceptor binding sites. However, these are embedded deep within the complex trimeric envelope structure and are inaccessible on the surface of the virions, only becoming exposed during the brief periods when the virus enters the cell. Furthermore, the surface of gp120 is cloaked in sugars that provide another mechanism for the virus to evade the effects of neutralising antibodies.

The induction of neutralising antibodies, together with a CTL response, is considered an essential property of an HIV vaccine. However, for the reasons above the ability to develop vaccines that stimulate neutralising antibodies has proved to be particularly difficult. Newer approaches are being investigated, including genetically modifying the envelope glycoproteins or mimicking structures that are targets for neutralising monoclonal antibodies. A greater challenge will be to induce such neutralising antibodies at the site of infection, namely the genital mucosa. Such approaches aim to block virus entry by preventing the engagement of gp120/41 with its cognate ligands on the cell surface providing sterilising immunity and protection from HIV infection.

Bibliography

BURTON DR, DESROSIERS RC, DOMS RW, KOFF WC, KWONG PD, MOORE JP, NABEL GJ, SODROSKI J, WILSON IA, WYATT RT. 'HIV vaccine design and the neutralizing antibody problem.' *Nature Immunology* 2004; 5: 233–236.

DAVIS CW, DOMS RW. 'HIV transmission: Closing all the doors.' *Journal of Experimental Medicine* 2004; 199: 1037–1040.

MELLORS JW, MUNOZ A, GIORGI JV, MARGOLICK JB, TASSONI CJ, GUPTA P, KINGSLEY LA, TODD JA, SAAH AJ, DETELS R, PHAIR JP, RINALDO CR JR 'Plasma viral load and CD4+ lymphocytes as prognostic markers of HIV-1 infection.' *Annals of Internal Medicine* 1997; 126: 946–954.

MOORE JP, DOMS RW. 'The entry of entry inhibitors: A fusion of science and medicine.' *Proceedings of the National Acadamy of Science USA* 2003; 100: 10598–10602.

SHATTOCK RJ, MOORE JP. 'Inhibiting sexual transmission of HIV-1 infection.' *Nature Reviews Microbiol* 2003; 1: 25–34.

SIMON V, HO DD. 'HIV-1 dynamics in vivo: Implications for therapy.' *Nature Reviews. Microbiology* 2003; 1: 81–190.

WEISS RA. 'Gulliver's travels in HIVland.' *Nature* 2001; 410: 963–967.

ZOLLA-PAZNER S. 'Identifying epitopes of HIV-1 that induce protective antibodies.' *Nature Reviews Immunology* 2004; 4: 199–210.

CHAPTER 6
HIV diagnostics

Adrian J Puren

KNOWLEDGE OF HIV STATUS is important in efforts to mitigate the effects of the disease, hence the interest in testing and diagnosis. The most common screening tests for HIV are the ELISAs and Simple/Rapid Assays. Assays that can use alternative body fluids such as saliva, whole blood and urine are also being developed. The choice of diagnostic test depends to some extent on the clinical stage of HIV infection because of the complexity of the infection process.

There are two approaches to the diagnosis of HIV – the detection of the virus itself and detection of an immunological response to the virus through the production of antibodies or cellular responses.

More recently, rapid testing is widely used and a novel advance is confirmatory rapid testing that contains multiple antigens. These tests are useful in clinic settings where sophisticated technology is not available and personnel may not be fully trained in other techniques.

The choice of diagnostic testing is determined by the diagnostic setting, eg early diagnosis relies on viral antigens, blood for transfusion on antibody and antigen testing and occupational exposure, baseline antibody testing and proviral DNA.

Population serosurveillance requires different approaches to testing depending on predicted population prevalence.

An HIV test should be considered positive only after screening and confirmatory tests are reactive. False-positives when both these tests are positive are rare. The clinical context is also important.

Participants in vaccine trials are a special case and different screening techniques are required to test for HIV positivity. Testing an infant in whom vertical transmission is suspected is another special situation and there is no universally accepted algorithm for testing the HIV infected infant in the absence of therapy.

History of HIV testing

There has been a rapid evolution in diagnostic technology since the first HIV antibody tests became commercially available in 1985. Today, a wide range of HIV antibody tests are available from both international and local diagnostic manufacturers for screening, confirming and monitoring HIV infection. The most common screening tests are the ELISAs and Simple/Rapid Assays. More recently, progress has been made in the development of assays that can utilise alternative body fluids to serum/plasma such as saliva, whole blood and urine. The most commonly used, but expensive, confirmatory test has been the Western Blot (WB). However, recently studies have shown that combinations of ELISAs or Simple/Rapid assays can provide results as reliable as the WB at a much lower cost. Some of the tests which assist in the establishment of the diagnosis of HIV infection may also be used to monitor the progress of the infection and the response to therapy, eg P24 antigen testing and nucleic acid amplification technologies.

Screening tests are used for initial testing because they are easier to perform than confirmatory tests, well suited to testing large numbers of samples, and less costly. They are highly sensitive and result in few false negatives (ie most infected people test positive). However, screening tests are not as specific as confirmatory tests, so in a small percentage of cases the test result will be positive even if the person is not infected. Therefore, providers should never give results from screening tests that have not been verified through a confirmatory test.

The Diagnosis of HIV infection

The diagnosis of HIV infection is not simply a matter of determining whether or not someone has been exposed to the virus or has responded to the presence of virus. The complexity of events after initial infection is such that there are recognised stages of HIV infection and these have a bearing on the choice of tests used for diagnosis of infection. Despite the wide array of diagnostic tools available, a serious and significant limitation is our inability to diagnose exposure to the virus during early infection or what is commonly referred to as the window period. Notwithstanding the technical limitations in terms of how rapidly we are able to detect presence of antibodies or virus the choice of which test to use when is guided by the most recent model of acute infection. Based on the reactivity of one or more assays, at least six sequential and consistent stages have been identified. These are based on the sensitivities of the various assays carried out in seroconverting plasma donors:

- Stage I: HIV is present in the circulation, reflected by the presence of RNA only
- Stage II: RNA and p24 antigen tests are positive and ELISA (EIA, enzyme immunoassay) test negative
- Stage III: RNA, p24 antigen, IgM-sensitive ELISA positive but Western blot without specific HIV bands
- Stage IV: as for Stage III but Western blot indeterminate
- Stage V as for Stage IV but Western blot positive except for p31
- Stage VI as for Stage V and including p31.

Stages I to IV are relatively short with mean durations of three to five days. The duration of Stage V is estimated to be 69.5 days and no endpoint is defined for Stage VI. Stage VI can be further divided into recent versus chronic infection.

Peak RNA levels coincide with antibody seroconversion (Stage III) followed by a decline coinciding with Western blot maturation (Stages V and VI). RNA may not decline to undetectable levels. HIV p24 antigen, on the other hand, is present during Stages II and III but slowly declines because of antigen-antibody complex formation.

Staging of HIV can be important. The process allows for selecting the most appropriate tools for diagnosis in particular settings, eg in the case of blood transfusion cases, or in resolving difficult or unusual cases. Staging can also allow stratification of clinical cases that could link to specific therapeutic interventions.

Why test for HIV?

Knowledge of individual HIV status is perhaps the single most important factor in any attempt to mitigate the effects of the disease. There are a number of specific settings in which HIV testing is indicated:

- when someone believes that they are at risk of infection through unprotected sexual activity, needle-stick injury or unsafe injection drug use
- when a pregnant women wishes to know her status to protect her unborn child
- when mother-to-child transmission of HIV is suspected
- for public health and infection control (for epidemiologic characterisation and public health policy implementation, blood banks)
- and as a requirement for certain types of short-term insurance.

What to test

Body fluids suitable for diagnosis include whole blood, serum, plasma, oral fluid (crevicular fluid) and urine. Crevicular fluid and urine have advantages because obtaining specimens is simple and non-invasive. However, there may be problems with the sensitivity and specificity of these assays, although most studies report that these may be comparable to standard ELISA or rapid tests. Measurement of HIV in cerebrospinal fluid and cervicovaginal lavage (CVL) is generally of clinical research interest only at present. However, it may be important when considering transmission of specific subspecies, or resistant varieties of virus.

HIV testing technology

The technologies used for diagnosing HIV vary in their levels of sensitivity and specificity. Because HIV often needs to be diagnosed at clinic level, these tests have also to be practical. How different types of technology are used for diagnosis may also depend on country-specific guidelines set up by clinical groups and regulatory authorities, or consensus documents from international bodies such as WHO. These often depend on diagnostic algorithms and may also be influenced by cost, availability of suitably trained staff and infrastructure and improvements in technology.

Tests may also be unsuited to particular settings or have been superseded by standard technologies. The Western blot is a case in point. Certain technologies have been revived as alternatives and may possibly be cheaper than newer methods. For example, the p24 antigen, used as a screening tool in blood banks, is also used in the diagnosis of mother-to-child HIV transmission and in monitoring responses to antiretroviral therapy.

There are two approaches to the diagnosis of HIV:

- The identification of the virus: viral culture, electron microscopy, production of antigen eg p24, detection of virus nucleic acids (nucleic acid testing, NAT) including integrated proviral DNA in cells or viral RNA in fluids.
- The detection of an immunological response to HIV that includes the production of antibodies including IgM, IgG, IgA or cellular responses including specific T helper (Th) and cytotoxic (Tc) cell responses.

The tools can be either qualitative, eg electron microscopy and proviral DNA or quantitative, such as viral culture or RNA viral loads. Sophisticated assays of Th and Tc are not practical in clinical practice and cell culture is also of limited use in clinical diagnostic work-ups.

The use of nucleic acid techniques (NAT) for diagnosis is not always clear and in certain instances may not be recommended. However, in difficult to diagnose cases where there is a high index of suspicion and antibody testing is negative, then it is possible to attempt to look for proviral DNA in peripheral blood mononuclear cells (PBMNC). Manufacturers do not always recommend the use of RNA viral load for diagnosis as false positives have been reported. This is the result of the lower specificity of certain viral load assays such as the branched DNA (bDNA, Bayer). The special cases where the use of nucleic acid testing is useful include looking back through samples for possible blood transfusion transmission or screening, vertical transmission, and misclassification of vaccine recipients. NAT may assist in earlier detection of infection in occupational exposure where a seroconversion event may have occurred. RNA may be detected within five days of infection.

The ELISA test is probably the best-known test of immunological response. Common features of all ELISAs are enzyme conjugates that bind to specific HIV antibodies and substrates/chromogens that produce colour in a reaction catalysed by the bound enzyme conjugate. The most common ELISA involves an indirect method in which HIV antigen is attached to one well of a 96-well microtitre plate, or to a macroscopic bead that is subsequently placed in a well of a plate. Antibody in the sample is allowed to react with the antigen-coated solid support, and after washing to remove unbound serum components, a conjugate is added (an antihuman immunoglobulin with a bound enzyme) that binds to the specific antibody that is attached to the antigens on the solid phase. Further washing after this step removes unbound antibody, and is followed by the addition of an appropriate substrate that results in colour development (detected by a spectrophotometer). Optical density values (OD) are produced as the coloured solution absorbs transmitted light and provides an indication of the amount of colour that is proportional to the amount of antibody bound (ie antibody concentration). A mathematical calculation, usually based on the OD of the negative controls multiplied by a factor, produces a cut-off value (CO) on which the OD of the sample is compared to determine the antibody status; samples with OD/CO values greater than 1.0 (in an indirect ELISA) are considered as antibody reactive (positive).

Alternative ELISA methodologies include a competitive format in which specific HIV antibody in the sample competes with an enzyme-bound antibody reagent for antigen sites on the solid phase. In this method, colour development is inversely proportional to specific HIV antibody concentration.

Another ELISA technology is the antigen sandwich method in which an enzyme (alkaline phosphatase or horseradish peroxidase) is conjugated to an HIV antigen (similar to the immobilised antigen on the solid phase). The antibody in the sample is 'sandwiched' between two antigen molecules; one immobilised on the solid phase and one containing the enzyme. Subsequently, the addition of substrate results in colour development in proportion to antibody concentration. The antigen sandwich ELISA is considered the most sensitive screening method, given its ability to detect all isotypes of antibody (including IgM). One disadvantage of this method is the relatively large volume (150 µl) of sample required, which may make repeat testing and testing of samples from infants difficult.

A new generation of combination ELISAs that simultaneously detects both antigen and antibody has been developed. These assays have demonstrated a high analytical sensitivity of detection that is the result of the combination of a third-generation format (antigen sandwich) for antibody detection and the ability to detect HIV p24 antigen simultaneously. Due to their ability to detect p24 antigen, the fourth generation ELISAs will be particularly useful for detecting early infection. Detecting early infection using antigen testing is of advantage in settings where patients could be considered for early initiation of treatment, counselling or interventions to reduce the risk of transmission. Individuals to be screened for infection in this way are generally from higher risk groups than the blood donor population, and thus require testing methodologies with high levels of analytical sensitivity to detect primary infection. A high level of analytical and epidemiological sensitivity has been demonstrated by most of the fourth generation assays with seroconversion and clade panels, as well as in a variety of patient populations, making them ideal for use in a variety of situations, including the diagnosis of early and established infection. In routine laboratory testing, HIV-infected samples that are identified via antigen detection would not have been identified by the usual screening antibody assays, since testing for antigens in patients is not commonly performed as a screening tool outside the blood banks.

Rapid testing

In the case of simple rapid test kits all reagents are contained in a flat cartridge, usually plastic or paper, including a strip which contains the antigens that will capture antibody in the sample. Whole blood, oral fluid, or serum is placed at the tip of the device and allowed to diffuse along the strip which is impregnated with reagents (often protein A colloidal gold), where reaction with the antigens occurs. Some use third generation technology (antigen sandwich). These tests can be completed in less than ten minutes (some within two minutes), require little or no addition of reagents, and contain a built-in-quality-control reagent to control for technical errors. Some can be stored at a wide range of temperatures (from 4–30 °C), and are easily transported. Rapid HIV tests are thus useful in certain settings because they are simple to perform and are reliable and robust. The use of fingerstick blood is less expensive, is less invasive, and is more suitable for collection in areas where specially trained phlebotomists may not be available; this collection method is easily taught to health care personnel (eg nurses) in outreach situations or mobile clinics. A comparison between laboratory-trained technologists and non-laboratory staff performing simple rapid assays has shown comparable results. A novel advance of the rapid kit is a confirmatory rapid kit that contains multiple antigens. These rapid, flow-through tests are performed in an identical manner to rapid screening tests (addition of several reagents in drop-wise fashion), and produce 'reaction profiles' similar to the Western blot tests and Line Immuno Assays.

Where to use which type of diagnostic technology

The choice of type of diagnostic technology is generally determined by the diagnostic setting, for example:
- early diagnosis, eg acute infection, would rely on detection of viral antigens or nucleic acids and/or antibody responses
- blood transfusion transmission screening, which relies on antibody testing, antigen testing, NAT
- occupational exposure can be tested using baseline antibody testing and proviral DNA where appropriate, eg symptoms suggestive of exposure
- participants in vaccine trials where specific ELISA design may distinguish between responses to vaccine constructs or breakthrough infections
- vertical transmission (mother-to-child transmission relies on nucleic acid testing, either proviral DNA or RNA viral load, or antibodies in the case of infants >15 or 18 months)
- assessments of prevalence would rely on antibody responses and of incidence on variations of antibody testing
- responses to antiretroviral treatment require monitoring of viral RNA levels.

Diagnosing HIV infection in adults

Factors that may influence the choice of testing in adults include the setting of testing, accuracy of the test, FDA or equivalent approval, complexity of the test, likelihood that the patient will return for the result, cost of the test and ease of sample collection. In routine laboratories, either an ELISA (EIA) or Western blot could be used. At least two or three ELISAs with different underlying principles or antigens could be used to make the diagnosis of HIV. The strategy can in part be determined by using the WHO guidelines for use of tests at a given prevalence and purpose.

The initial screening test should be one of high sensitivity and the confirmatory or supplementary test(s) may have a lower sensitivity, remembering however, that the requirement is one of high specificity.

Population serosurveillance

Population serosurveillance is used to establish the epidemiology of the disease, to implement public health programmes, to target prevention programmes and resources, to evaluate the effectiveness of prevention and control programmes, and to project the future numbers of cases of disease. It could be argued that the most important guide in HIV prevention programmes is not prevalence but incidence, ie the number and distribution of new cases (refer to CHAPTER 4 for details on incidence in South Africa). New cases of HIV infection would reflect a failure of public health programmes and the requirement to either refine existing programmes or introduce other approaches. In mature epidemics incidence is best measured directly rather than being derived from prevalence data.

The performance of assays under various conditions of prevalence can be determined by using the formulae for PPV (positive predictive value) and NPV (negative predictive value). The UNAIDS and WHO criteria stipulate that two tests are to be used for diagnosis at a prevalence of >10% in asymptomatic cases and three ELISAs if the prevalence is <10%. It is recommended that testing be performed on whole blood, serum, or plasma. An additional practical approach would be the use of dried blood spots (DBS). DBS have certain advantages in, for example, remote areas. An alternative in remote areas or where laboratory infrastructure is not readily available is the use of rapid HIV tests.

There is evidence that HIV subtype (clade) does not influence the sensitivity and specificity of ELISAs and simple rapid devices. However, it is recommended that before using such devices an in-country evaluation be performed. In the case of second-generation surveillance that relies on biological surveillance ie serology, data on behaviour and other factors are included to obtain a global picture of an epidemic. If an epidemic is generalised, antenatal clinics are the preferred sites for serosurveillance. By contrast, surveillance in concentrated or low level epidemics should focus on populations at risk. Serosurveillance data give an estimate of HIV prevalence rates, geographic distribution, trends over time in specific populations, eg by age and sex, and identifies populations at risk. The reliability of surveillance of HIV prevalence or incidence rate estimates is dependent on the accuracy of the HIV tests used, the frequency and timing of the survey, the appropriateness of the group(s) chosen for screening, the underlying prevalence in the population, the mode of transmission, consistency in methodology used both in terms of sampling and tests used, and representativeness of the site/or population included in the survey.

Interpretation of results

An HIV test should be considered positive only after screening and confirmatory tests are reactive. False-positive results when both screening and confirmatory tests are reactive are rare. The results should always be considered in the context of the clinical picture. Thus, the possibility of a mislabelled sample or laboratory error must be considered, especially if there is no identifiable risk for HIV infection.

A negative ELISA or simple rapid test result indicates the likely absence of HIV infection. However, if there is a clinical suspicion or in the case of occupational exposure, the test could be repeated within three to four weeks.

A result is indeterminate when, for example, two or three ELISAs or two simple rapid results are discordant. Under these circumstances testing should be repeated in two to four weeks. In the case of simple rapid tests it may be possible to use a third (tie breaker) simple rapid kit, or to forward a specimen to a laboratory that performs HIV ELISA testing if no technical problems with the S/R devices are suspected.

Participants in HIV vaccine trials

HIV vaccine-induced antibodies may be detected by current tests and may cause a false-positive result. People whose test results are HIV-positive and who are identified as vaccine trial participants should be encouraged to contact or return to their trial site for HIV counselling and testing. A similar approach could be adopted when using simple rapid devices. More than 10 000 individuals are estimated to have participated in HIV vaccine trials. The vaccine constructs are able to elicit responses that can be detected by standard ELISAs, rapid assays and Western blots.

A vaccine recipient who is misclassified may undergo unnecessary and costly testing. There is also the potential for misclassification of vaccine recipients and the social harm this may cause to an individual. On a population level, collection of serosurveilance data that includes misclassified vaccine recipients may result in overestimation or distortion of the prevalence of HIV. Those participating in vaccine trials need to know that this misclassification may result. It is also possible that a vaccine trial participant may engage in risky behaviour under the false belief that they are on the vaccine arm of the trial and therefore protected from acquiring infection with HIV. It may be necessary to alter testing strategies and algorithms and to identify participants of vaccine trials to maintain blinding. Testing of algorithms could include repeating indeterminate tests later or including a serological marker in the vaccine construct. This approach raises some ethical dilemmas as testing positive may lead to, amongst others, stigma, discrimination or loss of job or social security. Alternatively, vaccine constructs that contain epitopes that are not immunogenic on standard testing strategies are an option. In this case, vaccine-specific tests would have to be designed. NAT testing certainly offers certain advantages but is not without its own problems in terms of personnel, equipment and cost. Nevertheless, improvements in NAT testing, as well as other tests, are essential.

Detection of recent infection in adults: PHI and incident cases

The identification of recent infections may have clinical as well as epidemiological significance. Clinically, it is possible to initiate therapy early with potential important consequences for immune regulation and progress. However, there is no consensus on the value of initiating therapy so early given its complexity and the need for life-long treatment. From a population perspective, identifying recent infections provides an opportunity to counsel on behaviour that may reduce HIV transmission. The identification of recent infection is also important for those researching the introduction of measures such as vaccines or antiretroviral programmes on transmission. There are two phases of early infection that will be considered; primary HIV infection in the absence of seroconversion and post seroconversion infections, which would include positive antibody testing, known to be of recent origin.

The tools to detect early primary HIV infection (PHI) in the absence of seroconversion include antigen detection such as p24 or RNA. Symptoms such as rash and fever together with the presence of antigen are highly suggestive of PHI. Such symptoms are included in acute retroviral syndrome. However, studies have shown that the clinical diagnosis of PHI is often missed. In addition, the p24 antigen was shown to have a low sensitivity of 79% despite a specificity of 99.5%. One possible explanation for this is that the antigen is complexed to antibody despite the failure of third-generation ELISAs to detect antibodies in PHI-defined cases. RNA has been found to be highly sensitive in PHI cases. RNA values were usually >10 000 copies/ml in individuals presenting with PHI. Individuals with viral loads <10 000 copies/ml could either be in the resolution phase or the results could be false positives as a result of lower specificity. A conservative estimate for cut-off value for false positives is thought to be <5000 copies/ml.

The most well-established programme for the detection of incident infections is the serologic testing algorithm for recent HIV seroconversion (STARHS). This uses two ELISAs with greater and lesser sensitivity or alternatively the 'detuned' ELISA. The first ELISA is highly sensitive and detects antibody. All positive tests are then subjected to a second ELISA that is less sensitive to low antibody concentrations. A specimen that is positive on the sensitive ELISA but negative on the second ELISA reflects early infection. The assay is made less sensitive by using a higher serum dilution (1/20 000 compared to 1/400). The dilution is based on the observation that antibody titres increase following seroconversion. The sensitive ELISA plateaus soon after seroconversion but the less sensitive ELISA has a longer dynamic range and the standardised optical density (SOD) indirectly reflects antibody titres. A predefined cut-off distinguishes specimens with titres lower than 1/20 000, ie recent infection, from those with titres higher than 1/20 000, ie established infections. Samples that are positive on the standard sensitive ELISA and with standardised optical density below a certain prescribed cut-off value (0.45 for subtype C), are classified as recent infections. It is estimated that those who are classified as recent infections have seroconverted within the last 129 days. The case definition for incident HIV infection would include individuals with acute retroviral syndrome, PHI, individuals with documented seroconversion and individuals positive on the sensitive/less-sensitive ELISA.

The calculated seroconversion period described above is based on the use of subtype B reagents. Recent studies have shown that the HIV subtype affects the performance characteristics of the 'detuned' assay. In Thailand where the prevalent HIV subtype is E, the seroconversion duration is approximately 270 days. It is therefore important that other subtype reagents be included in the assay. Only one study in South Africa has reported formally on the use of the STARHS method and a window period of 200 days was used. However, more research is needed to validate this period and explore the applicability of the technique in countries with subtype C infection.

Other approaches to defining recent infection are based on qualitative and quantitative changes that occur in the antibody responses. These changes include, for example, antibody isotype, antibody avidity/affinity, antibody titre, conformation dependence of antibodies and the proportion of HIV IgG. The results of at least the antibody avidity and proportion of HIV IgG testing are promising. The proportion of anti-HIV IgG in total IgG increases following seroconversion. ELISAs that utilise antigen-coated wells detect HIV antibodies but are not quantitative and plateau soon after seroconversion. A competitive IgG capture ELISA has been developed to detect the increasing proportion of HIV IgG in serum following seroconversion. The assay captures HIV and non-HIV IgG, present in serum, in the same proportion. HIV IgG is then detected by a branched gp41 peptide, incorporating sequences from subtypes B, E and D. Initial validations have shown that the number of incident cases was within 10% of the expected number of cases. The ideal assay would be a combination of assay principles that takes into account factors such as subtype and possible misclassification.

Misclassification of AIDS cases as incident cases is possible in both the 'detuned' assay and the capture ELISA, and possibly the affinity assay. It is thought that, in the presence of a declining immune system and high antigen levels, the antibodies are complexed to antigen, reducing availability in both assays. Misclassification has been calculated to be about 2–5%. In addition, since the capture assay relies on proportion of IgG, conditions with hypergammaglobulinaemia, eg co-infections, may result in false high incidence. Incidence per 100 persons per year is calculated as the total number tested (seronegative plus recent infections) and corrected for the year using the factor 365/T, where T is the seroconversion duration.

Diagnosis of mother-to-child (MTCT) transmission of HIV

Transmission of HIV from mother to child could occur at the following times: *in utero*, intrapartum and postpartum.

Diagnosis of infection in the mother

With the introduction of various antiretroviral regimes that range from highly active antiretroviral therapy (HAART) to single dose nevirapine and AZT (zidovudine) it is imperative that the mother's status be established through voluntary counselling and testing. Establishing infection is through either ELISAs or on-site rapid testing. If antiretroviral therapy is to continue after the pregnancy, establishing the RNA viral load is useful.

Diagnosis of HIV infection in the infant

One of the factors that contributes to vertical transmission is the HIV viral load, although this is not absolute and there may be other factors that cause transmission even in the presence of antiretroviral treatment. There is a suggestion that the subtype (clade) of the virus may play a role in the timing of transmission. Nevertheless, antiretro-viral treatment is effective in reducing transmission rates. However, it is not yet clear whether knowledge of subtype would necessarily influence the mode of intervention.

In utero transmission accounts for approximately 30% of all cases. The remainder of the cases could be intrapartum exposure or the result of breastfeeding. The diagnosis of HIV infection under any of these three scenarios would rely on nucleic acid detection. NAT testing would detect proviral DNA in human peripheral blood mononuclear (PBMNC) cultures. The detection of proviral DNA within 48 hours to ten days would suggest *in utero* infection. The sensitivity of the test at 48 hours is probably approximately 50% but a high specificity is possible. The sensitivity and specificity increase to >90% at one month and are close to 98% by three and six months. The algorithm for confirming HIV infection in infants is partly set around the sensitivity of the assay, the role of breastfeeding and the cost of performing the test. There are reported cases of false negatives; the likely result of primer design not matching circulating subtypes. Overall, the false positive and negative rates for HIV DNA PCR are 1.5%.

There is no universal algorithm for testing the HIV-infected infant in the absence of therapy. One approach is to perform at least three PCRs spaced at least one to two months apart. If the first two PCRs are negative then re-testing may not be required. However, in the presence of breastfeeding, additional testing may be required. Seroconversion can be documented after the age of 15–18 months. The frequency of testing under such circumstances may be every three months. An alternative means of identifying vertical trans-mission is by using RNA viral load assays. In general, the RNA assays appear to be equally as effective and, in certain case reports, superior to proviral DNA PCR detection. The sensitivity of RNA increased from

34% at birth to between 95% and 99% at two, four and six months of age.

The detection of p24 has been suggested as an alternative means of diagnosing vertical transmission. Evaluation of an ultrasensitive p24 antigen assay (UPTA) for use in the diagnosis of paediatric HIV infection has been reported. The p24 antigen assays are a modification of the assay using standard kit reagents (PerkinElmer). The modifications include disruption of the antigen-antibody complex and increased sensitivity of the detection of the antigen. More widespread evaluation of the assay would be important to determine its usefulness. The early detection of HIV infection in infants should afford the opportunity to institute antiretroviral therapy. However, where therapy is not provided the viral load can be a possible predictor of progression to AIDS.

Monitoring disease progression and responses to antiretroviral therapy

The mainstay of monitoring antiretroviral therapy is the HIV viral load. The measurement of the HIV viral load is important in terms of assessing disease progression, initiating therapy before onset of symptoms, eg PHI, responses to therapy, the testing of new therapies, and drug failure. Currently there are three FDA-approved viral load assays that are commonly used, but additional assays are available, eg LCX HIV RNA Quantitative assay (Abbott Diagnostics). The three are NucliSens HIV-1 QT (Organon Technica), RT-PCR (Roche) and branched DNA (bDNA, Bayer).

The RNA viral load is an important predictor of the progression to AIDS and is usually measured in conjunction with the CD4 count. In the early days of antiretroviral therapy the concept was to 'hit early, hit hard' based on particular RNA viral load levels. However, initiating therapy based on viral load alone has been shown sometimes to be inappropriate and the emphasis has shifted to considering starting therapy based on the CD4 count. These guidelines vary from starting therapy at CD4 counts of 350 cells/µl (DHSS guidelines) to the WHO guideline of 200 cells/µl. Despite the change in guidelines, HIV RNA viral load is the standard to assess the effectiveness of therapy and disease progression.

A reduction in plasma HIV RNA of two-fold (0.3 log10) reduces the risk of disease progression and death by approximately 30%. A four-fold (0.6 log10) and ten-fold (1 log10) decrease of viral load reduces the risk of disease progression by 55% and 65% respectively. The reduction in risk of disease progression or death is independent of baseline plasma HIV RNA and CD4 counts. Moreover, the reduction in risk of disease progression or death is independent of an increased CD4 cell count that results from therapy. Nevertheless, the amount of virus in circulation is linked to the rate of virus production that in turn determines the rate of CD4 cell destruction. Thus, a primary feature of HIV infection is the progressive loss of CD4 cells. On average 30 to 60 CD4 cells are lost per year but it is not unusual for many patients to have relatively stable CD4 cell counts for several years followed by a period of decline. Progression to AIDS within one to two years of PHI occurs in approximately 5% of patients.

The CD4 cell count is an indicator of current immunological status and risk of opportunistic infection and a less useful marker of future progression of healthy patients. The CD4 cell count should increase rapidly following antiretroviral drug therapy as it is a reflection of the extent of suppression of viral replication. CD4 cell counts, as well as CD8 cell counts, can be determined by flow cytometry using either dual or single platform technologies. In the dual technology platform (DTP), a haematology analyser is used to obtain the total white cell counts and absolute lymphocyte count. The CD4 and CD8 cell count is then calculated from the CD4 and CD8 percentage positive cells obtained from the flow cytometer. Single-platform technologies (SPT) use latex beads of specific concentrations added to a control blood sample before flow cytometric analysis and therefore eliminates the use of a haematology analyser. The SPT allows for the enumeration of absolute and percentage lymphocyte subset values. Using SPT increases confidence in the results; the results are more reproducible and improved interlaboratory coefficients of variation are achieved.

The principles of the viral load assays are either based on target amplification, ie PCR in the case of NucliSens HIV-1 QT and RT-PCR or signal amplification in the bDNA assay. The anticoagulant is important in the performance of the assay. In the case of the NucliSens and Roche assays, EDTA and citrate are acceptable while EDTA is the preferred anticoagulant for bDNA. Heparin is not recommended for the former assays as it interferes with enzyme function.

The NucliSens HIV-1 QT assay requires the extraction of RNA using the Boom technology from a plasma sample. The RNA is of high quality and can be used for other applications such as sequencing (genotyping). The enzymatic amplification includes two HIV sequence-specific primers for the *Pol* gene, RNase H, T7 RNA polymerase and DNA polymerase. All reactions are performed at the same temperature. There have been improvements in assay including a degree of automation that improves on throughput. The dynamic range is 176–3 470 000 copies/ml. Nevertheless, criticisms include the possibility of non-specific amplification given the annealing temperature and variation in amplification efficiency.

RT-PCR (Roche) is a sensitive HIV viral load assay and improvements, such as the closed automated extraction system (Ampliprep), allows for high throughput. The dynamic range is 50–100 000 copies/ml (ultrasensitive format) or 400–750 000 copies in the case of the standard assay. The assay primers SK145 and SKCC1B amplify a conserved region in the *Gag* gene. The optimised hybridisation conditions and primer sequence allow for the detection of HIV group M subtypes. An internal quantitation control serves as a control for optimal reaction conditions. The control can be used to identify problems with RNA extraction, the presence of inhibitors or improper techniques. One of the major problems with PCR is that of contamination which can give rise to false positive results. An additional disadvantage is that only one set of primers derived from the *Gag* gene may result in inefficient amplification in the case of, for example, mutations in the 3' primer attachment region with resultant possible underdetection or false negative results.

bDNA technology differs from the two technologies above in that it is based on signal amplification and therefore does not affect the concentration of starting material, reducing the possibility of contamination. The dynamic range is 50 or 75–500 000 copies/ml. The FDA sets a lower limit of 75 copies/ml. The bDNA assay is a hybridisation-based technology that comprises 81 target probes that anneal to the *Pol* gene and 17 different capture probes that allow for solid phase hybridisation during the incubation step in wells of a 96-well plate. The semi-automated system has a high throughput and 168 specimens can be processed per day. A disadvantage of the bDNA assay is that there is no internal control within the sample and therefore it is not possible to state whether a negative sample is truly negative or whether the test was inhibited.

The assays do have excellent inter-laboratory reproducibility. The biological variation of HIV RNA in plasma in clinically stable individuals is approximately three-fold (0.5 log) and the variation is not associated with diurnal fluctuations. Thus viral loads above 0.5 logs are regarded as being significant. In general there is a good correlation between the assays. However, there could be variations of >0.5 log between assays. A major concern is that the assays have been developed and standardised in settings of HIV subtype B. Subtype B infection accounts for approximately 3% of all HIV infections. In addition, there is no universal standard for comparison between assays for quality control. How feasible and cost-effective such a standard is requires investigation. It is advisable that once a choice of assay has been made, monitoring be performed on the same assay. It is possible to perform recalibrations on a different assay if the same assay can no longer be used. Such recalibrations have not been widely reported in the literature. With the evolving epidemic, ie the increased diversity of HIV as reflected by recombinant forms, quasi species, and the increased availability of antiretroviral treatment, assays would be required to accurately determine the HIV RNA viral loads. The role of HIV subtyping may be a consideration where there is a mismatch between clinical assessment and viral load. For example, it has been reported that assay performance with different subtypes could vary by up to more than one log between bDNA and Roche. By contrast, a recent study performed in a HIV subtype C prevalent population did not reveal marked differences in viral load assessment in three commercial assays. It is thus critical to ensure that improvements are made to existing assays that take into account the factors listed, or to develop assays that are independent of marked variation.

Alternative cost-effective testing technologies are needed for monitoring HIV viral loads. Non-specific markers of inflammation such as β2 microglobulin and neopterin have not gained widespread favour. An example of technologies that could well fit the criteria would be the enzyme-dependent assays such as Cavidi Tech ExaVir LOAD reverse transcriptase assay where measurement of viral load is dependent on active enzyme. Enzyme activity is correlated to viral copies for ease of reporting. The assay would work regardless of HIV subtype. However, it would not be able to distinguish between HIV-1 and HIV-2 infections. In addition, debate around whether to have centralised laboratories perform assays to ensure quality of the results or to decentralise the testing and have 'low technology' but robust assays available at peripheral sites requires attention and evaluation, especially in resource-constrained countries.

Alternatives to HIV viral loads include p24 measurements. The boosted p24 antigen can be measured using a commercially available kit from PerkinElmer Life Sciences. However, there is no clear consensus as to the value of the p24 assay and its interpretation. The production of p24 is a reflection of protein synthesis but how this relates to viral replication and therefore how to interpret p24 production requires clarification. It may well be that p24 is more informative than viral load. For example, studies have shown that while there was a steady decline in the p24 production associated with an increase in CD4 count, the viral load was not affected. Moreover, studies of predictions of clinical progression have shown that a combination of p24 antigen and CD4 count gave almost equally good results to a combination of viral load and CD4 count. More work is required to validate the observations, including testing in populations infected with non-subtype B viruses.

Monitoring Quality of Testing

In addition to accuracy, the validity of diagnostic test results depends on the quality of a number of measures used before, during, and after the test is performed. To ensure the quality of test results, a programme of quality assurance, quality control, and quality assessment is necessary.

Quality assurance entails all aspects of quality control, from receipt of specimens through to final reporting, to ensure that the final results are as accurate as the assays allow. Specimens must be inspected on arrival for suitability; logging, processing, and all accompanying paperwork must be carefully reviewed and monitored. Also included in quality assurance are organised record-keeping systems, standard operating procedure manuals that act as references, a continuing education programme, supervisory review of results, a system for evaluation of laboratory personnel, use of the most appropriate tests/strategies, a mechanism for timely reporting, compliance with regulatory requirements, storage of specimens for follow-up testing, appropriate reporting forms, variance reporting for errors/inconsistencies, a good management system, and a good quality control and quality assessment programme.

Quality control refers to those specific measures that ensure that the test is performing as expected. Such measures include careful inspection of internal (kit) control values that validate the test, monitoring of physical parameters (temperatures, functioning of equipment), validation of new reagents (different kit lots), and use of external controls to verify the manufacturer's claims. The use of external controls, while recommended, is not required or compulsory. In the latter case, this may be dependent on the regulatory authority for accreditation.

Quality assessment is a means to challenge the overall performance of the laboratory. The process usually involves testing a panel of samples with known reactivity provided by an external source. Such assessment usually provides some information about the overall quality of the laboratory's performance. Results from each laboratory are compiled and feedback is provided. Other measures of assessment include internal audits (ie self-inspections of the laboratory and testing process), specimens provided by the laboratory quality assurance manager or supervisor, for blinded testing by personnel, and review of the total operation by an external agency. The ultimate challenge in assessing the ability of a laboratory to produce accurate results is to provide these panels of specimens in a blinded manner so that personnel are unaware that they are being monitored.

Bibliography

ACKERS ML, PAREKH B, EVANS TG, BERMAN P, PHILLIPS S, ALLEN M, McDOUGAL JS. 'Human immunodeficiency virus (HIV) seropositivity among uninfected HIV vaccine recipients'. *Journal of Infectious Diseases* 2003; 187: 879–886.

BARNETT D, GRANGER V, WHITBY L, STORIE I, REILLY JT. 'Absolute CD4+ T-lymphocyte and CD34+ stem cell counts by single-platform flow cytometry: The way forward'. *British Journal of Haematology* 1999; 106: 1059–1062.

BENJAMIN DK JR, MILLER WC, FISCUS SA, BENJAMIN DK, MORSE M, VALENTINE M, McKINNEY RE JR. 'Rational testing of the HIV-exposed infant'. *Pediatrics* 2001; 108:E3.

CERVIA J, KAPLAN B, SCHUVAL S, WEISS S. 'Virologic testing in the management of perinatal HIV exposure'. *AIDS Reader* 2003; 13: 39–47.

CENTERS FOR DISEASE CONTROL AND PREVENTION. REVISED GUIDELINES FOR HIV COUNSELING, TESTING, AND REFERRAL. *Morbidity and Mortality Weekly Report Recomm Rep* 2001; 50(RR-19): 1–57.

CLARKE JR. 'Molecular diagnosis of HIV'. *Expert review of molecular diagnostics* 2002; 2: 233–239.

CONSTANTINE NT, KETEMA F. 'Rapid confirmation of HIV infection'. *International Journal of Infectious Diseases* 2002; 6: 170–177.

CROWE S, TURNBULL S, OELRICHS R, DUNNE A. 'Monitoring of human immunodeficiency virus infection in resource-constrained countries'. *Clinical infectious diseases* 2003; 37(Suppl 1): S25–35.

ELBEIK T, LOFTUS RA, BERINGER S. 'Health care industries' perspective of viral load assays: The VERSANT HIV-1 RNA 3.0 assay'. *Expert review of molecular diagnostics* 2002; 2: 275–285.

FIEBIG EW, WRIGHT DJ, RAWAL BD, GARRETT PE, SCHUMACHER RT, PEDDADA L, HELDEBRANT C, SMITH R, CONRAD A, KLEINMAN SH, BUSCH MP. 'Dynamics of HIV viremia and antibody seroconversion in plasma donors: Implications for diagnosis and staging of primary HIV infection'. *AIDS* 2003; 17: 1871–1879.

JANSSEN RS, SATTEN GA, STRAMER SL, RAWAL BD, O'BRIEN TR, WEIBLEN BJ, HECHT FM, JACK N, CLEGHORN FR, KAHN JO, CHESNEY MA, BUSCH MP. 'New testing strategy to detect early HIV-1 infection for use in incidence estimates and for clinical and prevention purposes'. *Journal of the American Medical Association* 1998; 280: 42–48.

MANDY FF, NICHOLSON JK, McDOUGAL JS; CDC. 'Guidelines for performing single-platform absolute CD4+ T-cell determinations with CD45 gating for persons infected with human immunodeficiency virus'. Centers for Disease Control and Prevention. *Morbidity and Mortality Weekly Report Recomm Rep* 2003; 52(RR-2): 1–13.

MURPHY DG, COTE L, FAUVEL M, RENE P, VINCELETTE J. 'Multicenter comparison of Roche COBAS AMPLICOR MONITOR version 1.5, Organon Teknika NucliSens QT with Extractor, and Bayer Quantiplex version 3.0 for quantification of human immunodeficiency virus type 1 RNA in plasma'. *Journal of Clinical Microbiology* 2000; 38: 4034–4041.

PAREKH BS, PAU CP, KENNEDY MS, DOBBS TL, McDOUGAL JS. 'Assessment of antibody assays for identifying and distinguishing recent from long-term HIV type 1 infection'. *AIDS Research and Human Retroviruses* 2001; 17: 137–146.

PHILLIPS S, GRANADE TC, PAU CP, CANDAL D, HU DJ, PAREKH BS. 'Diagnosis of human immunodeficiency virus type 1 infection with different subtypes using rapid tests'. *Clinical and Diagnostic Laboratory Immunology* 2000; 7: 698–689.

PISANI E, LAZZARI S, WALKER N, SCHWARTLANDER B. 'HIV surveillance: A global perspective'. *Journal of Acquired Immune Deficiency Syndrome* 2003; 32(Suppl 1): S3–11.

SAVILLE RD, CONSTANTINE NT, CLEGHORN FR, JACK N, BARTHOLOMEW C, EDWARDS J, GOMEZ P, BLATTNER WA. 'Fourth-generation enzyme-linked immunosorbent assay for the simultaneous detection of human immunodeficiency virus antigen and antibody'. *Journal of Clinical Microbiology* 2001; 39: 2518–2524.

WALKER N, GARCIA-CALLEJA JM, HEATON L, ASAMOAH-ODEI E, POUMEROL G, LAZZARI S, GHYS PD, SCHWARTLANDER B, STANECKI KA. 'Epidemiological analysis of the quality of HIV sero-surveillance in the world: How well do we track the epidemic?' *AIDS* 2001; 15: 1545–1554.

CHAPTER 7
HIV-1 Genetic Diversity

Carolyn Williamson and Darren P Martin

HIV IS A MEMBER of a group of viruses referred to as the primate infecting lentiviruses of the family Retroviridae. There are two HIV types: HIV-1 (including three lineages called the M, N and O groups) and HIV-2 (including three lineages called the A, B and G groups). Viruses within the HIV-1 M group are primarily responsible for the global AIDS epidemic. The epidemic probably began when an ancestral HIV-1 M virus was transmitted to humans from chimpanzees in equatorial West Africa at some time during the 1930s. The HIV-1 M genetic diversity that has subsequently arisen has required subdivision of the group into 11 subtypes (called A1, A2, B, C, D, F1, F2, G, H, J, and K). Subtype C viruses overwhelmingly dominate the South African epidemic. Evidence suggests that multiple subtype C incursions into South Africa have occurred from elsewhere in Africa.

Extreme genetic diversity, a consequence of the error-prone and recombinogenic nature of HIV replication, seriously threatens our chances of containing the AIDS epidemic. Viruses within an infected person can rapidly evolve to evade immune responses (both natural and vaccine induced) and antiretroviral drugs. Despite the South African epidemic being characterised by lower HIV diversity than elsewhere in Africa, effective control of HIV using vaccines and drug therapy here may be compromised by the massive evolutionary potential of this virus.

HIV classification and diversity

HIV belongs to the family Retroviridae and the genus lentivirus: Lenti meaning slow and reflecting the long time it takes from infection to disease. HIV has been divided into two types, HIV Type 1 (HIV-1) and HIV Type 2 (HIV-2) (FIGURE 7.1).

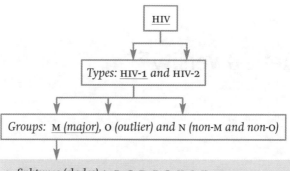

FIGURE 7.1 HIV classification

HIV-2 is less pathogenic than HIV-1 and largely restricted to West Africa, with limited spread to other countries. For historical reasons, all lentiviruses isolated from humans are called human immunodeficiency viruses or HIV and those isolated from simian primates are called simian immunodeficiency viruses or SIV. SIV has been isolated from a number of primates including the chimpanzee, sooty mangabey, *Macaca mulata*, African green monkey and Sykes monkey (FIGURE 7.2A).

HIV has been classified into three groups, M, N and O. The group M or major group are the viruses that are currently dominating the global AIDS epidemic and will be the focus of this chapter. Of lower prevalence in the epidemic are the outliers group (group O) and the non-M non-O group (group N).

Group M HIVs can be subdivided into subtypes or clades based on their phylogenetic relatedness. Currently there are nine described subtypes named A, B, C, D, F, G, H, J and K. Two of these subtypes A and F have been further subdivided into subtypes (referred to as A1, A2 and F1, F2 respectively). Two groups of viruses that were originally thought to be unique subtypes (E and I) have since been shown to possess recombinant genomes with regions originating from two or more subtypes. These so-called circulating recombinant forms (or CRFs) are now named CRF01_AE and CRF04_cpx respectively. Besides these two groups of recombinant viruses there are currently ten other described CRFs.

Although the currently classified HIV subtypes and CRFs are representative of the viruses primarily responsible for the AIDS epidemic, they do not give a complete view of HIV diversity. There are many fully sequenced group M HIVs that are too highly diverged to be placed within any existing subtype or CRF grouping and these have remained unique unclassified recombinants. In addition, certain inter-subtype recombinant viruses contain sequences that are of indeterminate origin, providing further evidence that HIV diversity is not fully represented under the current classification system. This implies that there is potentially a less prominent but far more diverse pool of HIV viruses circulating among humans than the classified subtypes and CRFs might suggest.

Whether fully representative of HIV diversity or not, full genome sequences determined over the last ten years have generated a reasonable snapshot of diversity at the critical exponential growth phase of HIV's population expansion. These data will be extremely useful in our attempt to understand how, in the face of whatever controls we attempt to exert on it, global HIV diversity will evolve in coming decades.

Mechanisms of HIV diversification

Extreme genetic diversity is the hallmark of HIV-1. The ability of HIV to rapidly evolve in response to environmental pressures enables continual adaptation and escape from selective forces such as immune responses and antiretroviral drugs. There are two mechanisms that HIV uses to generate diversity: firstly, mutations are introduced into viral genomes during replication, and secondly, recombination between viral genomes shuffles these mutations (FIGURE 7.3).

Mutations are introduced into the viral genome primarily because of the error-prone nature of the viral replication enzyme, reverse transcriptase. This enzyme introduces approximately one error for every 2000 nucleotides it incorporates (FIGURE 7.3A). In addition, unlike the human polymerases, reverse transcriptase is unable to correct these errors. With a genome of 10 000 nucleotides this means that every new genome that is produced during replication will contain up to five errors. As a consequence, within an infected individual no two viruses are identical. This assemblage of unique individual mutants are referred to as quasispecies. By infecting individuals with a swarm of mutant viruses, HIV has unique biological and evolutionary advantages over other viruses that infect with more clonal populations. Among these is the ability to rapidly adapt to fluctuating selection pressures, such as immune responses and anti-retroviral drugs.

However, the extremely high mutation rate of HIV also presents the virus with some problems: firstly, a large proportion of mutations will reduce viral fitness; secondly, potentially useful mutations may have no immediate value and could only become valuable if appropriate selection pressures were applied, and finally valuable

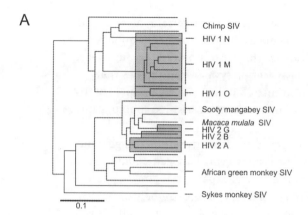

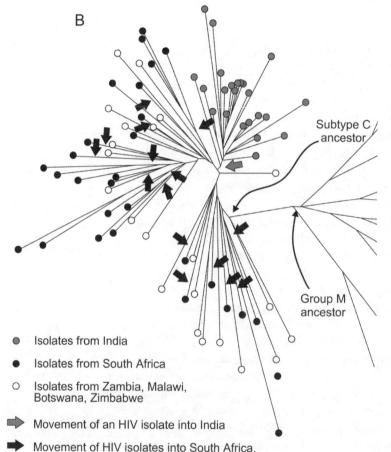

FIGURE 7.2 HIV diversity
A: Primate lentivirus diversity illustrated by an UPGMA dendrogram constructed from the full genome sequences of a virus representing the major HIV and SIV lineages. The six evolutionarily distinct groups of sequences isolated from humans are shaded

B: An expanded view of group M HIV diversity indicating the subtype and circular recombinant form (CRF) groupings. Also represented are unclassified sequences (US) and unclassified unique recombinant sequences (UUR). Horizontal distances indicate degrees of nucleotide sequence divergence (see scale bars) and vertical distances are arbitrary.

- Isolates from India
- Isolates from South Africa
- Isolates from Zambia, Malawi, Botswana, Zimbabwe
- Movement of an HIV isolate into India
- Movement of HIV isolates into South Africa.

Subtype C

Other group M subtypes

mutations may occur in genomes which contain other mutations that are harmful.

HIV can use recombination (FIGURE 7.3B) to overcome potentially harmful combinations of mutations. Recombination provides the virus with a very powerful mechanism whereby beneficial mutations can be uncoupled from harmful mutations. Recombination occurs during replication where the reverse transcriptase enzyme frequently switches between any HIV RNAs that are in close proximity. The resulting proviral DNAs that are generated, and eventually integrated, will almost invariably be recombinant. Recombination is so rife that it is believed that at least half of observable genomic diversity within an infected individual is generated through recombinational reassortment of mutationally derived diversity. The two features of HIV's molecular biology that encourage recombinational rearrangement of mutations are (1) the packaging of two separate genomes into every virion and (2) the infection of individual cells with more than one virion.

A Mechanisms of Diversification 1: Mutations introduced due to error-prone viral enzyme reverse transcriptase. Mutations introduced during replication. Reverse transcriptase introduces approximately one error for every 2 000 nucleotides. The viral RNA is approximately 10 000 nucleotides in length so approximately five errors are introduced every time the virus replicates

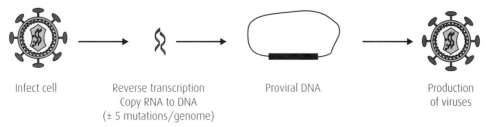

| Infect cell | Reverse transcription Copy RNA to DNA (± 5 mutations/genome) | Proviral DNA | Production of viruses |

B Mechanisms of Diversification 2: Generation of recombinant viruses occurs when two viruses enter the same cell resulting in the co-packaging of RNA of different origins. During reverse transcription of these RNAs the enzyme switches between RNA strands generating a proviral genome comprising of parts from the two viruses (so called mosiac or recombinant genomes)

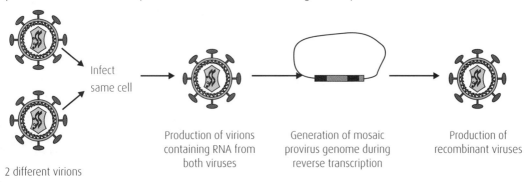

Infect same cell

2 different virions

| | Production of virions containing RNA from both viruses | Generation of mosaic provirus genome during reverse transcription | Production of recombinant viruses |

FIGURE 7.3

The Origin of HIV

In an attempt to discover the origin of HIV, samples have been collected from a number of primate species. Sequence comparisons between different HIV and SIV sequences indicate that an ancestral group M HIV was probably transmitted to a human from a chimpanzee (FIGURE 7.2A). Using the most reliable estimates of sequence evolution rate and extrapolating current diversity estimates backwards in time, it has been estimated that this interspecies transmission event occurred at some time in the 1930s. The chimpanzee SIV isolates most closely related to Group M HIVs have all been obtained from Equatorial West Africa and this is probably the region where a human first became infected with an ancestral HIV.

It is worth noting that the other five major HIV groupings (HIV-1 groups N and O and HIV-2 groups A, B and G; (FIGURE 7.2A), have all apparently evolved from different SIVs independently transmitted into humans. It would be careless to suppose that the global spread of group M HIVs was an exceptional event, and unlikely to be repeated. The continual transmission of SIVs into humans and the potential emergence of new HIV epidemics should be considered a serious global health threat.

Subtype distribution in Africa

The region with the greatest assemblage of HIV subtypes, circulating recombinant forms, and unique recombinants of any other region in the world is Equatorial West Africa/Central Africa (TABLE 7.1). This is not surprising as evidence points to this region being the origin of the epidemic and thus the virus would have been circulating and evolving within the human population there longer than anywhere else. This rampant and potentially uncontrollable proliferation of HIV diversification is worrying as there is the potential for new and more pathogenic HIV variants to emerge from the region.

In other regions of Africa, certain subtypes have dominated. Subtype C dominates in southern Africa and Ethiopia but is less prevalent in East Africa. The AG recombinant (CRF02) is dominant in many countries in West and Central Africa. Subtype A is common to East and West Africa whereas Subtype D is dominant in certain regions of East Africa. The associations of certain subtypes with specific regions of Africa are becoming less clearly defined over time. This is in part due to migration. In addition, an increasing number of recombinant viruses are being detected, especially in regions with genetically diverse epidemics.

South Africa has an overwhelmingly dominant subtype C epidemic with over 95% of viruses classified as subtype C. Minor subtypes present include subtype A, B, D, G and recombinant viruses.

Region	Country sampled	Dominant subtype(s) or CRF(s)	Diversity
Southern Africa	South Africa, Zimbabwe, Malawi, Botswana	C	Low
East Africa	Kenya, Uganda, Tanzania	A, D, C, recombinants	Medium
West Africa	Benin, Burkina Faso, Ivory Coast, Ghana, Gambia, Senegal, Guinea-Bissau, Guinea, Mali, Mauritania, Sierra Leone	A, AG	Medium
Equatorial West Africa/Central Africa	Democratic Republic of Congo, Cameroon, Equatorial Guinea	A, D, G, F, H, AE, H, AG, unclassified	High

TABLE 7.1 Distribution of HIV subtypes in Africa

Tracking the spread of HIV to South Africa

There have been two patterns of infection in South Africa on two different time scales. The first cases of AIDS in South Africa were diagnosed in men infected through homosexual contact in the early 1980s. At this time HIV was largely absent in the general population as demonstrated by several large surveys screening for HIV antibodies in miners, sex workers, outpatients and rural communities. A second epidemic driven by heterosexual transmission only became evident in South Africa in the late 1980s and early 1990s.

It is possible to use sequence diversity to track HIV transmission and spread. Molecular epidemiology studies have shown that the first epidemic in South Africa in homosexual men was associated with subtype B. This subtype is rarely found in Africa but is common in North America and Europe. This would imply that HIV first entered South Africa from another continent. In contrast, the second epidemic in the heterosexual population was associated with subtype C. This subtype is dominant in southern Africa and it is therefore likely that the second epidemic originated from regional spread from other countries in Africa and was not a consequence of the first epidemic.

The explosive epidemic in South Africa in the early 1990s was in fact a result of multiple introductions of HIV into the country. This can be illustrated by analysing the phylogenetic relationship between viruses. Explosive epidemics associated with single introductions and rapid spread of HIV (clonal epidemics) such as India, harbour viruses that are closely related and cluster together in phylogenetic trees (FIGURE 7.2B). However, viruses from South Africa show the opposite pattern with no major groupings. In fact, South African viruses are interspersed among sequences from Zambia, Malawi, Botswana and Zimbabwe (FIGURE 7.2B).

Implications of the extreme diversity of HIV

Both the epidemiological and treatment implications of high HIV diversity are as yet unclear. For example, while some evidence exists that progression to AIDS occurs more quickly with certain subtypes than it does with others, no convincing evidence has yet been obtained to prove that one subtype is significantly more virulent than another.

HIV diversity and its potential impact on vaccine efficacy has been a central focus of worldwide efforts to produce HIV vaccines. Consequently all HIV vaccines under development are only being designed to target individual group M subtypes. These subtype-specific vaccines aim to induce strong immune responses directed at conserved HIV proteins, conserved immunogenic epitopes within these proteins or predicted ancestral and consensus sequences that are more closely related to the proteins of circulating viruses than the circulating viral proteins are with one another. These vaccine projects derive hope from the fact that, despite the incredible rate at which HIV sequences can evolve, it is apparent that there are regions of the genome where sequences are quite significantly conserved. It is believed that many of these sequences are under strong selection constraints and cannot change too significantly without compromising their functionality.

There is also some concern, however, that many conserved sequences may simply be poor immune targets that have not been pressured by immune systems to change and that these sequences may therefore make poor vaccine targets. HIV proteins targeted by antiretroviral drugs are all encoded in the more conserved regions of the HIV genome. However, a range of drug resistance mutations have been observed for every widely used antiretroviral drug indicating that, given enough motivation, HIV will undergo and survive substantial mutational modification of its most conserved genes.

The question of how much viral diversity can be controlled by an effective HIV vaccine has, quite appropriately, become something of an obsession among researchers hoping to develop such vaccines. Rather sobering results from animal studies have suggested that even a perfect match between vaccine strain and virus is not sufficient to guarantee vaccine success. In a well-documented case study of a rhesus monkey inoculated with a multiple CTL epitope vaccine derived from the same virus strain it was subsequently challenged with, mutant viruses arose within 20 weeks post-challenge that were capable of escaping a potent vaccine-induced CTL response. This study has two very worrying implications. The first is that even the relatively small amount of viral diversification that occurs during the short time lag between infection and clearance by an optimal immune response may be sufficient to produce escape mutants. The second is that if, as is the likely situation with all HIV vaccines under development, vaccine-induced immunity is not sterilising and a virus can continue replicating at very low levels, it is probable that eventually enough diversity will be generated for escape mutants to emerge.

The range of subtypes and the amount of intrasubtype diversity within any geographical region will have a significant impact on the vaccine and drug management of HIV in that region. It is unlikely that reasonably effective subtype-specific HIV vaccines will provide full protection against all possible variants within the subtypes they are targeting, and it is almost certain that they will not fully protect against subtypes they are not targeting. Consequently, diversity and vaccine efficacy variables have been factored into models predicting the effectiveness of future HIV vaccination and drug administration programmes. These models suggest that, in the short term at least, a vaccine with low efficacy would still be better than no vaccine at all and that antiretroviral treatment of even a small proportion of infected individuals could have a large positive impact on the course of the epidemic. What no model can predict, however, is how global HIV population diversity will respond when confronted with partially protective vaccines and drug therapies that are incapable of decisively curing people.

It still remains to be seen whether the global HIV population can be controlled at its present diversity level. Given the extraordinary evolutionary potential that HIV has displayed in the past 70 years, it will be an enormous challenge to maintain whatever control over HIV we do achieve during the inevitable future diversification of the virus.

Bibliography

BAROUCH DH, KUNSTMAN J, KURODA MJ, SCHMITZ JE, SANTRA S, PEYERL FW, KRIVULKA GR, BEAUDRY K, LIFTON MA, GORGONE DA, MONTEFIORI DC, LEWIS MG, WOLINSKY SM, LETVIN NL. 'Eventual AIDS vaccine failure in a rhesus monkey by viral escape from cytotoxic T lymphocytes'. *Nature* 2002; 415: 335–339.

GAO F, BAILES E, ROBERTSON DL, CHEN Y, RODENBURG CM, MICHAEL SF, CUMMINS LB, ARTHUR LO, PEETERS M, SHAW GM, SHARP PM, HAHN BH. 'Origin of HIV-1 in the chimpanzee *Pan troglodytes troglodytes*'. *Nature* 1999; 397: 436–441.

GASCHEN B, TAYLOR J, YUSIM K, FOLEY B, GAO F, LANG D, NOVITSKY V, HAYNES B, HAHN BH, BHATTACHARYA T, KORBER B. 'Diversity considerations in HIV-1 vaccine selection'. *Science* 2002; 296: 2354–2360.

GRAY RH, LI X, WAWER MJ, GANGE SJ, SERWADDA D, SEWANKAMBO NK, MOORE R, WABWIRE-MANGEN F, LUTALO T, QUINN TC. 'Stochastic simulation of the impact of antiretroviral therapy and HIV vaccines on HIV transmission; Rakai, Uganda'. *AIDS* 2003; 17: 1941–1951.

MCCUTCHAN FE. 'Understanding the genetic diversity of HIV-1'. *AIDS* 2000; 14: S31–S44.

PAPATHANASOPOULOS MA, HUNT GM, TIEMESSEN CT. 'Evolution and Diversity of HIV-1 in Africa – a Review'. *Virus Genes* 2003; 26: 151–163.

THOMSON MM, PEREZ-ALVAREZ L, NAJERA R. 'Molecular epidemiology of HIV-1 genetic forms and its significance for vaccine development and therapy'. *Lancet Infectious Diseases* 2002; 2: 461–471.

VAN HARMELEN J, WOOD R, LAMBRICK M, RYBICKI EP, WILLIAMSON AL, WILLIAMSON C. 'An association between HIV-1 subtypes and mode of transmission in Cape Town, South Africa'. *AIDS* 1997; 11: 81–87.

WEI X, DECKER JM, WANG S, HUI H, KAPPES JC, WU X, SALAZAR-GONZALEZ JF, SALAZAR MG, KILBY JM, SAAG MS, KOMAROVA NL, NOWAK MA, HAHN BH, KWONG PD, SHAW GM. 'Antibody neutralization and escape by HIV-1'. *Nature* 2003; 422: 307–312.

YANG OO, SARKIS PT, ALI A, HARLOW JD, BRANDER C, KALAMS SA, WALKER BD. 'Determinant of HIV-1 mutational escape from cytotoxic T lymphocytes'. *The Journal of Experimental Medicine* 2003; 197: 1365–1375.

CHAPTER 8

Cellular immunity in HIV: A synthesis of responses to preserve self

Clive Gray

IN THIS CHAPTER salient points are brought into focus concerning general immunity and immunity to HIV-1 infection. An effective and efficient immune response develops to preserve self from non-self and a discriminating recognition process has evolved to ensure this. HIV-1 has successfully undermined the discriminating process and leaves the infected host open to many diseases where there is no longer an ability to preserve self. However, some HIV-1 infected individuals do not progress to AIDS and others appear to be resistant to infection. These individuals are thought to mount highly effective immune responses that provide some form of protection. The objective of many research efforts has been and will be to determine what type of immunity these individuals develop.

There are already some clues that certain HLA backgrounds are important and that strong T-cell immunity develops in people who progress slowly. Additionally, it is thought that events in the first few months of HIV-1 infection are crucial to emulate with a vaccine – as it is the T-cell responses to recently transmitted viruses that are the most effective at controlling viral replication. It is likely that the most important point at which pathogenesis takes hold and there is a 'point of no return', is when HIV-1 seeds to the lymphoid depots and begins to precipitate lymphoid structure degeneration. At this point, drug intervention is the only mechanism that would allow the immune system to restore, as drug-induced viral suppression would allow lymphoid structures to regenerate.

The nature of preventive vaccines will need to steer T-cell immunity in healthy individuals to recognise a series of epitopes that will prevent HIV replication from taking hold. The challenge will be to elicit these responses and to maintain the magnitude of response with effective priming and boosting using a mixture of effective immunogens and adjuvants. The nature of therapeutic vaccines will probably entail drug-mediated suppression of actively replicating virus, whilst allowing vaccine-elicited immunity to re-direct immunity away from immunodominance.

An introduction to the general principles underlying the immune response is provided in Part I and Part II and the chapter then proceeds to describe immune responses activated specifically in response to HIV infection. Parts 3 and 4 describe the implications of the immune response in relation to natural protection observed in a cohort of sex workers and the implications of this natural protection to vaccine development.

Part I: The immune response

The human body is constantly bombarded by infectious agents such as viruses, bacteria, protozoa and non-infectious agents such as dust, pollen and pollution. These enter the body through numerous portals. The first barrier is skin and the epithelial lining of the airways, gut and mucosal areas. Any break or loss of integrity in these physical protective barriers would allow introduction of foreign material into the internal world of the body.

The bulk of infectious agents that breaks through into the internal body are dealt with swiftly by the **innate immune response**. Innate immunity is the protection offered by specialised cells that engulf whole particles or release toxic substances that may kill offending pathogens. This line of defence is a primitive form of the immune response and has parallels with defence mechanisms in lower vertebrates. Organisms that survive the innate immune response are dealt with by the more specific **acquired immune response**. Acquired immunity has three central principles:

- specificity – recognition of fine detail via the interaction of receptors and ligands
- tolerance – where fine detail is not recognised by the immune system
- memory – where there is an unforgettable imprint of fine detail and this recognition can be recalled at a later stage.

The central function of the immune system is to protect the host from invading pathogens and preserve the integrity of the internal body. The internal world is known immunologically as 'self' and potential infectious agents that could be recognised by the immune system from the external world are known as 'non-self'. The central paradigm of immunity is recognition of non-self and the preservation of self.

Specialised lymphoid tissues of the immune system serve as primary and secondary depots of cells involved in the immune response. Cells of the immune system migrate from lymphoid tissue to the blood and lymph circulation and back to lymphoid tissue. Bone marrow is the primary lymphoid organ, where the precursors to all mature immunocompetent cells are derived as pluripotential progenitor cells.

T-cells develop into mature immunocompetent cells in the thymus. The thymus gland is very active in newborns and is responsible for the selection of T-cells in the body that can provide protection during life. The T-cells that leave the thymus are 'naïve' cells and have yet to encounter invading pathogens. During life, the thymus gland becomes smaller and atrophies and until recently it was thought that it became inactive during the third decade. However recent evidence has shown that the thymus is probably active throughout life.

The lymph nodes serve as platforms for the initiation of immune responses and are structurally arranged into discrete anatomical compartments of tissue and cells. Cells arrive in the lymph node from the peripheral circulation through the afferent blood vessels where B-cells develop and encounter antigens within the germinal centres, while T-cells encounter them in the paracortical region. The microenvironment of the lymph node allows B- and T-cells to encounter either whole 'or pieces' of invading pathogens, ensuring that immune response can occur. Any disruption to the architecture of the lymphoid tissue would affect the way in which B- and T-cells can be primed to new invading pathogens.

Cells of the immune system

Immune cells are in constant dynamic movement from one lymphoid region to another with cell migration taking place through the blood stream as well as the lymphatic system.

FIGURE 8.1 shows the relationship between the blood circulation, lymphatic circulation, lymph nodes and the initiation of the immune response. Here, naïve T-cells will circulate through the afferent vessel into the lymph nodes, where both CD4+ and CD8+ T-cells encounter antigen in the paracortical region of the lymph node. CD8+ T-cells, for example, will engage with antigen via the TCR and MHC-epitope complex and clonally expand. The resulting effector CD8+ T-cells leave via the efferent vessel and are able to migrate to peripheral non-lymphoid tissue and eliminate invading pathogens. Most of the effector cells will die through apoptosis, leaving a small residual of memory CD8+ T-cells that recirculate through the lymphatic and

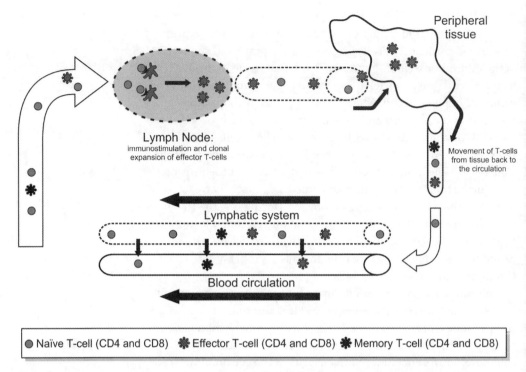

FIGURE 8.1 The relationship between the blood circulation, lymphatic circulation, lymph nodes and the initiation of a T-cell response. The arrows depict constant movement of naïve, effector and memory T-cells from the blood circulation to the lymphatic circulation and into the lymph nodes. Antigen-primed effector T-cells migrate within the circulation to areas of peripheral tissue damage (for example) where they are responsible for removing invading pathogen from these sites. In the case of HIV-1 infection, effector T-cells will migrate to areas of HIV-1 infection. Clonal expansion of T-cells occurs within the lymph nodes at the early stage of the immune response and is responsible for the clinical symptoms of lymphadenopathy during acute HIV-1 infection

blood circulation. The system should be viewed as closed, with many rounds of circulation through lymphoid and non-lymphoid tissue.

The lymphatic vessel system runs parallel to blood vessels and ensures that cells of the immune system are able to migrate from non-lymphoid tissues to lymphoid depots, allowing communication between portals where pathogens may enter the immune system.

One of the most important immune cell types is the dendritic cell (DC). These cells are known as 'nature's adjuvant', and are able to prime the immune system to new infections. Without the ability to prime T-cells to respond to invading antigens, the host is at risk of becoming immunocompromised and losing the ability to respond to infections. Dendritic cells are found not only in lymphoid tissues, but also in non-lymphoid tissues, such as the lungs, brain and skin. Here they function by engulfing invading pathogens; they present pieces of protein (antigen – see below) on the surface of the cell and migrate

from non-lymphoid areas of the body to lymphoid depots – such as
the lymph nodes. This process can be thought of as a 'kick-start' to get
the immune system going. FIGURE 8.2 shows the relationship between
DC priming and clonal expansion of T-cells. In this example, CD8+
T-cells clonally expand upon immunostimulation by DC to a specific
epitope, derived from an infectious agent.

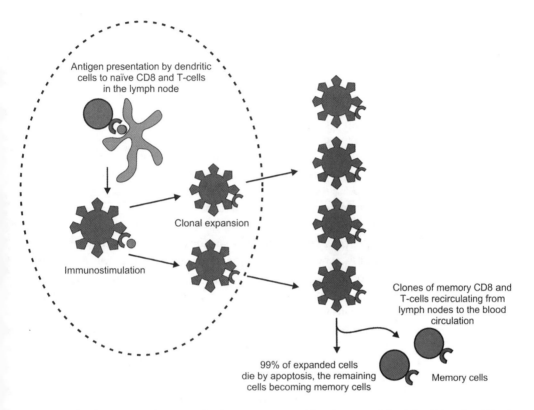

FIGURE 8.2 Clonal expansion of CD8+ T-cells after engagement with antigen. Specialised dendritic cells within the
lymph node (these cells are known as interdigitating cells) provide presentation of processed antigen to naïve
CD8+ T-cells in the paracortical region. The resulting immunostimulation of CD8+ T-cells is followed by clonal
expansion after the CD8+ T-cell re-encounters antigen. The clonal expansion of CD8+ T-cells result in clones of
effector CD8+ T-cells that leave the lymph node via the efferent vessel. The hallmark of the CD8+ T-cell clones is
that they express identical T-cell receptors and will consequently interact with the same epitope presented by
HLA molecules

T-cells all express CD3 on the surface along with the T-cell receptor
(TCR). Subsets of CD3+ T-cells express CD4, and in humans these are
the major T-cell subset. CD4+ T-cells are involved with coordinating
and helping the immune response to proceed smoothly, and are
hence also known as T-helper cells. FIGURE 8.3 shows the relationship
between CD4+ T-cells and the immune system.

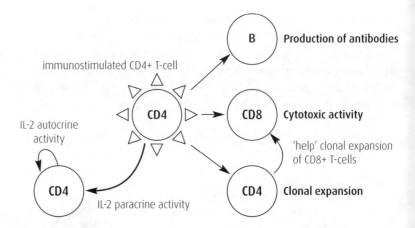

FIGURE 8.3 The CD4+ T-cell plays a central role in 'conducting' the immune orchestra. Through the liberation of cytokines, such as IL-2, the CD4 cell facilitates clonal expansion of other CD4+ T-cells and CD8+ T-cells. CD4+ T-cells also facilitate development of B cells and the production of antibodies. Depletion and disabling of CD4+ T-cells in HIV-1 infection results in removal of the 'conductor' and is one of the main reasons for precipitating an immunocompromised state

T-helper cells can be thought of as the conductors of the immune orchestra, where they coordinate the immune response as a movement of cells with different functions leading to removal of foreign pathogens. Thus, any disease or infection that impedes or destroys CD4+ T-cells will cause the immune system to lose order and enter chaos and eventually degenerate. In healthy humans, CD8+ T-cells make up the smaller proportion of CD3+ T-cells and are involved in protecting the host from invading pathogens. These cells are also known as cytotoxic T-lymphocytes (CTL) and function by killing cells marked with foreign pathogen. It is generally thought that CTL can only function with the help of CD4+ T-helper cells, but there are some reports which show that CD8+ T-cells can function independently of CD4+ T-cells. The killing potential of CD8+ T-cells is effected through perforin: on contact with the target cells, CD8+ T-cells release perforin which punches holes into the target cell – leading to cell death and removal from the circulation. Another mechanism used for CD8+ T-cell killing potential is the Fas-FasL (ligand) interaction.

Cytokines and Th1- and Th2-profiles

CD4+ T-cells communicate with other cell types, for example with B-cells and CD8+ T-cells, through cell contact and liberation of cytokines. There are a host of different cytokines with discrete functions, some that facilitate the switching on of immunity and others that help switch off immune responses. First identified in mouse models, different cytokines can be placed into a network model of a Th1-type and Th2-type system. A Th1-type response consists of CD4+ T-cells liberating a profile of cytokines that direct T-cell immunity and involve, for example, IL-1, IL-2, IL-6, IL-12, IL-15, TNFa and IFNg. A Th-2 type response consists of CD4+ T-cells liberating a profile of cytokines that direct humoral immuninty and are involved in switching on B cell immunity. These cytokines include IL-4, IL-5, IL-10 for example. FIGURE 8.4 shows the Th1 and Th2 model and how IL-12 and IL-4 steer immunity to cellular or humoral immunity. In humans, the model is not as clear cut – although elements of the model are useful in interpreting immunity and deciding how to measure immune responses to different pathogens.

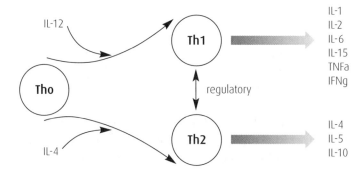

FIGURE 8.4 Multiple cytokines are liberated by many different cell types of the immune system. For CD4+ T-cells, many of the cytokines that have been identified can be placed into a Th1/Th2 model. It is postulated that precursor Th0 cells have the ability to secrete all cytokines and are naïve (ie they have not encountered antigen). Upon encounter with different types of pathogen, either IL-12 or IL-4 will facilitate steering towards a Th1 or Th2 cytokine phenotype. A Th1 type CD4+ T-cell will liberate cytokines promoting cellular immunity and a cytolytic CD8+ T-cell response. A Th2 type CD4+ T-cell will liberate cytokines promoting more of an antibody response. There is likely to be a balance between Th1/Th2 cytokines in an immune response and it has been reported that during HIV-1 disease progression, Th2 type responses predominate which accounts for loss of cellular immunity and progression of disease to AIDS

Antigens, epitopes and antigen presentation

The crucial feature of the immune system in the successful clearance of invading pathogen is specificity. In this context specifity means that T-cells can recognise short linear protein fragments of the invading pathogen. The regions recognised are known as antigens and the short linear fragments within the antigen, usually consisting of 8–18 amino-acids are known as epitopes. Thus, the T-cell receptor

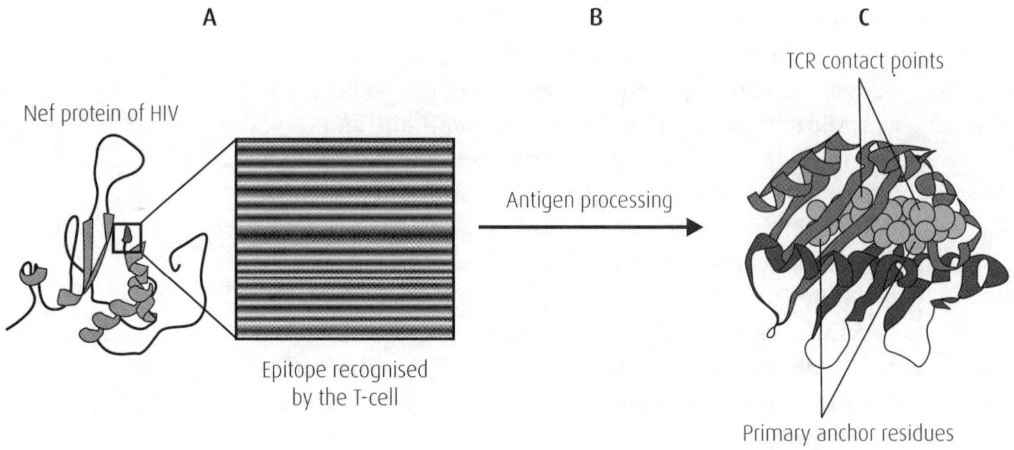

A B C

FIGURE 8.5 One of the hallmarks of immunity is specificity, where this is represented as recognition of 8-16 amino-acid length epitopes by the T-cell receptor. 8.5A shows an example of an epitope embedded within the Nef protein of subtype C HIV-1 (yellow represents the epitope). After antigen processing (B), the epitope is bound in the groove of the HLA (C). The ends of the epitope are bound in the peptide groove and the mid region of the epitope contain amino-acids which serve as contact residues for the T-cell receptor

(TCR) expressed on the surface of the T-cell can recognise a series of epitopes derived from antigens, which in turn, are derived from the invading pathogen. The epitopes recognised by TCRs are invariably derived from regions embedded within the secondary and tertiary protein structure. For the epitopes to be exposed and presented to the TCR, proteins from the pathogen are first degraded and broken down. This process is known as antigen processing and presentation. FIGURE 8.5 shows an epitope found in the HIV Nef protein. It is nine amino-acids in length and the fine nature of TCR recognition of this epitope defines immune specificity. The epitope is presented in the groove of an MHC class I molecule (FIGURE 8.5C), allowing the TCR to recognise the part of the invading pathogen, via the TCR-peptide-MHC interaction (FIGURE 8.6).

Specialised cells, such as dendritic cells and macrophages, have the ability to process antigens. A simple scenario would be that invading pathogens, such as bacteria, are engulfed by phagocytic cells and digested by lysosomal and proteosomal enzymes. The degraded proteins are processed to become epitopes within the cytosol of the cell and presented on the surface of the cell by class II MHC molecules. In the case of viral infections, endogenously processed epitopes, derived from the transcription of viral genes, are presented on the surface of the cell by class I MHC molecules. It is also possible that when virally infected cells die, the effete cells are engulfed by dendritic cells and virally derived epitopes are presented by class II MHC molecules. This is known as cross-presentation. FIGURE 8.6 shows a cartoon of epitope presentation and recognition by the TCR from a CD8+ T-cell.

CD4+ T-cells possess a set of TCRs that recognise epitopes presented by class II MHC. CD8+ T-cells possess a set of TCRs that recognise epitopes presented by class I MHC. These T-cells can only become functional when the TCR engages with the epitope presented by the MHC. The specific nature of immunity lies in the ability of one T-cell to express a TCR that can bind to one epitope. TCR-epitope interactions lead to expansion of T-cells (see clonal expansion) leading to multiple clones, or copies, of T-cells expressing the same TCR.

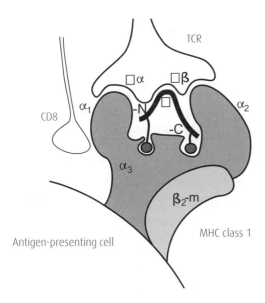

FIGURE 8.6 A side view of an epitope bound to the MHC (HLA), where the ends of the epitope are anchored to the floor of the MHC molecule. The T-cell receptor (TCR) is shown to make a snug fit making contact with the sides of the MHC molecule and the kinked region of the mid-part of the bound epitope. Upon engagement of the TCR and epitope bound in the MHC groove, the CD8+ T-cell becomes activated

The T-cell receptor

The structure of the TCR on the surface of the CD4+ or CD8+ T-cell allows it to engage with regions of the epitope presented by the MHC molecule on the surface of the antigen-presenting cell. The structure of the TCR belongs to the superimmunoglobulin class and the variable portion of the receptor resembles an immunoglobulin structure. As will be discussed below, there is a series of events that enables T-cells to clonally expand directed to specific epitopes. During the early stages of an immune response, numerous T-cells will engage with epitopes via a selection of TCRs and the receptor that has the highest avidity to an epitope will be selected for expansion into a single population of T-cells expressing the TCR that has the 'best fit'. Clonality of T-cells can be measured by assessing the length of the complementary determining region 3 (CDR3) gene that will indicate which V beta structure is expressed that constitutes the TCR.

Major histocompatibility complex (MHC)

The MHC is a set of genes that code for proteins that direct T-cell immunity. As discussed in the previous section, two important classes of MHC are involved in T-cell recognition of epitopes – class I and class II.

The MHC in humans is known as the human leukocyte antigen (HLA) system and is one of the most polymorphic proteins in the human population. The uniqueness of individuals is partly defined by HLA, where each person has a defined HLA type consisting of pairs of inherited genes. The HLA system was originally known as transplantation antigens, as transplantation of organs between two HLA incompatible individuals resulted in rejection of the transplanted tissue. Identical twins have 100% HLA compatibility and it was found originally in monozygotic cattle that no rejection of transplanted tissue took place.

Certain HLA types have been associated with various diseases, such as rheumatoid arthritis, spondalysing ankylosis, type I diabetes and other such auto-immune diseases. As the sole function of class I and II HLA is to present epitopes to circulating T-cells, possible aberrant T-cell function and recognition of self, as in autoimmunity, will thus involve the HLA. Likewise, certain HLA types are involved with doing well or badly after being infected with HIV-1. This will be explored in more detail in Part II.

FIGURE 8.6 shows how epitopes are bound in the HLA groove. There are certain rules that govern how epitopes are bound and hence presented by the HLA, where class I molecules bind epitopes ranging from eight to 11 amino-acids in length. Class II HLA can bind epitopes that are longer, 12 to 18 amino-acids, and are not constrained by the tight space of the binding groove found in class I HLA molecules.

The amino-acid residues found within the middle of the epitope are orientated toward the TCR and certain amino-acids are contact residues with the TCR. For full recognition of the epitope, restricted by a particular HLA molecule, the TCR recognises the contact residues of the epitope as well as parts of the alpha 1 and 2 helices of the MHC (FIGURE 8.6).

The T-cell response and clonal expansion

So far, this chapter has discussed cells of the immune system, antigens and epitopes, presentation of epitopes and recognition of epitopes through the TCR-MHC interaction. This section will attempt to synthesise these events into the physiological process of an ongoing immune response.

After engaging and processing antigen in the peripheral tissue, DCs will migrate to the secondary lymphoid depots, such as the lymph nodes. Within the microenvironment of the lymph node, DC will present antigen to naïve CD4+ and CD8+ T-cells and provide a situation of immunostimulation – priming and cell activation. Selection of T-cells via TCR engagement with epitopes presented either by class I (CD8+ T-cells) or class II (CD4+ T-cells) HLA will occur. Selected T-cells will expand in a clonal manner into effector T-cells, and clones of effector T-cells will express TCRs that will recognise epitopes originally presented to naïve T-cells by DC in the lymph node. Typically during an immune response, there is a polyclonal T-cell response; where there is a mixture of T-cells expressing TCRs capable of recognising multiple epitopes. If there is a situation where there is persistence of antigen, there may be skewing of the T-cell response to a set of TCRs recognising a limited number of epitopes, producing an oligoclonal response.

The role of clonally expanded CD4+ and CD8+ effector cells is ultimately to remove invading antigen from the host and allow 'self' to survive. Approximately 99% of effector clones die from apoptosis and the remaining 1% become quiescent memory T-cells, capable of responding to re-exposure to antigen and mounting a more rapid secondary response. FIGURE 8.2 depicts the series of events leading to clonally expanded CD8+ T-cells that can interact with an epitope on infected cells.

Part II: What happens to the immune system during HIV-1 infection

This section will focus on specific T-cell immunity and HIV infection. It is known that HIV infects CD4+ T-cells and causes immunosuppression in the host, often measured as a depressed CD4 count, which in turn is proportional to the level of immunopathology caused by HIV infection. For this reason CD4 counts are used clinically as a measure of disease prognosis, effectiveness of antiretroviral therapy and disease staging for provision of therapy. However, there are many events that build up to CD4 depression and, in a sense, such a measurement is a gross representation of immune degradation caused by HIV infection. This section will deal with the battle between the immune response and HIV replication and persistence, which ultimately leads to the collapse of the immune system.

HIV-1 infects cells bearing CD4 and chemokine co-receptors, but also monopolises lymphoid structures and the anatomical platform required to mount effective immunity. After initial transmission of HIV-1, the virus 'seeds' to the lymphoid depots which coincides with a fall in plasma viral copies. The transient rise and fall in viraemia also coincides with very active immunity and specifically CD8+ T-cells imparting cytotoxic T-lymphocyte (CTL) activity.

Within the lymphoid depots, HIV-1 resides within the germinal centres of the lymph nodes, spleen, tonsils and thymus and exists, in the main, as whole virus on the surface of follicular dendritic cells (FDC) in the lymph node. As a result, the normal function of FDC in presenting antigen is thought to be overriden. How does HIV-1 get to the lymph nodes, bearing in mind that the most frequent entry point of virus into an infected host is through mucosal surfaces around the cervix and rectum? Viral transmission is thought to be cell-associated (ie free virus is not passed from one person to another) and there is probably cell contact between the dendritic cells from the newly infected recipient with cells harbouring HIV-1. This interaction probably takes place in lymphoid structures in close proximity to the cervix and rectum, and dendritic cells from the newly infected individual migrate from the cervical region to lymph nodes elsewhere in the body. Virus has been shown to be carried on dendritic cells by DC-SIGN to lymph nodes distal to the point of viral transmission. Once HIV-1 resides in the lymph nodes, an explosion of immune activity occurs which initially may partially control viral replication, but in the majority of individuals immunity eventually collapses leading to AIDS. This process may take from two to ten years and the length of the process underlies how successful immunity can be in the early stage of infection.

A closer look at the T-cell response to HIV-1 infection

During the initial burst of immunity to HIV-1 infection, CD8+ CTL are thought to play an important role in the initial containment of viral replication. The important role that CD8+ CTL and CD4+ T-helper responses might play in providing protection is emphasised by their role in long-term non-progressors (no disease progression) and CTL-presence in highly exposed persistently seronegative individuals (HEPS).

CD8+ CTL are cells that recognise class I HLA restricted epitopes and are thought to play a crucial role in slowing HIV replication and protecting HIV-infected individuals from disease progression. The emergence of these cells during HIV infection is rapid, and within hours they are active within the body. CD8+ CTL activity has been shown to be very effective in controlling viral infections in mouse models, such as with lymphocyte chorionic myelitis virus (LCMV) and in humans, such as EBV. Experiments in monkeys have shown that when CD8+ T-cells are depleted from the periphery, these animals cannot control SIV infection: direct evidence that CD8+ T-cells are involved in viral containment.

In HIV infection, associations between certain class I HLA alleles and rapidity or slowness of disease progression implicate the role of CD8+ CTL. CD8+ CTL are implicated in controlling the initial burst of viraemia; individuals who rapidly progress to AIDS do not control HIV replication and have possibly never mounted protective immune responses. It may be argued that effective CTL and T-helper cell responses elicited at the primary stage of infection are important for determining whether viral burden is to be controlled. Failure to mount sustained CTL and T-helper responses from the early stage of infection may be due to an inability to develop immunodominant CTL responses or because responses may be targeting variable protein regions precipitating HIV-1 escape. In this situation, there would be uncontrolled viral replication and a higher probability of disease progression.

Establishing persistence – antigen overload

One of the hallmarks of HIV infection is that it establishes persistent infection in the individual. This leads to profound immunological imbalances as the infected host attempts to control virus and eliminate antigen. Persistence of HIV antigens leads to continued T-cell activation into a hyperactivated state. It is quite possible that the immune degradation observed during HIV disease progression is the result of the hyperactivated state of the immune system, which is maintained by persistent viraemia. Immune-mediated pathology is not unique to other viral infections; this has been observed with respiratory syncitial virus infection.

How does HIV escape immunity?

Despite persistent infection, and the inability of the immune response to clear infection, specific T-cell immunity has been correlated with mutations occurring in epitopes. This is partly a measure of the strength of immune pressure and a collection of viral escape mutations in the virus is thought, in part, to shape viral diversity.

Immune-driven viral diversity

Viral escape from CTL pressure has been demonstrated in murine responses to LCMV, SIV-infected and SHIV-challenged macaques and in HIV-1 infection. Accumulation of CTL epitope variants has been associated with increased viral load and pathogenesis in HIV leading to death in macaques. Following transmission, the virus replicates exponentially prior to control of replication, presumably due to CTL responses. Studies in macaques have shown that CTL pressure is one of the major forces driving sequence change in acute infections. In this study they found that the *tat* gene was the first region to evolve, and was the only region associated with escape from CTL responses. A number of other human studies have shown that CTL epitopes change in relation to CTL responses and can occur early or late in infection. It is thus intriguing to speculate that HIV-1 diversity is a result of selective pressures exerted by host immunity, which in turn is directed by the HLA background of a given population. Continuous selective pressures are exerted on HIV-1 as one infected person transmits the product of immune selected virus to the next person, who in turn exerts immune pressure. In this manner, continued viral diversity is transmitted through the population, where the host genes and immune responses 'imprint' continued viral diversity.

HIV establishes immunodominance

There are several regions of the HIV-1 genome that are highly conserved. For example, the central region of the *Nef* protein tends to be invariant between clades of HIV-1 and between infected individuals. Areas of high protein conservation tend to equate with important functional regions for the virus and contain domains encoding critical proteins, such as enzymes. As HIV-1 infection results in persistent viral replication, and is not cleared by the host, there is a continuous abundance of virally-derived proteins expressed in lymphoid depots and on the surface of antigen processing cells (APC). This results in chronic T-cell activation leading to a focus of specific T-cell immunity on selected epitopes presented within the individual. This in turn results in immunodominance, where within individuals there is a high frequency of HIV-1 specific T-cells recognising one epitope, which dominates all other responses. It is not clear whether immunodominance is good or bad for the infected individual. It may be bad from the perspective that immunity is focused on a series of epitopes that precludes the immune response from 'seeing' other regions of the expressed genome. However, as these epitopes usually lie within highly conserved domains of the viral genome, there is a low probability of escape from the immune response.

There are several decoy mechanisms that HIV-1 employs to 'out-wit' host immunity. These include mutations leading to epitope escape (discussed above), down-regulation of CD4 and Class I MHC expression and sequestration to lymphoid depots. It is possible that establishment of immunodominance may be another type of immune decoy. It is possible too that abundantly expressed proteins may skew immunity to recognition of dominantly expressed epitopes that could be redundant in terms of maintaining viral fitness and replication competency.

Part III: Immunity associated with protection from HIV-1 Infection: The case of commercial sex workers

A rare number of individuals exist who appear to have natural resistance to HIV-1 infection. Cases have emerged of individuals reporting multiple exposures to HIV-1 but who appear not to be susceptible to infection and who are persistantly seronegative. These individuals may provide us with important clues to protective immune responses, which can inform HIV vaccine development. They are variously called exposed seronegatives or highly exposed persistantly seronegatives (HEPS). We will use the term HEPS.

Multiple factors, involving host factors and viral fitness, are likely to contribute to possible protection from HIV-1 infection. Polymorphisms in host chemokine receptor/ligand genes have been shown to play a role in protection. Associations between HLA and protection have also been described, which as discussed in Part I, ultimately play a role in directing the type of immune responses that can result in protection.

CTL activities have been demonstrated in high-risk uninfected men who have sex with men (MSM), heterosexual partners of infected men and women, female sex workers and individuals with occupational HIV-1 exposures. In many of the studies reported, approximately one third of HEPS individuals display CTL activity. To date, the best-characterised HEPS cohort of female sex workers has been from Nairobi, Kenya, where a small number of these women have remained uninfected for up to 12 years. Approximately half of these women possess CTL that recognise multiple conserved HIV epitopes. Many of these epitopes were no longer recognised in a small fraction of women who became HIV-1 infected after temporary cessation of sexwork, inferring that switching in epitope specificity resulted in loss of protection. Earlier experiments that explored the hypothesis that CTL identified in HEPS individuals can provide protection was accomplished by transferring CD8+ lymphocytes from HEPS individuals to SCID/beige mice, which then provided protection against subsequent systemic HIV-1 challenge. Other murine experiments have shown that mucosal, rather than systemic, HIV-specific CTL are necessary to confer resistance to mucosal transmission. This has been further supported in rhesus macaques where transient infection of the colonic mucosa elicited class I HLA-restricted anti-SIV Env CTL and there was presence of mucosal CTL correlated with protection against further colonic viral challenge. Mucosal CTL may play a major role in protection at the site of HIV-1 transmission.

Evidence for low levels of HIV-1 infection in HEPS

Although acquired immunity may play a role in the control of HIV-1 infection and in an exposed seronegative scenario, it cannot be discounted that T-cell responses in HEPS individuals denote prior HIV-1 exposure, perhaps due to cross-priming from HIV-1 infected cells acquired from their partner. This has led to the hypothesis that HEPS individuals may have latent infection in quiescent cells after initial HIV-1 infection. This hypothesis was derived from the finding that HIV-1 reservoirs have been identified in resting CD4+ T-cells as early as ten days after infection and may persist for up to 60 years, even with current treatment modalities of highly active antiretro-viral treatment. Recent studies have identified extremely low levels of HIV-1 DNA in resting CD4+ T-cells in a group of HEPS individuals and found 2×10^2–10^8-fold lower DNA copies than in HIV-1 infected individuals. The infected cells resided primarily in the subcapsular and parafollicular cortex of lymph nodes, suggesting the possibility that extremely low levels of HIV-1 antigen presentation and priming in HEPS individuals may be the driving factor behind detectable T-cell responses in these individuals.

The role of HLA in protection

As certain HLA backgrounds have been found to be associated with HEPS sex workers, this would suggest that certain dominant T-cell responses might play a significant role in protection. An increased frequency of HLA-B18 and HLA-A11 has been found in HEPS sex workers in Thailand. HLA-B18 has also been found to associate with resistance to HIV-1 infection in the Nairobi HEPS cohort. In addition, HLA-B18 has been reported to be associated with slow or non-progres-sion to AIDS in HIV-1 infected Caucasians. Studies performed in The Gambia have shown that the most prevalent HLA allele associated with HEPS individuals was HLA-B35 and additionally HLA-A6802 and –B18 have been strongly associated with HEPS CSW in Kenya. A subse-quent study showed that an HLA-A2/68 super haplotype, significantly associated with expression of both A*0202 and A*6802 allele sub-types, was identified with protection in this cohort. This information has important implications for design of vaccines, as it indirectly links plausible CTL responses with HLA families.

The influence of HLA on HIV-1 infection

A number of studies have found an association between HLA class I allele expression and HIV-1 disease progression. Certain HLA mole-cules are associated with an immunodominant state as discussed above. For example, HLA-B27 and HLA-B14 have been associated with slow progression to AIDS. Conversely, HLA-A29 and HLA-B22 have been significantly associated with rapid progression to AIDS. It may be thought that those HLA alleles that are associated with slow disease progression may steer immunity to recognise immunodominant epitopes found within conserved regions of HIV-1. The resulting CTL responsiveness could then reduce viral antigenic diversity and viral burden and result in a lower viral set-point. Conversely, disease progression has been associated with HLA homozygosity, especially within either the A and B loci and may be a result of limited antigen presentation. Recent compelling evidence for the role of HLA in control of HIV-1 replication includes the description of a highly focused CTL response in a subgroup of long-term non-progressors (LTNP) where there was a significant association with HLA B*57. HLA associations with control of viral replication have been extended to include further alleles of the Bw4 family. There are two families of HLA-B locus alleles that share 'public epitopes', Bw4 and Bw6, and an individual who is heterozygous for two different HLA-B alleles may be homozygous with respect to HLA-Bw4 or -Bw6. For example, a select group of LTNP who were homozygous for Bw4 was associated with control of viraemia and delaying the onset of development of AIDS. Further related was the association of the A2/A68 supertype with resistance to HIV-1 infection in Kenyan female sex workers. However, this supertype was not observed in a population study in Botswana, nor in a group of HEPS individuals from KwaZulu-Natal, although there was evidence of a higher frequency of HLA-A68 in non-infected or HEPS individuals. There is also evidence that HLA class II alleles/ haplotypes play a crucial role in the control in viral replication and resistance. Thus, for example, the DRB1*13-DQB1*06 haplotype has been associated with maintaining viral suppression in a group of HIV-1 patients receiving antiretroviral therapy as well as in a group of LTNP. In the case of the female sex workers, the DRB1*01 allele was independently associated with resistance to infection.

Alternative mechanisms of natural resistance to HIV-1 infection

The failure to detect HIV-1 specific T-cell responses in all HEPS individuals suggests the existence of additional protective mechanisms in these individuals. Understanding alternative mechanisms of natural resistance is important for devising innovative vaccine design. Some studies of HEPS women have suggested that resistance involves the reduced surface expression of essential co-receptors or increased production of β-chemokines, MIP-1α, MIP-1β or RANTES. Other studies have suggested that suppressive factors produced by CD8+ cells are an important component of HEPS protection and that maintenance of this suppressive activity depends on periodic exposure, either to HIV-1 or to alloantigens. The elusive nature of protection in these women indicates that correlates of protection may not lie in the areas of investigation that so much effort and data have generated. It is perhaps likely that novel genes, with unknown function, may be associated with protection in these individuals.

Part IV: Vaccines and immunogenicity

A vaccine is of paramount importance to develop and implement as a public health preventive measure for South Africa and other regions worst affected by the epidemic. Many aspects of vaccine research take cues from HIV-1 infected individuals at the acute stage of infection and also from HEPS individuals. It is important to identify epitopes within HIV-1 proteins that may correlate with control of viraemia. An effective preventive vaccine will need to evoke both cellular and humoral immunity and vaccine efficacy will be measured not only by precluding HIV-1 infection, but also by preventing or slowing disease progression and transmission. Thus, viral load is a critical endpoint of vaccine studies. The main determinant of disease progression in an individual is high plasma HIV-1 viral load and the level of infectiousness is directly proportional to the magnitude of viraemia in plasma, genital tract secretions and breast-milk. If a vaccine were capable of controlling viral replication, the rate of disease progression and HIV-1 transmission would potentially be lowered. This is an essential point of preventive vaccine research with vaccines that are designed to elicit specific T-cell immunity. The first stage is to design a vaccine candidate that is immunogenic.

The immunogenic capacity of a candidate HIV-1 vaccine is how well it can cause the vaccine recipient immune system to either produce anti-HIV antibodies (humoral immunity) and/or anti-HIV T-cell responses (cellular immunity). This means that an immunogenic vaccine will induce immune responses specifically directed at the proteins, or antigens, expressed by the genes in the vaccine. Hopefully, these responses will provide primed immunity that will cross-react with the live pathogen in the event that the vaccine recipient ever becomes exposed or infected with HIV-1. Phase I and II clinical trials measure safety and the degree of immune priming.

There are a multitude of vaccine candidates that are either in early clinical trials or in the development pipeline. The most promising candidates are attenuated live vectors containing HIV-1 genes. Such vectors include Sindbis, adenovirus, associated adenovirus, Venezuelan Equine Encaphalitis virus as examples. These vectors have been attenuated so that no infection by the vector can take place after administering the formulated vaccine. In addition to these vectors, a host of recombinant DNA constructs are available using HIV-1 genes from various clades. It is envisioned that a prime-boost strategy be adopted where DNA vaccines are used to prime immunity and the vector is used to boost specific T-cell immune responses at a later time, which will serve to focus CD8+ T-cells to recognise an array of epitopes. The importance of using DNA-based vaccines is that to efficiently elicit CD8+ T-cell responses, endogenous antigen processing is required in the vaccine recipient.

How do we measure CD8+ T-cell immunogenicity?

Three different methodologies can be used to measure CD8+ T-cell responses in vaccine recipients. The first method is the IFNγ ELISPOT assay, an endpoint measurement now used for virtually all vaccine candidates designed to elicit T-cell immune responses. The ELISPOT assay is highly sensitive and quick to perform and measures T-cell cytokine secretion in response to the vaccine candidate. The assay is based on the same principle as the ELISA, although the ELISPOT measures the number of cytokine-secreting cells, rather than the concentration of the cytokine produced. The quantity of cytokine-secreting cells is measured by counting the imprint of cells after short-term stimulation with peptides matching proteins expressed by the vaccine. The imprint remaining is counted as a spot on the membrane of the ELISA plate and using a specialised digital counting system, we can quantify the IFNγ spots. This will provide an *ex vivo* frequency of T-cells elicited in response to the vaccine candidate and is now used as the primary end-point assay for HIV-1 vaccine trials. One important feature of this assay is that it can be subjected to quality control and assurance and allows different laboratories to be validated with each other as well as specifically for each vaccine trial.

The second method involves measuring CTL activity as a measure of the functional killing capacity of CD8+ T-cells, using radioactive ^{51}Cr release. This assay is based on culturing peripheral blood cells with vaccine-matched proteins so that any priming of CTL by the vaccine can be detected after expanding these cells *in vitro*. These CTL assays are used to measure the frequency of vaccine-specific T-cell populations using ^{51}Cr-labelled vaccine recipient immortalised B-cell lines as surrogate target cells. The basis for this assay is a nine to 14 day *in vitro* stimulation using vaccinia-infected peripheral blood cells and interleukin-2 and -7.

The third method is the use of flow cytometry and intracellular cytokine staining. Similar to the ELISPOT assay, peripheral blood is stimulated for a short time with vaccine-matched peptides and T-cell subsets expressing cytokines (IFNγ for example) are identified using fluorochrome-conjugated monoclonal antibodies to CD4 or CD8 cells. This method has been used successfully to identify the magnitude and breadth of antigen-specific CD4+ and CD8+ T-cells in HIV-1-infected individuals. The major disadvantage of this method is that the lowest threshold of the flow cytometry-based assay is approximately 0.05% (or 1/2000 CD8+ T cells), whereas it is possible to detect 1/50 000 cells using the ELISPOT assay. This may be a very important limitation of the method if the vaccine elicits low frequency of responses.

The vaccine is considered immunogenic if any one of the immunology end-point assays are positive. Once a vaccine has been found to be immunogenic in a phase I trial, it will advance to the next stage of phase II clinical trials and ultimately a phase III efficacy trial.

The significance of CTL and HLA in vaccine design

One of the aims of developing a preventative vaccine is to elicit protective T-cell responses in individuals who might be at risk of becoming HIV-1 infected. In this context it is important to identify epitopes that are firstly associated with protection and secondly, cover a wide number of individuals within a population. The finding that epitopes can be shared within families of HLA supertypes (see below) may greatly facilitate selection of candidate epitopes that have wide population cover. Additionally, the design of a vaccine that can elicit both immunodominant and subdominant CTL responses may limit uncontrolled breakthrough infections. The hazard of eliciting a single immunodominant response in a vaccinee may predispose that individual to viral escape in the event of a breakthrough infection (a vaccine volunteer who becomes HIV-1 infected whilst on the vaccine trial).

HLA supertypes

The high degree of class I HLA polymorphism within populations has evolved to protect against continual viral exposure and to ensure that specific host immunity can target potentially multiple viral antigens and prevent virion spread within a host. For some reason, HIV-1 circumvents this evolutionary mechanism in the majority of infected individuals. Whether this is related to the inability of infected individuals to mount broad enough CTL responses, that use more than one HLA allele, is unclear. To deconvolute the complexity of HLA polymorphism for understanding how immunity targets specific epitopes of HIV is a goal of preventive vaccine design. It is possible to simplify epitope selection for inclusion into a vaccine by identifying peptides capable of binding multiple HLA molecules because of overlapping peptide-binding motifs. For example, it would be possible to identify protein sequences that contain overlapping epitopes capable of binding multiple HLA molecules. Identity of single peptides that can bind multiple HLA molecules is thus an attractive method of ensuring that regions of HIV-1 can be targeted by a wide number of individuals. Thus, approximately 66% of peptides that bind to HLA-A*0201 will bind in a cross-reactive manner to three or more other HLA-A2 supertype alleles: HLA-A*0201, -A*0202, -A*0203, -A*0204, -A*0205, -A*0206, -A*0207, -A*6802 and -A*6901. The HLA-A3 supertype includes, minimally, HLA-A*03, -A*11, -A*3101, -A*3301 and -A*6801 alleles. Approximately 40% of peptides bearing the HLA-A3 super-motif are capable of binding HLA-A*03, the most common allele of this supertype, and will bind in a cross-reactive manner with at least three of the five most common HLA-A3 supertype family members. The HLA-B7 supertype was originally described as HLA-B*0702, -B*3501-03, -B*51, -B*5301 and -B*5401. However, published motifs for HLA-B*0703-05, -B*1508, -B*5501-02, -B*5601-02, -B*6701 and -B*7801 suggest that these additional alleles are also members of the B7 supertype family. A significant degree of binding cross-reactivity exists and about 20% of the peptides that bind to HLA-B*0702, the most frequent allele of this family, also bind three or more of the five most common HLA-B7 supertype molecules. For the HLA-24 supertype family, there is sequence homology in binding motifs for HLA-A*2402 and -A*3001. For the HLA-B27 supertype family, motifs for HLA-B*14, -B*1509, -B*38, -B*3901, -B*3902, -B*73 share specificity for peptides and HLA-B*1503, -B*1510, -B*1518, -B*2701, -B*2708, -B*4841, and -B*4802 possess the B27-supertype B pocket consensus motif.

Is the immune response to HIV-1 good or bad?

The strong robust immune response to HIV-1 is thought be effective in the early stage of infection. However, as HIV mutates and there is continual immune evasion, it is possible that the side-effect of host immunity is the destruction of self. These are questions unanswered, but the hypothesis would be that an unchecked immune response that continues unabated will lead to immune destruction. Could it be possible that HIV-1 has successfully redirected immunity to precipitate its own demise and by the time this happens, enough virus has been transmitted to ensure its survival?

Bibliography

APPAY, V. ET AL. 'Dynamics of T-cell responses in HIV infection.' *Journal of Immunology* 2002; 168: 3660–3666.

BORROW P ET AL. 'Virus-specific CD8+ cytotoxic T-lymphocyte activity associated with control of viremia in primary human immunodeficiency virus type 1 infection.' *Journal of Virology* 1994; 68: 6103–6110.

DETELS R ET AL. 'Persistently seronegative men from whom HIV-1 has been isolated are genetically and immunologically distinct.' *Immunology Letters* 1996; 51: 29–33.

GASCHEN B ET AL. 'Diversity considerations in HIV-1 vaccine selection.' *Science* 2002; 296: 2354–2360.

GOULDER PJ ET AL. 'Late escape from an immunodominant cytotoxic T-lymphocyte response associated with progression to AIDS.' *Nature Medicine* 1997; 3: 212–217.

GRANT AD, DJOMAND G, DE COCK KM. 'Natural history and spectrum of disease in adults with HIV/AIDS in Africa.' *Aids* 1997; 11(Suppl B): S43–54.

KASLOW RA ET AL. 'Influence of combinations of human major histocompatibility complex genes on the course of HIV-1 infection [see comments].' *Nature Medicine* 1996; 2: 405–411.

KAUL R ET AL. 'HIV-1-specific mucosal CD8+ lymphocyte responses in the cervix of HIV-1-resistant prostitutes in Nairobi.' *Journal of Immunology* 2000; 164: 1602–1611.

KLENERMAN P, ZINKERNAGEL RM. 'What can we learn about human immunodeficnecy virus infection from a study of lymphocytic choriomeningitis virus?' *Immunology Review* 1997; 159: 5–16.

KORBER BTM ET AL. *HIV Molecular Immunology 2001.* Los Alamos National Laboratory, Theoretical Biology and Biophysics Los Alamos, New Mexico. 2001.

KOUP RA ET AL. 'Temporal association of cellular immune responses with the initial control of viremia in primary human immunodeficiency virus type 1 syndrome.' *Journal of Virology* 1994; 68: 4650–4655.

KURODA MJ ET AL. 'Emergence of CTL coincides with clearance of virus during primary simian immunodeficiency virus infection in rhesus monkeys.' *Journal of Immunology* 1999; 162: 5127–5133.

MASHISHI T, GRAY CM. 'The elispot assay: an easily transferable method for measuring cellular responses and identifying T-cell epitopes.' *Clinical Chemical Laboratory Methods* 2002; 40: 903–10.

PANTALEO G ET AL. 'Accumulation of human immunodeficiency virus-specific cytotoxic T lymphocytes away from the predominant site of virus replication during primary infection. *European Journal of Immunology* 1997; 27: 3166–3173.

PLOTKIN SA. 'Immunologic correlates of protection induced by vaccination.'*Pediatric Infectious Diseases Journal* 2001; 20: 63–75.

ROWLAND-JONES SL ET AL. 'Cytotoxic T-cell responses to multiple conserved HIV epitopes in HIV-resistant prostitutes in nairobi [In Process Citation].' *Journal of Clinical Investigation* 1998; 102: 1758–1765.

SCHMITZ JE ET AL. 'Control of viremia in simian immunodeficiency virus infection by CD8+ lymphocytes.' *Science* 1999; 283: 857–60.

SANDSTROM E, BIRX D. 'HIV vaccine trials in Africa.' *Aids* 2002; 16 (Suppl 4): S89–95.

ROBINSON HL. 'New hope for an AIDS vaccine.' *Nature Reviews. Immunology* 2002; 2: 239–50.

HIV risk factors and prevention strategies

CHAPTER 9

Reducing sexual risk behaviours: Theory and research, successes and challenges

Catherine Mathews

SEXUAL BEHAVIOUR IS THE main driver of the South African HIV epidemic. The median age at first sexual intercourse among South Africans is 18 years, and 8% of women who have ever had sexual intercourse have done so by the age of 15. Among sexually active men aged 15 to 24 years, 23% reported multiple partners in the preceding 12 months. Among sexually active women and men, condoms were not used during 43%–80% of the most recent incidents of sexual intercourse. Sexual behaviour is shaped by personal, interpersonal, environmental, cultural and structural forces. The personal factors influencing sexual risk behaviour include feelings and cognitions related to sexuality, HIV/AIDS, and the self. Factors related to inter-personal relationships, such as negotiating condom use, coercive male-dominated sexual partnerships and peer pressure to be sexually active, are also important. Cultural factors, such as traditions, shared beliefs, and the norms of the larger society, also play a role. Unfortunately, these often support an unequal distribution of sexual power between men and women and subordinate women's needs and rights.

Structural factors, such as the legal, political and economic elements of society also have an important influence in sexual behaviour. 'Soul City' and 'Mothusimpilo' are two South African HIV prevention projects that address the personal, social, economic and political forces that cause and maintain the HIV epidemic. The first, Soul City, uses edutainment and advocacy, and has met with some success at both the individual and broader societal levels. The second, Mothusimpilo, South Africa's first attempt to reduce HIV at a community level, used participatory peer education, community mobilisation, condom promotion, and STI management among mineworkers, commercial sex workers and community residents. The relative successes and failures of these two projects provide valuable insights about how to alter the vulnerability to HIV of South Africans. They demonstrate the need for a commitment to develop and sustain long-term interventions that address social factors, including poverty and gender inequalities.

In South Africa, the HIV/AIDS epidemic is driven primarily by sexual behaviours that expose individuals to the risk of infection. In tackling the epidemic, the deepest and most difficult problem of all is trying to change sexual risk behaviour. This chapter describes the prevalence of key sexual risk behaviours – plainly underlining the gravity of the problem – and considers ways in which South African initiatives can confront, and have confronted, the huge and difficult challenge of reducing sexual risk behaviour. Four principal questions guide our considerations. What are the forces shaping an individual's sexual risk behaviour? Is there a role for theory in tackling the forces shaping sexual risk behaviour? Is it possible to change sexual behaviour? What are the challenges in measuring the successes and failures of initiatives that attempt to reduce risk behaviour? In particular, two ground-breaking South African HIV prevention initiatives present us with instructive case studies: 'Soul City' and 'Mothusimpilo', both of them research- and theory-based, multi-million Rand projects with high-level national and international support and commitment. One appears to have been effective, the other not and the chapter reviews their relative successes and failures for possible indicators of what it takes to reduce sexual risk behaviour in South Africa.

The prevalence of risky sexual behaviour

To what extent do South Africans expose themselves to the risk of HIV infection through their sexual behaviour? TABLES 9.1–9.3 draw on the findings of two South African national surveys, the Demographic and Health Survey of 1998 (SADHS), and the Nelson Mandela Human Sciences Research Council Survey of 2000 (HSRC survey).

TABLE 9.1 shows that the age by which one half of South Africans report having had penetrative sexual intercourse is 18 years (median age). The SADHS found that 8% of women aged 25 to 49 (at the time of

TABLE 9.1 Median age at first sexual experience of those surveyed who had ever had sexual intercourse

Study and Year	Age Group	Median: male	Median: female
SADHS 1998	25–49 years		18 years*
HSRC 2002	25–59 years	18**	18**

* 99% of women in this age group had ever had sexual intercourse

** The proportion of respondents in this age group that had ever had sexual intercourse is not reported

the survey), who had ever had sexual intercourse, had done so by the age of 15. The SADHS collected data only on the age at sexual debut of women in the reproductive ages. The HSRC survey found that fewer than 2% of children in the 12 to 14 year age group reported having had previous sexual intercourse.

TABLE 9.2 describes the proportion of respondents who reported multiple sexual partnerships (those reporting more than one sexual partner) during the 12 months prior to the survey. The HSRC survey found that men were more likely than women to report multiple partnerships.

Study and Year	Age Group	Male	Female
SADHS 1998	15–49 years		4%
HSRC 2002	15–24 years	23%	9%
HSRC 2002	25–49 years	12%	3%

TABLE 9.2 Multiple sexual partners in the 12 months prior to the survey, among those who had sexual intercourse during the time period

Both surveys found that sizeable proportions of respondents reported no sexual intercourse during the previous 12 months (sometimes referred to as 'secondary abstinence'). The SADHS survey found that 23% of women aged 15 to 49 reported no sexual partners during the 12-month period. The HSRC found that 18% of men aged 15 to 24, 9% of men aged 25 to 49, 14% of women aged 15 to 24 and 17% of women aged 25 to 49 reported no sexual intercourse in the 12-month period.

TABLE 9.3 describes condom use during the respondent's last sexual intercourse. Both surveys found that younger respondents and those in urban areas (as opposed to non-urban areas) reported significantly higher rates of condom use. A comparison of the SADHS and HSRC surveys suggests that condom use has increased between 1998 to 2002. For example, the SADHS found that only 19.5% of women aged 15 to 19 years reported condom use at last sexual intercourse. Four years later, the HSRC survey found that 48.9% of women in this age group reported condom use at last sex. The increase was consistent across all age groups.

Study and Year	Age Group	Male	Female
SADHS 1998	15–49 years		8%
HSRC 2002	15–49 years		29%
HSRC 2002	15–24 years	57.1%	46.1%
HSRC 2002	25–49 years	26.7%*	19.7%

TABLE 9.3 Condom use during last sexual inter-course, among those who were sexually active during the 12 months prior to the survey

These two national surveys paint an overarching (albeit incomplete) picture of the extent to which South Africans are exposed to the risk of HIV through sexual behaviour. This picture will vary to an extent from place to place, by age, by education and by socioeconomic status, but overall it shows that young South Africans begin to be sexually active between the ages of 12 to 14, and that by age 18 half will have had sexual intercourse. Some South Africans (9%–23%) who have previously been sexually active, report 'secondary abstinence' (abstaining from intercourse over a 12-month period). However, among those not abstaining, 3%–23% have multiple sexual partnerships. Condom use, while increasing, is not widespread. Judging from the HSRC survey, condoms were not used during 43%–80% of the most recent incidents of sexual intercourse (varying by age and gender). These surveys provide sufficient evidence of the extreme urgency of reducing sexual risk behaviour, evidence that is reinforced by many smaller, local South African surveys.

The forces shaping sexual risk behaviour

Why do South Africans continue to expose themselves to the risk of HIV infection through their sexual behaviour? Explanations of sexual behaviour that focus primarily on personal and interpersonal factors give us only part of the picture. It is very important that we also extend our view to broader contextual factors of structure and environment and the way these shape the possibilities for safe sexual behaviour. This is particularly important in South Africa, where health problems of poor communities stem very largely from economic, political and social condition, and where individual choices about adopting healthy behaviours are constrained by these broader conditions.

Eaton, Flisher and Aarø from the University of Cape Town, in their review of unsafe sexual behaviour in South African youth, have developed a conceptual framework for the factors that promote sexual risk behaviour, or that cause barriers to safer practices. Their model distinguishes between three levels of factors or domains of analysis (domains which to a certain extent overlap and reciprocally influence each other): **personal** factors; factors in the **proximal** context (including interpersonal factors and factors related to the immediate living environment); and factors in the **distal** context (including structural and cultural factors). In the following section, their framework is used to describe some of the important South African influences on sexual risk behaviour.

Personal factors

Personal factors are those that reside within the individual person, such as cognitions and feelings related to sexual behaviour and HIV/AIDS and thoughts about one's self. Personal factors influence sexual behaviour and HIV risk. For example, the Eaton, Flisher, Aarø review shows that among South African youth, self-efficacy (the confidence a person feels about performing a particular activity) for condom use is associated with higher self-reported condom use. It also shows that low self-esteem is associated with earlier sexual debut, having more sexual partners, and having a negative attitude towards condom use. The HSRC national survey showed that correct knowledge about HIV/AIDS (that HIV caused AIDS, and that HIV is not transmitted through touch and kissing) was associated with self-reported adoption of HIV preventive behaviour over the years prior to the survey, and with condom use during the last sexual intercourse.

The proximal context

The 'proximal' context encompasses features of relationships and the environment that intimately impinge upon an individual. Proximal factors include those related to interpersonal relationships: negotiating condom use; coercive, male-dominated sexual relationships; peer pressure to be sexually active; relationships with parents and health workers, etc. The proximal context also embraces the physical and organisational living environment: where one lives (urban or rural, on the streets, in prison, etc); the quality and quantity of health services; access to condoms, to the media, to recreational facilities.

Gender inequality is an important feature of many sexual relationships, and one associated with HIV risk. Jewkes and colleagues have demonstrated in a study among teenage girls in the Eastern Cape, the 'Stepping Stones behavioural intervention for HIV', that having a male partner more than five years older (a marker of gender inequality) was associated with a significantly higher risk of being HIV positive. They also found that communication was poorer in relationships marked by a substantial age difference, and the likelihood of the woman being able to suggest condom use was lower. The peak age-specific HIV prevalence for women in South Africa is 25 to 29 years of age, five years earlier than the peak for men (30 to 34 years), and teenage boys have a very low HIV prevalence (CHAPTER 4 and CHAPTER 16). This indicates that HIV infections in teenage girls are almost entirely due to having sex with men who are on averagefive years older than they are.

Women with violent or controlling male partners are at increased risk for HIV infection. This has been demonstrated by Dunkle and colleagues in a cross-sectional study among 1366 women presenting for antenatal care at four health centres in Soweto. Consistent with prior research, they found that intimate partner violence was associated with an increased likelihood of women engaging in HIV risk behaviour (having multiple partners, having concurrent partners, engaging in transactional sex and having problems with substance use). They also found that, after adjustment for women's HIV risk behaviour, intimate partner violence and high levels of male dominance and control in a woman's current relationship were associated with HIV seropositivity.

The institutional climate of both health services and schools has a significant effect on sexual risk behaviour. For example, Abdool Karim and colleagues have shown that young people's access to free condoms provided by clinics is restricted by the negative attitudes of clinic staff, or by clinics running out of supplies. Campbell and MacPhail have shown how the institutional environment of the school can promote gender inequalities and undermine effective, student-led HIV prevention programmes. Schools in poor areas are usually poorly resourced with high levels of disorganisation. Teachers lack training and they feel uncomfortable taking HIV discussions beyond the biomedical sphere to discuss relationships, sexuality and emotions. Authoritarian and didactic education approaches are still common, and these undermine students' own peer education initiatives and their capacity to challenge norms around gender inequality and violence. A review of international research on the impact that schools have on adolescent sexual behaviour by Kirby confirms the effect of the institutional climate of schools on risk behaviour. It shows that girls in schools with high rates of poverty and social disorganisation are more likely to become pregnant. It also shows that school programmes addressing problems in the school environment not related to sexuality (such as increasing student attachment to the school and reducing dropout) effectively delay sexual initiation and reduce pregnancy rates among students.

The distal context

The distal context encompasses the less immediate elements of a person's environment. These include both cultural factors, such as traditions, the norms of the larger society, the social discourse within a society and shared beliefs and values, and structural factors, such as the legal, political, economic and organisational elements of a society.

Discourses that support the unequal distribution of sexual power between men and women, and the subordination of women's needs and rights have an important influence on sexual behaviour and HIV risk. Research has shown, for example, that condemnation of young women's premarital sexual activity causes barriers to their adoption of preventive practices, while ideas about masculinity, risk taking and sexual conquest increase men's HIV risk behaviours. Norms around intimate partner violence make women vulnerable to HIV infection through coercive sex and sex without a condom. Similarly, racist and homophobic discourse may increase the risk of HIV in those targeted.

The myth that sex with a virgin will cure HIV has been thought to be common in South Africa, and to play a role in child rape and the transmission of HIV to girls and young women. Recently, Jewkes (in Richter et al.) has reviewed the available evidence for the prevalence of this belief in South Africa and its relationship to HIV risk behaviour. The research findings are contradictory, with some studies (including the HSRC national survey) finding scant evidence of the existence of such a belief, and others (a qualitative study in KwaZulu-Natal and a survey at a motor industry in the Eastern Cape) finding it to be highly prevalent. Jewkes suggests that while there have been isolated cases where the practice of 'virgin cleansing' has definitely been the motivation for child rape it is unlikely that it is a common motivation, given the infrequency with which service providers see such cases, and given that the number of child rape cases has not been increasing nationally over the last five years during which the HIV epidemic has spiralled.

The country's migrant labour practices are highly significant among the structural elements of the South African context that affect sexual behaviour and HIV risk. A century of laws curtailing the free movement of the majority of the population, together with more specific mining and industrial employment practices, have shaped a labour system in which circular migration has been and remains a way of life for millions, severely disrupting family lives. Lurie and others have shown that, compared with non-migrant men, migrants reported a higher total number of casual partners and were more likely to be HIV positive. Their work has also demonstrated that a history of repeated relocation (often a result of apartheid policies and political violence) is an independent risk factor for HIV (CHAPTER 19). Work conditions for migrants employed in South African mines are extremely harsh and dangerous; living conditions in the mine hostels are crowded and unpleasant, and miners are away from their families for long periods. Campbell's qualitative study of migrant miners in two Gauteng mining houses describes their sense of powerlessness in the face of these conditions, given their low level of education, the poverty of their communities, and the current levels of unemployment countrywide. She illuminates the link between structural and environmental conditions and sexual behaviour, showing how sexual relationships and sexual risk-taking provide one of the few opportunities for assertion of miners' masculine identities, in an environment where they have little control over important aspects of their life.

Poverty and social marginalisation are pervasive factors in the lives of the majority of South Africans, exerting a powerful influence on sexual behaviour. No explanation of HIV risk behaviour will be adequate without referring to them. Kelly and Parker of CADRE, in their investigation of youth response to HIV/AIDS in six sentinel sites across South Africa found that among 15 to 19 year olds, those from homes where there was not enough money for even food and clothes were almost twice as likely to have had sexual intercourse than those from homes where there was money for holidays and some luxury goods. They identified three main explanations for the association between poverty and increased sexual activity among young people: the exchange of material and financial resources for sex plays a more important role in sexual decision making in poorer communities; there is a marked breakdown of parental authority in poor (especially rural) areas with one or both parents being migrant labourers; and there are few youth recreational facilities.

Parker, Easton and Klein observe that social factors such as poverty, instability, gender inequalities, sexual oppression and racism often have interactive and synergistic effects, directly determining the vulnerability to HIV of groups and individuals. They describe this as 'structural violence', and the concept is particularly relevant in South Africa where historically constituted political and economic marginalisation, based on racist ideology, has shaped the vulnerability of the vast majority of the population.

Theories about health behaviour and their role in tackling the forces shaping sexual risk behaviour

Theories are the conceptual frameworks within which we seek to explain why people behave in ways that put their health at risk, and why they adopt health-protective behaviour. They point us towards key constructs, key processes, key mechanisms that hypothetically influence health behaviour. Theory-driven interventions attempt to impact on these constructs and processes, and theory-driven evaluations measure the specific extent of the impact. Theories with a superior ability to identify the factors influencing risk behaviour will lead to more efficacious interventions and the development and application of behavioural and social theory has the potential to contribute to reducing sexual risk behaviour and improving public health.

In a 1991 National Institutes of Health workshop in the USA, the developers and/or leading proponents of five theories commonly used in health promotion (and HIV prevention) were brought together to attempt to identify a common set of factors to be considered in any behavioural analysis. The theories all focused primarily on the personal and interpersonal factors influencing health behaviour, and included the Health Belief Model, Social Cognitive Learning Theory, the Theory of Reasoned Action, the Theory of Self-Regulation and

Self-Control, and the Theory of Subjective Culture and Interpersonal Relations. The workshop outcome, reported by Fishbein and colleagues, was the identification of a limited number of variables that were potential determinants of any given behaviour. There was consensus that changed behaviour was more likely to occur if the individual: (a) has a strong positive intention to perform it; (b) is not impeded by constraints, either external or internal to the person, that make the behaviour difficult to achieve; (c) perceives more social or normative pressure from relevant referents to perform the behaviour than not to perform the behaviour; (d) has the necessary skills to perform the behaviour; (e) believes that the perceived advantages outweigh the perceived costs, ie the person has a positive attitude toward performing the behaviour; (f) perceives the performance of the behaviour to be consistent with his/her self-image; (g) has an emotional reaction to performing the behaviour that is more positive than negative and (h) perceives that he/she has the capabilities to perform the behaviour under a number of different circumstances. Recent research by Vergnani, Flisher and Blignaut among a representative sample of 1884 Grade 11 students at Cape Town high schools, demonstrated the relevance of each one of these constructs, confirming that all these variables were associated with condom use and intended condom use.

We have already noted how sexual behaviour is influenced by an array of factors operating at the personal, proximal and distal levels, presenting a level of complexity beyond possible explanation by any single theory. More importantly, we cannot limit ourselves to theories that focus only on individual level and interpersonal determinants of sexual behaviour and HIV risk. Yet individual and interpersonal theories (such as the Health Belief Model and the other theories included in Fishbein's report) have so far been the ones most influential in the development of HIV prevention interventions, even in less developed countries where the impact of social and environmental factors on sexuality is most evident and the need to effect change in the distal context is most pressing. In South Africa, it is crucial for prevention initiatives to follow theoretical approaches that do take account of the broader social and environmental factors – where the premise is that the collective health of communities can be enhanced by processes, structures and policies that foster individual health-promoting actions or reduce or eliminate health hazards in the social and physical environment. We can note here three such lines of approach that have guided recent South African prevention projects: *Community organisation*, *social capital theory*, and *media advocacy*.

Community organisation is a fairly broad conceptual framework for interventions based on social science theories well described by Glanz and colleagues. It indicates processes by which community groups are helped to collectively identify common problems or goals, mobilise resources, and develop and implement strategies for reaching their goals. There is no single unified model of community organisation, but a common set of theoretical and conceptual principles include:

- *Empowerment:* A central tenet of community organisation practice; the process by which individuals and communities are enabled to take power and act effectively in transforming their lives and environments.
- *Community competence:* Increasing the ability of the community to function effectively as a problem-solving unit.
- *Community participation:* An important focus of attention in the health world since the Alma Ata Conference in 1998; there is a large literature on community participation in health.
- *Creating 'critical consciousness':* Concept and methodology developed by Paulo Freire, and used for teaching illiterate people to read while at the same time developing their insight into the political and social situation in which they found themselves. The process involves working with people to elucidate the root causes of their problems and challenging them to devise action plans based on critical reflection to transform their social circumstances. This method has been used widely in health education and the Mothusimpilo project is a particular instance of its application.

Social capital theory is one of the emerging theories in health promotion described by DiClemente and colleagues. It has only recently become established in health promotion research, stimulated by Putnam's research on the performance of regional governments in Italy. This research found that those with superior governance had more social capital (a public spiritedness among citizens), higher levels of civic participation, and the tendency to form collaborative, often non-political organisations. Social capital, in Putnam's terms, refers to 'the features of social life – networks, norms and trust – that enable participants to act together more effectively to pursue shared objectives'. Putnam suggested that the core elements of social capital (trust and cooperation) could be developed over time by repeated interaction of individuals and groups in longstanding relationships supported by community institutions. Fran Banm (in Campbell) has described the application of this theory to health promotion, this theory proposes that people are more likely to embrace health-enhancing behaviour change if they live in communities with raised levels of social capital: high levels of participation in local organisations, with associated enhancement of trust and reciprocal help and support, and a positive local community identity.

Putnam distinguishes between two operational levels of social capital: *bonding* social capital and *bridging* social capital. These concepts, and their application, are clearly described in Campbell's evaluation of the Mothusimpilo project. Bonding social capital refers to relationships in which homogeneous groups are bonded in trusting, reciprocally supportive relationships with a positive common identity, such as group solidarity in close neighbourhoods. Bridging social capital operates at the organisational level and refers to the linking together of different organisations around a common purpose to access resources and assets from outside the community. For example, it refers to the links between small local groups and more powerful local groups, or networks of influence beyond their geographical location, or more powerful extracommunity agencies. The concept of bridging social capital is particularly and intuitively relevant in poor, marginalisd communities, where the resources within communities are not sufficient to tackle HIV. It puts the focus on processes of accessing extra-community resources which do not undermine the participation and control of the community in question. The Mothusimpilo project is an example of a project that attempted to prevent HIV through harnessing the potential of both bonding and bridging social capital.

There already exist valid instruments for measuring the theoretical constructs of social capital at the macro-level (trust in government, political engagement, connections with and perceptions of community associations). In health promotion, assessing constructs such as bridging social capital may provide valuable insights into the successes and failures of community-based health promotion initiatives. The Mothusimpilo project is, again, a case in point, where qualitative evaluation within the social capital paradigm has yielded valuable insight into why the project failed to have an impact on STIs.

Media advocacy is an important new approach to promoting health through mass communication. The traditional way in which the mass communication system has been used to promote health has been through public communication campaigns and social marketing aiming to have an impact on individual-level influences on health behaviour. Media advocacy theory indicates alternative approaches that use 'issue-framing' strategies, more usually associated with political campaigns, to affect community- and distal-level factors in health behaviour. Michael Pertschuk (in Glanz), one of the founders of this approach, defines it as 'the strategic use of mass media for advancing a social or public policy initiative'. Media advocacy strategies aim to increase public support for more effective policy-level approaches to public health problems. To achieve this, they stimulate media coverage to draw attention to the role of those who shape the environment in which individual health-related decisions are made. They aim to empower the public to take action to change the social and political environment. The Soul City initiative provides a case study in the application of this approach.

Can sexual behaviour be changed?

HIV prevention interventions **can** reduce sexual risk behaviour. This has been well established by numerous methodologically sound evaluations of risk reduction interventions. Some of these studies have also measured and shown consequential reductions in STI incidence. Several systematic reviews of HIV prevention intervention research have confirmed that prevention programmes can work, some using meta-analyses to quantify the protective effects of the reviewed interventions. For example, The HIV/AIDS Prevention Research Synthesis study showed that among heterosexual adults in the USA, the interventions reduced sexual risk behaviours by about 19%, and reduced STIs by about 26%. Among sexually active adolescents in the USA, the interventions reduced unprotected sex by about 34%.

Some of the HIV prevention interventions that have been shown to be effective have focused on personal and interpersonal risk factors, directing interventions to individuals, couples or small groups. Other effective interventions go beyond individual behaviour change goals and target change at the immediate community level (proximal context). Another category of intervention aims to change individual behaviours, the community environment, or both, through structural and environmental change (change in the distal context).

Addressing the personal and interpersonal influences on sexual risk behaviour

The two following examples describe effective interventions that focus primarily on the personal and interpersonal forces influencing sexual risk behaviour. The interventions are delivered by health service providers to their clients, face-to-face.

Project RESPECT was a large trial of an HIV risk reduction intervention conducted in public STI clinics in the USA. Through this trial, Kamb and colleagues demonstrated that brief, interactive, client-centred counselling interventions using personalised risk reduction plans, together with HIV testing, increased condom use and prevented new STIs. They compared the effects of two interactive HIV/STI counselling interventions, 'enhanced counselling' and 'brief counselling', with (then current) conventionally didactic prevention messages in a randomised controlled trial among

5758 patients attending five public STI clinics in the USA.

The enhanced counselling involved HIV testing in the context of four counselling sessions based on the theories of *reasoned action* and *social learning*, and aimed at changing self-efficacy, attitudes, and perceived norms underlying condom use. The brief counselling involved HIV testing in the context of two counselling sessions which aimed to assess actual and self-perceived HIV/STI risk, help the participant recognise barriers to risk reduction, negotiate an acceptable and achievable risk reduction plan, and support patient-initiated behaviour change. At both three and six month follow-up visits, self-reported 100% condom use was significantly higher among the participants in both the enhanced counselling and brief counselling arms of the study compared with the participants receiving the didactic messages. At the six-month follow-up 30% fewer participants in the enhanced counselling and brief counselling arms had new STIs, compared with those in the arms receiving didactic messages. At the twelve-month follow up, 20% fewer participants in the counselling arms had new STIs.

HIV voluntary counselling and testing has been shown to be feasible in both developed and less developed countries, and effective in reducing HIV-related risk behaviour.

The VCT Efficacy Study in Tanzania, Kenya and Trinidad was a randomised clinical trial that assessed whether VCT, given to individuals or couples, was effective in reducing risk behaviour associated with the sexual transmission of HIV. Prior to this study, several literature reviews, based primarily on observational studies, had indicated that VCT was especially effective in reducing risk among those diagnosed with HIV and for serodiscordant couples.

In this study, 3120 individuals and 586 couples in the three countries were randomised to receive VCT or health education and followed up at an average of 7.3 months for the first follow-up and 13.9 months for the second follow-up with retention rates in excess of 70% for all groups. This study found substantial and significant behaviour changes among both men and women receiving the VCT intervention compared with those receiving basic health information. For example, among individuals assigned VCT, there was a 35% reduction among men and a 39% reduction among women, in the proportion reporting unprotected intercourse with non-primary partners, while in the control arm the reductions were 13% and 17% respectively. Couples assigned VCT reduced unprotected intercourse with their enrolment partners significantly more than couples assigned health education, although no differences were found in unprotected intercourse with their non-enrolment partners. These changes were maintained at the second follow-up and also replicated when the control group was offered VCT. The effect of the intervention on HIV incidence was not measured.

Intervening in the proximal context to bring about community-level change

Studies focusing on changing social norms through the selection, recruitment and training of 'opinion leaders', based on the *Diffusion of Innovations* theory, have been successful in a wide variety of health interventions. This theory addresses the process by which new risk-reducing behaviours and other innovations diffuse through community networks to individuals, leading to social change. Kelly and colleagues conducted a seminal series of studies in the USA, showing that this approach reduced HIV risk behaviour in gay communities. In a randomised controlled trial among gay bar patrons in eight small American cities, they demonstrated that strategically selected, respected, influential opinion leaders, trained to promote risk-reduction to their peers, produced community-wide decreases in self-reported risk behaviours. Opinion leader interventions are potentially compatible with community-based participatory peer education approaches, such as those used in the Mothusimpilo project, and they have considerable potential in less developed countries and among adolescents (peer influence is among the most influential factors in determining adolescent behaviour).

There are local examples of programmes aiming at community-level change which have successfully demonstrated individual-level change. In KwaZulu-Natal, Harvey, Stuart and Swan conducted a randomised controlled trial, to evaluate the effects of DramAidE, a school-based lifeskills and HIV/AIDS programme, which was founded on the participatory learning methods of Paulo Freire and the drama techniques of Augusto Boal. The evaluation showed the programme to be effective at the individual level, improving students' knowledge and attitudes and increasing condom use. In Zimbabwe, Katzenstein and colleagues have shown that peer-education programmes among factory workers led to a 34% lower rate of new HIV infections than in comparable factories with no such programmes.

Building health enabling environments – the distal context

It is more difficult to get evidence for the success of programmes focusing primarily on impacting community-level processes and structural and environmental barriers. The randomised controlled trial is the existing standard in research design and it is not always compatible with the evaluation of community- or society-level interventions. Evaluation methodologies for interventions that address change in factors in the distal context are still under development.

Thailand's 100% Condom Programme is an example of an intervention that addresses the structural barriers to condom use. In 1989 the Thai government piloted this programme and in 1991 it was adopted as the official policy to ensure that men could not obtain commercial sex without using a condom. Free condoms were supplied for commercial sex. Brothels were threatened with closure if any evidence of the transmission of STIs to male clients was obtained from the STI treatment services. Sex workers were examined periodically for STIs, and mass advertising on television and radio stressed that men should use condoms with sex workers.

There is strong (but not conclusive) evidence that the programme has been effective and it is estimated to have averted about two million HIV infections and over 200 000 cases of STIs annually and played a central role in containing the HIV epidemic in Thailand. Hannenberg and colleagues described an increase in condom use during commercial sex from 14% in 1989 to 94% in 1993. Between 1989 and 1993, new cases of STIs among men declined by 79%. This was in contrast to a steady increase in STI cases from the 1960s. This type of intervention is probably not transferable to countries where the HIV epidemic is not generated by an easily identifiable or organised 'core group' such as sex workers in brothels, or where the policing of commercial sex would be incompatible with the sociopolitical climate, or where sex work is illegal.

The Soul City and Mothusimpilo projects are South African examples of interventions focusing on the distal context.

Implementing and evaluating prevention programmes: Some challenges

Interventions that aim to change behaviour and reduce HIV can be difficult to evaluate. Outcome measures such as HIV and STI reduction are the most convincing indicators of programme impact as they are the primary goal of the intervention in the context of HIV risk reduction, but the sample sizes required for demonstrating a reduction in the incidence of HIV or other STIs may exceed the available evaluation resources. Many evaluations attempt to show a change in self-reported sexual behaviour but not much research has been done on the validity of self-reported measures. Nevertheless, a good deal of evidence from South African research does lend support to their acceptance: associations have been documented between sexual behaviour and other risk behaviours, and internal consistency in the data from various studies has been observed, with, for example, consistent age and gender differences present. However, there is evidence from two studies, conducted in other settings, of potential problems in relying on self-reports. A prospective cohort study conducted in the USA by Zenilman and colleagues has demonstrated that self-reported condom use was not associated with lower STI incidence. Another study conducted by Cowan and colleagues, among Zimbabwean high school students, found poor correlation between STI prevalence and reported sexual experience, due to students' concerns about the confidentiality of the data collection methods.

The individually or cluster-randomised control trial undoubtedly provides the soundest evidence of intervention effects. However, randomised controlled trials are often not feasible when evaluating HIV prevention interventions that attempt to effect changes at community or societal level. Another challenge in evaluating interventions that aim for community level and broader social change is that their impact on communities, society and HIV may take years to manifest.

Outcome measures, such as reductions in risk behaviour or STIs, contribute little to an understanding of why a programme succeeds or fails. Process evaluations, on the other hand, are able to examine what it is about a particular programme that determines its success or failure, enabling others to understand the processes that lead to success. The value of a qualitative, process evaluation is illustrated in the Mothusimpilo case study, where it provides insight into why a comprehensive, carefully conceived and apparently well-resourced HIV prevention programme had no impact on STI incidence.

Preventing HIV in South Africa poses the ultimate challenge to our society. Based on the experiences of the Mothusimpilo project, Campbell insists that the HIV epidemic is extraordinary, requiring extraordinary approaches to prevention. Small-scale, short-term HIV prevention projects are important, but they need to be part of a broader commitment to develop and sustain long-term, large-scale, well-resourced interventions capable of altering the historically constituted, political, economic conditions that have been identified as shaping vulnerability and risk behaviour. These comprehensive approaches require long-term vision, coordinated planning across sectors, and strong political commitment.

Case Study

The Soul City Institute for Health and Development Communication is a South African non-governmental organisation that uses the mass media to improve health and well-being. Soul City is an extremely popular national, multi-media 'edutainment' vehicle that integrates health and development issues into prime time television and radio dramas, supported by print material. Soul City reaches approximately 17 million South Africans. Advocacy (including community

mobilisation and media advocacy) complements the edutainment
media. This case study focuses on one of the Soul City series.

How does Soul City attempt to reduce sexual risk behaviour?

Soul City series 4 comprised a 13-part prime-time television drama, a
45-part radio drama transmitted in nine languages through the
public broadcaster, three full-colour booklets distributed through ten
newspapers nationally, a national advocacy strategy involving lobbying of Government and decision makers, and community mobilisation. It set out to achieve reductions in sexual risk behaviour,
domestic violence and sexual harassment by:

- **Affecting the individual determinants of health**. Soul City uses
  concepts from selected socialpsychological theories to accomplish
  individual behaviour change. For example, the television drama
  features Pinki, a young woman who escapes a situation in which
  she was becoming financially and emotionally dependent on a
  sexual partner and in which she was at risk of abuse and HIV infection. She then models self-confidence and independence in relation
  to men and her story demonstrates the benefits of sustaining
  one's independence through personal savings. The story provides
  viewers with a learning opportunity as they follow the behaviour
  of this protagonist, successes and mistakes included. It aims to
  build viewers' confidence (self-efficacy) in their ability to achieve
  their aspirations through personal savings and entrepreneurship
  (as opposed to dependence on sexual partners).
- **Creating a supportive interpersonal environment**. The drama
  portrays respected community elders, traditional leaders, nurses,
  and priests as role models who take a stand against violence
  against women, and have caring, supportive attitudes about HIV.
- **Creating a supportive social and political environment**. Media
  advocacy aims to increase public support for more effective public
  health policies: policies to create a supportive social and political
  environment in which individual decisions about health behaviours are made. Soul City advocates joining forces with the
  National Network on Violence Against Women (NNVAW) to provide
  grassroots support to Soul City audiences and to mobilise individuals and communities to take action to end the abuse of women.
  Soul City and NNVAW launched a campaign to advocate for and
  ensure the speedy and effective implementation of the new
  Domestic Violence Act, aimed at protecting women from abuse.

Evidence of Soul City's effects

- **At the individual level**: Scheepers and colleagues, based on the findings of two consecutive, national, cross-sectional surveys, each including 2000 participants, reported that Soul City exposure was associated with:
  - increasing awareness and more accurate knowledge
  - stimulating interpersonal dialogue within families and other social networks
  - increasing self-efficacy and a sense of empowerment (particularly among women)
  - decreasing experience of negative social or peer pressure
  - shifting attitudes, intentions and intermediate practice towards sustaining healthier choices (ie health-seeking / support-seeking behaviour as well as support-giving behaviour)
- **In the immediate interpersonal environment**: Soul City commissioned a qualitative study in two sentinel sites (a rural and an urban community), comprising 30 interviews with community leaders, and representatives of social and health services. Goldstein and Scheepers and colleagues illustrated how Soul City messages had influenced many of the respondents to address the problem of HIV more effectively and sensitively. For example, nurses described how they had been influenced to care more about patients and to change clinic policy to make condoms more accessible. Religious leaders used Soul City as an example in sermons, and were moved to overcome the taboos around dealing with youth sexuality.
- **In the broader social environment**: Soul City commissioned a qualitative evaluation consisting of 97 interviews and focus

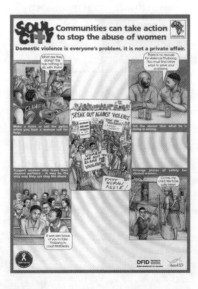

Soul City: an exceptionally popular drama grounded in local contexts, developed through thorough formative research, addressing personal, proximal and distal factors related to HIV risk behaviour, and committed to evaluation groups with National and Provincial Government, service providers, NGOs, institutions, and community members, to assess their role in facilitating the implementation of the Domestic Violence Act. The study indicates that Soul City played a role in public protests and community mobilisation against violence against women. For example, one respondent said, 'Soul City influenced us to organise the march ...' (This was consistent with the survey finding that exposure to Soul City television and radio broadcasts was associated with reported participation in public protests against violence against women.) The study also illustrated the role played by Soul City and the NNVAW in both pressurising and supporting the police to implement the Act.

Case study

The Mothusimpilo (working-together-for-health) project was started in 1998 in the Carltonville mining community near Johannesburg. Carltonville is the site of the largest gold-mining complex in the world.

Intervention

The project aimed to reduce the STI and HIV prevalence among miners living in twelve single-sex mine hostels, commercial sex workers living in informal settlements close to the mine hostels, and the residents of the nearby township. Based on the premise that the impact of health programmes is likely to be maximised by the participation and representation of 'grassroots' communities in planning and implementation, the project sought to achieve two forms of local community participation:

- Community-led peer education, by recruiting and training peer educators among mineworkers, sex workers and young people in and out of school; and
- the establishment of a multi-stakeholder committee, to draw in, and create partnerships among a broad range of local community representatives (mine management, trade unions, grassroots community organisations, academics, funders, and representatives from provincial and national health services) in collaborative project management and implementation.

The project also:
- distributed condoms through peer educators and clinics
- trained nurses, general practitioners and traditional healers in syndromic management of STIs; and
- instituted periodic (monthly) presumptive treatment for curable STIs among sex workers (which only started in February 2000).

Theoretical approach

In its desire to move beyond individualistic biomedical and behavioural policies and interventions, the project attempted to have an impact on a range of community-level factors and relationships assumed to play a key role in the success or failure of health promotion interventions. Specifically, the project attempted to mobilise and build *bonding* and *bridging* social capital. The peer education initiatives sought to build bonding social capital by supporting the development of homogenous groups, such as sex workers, miners and school students, bonded in trusting, reciprocally supportive relationships with a positive common identity. These relationships were to provide the context for the development of a *critical consciousness* of the way in which gender relations and poverty serve as obstacles to behaviour change, a collective renegotiation of sexual and social identities in ways that are less damaging to sexual health, and the development of confidence and empowerment to be able to engage in safer sexual behaviour. Bridging social capital was identified in relationships of trust and support among groups of people with an overlapping mutual interest (the prevention of HIV) whose access to varying resources may in turn be mobilised to benefit the community in question. The project recognised that the HIV prevention efforts of socially and economically marginalised communities such as miners and sex workers needed to be supported and reinforced by those of more powerful stakeholder groups. It sought to build bridging social capital through the multi-stakeholder committee, so that an array of resources along with various sources of power and expertise could be brought to bear on the HIV problem in the mining community.

Was the project effective?

The quantitative outcome evaluation, conducted by Williams and colleagues, comprising cross-sectional surveys (a randomised controlled trial was considered to be unethical and not logistically possible) in 1998 and 2000 among mineworkers, sex workers and adults in the community, demonstrated some changes in reported sexual behaviour. For example, among miners, the prevalence of reported consistent condom use with casual partners increased from 13% to 27%, a statistically significant difference. However, the prevalence of all three curable STIs either remained steady or increased over the two years, across all groups. For example, among miners, the prevalence of chlamydia increased from 4% to 14%, syphilis increased from 6% to 8% and gonorrhoea from 3% to 7%. The prevalence of HIV at baseline among men and women in the general population, mineworkers, and sex workers, was 20%, 37%, 29% and 69%, respectively. The HIV prevalence in 2000 was not available at the time of writing.

Why did the project fail to reduce STI prevalence?

The qualitative process evaluation conducted by Campbell sheds light on the factors that may have been responsible. It comprised ongoing in-depth interviews over the course of five years with miners, sex workers, young community residents, project workers and stakeholders, and a review of project documentation. It illustrates how, in a context of overwhelming poverty and brutal competition for very limited resources, the project succeeded in mobilising bonding social capital and building cohesive sex worker-led peer groups, with a commitment to condom use. Yet, the project failed to effectively build bridging social capital through the multi-stakeholder committee. The quality and quantity of the stakeholders' commitment to the project varied, and some of the more powerful stakeholders failed to support efforts to develop health-enabling social conditions in the mining community, preferring to devote their energies to STI management. One consequence was that the project was unable to establish adequate peer groups among male miners, who hold the economic and psychological power to undermine condom use in encounters with sex workers. A major consequence of the failure of the multi-stakeholder committee was that economically and socially marginalised community members were isolated from those with power to impact on the economic, political and social conditions in their environment.

Bibliography

ABDOOL KARIM Q, PRESTON-WHYTE E, ABDOOL KARIM SS. 'Teenagers seeking condoms at family planning services, Part 1: A user's perspective.' *South African Medical Journal* 1992; 82: 107–110.

ABDOOL KARIM SS, ABDOOL KARIM Q, PRESTON-WHYTE E, SANKAR N. 1992. 'Reasons for lack of condom use among high school students.' *South African Medical Journal* 1992; 82: 107–110.

CAMPBELL C. *'Letting them Die.' How HIV/AIDS prevention programmes often fail.* 2003 Cape Town: Double Storey Books.

COWAN FM, LANGHAUG LF, MASHUNGUPA GP, NYAMURERA T, HARGROVE J, JAFFAR S, ET AL. 'School based HIV prevention in Zimbabwe: Feasibility and acceptability of evaluation trials using biological outcomes.' *AIDS* 2002; 16: 1673–1678.

DICLEMENTE RJ, CROSBY RA, KEGLER MC (EDS). 2002. *Emerging Theories in Health Promotion Practice and Research. Strategies for Improving Public Health.* San Francisco: Jossey-Bass Publishers.

DUNKLE KL, JEWKES RK, BROWN HC, GRAY GE, MCINTYRE JA, HARLOW SD. 'Gender-based violence, relationship power and risk of HIV infection in women attending antenatal clinics in South Africa.' *Lancet* 2004; 363: 1415–1421.

EATON L, FLISHER AJ, AARØ LE. 'Unsafe sexual behaviour in South African youth.' *Social Science and Medicine* 2003; 56: 149–165.

FISHBEIN M, BANDURA A, TRIANDIS HC, KANFER FH, BECKER, MH AND MIDDLESTADT, SE. *Factors influencing behavior and behavior change. Final report:* Theorist's workshop. Washington, October 3–5. 1991.

GLANZ K, LEWIS FM, RIMER BK (EDS). 1990. *Health Behavior and Health Education. Theory, Research and Practice.* San Francisco: Jossey-Bass Publishers.

GOLDSTEIN S, USDIN S, SCHEEPERS E, JAPHET G. *Communicating HIV and AIDS, what works? A report on the impact evaluation of Soul City's fourth series.* Unpublished report available from Soul City. www.soulcity.org.za

HANNENBERG RS, ROJANAPITHAYAKORN W, KUNASOL P, SOKAL DC. 'Impact of Thailand's HIV-control programme as indicated by the decline of sexually transmitted diseases.' *Lancet* 1994; 344: 243–245.

HARVEY B, STUART J, SWAN T. 'Evaluation of a drama-in-education programme to increase AIDS awareness in South African high schools: A randomized community intervention trial.' *International Journal of STD and AIDS* 2000; 11: 105–111.

JEWKES R. 'Child sexual abuse and HIV infection.' 2004. In: Richter L, Dawes A. and Higson-Smith C. *The sexual abuse of young children in Southern Africa* Pretoria: HSRC Press. pp 130–142.

KAMB ML, FISHBEIN M, DOUGLAS JM, RHODES F, ROGERS J, BOLAN G, ET AL. 'Efficacy of Risk-Reduction Counseling to Prevent Human Immunodeficiency Virus and other Sexually Transmitted Diseases. A Randomized Controlled Trial.' *Journal of the American Medical Association* 1998; 20: 1161–1167.

KATZENSTEIN D ET AL. 'Peer education among factory workers in Zimbabwe: Providing a sustainable HIV prevention intervention.' Abstract No. 33514, XII International Conference on AIDS, Geneva, 1998.

KELLY JA, MURPHY DA, SIKKEMA KJ, MCAULIFFE TL, ROFFMAN RA, SOLOMAN LJ, WINETT RA, KALICHMAN SC, AND THE COMMUNITY HIV PREVENTION RESEARCH COLLABORATIVE. 'Randomized, controlled, community-level HIV-prevention intervention for sexual-risk behavior among homosexual men in US cities.' *Lancet* 1997; 350: 1500–1504.

KELLY K, PARKER W. *Communities of Practice. Contextual mediators of youth response to HIV/AIDS. Sentinel site monitoring and evaluation project.* Centre for AIDS Development, Research and Evaluation. 2000. www.cadre.org.za.

KIRBY D. 'The impact of schools and school programs upon adolescent sexual behavior.' *Journal of Sex Research* 2002; 39: 27–33.

LURIE MN, WILLIAMS BG, ZUMA K, MKAYA-MWAMBURI D, GARNETT G, STURM AW, SWEAT MD, GITTELSOHN J, ABDOOL KARIM SS. 'The impact of migration on HIV-1 transmission in South Africa: A study of migrant and nonmigrant men and their partners.' *Sexually Transmitted Diseases* 2003; 30: 149–156.

MULLEN PD, RAMIREZ G, STROUSE D, HEDGES LV, SOGOLOW E. 'Meta-analysis of the effects of behavioral HIV prevention interventions on the sexual risk behavior of sexually experienced adolescents in controlled studies in the United States.' *Journal of Acquired Immune Deficiency Syndrromes* 2002; 30 Suppl 1: S94–S105.

SHISANA O, BEZUIDENHOUT F, BROOKES HJ, CHAUVEAU J, COLVIN M, CONNOLLY C, DITLOPO P, KELLY K, MOATTI JP, LOUNDOU DA, PARKER W, RICHTER L, SCHWABE C, SIMBAYI LC, DAVID STOKER D, TOEFY Y, VAN ZYL J. 2002. *Nelson Mandela/HSRC Study on HIV/AIDS.* Cape Town: Human Sciences Research Council.

NEUMANN MS, JOHNSON WD, SEMAAN S, FLORES SA, PEERSMAN G, HEDGES LV, SOGOLOW E. 'Review and Meta-analysis of HIV Prevention Intervention Research for Heteroexual Adult Populations in the United States.' *Journal of Acquired Immune Deficiency Syndromes* 2002; 30 Suppl 1: S106–S117.

PARKER RG, EASON D, KLEIN CH. 'Structural barriers and facilitators in HIV prevention: A review of international research.' *AIDS* 2000; 14 (suppl 1): S22–S32.

RICHTER L, DAWES A, HIGSON-SMITH C. 2004. *The sexual abuse of young children in Southern Africa.* Pretoria: HSRC Press.

SCHEEPERS E, CHRISTOFIDES NJ, GOLDSTEIN S, USDIN S, PATEL DS , JAPHET G. *Evaluating health communication – a holistic overview of the impact of Soul City IV.* Health Promotion Journal of Australia. 2004; 2: 121–133.

VERGNANI T, FLISHER AJ, BLIGNAUT R. 'Factors affecting condom use by South African adolescents.' 14th International AIDS Conference, Barcelona, Spain, 7–12 July 2002.

VOLUNTARY HIV-1 COUNSELING AND TESTING EFFICACY STUDY GROUP. 'Efficacy of voluntary HIV-1 counselling and testing in individuals and couples in Kenya, Tanzania, and Trinidad: A randomised trial.' *Lancet* 2000; 356: 103–12.

WILLIAMS BG, TALJAARD D, CAMPBELL CM, GOUWS E, NDHLOVU L, VAN DAM J, CARAËL M, AUVERT B. 'Changing patterns of knowledge, reported behaviour and sexually transmitted infections in a South African gold mining community.' *AIDS* 2003; 17: 2099–2107.

ZENILMAN JM, WEISMAN CS, ROMPALO AM, ELLISH N, UPCHURCH DM, HOOK EW, CELENTANO D. 'Condom use to prevent incident STDs: The validity of self-reported condom use.' *Sexually Transmited Diseases* 1995; 22: 15–21.

CHAPTER 10
Barrier methods

Landon Myer

CONDOMS REMAIN AN EFFECTIVE way to prevent pregnancy and the transmission of sexually transmitted infections, including HIV. They have a long history, first recorded in ancient Egypt.

Most condoms today are made of latex, but newer materials such as polyurethane are being used, particularly for female condoms. Condoms are often packaged with either a non-allergenic powder or a silicone-based lubricant that may contain a spermicide.

Used correctly, condoms are highly effective in preventing the transmission of HIV and other STIs. Studies of serodiscordant couples show that the transmission of HIV is substantially reduced with 100% condom use. Female condoms, used correctly, are as effective in preventing disease transmission as male condoms.

There are three main sources of male and female condoms in South Africa: free through the public sector, through social marketing programmes and through commercial distributors.

Levels of condom use vary widely between groups, but are thought generally to be low in South Africa. Barriers to condom use include perceptions that their use means lack of trust and infidelity, and the social and economic disempowerment of women.

Despite recent advances in other areas of HIV prevention, including behavioural interventions, microbicides and vaccines, condoms remain a pivotal part of the fight against HIV/AIDS. Condoms are inexpensive and relatively easy to use. They provide protection against transmission of HIV and a wide range of other sexually transmitted infections (STIs) as well as pregnancy. Although there are a number of significant barriers to condom use, these are not insurmountable, and there are a range of interventions that seek to address the most prominent barriers to condom use in the South African context.

The first record of condom use comes from Egypt, where hieroglyphics recorded before 1000 BC showed men wearing sheaths over their erect penises. Condoms were used during the Roman Empire, and the word condom is probably derived from the Latin *condon*, meaning receptacle. In Europe during the seventeenth and eighteenth century, condoms made from linen or animal intestine were available for both pregnancy prevention as well as prophylaxis against STIs. The rubber condom as we know it today was first widely produced after the vulcanisation of rubber was patented in 1844. Through the first half of the twentieth century, condoms remained the most widely available form of contraception and STI prevention. But as effective treatment for many STIs and alternative forms of contraception became widely available, condom use declined in much of the world in the 1950s through 1970s; it has only been in the 1980s and 1990s that condoms regained widespread attention in response to the HIV/AIDS epidemic.

Today, most condoms are made from latex harvested from the tropical rubber tree. During the manufacturing process the raw latex is mixed with various chemicals to improve its durability and flexibility. To create the appropriate shape, steel or glass models are dipped into liquid rubber and allowed to dry. By repeating this dipping and drying process a number of times, a condom of appropriate thickness is created. The completed condom is sealed within a light- and heat-resistant plastic package to improve its durability under various storage conditions. Condoms are often packaged with either a fine non-allergenic powder or a silicone-based lubricant that may contain a spermicide (oil-based lubricants are avoided as they facilitate the degradation of latex). Although the vast majority of male condoms available today are made of latex rubber, condoms made of animal intestine (often referred to as 'natural skin' condoms) are still manufactured by some commercial companies. There are also a number of plastics and other artificial materials, most notably different types of polyurethane, that are used in female condoms and increasingly some types of male condoms.

Efficacy of condoms

When used correctly, the modern condom is highly effective in preventing the sexual transmission of HIV and several other sexually transmitted infections. As FIGURE 10.1 shows, the HIV particle is substantially smaller than bacterial STIs and human sperm; thus, condoms designed to prevent the transmission of HIV will also prevent the passage of other organisms (condoms can even prevent the transmission of the Hepatitis B virus, which at approximately 0.00004 mm in size, is substantially smaller than HIV).

Relative Cell Sizes

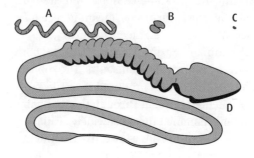

FIGURE 10.1 Relative sizes of human sperm and various pathogens that are blocked by male latex condoms *Source: Family Health International/Hill Studio. This illustration appeared in the monograph: The Male Latex Condom: Recent Advances, Future Directions*

A. *Treponema pallidum* (syphilis)
B. *Neisseria gonorrhoea* (gonorrhoea)
C. Human immunodeficiency virus (HIV)
D. Human sperm

Male condoms have demonstrated efficacy in preventing transmission of a wide range of bacterial STIs, including *Treponema pallidum* (syphilis), *Neisseria gonorrhoea* (gonorrhoea), *Trichomonas vaginalis* (trichomoniasis) and *Chlamydia trachomatis* (chlamydia). The role of condoms in preventing bacterial vaginosis in women is less clear, as it is difficult to discern any protective effect of condoms from the increased risk of bacterial vaginosis associated with both sexual intercourse and the insertion of foreign substances into the vagina. The role of male condoms in preventing viral infections other than HIV is also well established, as strong data exist to show that male condoms reduce the sexual transmission of herpes simplex, hepatitis B, and human papilloma viruses. Interestingly, there has been some question as to whether the protective efficacy of the male condom may differ for female-to-male transmission versus male-to-female transmission for some infections, particularly those such as herpes simplex virus in which infectious lesions may be found in genital areas not covered by a condom. This possibility is biologically plausible; however, there are no strong data to support appreciable gender differences in the protection conferred by condoms.

The strongest evidence for the role of condoms in preventing the transmission of HIV comes from serodiscordant couples studies which uniformly show that increased condom use is associated with substantially reduced risk of HIV transmission. However, there are still important questions regarding whether inconsistent condom use (that is, condom use in less than 100% of sexual contacts) is protective. While some studies have suggested that inconsistent condom use may offer more protection than no condom use whatsoever, others have demonstrated that the transmission of HIV among irregular condom users is similar to that of individuals who do not use condoms. For instance, in a study of self-reported condom use and HIV incidence among 17 264 individuals in rural Uganda, inconsistent condom use was associated with a similar incidence of HIV as no condom use. In the same study, consistent condom use was associated with a dramatically reduced risk of incident HIV infection compared with no condom use. Furthermore, how imperfect condom use (for instance, some vaginal penetration prior to the condom being put onto the penis) may affect condom efficacy against HIV is not well understood.

Compared with the male condom, there are generally fewer epidemiological data regarding the efficacy of the female condom in preventing HIV and other STIs. However, the female condom protects essentially the same mucosal surface area as the male condom, and the polyurethane and other materials used in the construction of the female condom are generally stronger and less permeable than the latex rubber used in most male condoms. As a result, it is generally accepted that the efficacy of the female condom, when used correctly, in preventing transmission of HIV and other STIs is at least comparable to that of male condoms. In addition, there has been some research into the question of whether female condoms can be reused (unlike the male condom if they are cleaned appropriately); while this practice is not widely recommended, it does seem feasible, as female condoms do not degrade appreciably after several washings.

Regarding the use of condoms for prophylaxis against unwanted pregnancy, few data on comparative contraceptive efficacy exist for South Africa and other developing countries. However, studies from the United States and Europe have shown that among couples using male condoms as their sole form of contraception, the proportion of women becoming pregnant in the first year of condom use range from 3% for perfectly consistent use to 14% for typical use; the corresponding proportions for female condoms range from 5% for perfect use to 21% for typical use. While these statistics are substantially lower than for most hormonal methods of contraception (for example, the combined oral contraceptive pill has a corresponding pregnancy proportion of 0.5% for perfect use, making it approximately 28 times more effective than typical condom use), they are broadly comparable to the efficacy of the diaphragm and withdrawal methods for pregnancy prevention. The contraceptive efficacy of condoms has important implications for 'dual protection' – the prophylaxis of both pregnancy and sexual infection – which may require more than condom use alone.

Public sector condom distribution in South Africa

Male and female condoms are available in South Africa through three general sources: free of charge through the public sector, through social marketing programmes operated by non-governmental organisations (NGOs), and through commercial distributors.

Public sector condoms are purchased by the National Department of Health and are distributed free of charge to the public. These condoms are made available largely through public sector health facilities such as primary care clinics, community health centres, or AIDS Training, Information and Counselling Centres (ATICCs) in each province. A substantial number of public sector condoms are also distributed through government offices and departments, as well as NGOs that work in HIV/AIDS prevention and reproductive health such as the Planned Parenthood Association of South Africa (PPASA). In addition, private individuals and organisations are allowed to procure and distribute public sector condoms from provincial and local supply stores free of charge; in this way, industry and other private businesses can make condoms available to their employees.

The distribution of public sector condoms has been a key part of the National Department of Health's HIV prevention strategy. In the early 1990s, a small condom procurement and distribution project was the principal activity of the national government's HIV/AIDS programme. However, the numbers of condoms distributed by the government has increased dramatically since 1994 as part of the expanded HIV/AIDS prevention efforts (see FIGURE 10.2). In 2002, approximately 350 million male condoms were distributed nationally at a cost of slightly more than 100 million rand (roughly 29 cents per condom). It is anticipated that the numbers of condoms distributed by the Department of Health will continue to rise, albeit at a slower rate, with an estimated 400 million male condoms to be distributed during the 2003/2004 financial year. Across much of sub-Saharan Africa, the 'condom gap' – the difference between the estimated need for condoms and the numbers actually distributed – has been cited as a fundamental barrier to HIV prevention efforts; in the case of South Africa, this gap appears to be closing.

In the past there have been widespread concerns regarding the quality of the condoms distributed by the government, with a number of recalls of specific batches of public sector condoms, as well as anecdotal reports of low-quality condoms leading to frequent breakage and tearing. In response to these trends, the Department of

Health updated its quality standards based on international technical guidelines and refined its procurement specifications considerably. Although public sector condoms are still sometimes stigmatised as inferior products, in part due to their generic packaging (in contrast to the specific brands of condoms that are available for sale), the condoms that are distributed through the Department of Health today are of a comparable quality to other sources of condoms in South Africa.

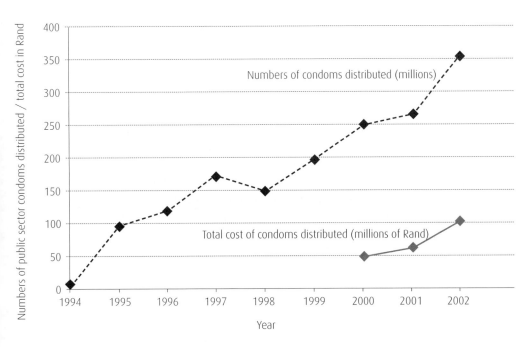

FIGURE 10.2 Public sector male condom distribution and costs in South Africa, 1994–2002. Note: Cost and distribution statistics for 2002 are best available estimates; cost data prior to 2000 is not available
Source: Mr John Wilson, National Department of Health Logistics

With a growing number of condoms distributed through the public sector, additional concerns have been raised around the possible wastage of free condoms. To address this question, a study undertaken during 1998 and 1999 followed individuals who had procured condoms from public sector health facilities around the country for up to six weeks in order to trace what actually happened to the individual condoms procured. Of the 384 individuals and 5528 condoms followed, this study found that 44% had been used during sex, 22% had been given away to other people, and less than 10% had been discarded; the remainder were still available for use. Extrapolating these findings to public sector condom distribution in 2002, at least 150 million male condoms were used during sex – or almost 14 condoms used in sex – for every South African man between the ages of 15 and 49.

The Department of Health's programme for the public sector distribution of female condoms was implemented in 1998 but has been substantially smaller than the male condom programme. This is attributable primarily to the increased cost of female condoms: in 2002, female condoms cost the national government R7.50 per condom, making them roughly 25 times more expensive than male condoms. There have been substantial operational challenges encountered in developing the female condom programme from scratch, and despite considerable interest from policy-makers and researchers, the long-term demand in the general population for this new prevention technology remains unclear. The female condom pilot programme has expanded from 27 sites across the country in 2000 distributing some 600 000 female condoms, to over 200 sites distributing approximately 2.5 million female condoms in 2002, and should continue to grow in the coming years. However, the rate of growth will be determined by the general population's acceptance of the female condom. A study undertaken by the Reproductive Health Research Unit indicates that partner reluctance, over-lubrication and size of the device may hinder its sustained growth.

Case study

In keeping with the growth in condom distribution nationally, condom distribution in the Western Cape has increased substantially in the last few years. In 1997, roughly 4.5 million male condoms were distributed free of charge to the public; during 2003, well over 20 million public sector condoms were distributed, representing about 6% of the national total. In order to facilitate all forms of condom distribution, public sector condoms can be procured from the provincial supply store by anyone, free of charge. Analysis of provincial supply records shows that in the year from June 2002 to May 2003, almost 1000 orders were placed for a total of 22 million public sector condoms from the provincial warehouse (or approximately 18 condoms distributed for every man in the province between the ages of 15 and 49). These were distributed in the following way:

- the majority (12.7 million condoms, or 60%) went to the public sector health care system (including primary, secondary and tertiary facilities);
- almost four million condoms (19% of the total) were ordered by NGOs such as the Planned Parenthood Association (PPA), the Triangle Project, Sex Worker Education and Advocacy Taskforce (SWEAT) and the Society for Family Health;

- 1.8 million (9%) were distributed through business and industry;
- 1.4 million (7%) were distributed through private medical care systems (including GPs, pharmacists, as well as private clinics and hospitals);
- more than 600 000 (3%) were distributed by universities and technikons; and
- approximately 500 000 (2%) were distributed through government offices.

Condom social marketing

While the growing public sector condom distribution programme represents an important element of the Department of Health's HIV prevention efforts, the sustainability of the programme has been questioned. Currently the national condom procurement and distribution logistics system is driven by international donor-funded consultants and it is unclear whether the current increases in public sector condom distribution will be able to continue into the coming years, particularly if there is a shift in donor support. It may be unrealistic to expect that the South African government could, or should, meet the growing demand for condoms (both male and female) across the country. Two alternative sources of condoms seek to fill continuing unmet needs.

Commercial condom brands, such as Durex and Contempo, are sold through a variety of different retail outlets. These brands are sold for profit, are targeted at those who can afford them, and are too expensive for the majority of South Africans to use regularly. A more affordable alternative is provided by condoms distributed through social marketing programmes. Like commercially marketed condoms, these are sold as a particular brand (in contrast to generic public sector condoms), however the prices are substantially lower than commercial brands. The principal social marketing male condom brand sold in South Africa is Lover's Plus, which is distributed by a Johannesburg-based NGO, the Society for Family Health. Lover's Plus has a substantially lower retail price and is available at a wide range of outlets around the country, including grocery and convenience stores, chemists, and a range of informal outlets. Lover's Plus has increased in popularity over the past several years, and a brand of female condoms (Care condoms), as well as another male condom social marketing brand (Trust condoms), have been introduced.

Part of the underlying rationale for the social marketing approach is the idea that health services and technologies that are available free of charge are less likely to be valued, and may be more likely to be wasted, than technologies for which individuals must pay even a nominal amount. In keeping with this idea, social marketing condoms aim to be inexpensive enough to be widely accessible, but still cost enough to be valued and associated with quality in the eyes of consumers. The distribution of social marketing condoms in South Africa has been accompanied by a series of popular advertising campaigns aimed at promoting both awareness of condoms in general, as well as particular social marketing brands. The numbers of male condoms distributed through social marketing across the country has recently increased substantially, from less than one million condoms sold in 1996 to more than 10-million in 2002; although condom social marketing programmes in South Africa are considerably smaller than the national public sector distribution programme, social marketing continues to fill a critical niche in improving condom accessibility and promoting condom use, particularly among young people.

Prevalence of condom use

Although the numbers of condoms distributed in South Africa has increased over the past decade, whether this has been paralleled by an increase in condom use remains unclear. There are no data, from either the general population or particular risk groups (such as young people or commercial sex workers), that allow a meaningful comparison of changing condom use patterns through time, and comparisons of the results of different studies are made more difficult by variability in the measures of condom use employed.

Probably the best available data on condom use nationally comes from the 1998 Demographic and Health Survey (DHS) conducted by the Department of Health and the Medical Research Council. In a nationally representative sample of women aged 15 to 49 years who were sexually active in the year prior to being interviewed, this study found that overall 22% of women reported having ever used a condom during sex, and 8% reported using a condom during their last sexual contact. However, there is substantial variation in condom use with age: 20% of women aged 15 to 19 years reported condom use at last sexual intercourse, compared with 3% of women aged 45 to 49. Levels of reported condom use were highest in urban populations; among provinces, women in Gauteng and the Free State reporting the highest levels of condom use, and women in the Eastern and Northern Cape the lowest. Across the country, only 2% of women surveyed reported using a condom for contraception.

Numerous other studies have reported the prevalence of condom use in particular study populations from different parts of the country. While the levels of condom use vary substantially depending on the group studied and the exact measures involved, the overall trends in the literature support the DHS finding that levels of condom use are generally low, though it is more common among young people and in urban settings. Moreover, consistent condom users appear to comprise only a fraction of all individuals reporting condom use – indicating that an even smaller proportion of at-risk individuals achieve maximal protection. And although to date no South African research has focused on the sexual behaviours of HIV-infected individuals, it is important to note that these low levels of condom use are likely to apply both to HIV-negative individuals who are susceptible to infection, as well as those who are infected and may potentially transmit the virus to others.

Condom use is often dependent on type of relationship or circum-stance, with evidence from a wide range of settings indicating that condoms are more likely to be used in casual or non-regular partner-ships, but remains unlikely at first sex for both men and women.

Barriers to condom use

A number of factors have been implicated as barriers to condom use, with the findings from South African research supporting evidence from elsewhere in sub-Saharan Africa. Probably the most common barrier to condom use is the widespread perception of condoms as representing high-risk sexual partnerships. In many sexual relation-ships, condoms are associated with infidelity, lack of trust, and the possibility of infection. As a result, attempts to introduce condom use into a sexual relationship can be fraught with confusion, awkward-ness and misunderstanding. Meanwhile, many men and women complain that wearing male condoms makes intercourse less pleasur-able – leading to popular analogies such as 'taking a shower while wearing a raincoat' or 'eating a sweet with the wrapper on'. Along with women's social and economic disempowerment in many South African communities, these factors render many women unlikely to be able to negotiate condoms with their partners, and many men unlikely to want to use condoms (and vice versa). As a result, many studies have shown that negative attitudes of both men and women towards condoms represent a basic barrier to their use.

In addition, a number of individual characteristics and behaviours are frequently linked to a lack of condom use among individuals at risk. Among psychological factors, individuals who perceive them-selves not to be at risk of becoming infected appear less likely to wear condoms, as do individuals who have less hope for their personal future. Among behavioural factors, condom use frequently varies with the type of sexual partner involved, with condom use between casual partners usually more common than between partners in a long-term monogamous relationship, a finding which emphasises the role of perceived risk in shaping behaviours. Several studies have demonstrated that alcohol consumption is associated with lack of condom use; this phenomenon is particularly problematic because many individuals meet high-risk sexual partners in social settings where alcohol is available. There are numerous data to suggest that condoms are also less likely to be used in partnerships where an effective form of contraception (usually injectable or oral hormonal contraceptives) is being used. This points to the need for interventions that promote dual method use (the simultaneous use of condoms with another form of contraception) among high-risk women.

One important predictor of condom use is previous experience using condoms. Several studies have suggested that individuals who have used condoms previously will be more likely to use them in the future. While this may seem self-evident, it points to the role of experience in facilitating condom use. It is likely that many of the complaints regarding condom use being less pleasurable for the male partner may be attributable to a lack of practical skills in condom use, particularly in putting condoms onto the penis correctly. Although public sector condoms do not come with instructions on their use, this suggests a need for more explicit user instructions accompanying condom distribution.

Probably the most fundamental barrier to condom use in South Africa is the poor availability and accessibility of condoms, despite the large numbers of condoms purchased for distribution by the national government. Shortages and stock-outs of public sector condoms have been common in previous years, though these are becoming less frequent as more condoms are purchased by the government and management of public sector distribution systems improve. For example, a 1998 survey of condom availability in KwaZulu-Natal found that 100% of public sector clinics and 55% of general practitioners had male condoms available. But even when condoms are available at a public sector health facility, their accessibility may be problematic. A 1992 study that used young men and women as simulated patients to assess the accessibility of condoms in 12 clinics around Durban found that in the ten clinics that had condoms available, actually accessing condoms proved difficult. Female patients were intimidated by clinic staff who disapproved of sexually active young women, and clinics distributed condoms in public spaces which did not allow for privacy. Issues of provider attitudes may have improved in recent years, particularly in urban areas. But in many settings, privacy and provider barriers continue to represent important hurdles to distributing condoms to those who may want them.

Interventions to promote condom use

Each of the barriers to condom use described above points to a particular form of intervention. Behavioural interventions often target many of these barriers in addressing sexual behaviour and risk-taking, described in detail as part of CHAPTER 9. There are two other categories of interventions that also seek to overcome specific barriers: interventions seeking to improve the accessibility of condoms, and developments in condom technology.

Improving accessibility

As mentioned above, the ability to access condoms is a basic hurdle to their use. For commercial and social marketing condoms, accessibility is largely a function of cost and availability for sale at retail outlets. Access is more complex in the case of public sector condoms that are distributed free of charge. Presuming an adequate supply of condoms through the public sector distribution system, condoms should be available at any public health facility. Although at one time condoms were distributed only through pharmacies, most facilities now use some form of open condom dispenser (if only in the form of an open box of condoms placed on a chair in a waiting area). Even so, many individuals are likely to feel awkward procuring condoms from a health facility, particularly young people. Others are likely to find accessing a health facility regularly to procure condoms difficult, particularly when the nearest facility has limited operating hours. To address these concerns, an increasing number of initiatives are underway to move public sector condom distribution away from health facilities. Some activities, such as using peer educators or community-health workers to distribute condoms (sometimes called community-based distribution), seek to make condoms more accessible to the general population. Other initiatives, often referred to as targeted distribution, seek to distribute condoms intensively among a particular group, such as commercial sex workers, which may be at increased risk. Another approach to targeted condom distribution is to make condoms accessible in places where people commonly meet casual sex partners (and thus are likely to need condoms), such as clubs, bars or shebeens. Usually these alternative forms of condom distribution are driven by NGOs, though the distribution of public-sector condoms by businesses to their workers, particularly common in industrial settings, may also be thought of as a form of targeted distribution.

Another way to increase the dissemination of condoms outside of public sector health facilities is via existing peer networks. One recent study of the passage of public sector condoms among peers showed that almost half of all individuals procuring public sector condoms had recent experience in either giving condoms to or receiving them from other people. This type of 'informal distribution' differs markedly by gender, with women more likely to be involved in giving or receiving condoms among family members, and men more likely to give or receive condoms among friends. Other research has considered the potential of traditional healers as possible distributors of condoms and behavioural risk-reduction messages. While more research is needed into these types of informal condom distribution, certainly this evidence demonstrates the potential for peer-based social networks for the distribution of condoms and other HIV prevention interventions.

One important system for targeted condom distribution that has not yet received adequate attention is condom availability at secondary schools. Intervening effectively among young people in educational settings is a critical challenge in HIV prevention, and adolescents have been the focus of numerous school-based interventions. Although condoms are widely available at most tertiary educational institutions, the notion of school-based condom distribution has been met with stiff resistance. Why there is no national policy to make public sector condoms available in schools remains unclear, however. There is strong evidence from elsewhere that the availability of condoms in schools does not promote sexual activity among young people, which has been suggested as a common concern. In fact, the opposite effect may result through the reinforcement of school-based sexual education messages. Although a small number of secondary schools have chosen to make condoms available to their students, school-based condom distribution remains largely unheard of in most parts of the country.

New technology

Recent improvements in condom technology seek to increase the comfort of condom use for both sexual partners while maintaining or improving the strength and efficacy of the condoms. Sometimes these aims are in direct opposition, seen most commonly in the thickness of condoms: the sensitivity of the condom decreases, but the strength of the condom increases, with increasing thickness of the latex used. Three other areas of technological advancement in condom design are size, shape and construction materials.

The size of the condom, as measured by the width of the condom as it is laid flat, is an important variable in condom construction. A condom that is too tight may be more difficult to put on and more likely to break during intercourse, while one that is too loose is more likely to slip off. Internationally condoms come in a range of sizes, from 47 to 55 millimetres, and recent evidence suggests that there may be considerable variation in erect penis sizes within and between populations. In South Africa, most public sector condoms are 52 to 53 millimetres in circumference and 170 to 180 millimetres long as part of a 'one size fits all' policy. Given the capacity of latex rubber to stretch while maintaining its strength, it is unlikely that a substantial number of individuals find these dimensions too small. Although there may be a need for variable condom sizing, particularly for sexually active youth who may benefit from slightly smaller condom sizes, there is little understanding of how penis sizes may vary across the South African population with age and even less idea of what size condoms are considered the most comfortable.

Different shapes of condoms are likely to have different characteristics of strength and comfort. Recent research suggests that condoms that are loose by design may allow greater sensation through friction than tighter condoms. Along these lines, different condom manufacturers are experimenting with a range of condom shapes to maximise comfort and pleasure (FIGURE 10.3). South African public sector condoms, and most versions available commercially in the country, are generally standard straight-sided condoms.

A third area of development in condom technology is in the materials used. Polyurethane male condoms (manufactured from the same material as the female condom) confer greater strength than

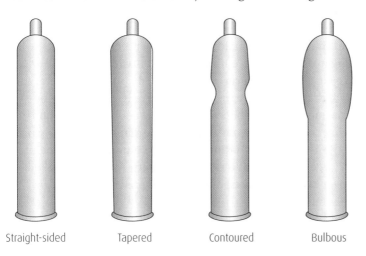

Straight-sided   Tapered   Contoured   Bulbous

FIGURE 10.3 Different condom shapes which may be used to maximise comfort during use *Source: Family Health International/Hill Studio. This illustration appeared in the monograph: The Male Latex Condom: Recent Advances, Future Directions*

their latex counterparts and avoid problems associated with latex allergies. Other developments focus on different kinds of lubricants, which will not compromise the structural strength of the condom; some, such as spermicidal and microbicidal lubricants, may enhance the protection provided by condoms against pregnancy and sexually transmitted infections. Various lubricants can be packaged into the condom during production, producing a pre-lubricated condom, or offered separately for individuals who prefer additional lubrication. In addition, opaque foil wrappers are likely to delay material degradation due to light exposure in comparison with translucent plastic packaging.

While the vast majority of South Africans would probably agree that sex protected with a condom is less pleasurable than unprotected sex, researchers have yet to document and disseminate different ways to improve the comfort of condom use. This could be a matter of size, of shape and/or of the materials involved, and may vary widely across a diverse population according to individual perceptions of pleasure. However, there are South Africans who have discovered ways of making condom use more comfortable. These are individuals who have used condoms regularly for a long period, such as commercial sex workers or couples who rely on condoms for family planning. Research among these groups can reveal different steps that can be taken to make condom use more comfortable – as has been demonstrated by research undertaken in developed countries. This in turn may inform a series of 'best practices' for comfortable condom use that can be incorporated into behavioural intervention materials promoting pleasurable and effective condom use to distribute alongside condoms. This represents an important area which has not yet been explored in South Africa.

Other barrier methods for HIV prevention

Besides the male and female condom, other methods which are being investigated for their potential to prevent HIV infection are devices that cover the cervix, eg cervical caps and diaphragms. Several studies indicate that the diaphragm, which is currently used as an inexpensive contraceptive method, could serve the additional function of reducing the risk of HIV transmission. The diaphragm is designed to cover the cervix, which is thought to be a vulnerable entry point to HIV. A large efficacy trial is planned in South Africa to assess the effectiveness of the vaginal diaphragm in preventing HIV.

Conclusion

Until alternative methods become available, male and female condoms will remain the principal technology for preventing the sexual transmission of HIV in South Africa. Although the gap between the need for condoms and the numbers actually distributed may be closing as a result of increases in the government's programme of distributing condoms free of charge, important barriers to condom use remain across the country. Ongoing interventions to improve the accessibility of condoms, as well as making condoms more comfortable to use, have the potential to increase condom use substantially.

Acknowledgements

The author would like to thank the following individuals for their assistance in the background research for this chapter: Brenda Smuts (Cape Metropole Health Department), Marleen Poolman (Provincial Administration of the Western Cape), David Nowitz (Society for Family Health), and John Wilson (consultant to the National Department of Health's HIV/AIDS & STD Directorate).

Bibliography

ABDOOL KARIM Q, ABDOOL KARIM SS, SOLDAN K, ZONDI M. 'Reducing the risk of HIV infection among South African sex workers: Socioeconomic and gender barriers'. *American Journal of Public Health* 1995; 85: 1521–1525.

ABDOOL KARIM Q, PRESTON-WHYTE E, ABDOOL KARIM SS. 'Teenagers seeking condoms at family planning services, part I: A user's perspective'. *South African Medical Journal* 1992; 82: 356–359.

ABDOOL KARIM Q, ABDOOL KARIM SS, PRESTON-WHYTE E. 'Teenagers seeking condoms at family planning services, part II: A provider's perspective'. *South African Medical Journal* 1992; 82: 360–362.

AHMED S, LUTALO T, WAWER M, SERWADDA D, SEWANKAMBO NK, NALUGODA F, MAKUMBI F, WABWIRE-MANGEN F, KIWANUKA N, KIGOZI G, KIDDUGAVU M, GRAY R. 'HIV incidence and sexually transmitted disease prevalence associated with condom use: A population study in Rakai, Uganda'. *AIDS* 2001; 15: 2171–2179.

BEKSINSKA ME, REES HV, DICKSON-TETTEH KE, MQOQI N, KLEINSCHMIDT I, MCINTYRE JA. 'Structural integrity of the female condom after multiple uses, washing, drying, and re-lubrication'. *Contraception* 2001; 63: 33–36.

DAVIS KR, WELLER SC. 'The effectiveness of condoms in reducing heterosexual transmission of HIV'. *Family Planning Perspectives* 1999; 31: 272–279.

GARDNER R, BLACKBURN RD, UPADHYAY, UD. 'Closing the Condom Gap'. *Population Reports*, Series H, Number 9. Baltimore, USA: Johns Hopkins University School of Public Health, Population Information Programme, 1999.

GILMOUR, E, ABDOOL KARIM SS, FOURIE HJ. 'Availability of condoms in urban and rural areas of KwaZulu-Natal, South Africa'. *Sexually Transmitted Diseases* 2000; 27: 353–357.

LAMPTEY PR, PRICE JE. 'Social marketing sexually transmitted disease and HIV prevention: A consumer-centred approach to achieving behaviour change'. *AIDS* 1998; 12(suppl 2): S1–S9.

LITTLE F, MYER L, MATHEWS C. 'Barriers to accessing free condoms at public health facilities across South Africa'. *South African Medical Journal* 2002; 92: 218–220.

McNEILL ET, GILMORE C, RINGER WE, LEWIS AH, SCHELLSTEDE WP. (EDS.). *'The Latex Condom: Recent Advances, Future Directions'*. North Carolina, USA: Family Health International, 1998.

MANTELL JE, SCHEEPERS E, ABDOOL KARIM Q. 'Introducing the female condom through the public sector: Experiences from South Africa'. *AIDS Care* 2000; 12: 589–601.

MYER L, MATHEWS C, LITTLE F, ABDOOL KARIM SS. 'The fate of free male condoms distributed to the public in South Africa'. *AIDS* 2001; 15: 789–793.

MYER L, MATHEWS C, LITTLE F. 'Improving the accessibility of condoms in South Africa: The role of informal distribution'. *AIDS Care* 2002; 14: 773–778.

SHELTON JD, JOHNSTON B. 'Condom gap in Africa: Evidence from donor agencies and key informants'. *British Medical Journal* 2001; 323: 139.

WORLD HEALTH ORGANISATION. *'The Male Latex Condom'*. Geneva: WHO, 1998.

CHAPTER 11

Mother-to-child transmission (MTCT) of HIV-1

Hoosen 'Jerry' Coovadia

MOST CHILDREN WITH HIV infection have contracted their disease through mother-to-child transmission and HIV/AIDS is a significant contributor to infant mortality in Africa.

MTCT occurs in utero, during labour and delivery and during breastfeeding. The overall transmission rates are between 25% and 45% of all children born to HIV positive women in Africa.

Maternal viral load has a direct effect on intrauterine, intrapartum and breastfeeding transmission; the higher the viral load the more likely is transmission. However, transmission may occur even at low viral loads and the relationship between viral load and breastfeeding is not absolute.

Obstetrical factors such as vaginal versus caesarian delivery, premature rupture of membranes and intervention during delivery contribute to HIV transmission. Infant factors such as prematurity and mucosal lesions also contribute.

There are various antiretroviral regimens that are known to prevent MTCT, the most effective involving more than one drug. However, many African countries, for reasons of cost, use only one drug. A much wider approach to the prevention of MTCT of HIV is needed that provides for the interests of the infected mother, her partner and their infected and uninfected children.

The scale of the problem

In all the plagues which have swept the world it is often women and children who are most affected. However, it is children who have to carry the promise of new life and the rebirth of nations in any catastrophe that has the potential to wipe out whole civilisations. HIV/AIDS is a pandemic whose impact is without precedent and this chapter deals with the crucial prevention of HIV infection in children and relevant aspects of maternal HIV/AIDS.

Year by year, as the pandemic spreads globally and threatens to engulf millions in India and China, the numbers of children infected and dying relentlessly increase. The toll is announced annually by UNAIDS. Since the initial recognition of the disease and the consequent pandemic, four million children under 15 years of age worldwide have been infected and in 2002 alone an estimated 800 000 children became newly infected. About 580 000 children died of HIV/AIDS in 2001. With few exceptions children acquire their HIV infection from their mothers. The prevalence of HIV in children will therefore be highest among populations in which the major route of transmission in adults is heterosexual. Africa bears 70% of the global burden of HIV in all age groups, but has at least 90% of all the HIV infected children in the world. Every day in Africa, about 2000 children acquire HIV infection from their mothers.

Without antiretrovirals, this is a lethal disease and progression to AIDS and death is much more rapid in children than in adults. In Africa, where deprivation and other social factors already dictate a high disease burden in poor children, the upper end of mortality in HIV-infected children is in the region of 55% by two years of age, 90% by three years, and 98% by five years. Childhood mortality rates are rising in many African countries. In the southern African region where HIV prevalences are the highest in the world, HIV/AIDS is a significant contributory factor to the deaths of children under five years of age.

Routes of transmission

Most, probably 90 to 95%, of HIV positive infants are infected through their mothers. Thus HIV prevalence figures from antenatal clinics are important indicators of the risk for infants and children. The remainder become HIV positive through unsafe procedures such as use of contaminated needles, medical equipment, blood and blood products. A small but unknown proportion may be due to practices which cause breaks in the skin or are victims of sexual coercion and abuse.

Mother-to-child transmission of HIV occurs in the intrauterine period, during labour and delivery and postnatally through breast-feeding. The proportion of transmission through each of these routes is shown in TABLE 11.1. The overall transmission rates (in the absence of known effective interventions) are between 25% to 45% of all children born to HIV positive women in Africa; higher than the range of 10% to 30% found in the industrialised countries. Intrauterine transmission may occur from early pregnancy, probably nearer the second trimester. The greatest likelihood, however, is during the last few months before delivery. HIV may be transmitted postnatally as long as breastfeeding continues. In the absence of breastfeeding, the virus can be detected up to four weeks to six weeks after birth. This is due to infection during labour and delivery, and a fraction from the intrauterine period.

Timing	Transmission Rate
During pregnancy	5–10%
During labour and delivery	10–20%
During breastfeeding	5–20%
Overall without breastfeeding	15–30%
Overall with breastfeeding till 6 months	25–35%
Overall with breastfeeding till 18 to 24 months	30–45%

TABLE 11.1 Timing and risks of transmission
Source: De Cock KM et al. JAMA 2000; 283: 1175-82

Risk factors for transmission

It is essential to understand the factors known to be associated with the passage of the virus from mother to infant to determine interventions that reduce this transmission. These may be maternal, viral and infant characteristics. The factors that have the strongest impact on the rate of HIV transmission are the severity of HIV disease in the mother (as reflected in the RNA viral load in plasma and in breastmilk, CD4 count, and in clinical progression), the route of delivery (caesarean section vs vaginal delivery), and the duration of breastfeeding.

Maternal viral load has a direct effect on intrauterine, intrapartum and breastfeeding transmission; the higher the viral load the greater the increase in the transmission rate. Women with newly acquired infection during pregnancy or postnatally, when viral loads are very high, are particularly likely to transmit virus to their infants. However, transmission may occur even at low viral loads while many infants remain uninfected despite high maternal viral loads. For breastfeeding in particular, there is at best an incomplete relationship between viral load and transmission, as the RNA load is highly variable between breasts and over time. This implies that other factors are also important for MTCT. The known risk factors and the strength of their association are given in TABLE 11.2.

Vaginal delivery increases the ingestion by the newborn of infected maternal blood, plasma and other secretions. Elective caesarean section decreases perinatal transmission by more than 50%.

Duration of breastfeeding has been shown by a number of studies from developing and industrialised countries to affect the rate of transmission. The estimated rate of HIV transmission over 24 months of breastfeeding is about 16%. In a recent meta-analysis of

Known Risk Factors	Inconclusive Risk Factors	Inconsistent Risk Factors
Severity of HIV	Host genetic factors	Primary HIV infection in mother
High maternal viral load	Immature immune system in infant	Prior HIV-infected sibling
Low maternal CD4	Viral genotype and/or phenotype	Older maternal age
Advanced maternal disease	Increased viral strain diversity	Primiparity
Delivery	Maternal neutralising antibody	Alcohol use during pregnancy
Duration of rupture of	Illicit drug use during pregnancy	History of abortions or stillbirths
membranes > 4 hours	Frequency of unprotected sexual	Duration of labour
Premature delivery < 37 weeks	intercourse	Low neonatal Apgar score
Breastfeeding	Multiple sex partners during	Low gastric acid secretion
Duration of breastfeeding	pregnancy	Immaturity of neonatal gastro-
Breastmilk viral load	Maternal nutritional status	intestinal tract
Mastitis	Anaemia during pregnancy	Infant gender
Cracked and bleeding nipples	Cigarette smoking	Season of birth
Breast abscess	Chorioamnionitis	Placental *P falciparum* infestation
	Abruptio placentae	Maternal vitamin A deficiency
	Sexually transmitted infections	Material tuberculosis and hepatitis
	(eg syphilis)	
	Use of foetal scalp electrodes	
	Episiotomy and vaginal tears	

TABLE 11.2 Risk Factors for Mother-To-Child-Transmission of HIV, according to strength of evidence
Adapted from Bulterys et al. AIDScience 2002; 2

breastfeeding studies from sub-Saharan Africa the cumulative probability of acquiring HIV infection after four weeks was about 3% at three months, 5% at six months, 9% at 12 months, and 15% at 18 months. The contribution of postnatal transmission to overall transmission after four weeks was estimated to be 42% in this study. As the optimum period for exclusive breastfeeding in all children (HIV+ and HIV-) is six months, it is worth noting the risk of transmission of about 6%–7% for this period.

There is uncertainty about the timing of breastfeeding transmission. Some studies have suggested that the highest rate of transmission occurs in the first six months (up to 75% of total transmission in a Kenyan randomised control trial), whilst the meta-analysis referred to above, found a constant risk of transmission throughout the breastfeeding period. Breast factors associated with MTCT include subclinical and overt mastitis, and cracked or bleeding nipples. The pattern of breastfeeding may also influence MTCT. In a study from Durban, South Africa, the rates of transmission by six months were similar (about 20%) in infants either exclusively breastfed or exclusively formula fed; this was lower than the rate (26.1%) in those given mixed feeding. At 15 months the rate remained lower in those exclusively breastfed compared with the mixed feed group. There is additional support for this finding but none sufficiently stringent to warrant acceptance of exclusive breastfeeding to reduce MTCT as public policy. There is no good evidence that maternal nutrition influences the transmission of HIV to infants.

Maternal HIV variants selected through immune pressure, and an MHC Class 1 gene uniquely expressed in the placental cytotrophoblast, may influence perinatal transmission. Chorioamnionitis has been associated with increased MTCT in some studies but not in others. A trial of pre- and intra-partum antibiotic prophylaxis of chorioamnionitis has shown no benefit.

Obstetric factors have an impact on perinatal transmission: vaginal delivery rather than caesarean section, and prolonged rupture of membranes (more than four hours), increase MTCT. Invasive procedures during labour and delivery may also increase the risk of perinatal transmission. These include foetal scalp monitoring, amniocentesis, foetal scalp electrodes, episiotomy, and instrumental delivery. However, this association has not been detected in all studies.

Infant factors such as prematurity and mucosal lesions due to thrush are associated with an increased risk of transmission.

Risky sexual behaviour before and during pregnancy (new sexual partner; sex without a condom with regular partner) may increase the risk of perinatal transmission. It is important to stress safe sex in women who are pregnant or who intend becoming pregnant to reduce MTCT during the perinatal period. Vaginal disinfection with antiseptics, treatment of sexually transmitted infections during pregnancy, and Vitamin A or multivitamin supplements, were ineffective in reducing MTCT, although these interventions may improve neonatal and infant outcomes.

Prevention of transmission

TABLES 11.3A and 11.3B summarise the trials of antiretroviral interventions to reduce mother-to-child transmission of HIV in non-breastfeeding and breastfeeding women respectively.

In February 1994, the Paediatric AIDS Clinical Trials Group (PACTG), using AZT in a protocol to decrease MTCT (076), showed that transmission was reduced from 25.5% to 8.3%. Since then there have been many major trials. The 076 protocol has been employed extensively in the industrialised countries, resulting in a dramatic reduction in the number of HIV-infected children. Among developing countries, the wide-scale introduction of some of the shorter regimens is expected to reduce the numbers of new HIV infant infections considerably. The diversity of protocols studied makes direct comparisons between trials difficult. In general, the longer the course of

TREATMENT

	Mother			Infant	Transmission rate: Active vs placebo	Relative efficacy
	Antepartum	Intrapartum	Postpartum			
PACTG 076 *Zidovudine*	100 mg 5x/day(po) (from week 14–34)	At onset: 2 mg/kg(iv) for 1 hr, then 1 mg/kg/hr	No	2 mg/kg 6 hourly (po) (for 6 weeks)	At 18 months: 8.3% vs 25.5%	68%
CDC Thai *Zidovudine*	300 mg 2x/day(po) (from week 36)	At onset: 300 mg, then 3 hourly (po)	No	No	At 6 months 9.4% vs 18.9%	50.1%
Harvard University – Thai					Kaplan Meier	
Arm LL *Zidovudine*	300 mg 2x/day(po) (from week 28)	300 mg 3 hourly	No	2 mg/kg qid (for 6 weeks)	6.5%	
Arm LS *Zidovudine*	300 mg 2x/day(po) (from week 28)	300 mg 3 hourly	No	2 mg/kg qid (for 3 days)	4.7%	
Arm SL *Zidovudine*	300 mg 2x/day(po) (from week 35)	300 mg 3 hourly	No	2 mg/kg qid (for 6 weeks)	8.6%	
Arm SS *Zidovudine*	300 mg 2x/day(po) (from week 35)	300 mg 3 hourly	No	2 mg/kg qid (for 3 days)	10.5%	

TABLE 11.3A Antiretroviral interventions to reduce mother-to-child transmission of HIV: Non-breastfeeding

antiretrovirals, the better the outcome. The main effect is on intrapartum and intrauterine routes of transmission; and the data suggest that these effects are mediated through reduction in maternal viral load, and pre- and post-exposure prophylaxis in the infant.

Combination antiretrovirals among breastfeeding women appear to be more effective in reducing the MTCT rates assessed in early infancy (at about two months). For example, the PETRA trial showed that AZT plus 3TC resulted in a 63% reduction in HIV transmission, and a 61% reduction in HIV transmission and mortality at six weeks. The logical extension of this is the finding in industrialised countries that the use of potent combinations of antiretrovirals, together with elective caesarean section, has decreased transmission to less than 2%. The simplest effective regimen is HIVNET 012, which uses single dose nevirapine for mother and newborn. The 012 regimen was shown to be equivalent to the intrapartum/postpartum arm of SAINT, the South African Intrapartum Nevirapine Trial. The main advantage of 012 is the ease of administration and low cost; the chief drawback is concern about resistance to the drug. Other antiretroviral regimens are costlier and more demanding of health services. Women with severe disease may require particular attention in choice of

TREATMENT

	Mother			Infant	Transmission rate: Active vs placebo	Relative efficacy
	Antepartum	Intrapartum	Postpartum			
Ivory Coast		At onset:			At 3 months	
Zidovudine	300 mg 2x/day (po) (from week 36)	300 mg, then 300 mg 3 hourly (po)	No	No	15.7% vs 24.9%	37%
Ivory Coast/ Burkina Faso		At onset			At 6 months	
Zidovudine	300 mg 2x/day (po) (from week 36–38)	600 mg single dose (po)	300 mg 2x/ day (po) (for 1 week)	No	17.1% vs 27.4% At 15 months 21.5% vs 30.6%	35% 30%
Petra Trial		At onset			At 6 weeks	
Arm A Zidovudine	300 mg 2x/day (po) (from week 36)	300 mg 3 hourly (po)	150 mg 2x/ day(po) (for 1 week)	4 mg/kg 2x/ day (po) (for 1 week)	5.7% vs 15.3%	57%
3TC Lamivudine	150 mg 2x/day (po) (from week 36)	150 mg 12 hourly (po)	300 mg 2x/ day (po) (for 1 week)	2 mg/kg 2x/ day(po) (for 1 week)	At 18 months 14.9% vs 22.2%	21%
Arm B Zidovudine	No	300 mg 3 hourly (po)	300 mg 2x/ day (po) (for 1 week)	4 mg/kg 2x/ day (po) (for 1 week)	At 6 weeks 8.9% vs 15.3%	36%
3TC Lamivudine	No	150 mg 12 hourly (po)	150 mg 2x/ day (po) (for 1 week)	2 mg/kg 2x/ day (po) (for 1 week)	At 18 months 18.1% vs 22.2% ZDV vs NVP	7%
HIVNET 012		At onset			At 14–16 weeks	
Nevirapine	No	200 mg (po)	No	2 mg/kg within 72 hours of birth	25.1% vs 13.1 %	47%
Zidovudine	No	600 mg (po), then 3 hourly until delivery	No No	4 mg/kg (po) BID for 7 days after deilvery	At 18 months 15.7% vs 24.1%	41%
SAINT		At onset:			ZDV/3 TC vs NVP At 8 weeks	
Arm Zidovudine	No	600 mg (po), then 300 mg 3 hourly until delivery	300 mg (po) BID for 1 week	>2kg: 12 mg (po) BID for I week <2kg: 4 mg/kg BID for 1 week		
3TC Lamivudine	No	150 mg (po), then 150 mg every 12 hours until delivery	150 mg (po) BID for 1 week	>2kg: 6 mg (po) BID for 1 week <2kg: 4 mg/kg BID for 1 week	9.3% vs	
Arm Nevirapine	No No	200 mg (po) (additional dose 48 hours later if still in labour)	200 mg (24–48 hrs)	6 mg – (24–48 hrs)	12.3%	

TABLE 11.3B Antiretroviral interventions to reduce mother-to-child transmission of HIV: Breastfeeding

antiretrovirals. Short-course AZT in the West African trials did not appear as effective in those with low CD4 counts. In contrast, the 012 trial showed no significant beneficial effect of nevirapine in mothers with viral load below 50 000 copies/ml.

The West African trials and HIVNET 012 established that the early efficacy in reducing transmission waned but was not lost between 18 months and 24 months of age; this was due to the accumulation of new infections from breastfeeding. In the PETRA study the efficacy in ARM A (the most effective regimen) was extinguished by 18 months in breastfeeding women.

Recent trials have shown that combination antiretrovirals given during pregnancy and through the perinatal period can reduce transmission to between 2% and 6% in formula feeding and breastfeeding infants respectively. The currently recommended regimen by WHO is short-course zidovudine plus single dose nevirapine to mother and newborn. Antiretrovirals, especially a combination of nevirapine and zidovudine, given after birth to the infants of women who had come too late in pregnancy to receive antenatal regimens, have also been shown to be effective.

The important point for public health is to retain the early efficacy and prevent any new infections. There are studies underway to examine ways to reduce breastfeeding transmission. In the richer countries, HIV positive mothers are advised to avoid breastfeeding. This is not a realistic choice for the majority of women in developing countries for the following reasons: high mortality from pneumonia and diarrhoea accompanying formula feeding; departure from established tradition of breastfeeding reveals HIV status and results in discrimination; cost of purchase and preparation of formula; loss of wide range of benefits consequent on breastfeeding. There is suggestive evidence from a few African studies that antiretrovirals given to the breastfeeding infant reduce postnatal transmission. For the present the recommendation from our centre is the following: use of an appropriate antiretroviral regimen and skilled counselling on feeding choices based on the WHO/UNICEF/UNAIDS guidelines; exclusive breastfeeding for six months for those who choose this option, and rapid weaning thereafter.

Improvement in obstetric practices, prompt treatment of oral thrush, lactation management, expressing and heat-treating breastmilk, condom use and avoidance of new sexual partners during pregnancy, are additional measures to reduce MTCT. Caesarean section is inappropriate as a public health intervention in developing countries.

Antiretrovirals are well tolerated by mothers and their infants in MTCT trials. The short and medium term safety for the key antiretrovirals used is reassuring. Neurologic disease and death among infants exposed to perinatal AZT/3TC reported in one study, have not been confirmed by careful review of very large numbers of infants exposed to nucleoside analogues. The main problem has been the emergence of resistance to the drugs used. AZT used among antiretroviral-naïve women is not associated with resistant viral strains. Resistance does occur with nevirapine and 3TC. In the HIVNET 012 trial 19% of the women developed resistance, and 46% of the HIV-infected infants developed resistance by six weeks of age. However, this resistance in both mothers and infants was transient and was undetectable by 18 months. Further work is required to assess outcomes if these antiretrovirals are used for future pregnancies or for chronic treatment. The benefits outweigh the drawbacks when these drugs are used for prevention of MTCT. The choices of antiretrovirals in women of childbearing potential are discussed in greater detail in CHAPTER 33.

Provision of services and implementation of research results

The translation of research into policy and practice was rapid in the industrialised countries and the 076 regimen quickly attained the status of 'standard of care'. This has dramatically reduced the number of new HIV infections in infants. In the US the 076 regimen was accepted by the appropriate government agency, a task force was established, guidelines drawn up, and universal voluntary counselling and testing services provided. The programme promptly became successful within a setting of adequate health and other social services. Mothers could avoid breastfeeding transmission and use formula.

There have been barriers to implementation in developing countries. These include a shortage of funds, infrastructural inadequacies (counsellors, laboratories for HIV tests, antenatal clinic services), stigma, and inappropriate regimens. The elements of success include community involvement, access to appropriate antenatal services, high-quality counselling, rapid tests for HIV, and sensible infant feeding policies applicable to populations and grounded in informed choice. Obstacles are being progressively overcome and many countries in Africa, Asia and Latin America have substantial programmes to reduce MTCT.

Comprehensive approach to MTCT services

The emphasis has been on the immediate measures to reduce transmission of HIV from the mother to the infant during the antenatal, intrapartum and postnatal periods. There is a compelling and ethical case to be made for a much wider view of the subject of MTCT that makes provision for the interests of the HIV-infected mothers and their partners and their HIV-infected infants and HIV-uninfected infants. The UN's comprehensive programme addresses this and has four components:

- prevention of HIV in women, young people, and in the general population
- prevention of unintended pregnancies, and free choice on termination of pregnancies in HIV infected women
- prevention of MTCT
- provision of care, treatment and support to HIV infected women, their infants, and families.

Infant feeding choices to maintain child health and to reduce MTCT are contained within the last two points.

Substantial price decreases of antiretrovirals, availability of global funding sources, increasing awareness of the benefits of these drugs, popular movements demanding better access to antiretrovirals, and support within governments in Africa, have improved prospects for providing antiretroviral therapy on a much larger scale.

Selected bibliography

DABIS F, EKPINI ER. 'HIV-1/AIDS and maternal and child health in Africa'. *Lancet* 2002; 359: 2097–104.

BULTERYS M, NOLAN ML, JAMIESON DJ ET AL. 'Advances in the prevention of mother-to-child HIV-1 transmission: Current issues, future challenges'. *AIDScience* 2002; 2: available online (www.Aidscience.org)

COOVADIA HM, COUTSOUDIS A. 'Problems and advances in reducing transmission of HIV-1 through breast-feeding in developing countries'. *AIDScience* 2001; 1: available online (www.Aidscience.org)

MOFENSON LM. 'Tale of Two Epidemics – The Continuing Challenge of Preventing Mother-to-Child Transmission of Human Immunodeficiency Virus'. *Journal of Infectious Diseases* 2003; 187: 721–724.

NOLAN M, FOWLER MG, MOFENSON LM. 'Antiretroviral prophylaxis of perinatal HIV-1 transmission and the potential impact of antiretroviral resistance'. *Journal of Acquired Immune Deficiency Syndrome* 2002; 30: 216–229.

UNICEF-UNAIDS-WHO-UNFPA. *HIV transmission through breastfeeding. A review of the available evidence.* World Health Organisation. Geneva. 2004

CHAPTER 12
Sexually transmitted infections

David Coetzee and Leigh Johnson

CLASSICAL SEXUALLY TRANSMITTED INFECTIONS (STIs) other than HIV are caused by bacteria, fungi, protozoa and viruses other than HIV. South Africa has one of the highest STI prevalence rates in the world.

Classical STIs contribute to infertility and pregnancy and birth complications in women. However, their main importance is the role of classical STIs in enhancing the transmission of HIV.

This enhancement of HIV transmission is a result of classical STIs causing inflammation of the genital tract, which increases the presence of T lymphocytes and macrophages. Ulcerative STIs also disrupt the genital epithelial barrier. Both increase susceptibility to HIV infection in the HIV-negative partner. An HIV-infected partner sheds more virus in the presence of a classical STI, so increasing the probability of HIV transmission.

Results of studies on the effect of treating classical STIs on HIV incidence are conflicting. Programmes to prevent HIV transmission by managing individuals presenting with STIs appropriately are most likely to be effective early in an HIV epidemic while presumptive treatment of individuals frequently infected with STIs may be more cost effective than programmes implemented in the general population. The principle of treating STIs syndromically has been established and implemented in public sector health services in South Africa.

Introduction

Infections by bacteria, fungi, protozoa and viruses other than HIV are transmitted by sexual contact and may cause a variety of clinical conditions. These are referred to as the classical Sexually Transmitted Infections (STIs) in contrast to infection with HIV. South Africa ranks as one of the countries with the highest prevalence of classical STIs in the world. The main factors that have contributed to the high prevalence of HIV have also contributed to the creation of a large pool of persons with STIs. These factors include the entrenched migrant labour system, socioeconomic and gender inequalities, the failure of prevention programmes, and apartheid and the political disturbances and violence of the last three decades. In addition, poor access to, and the low quality of, STI treatment and poor health-seeking behaviour have aggravated the problem.

The commonest symptoms of STIs are penile discharges in men, abnormal vaginal discharges in women and anogenital ulcers in men and women. Less common symptoms include anogenital warts, scrotal pain or swelling, inguinal swelling and lower abdominal pain in women.

Classical STIs cause many complications, including infertility in women, along with scarring of the fallopian tubes that can result in ectopic pregnancy. Infection with an STI can lead to spontaneous abortion, premature rupture of membranes, intra-uterine death and still-births. Potential effects on the infant include low birth weight, infant blindness, neonatal pneumonia and mental retardation. However, it is the interaction between the classical STIs and HIV that has re-emphasised the importance of classical STIs because their presence enhances the transmission of HIV.

The interaction between HIV and other STIs

There are a number of reasons for the differences in HIV prevalence observed globally and the interaction with classical STIs. First, both HIV and the classical STIs have the same mode of transmission; unprotected sexual intercourse. Secondly there is an epidemiological interaction between HIV and other STIs, which are very prevalent in countries with weak health systems and poor socioeconomic conditions. These interactions are numerous and complex, and it is important to understand the global HIV/AIDS epidemic in the context of its interaction with classical STIs.

Discharges caused by STIs cause inflammation of the genital tract, which increases the presence of T lymphocytes and macrophages. Ulcerative STIs lead to disruption in the genital epithelial barrier and both these factors result in increased susceptibility to HIV infection in the HIV-negative partner. In addition, the HIV-infected partner is more infectious in the presence of an STI as there is increased HIV viral shedding when an HIV-positive partner has an STI and hence an increased probability of HIV transmission. Numerous studies have confirmed this effect. The strength of association appears to be strongest for classical STIs that cause genital ulcers (ie chancroid, syphilis and herpes), and weaker for STIs that cause discharges (ie gonorrhoea, chlamydia and trichomoniasis). Although not usually regarded as STIs, reproductive tract infections such as bacterial vaginosis and candidiasis have also been shown to increase susceptibility to HIV infection.

There remains much uncertainty regarding the relative significance of asymptomatic infections. The question is pertinent in the design of HIV prevention programmes, as studies show a large proportion of classical STIs are asymptomatic. For example, a study in rural Uganda showed that over 70% of non-ulcerative STIs were asymptomatic for both men and women in the general population.

HIV viral shedding is more common in men with asymptomatic urethritis than in men without urethritis, independent of antiretroviral therapy, suggesting that asymptomatic infections play some role in HIV transmission, but the evidence is inconclusive. There are numerous factors complicating the assessment of STIs as a co-factor for HIV transmission especially in cross-sectional studies. In addition, it is ethically difficult to assess the significance of these effects.

On the strength of the available evidence, it appears that STIs have a greater effect on the risk of female-to-male HIV transmission than on the risk of male-to-female transmission. Studies also suggest that STIs are more likely to increase the risk of HIV transmission when present in the HIV-negative partner than when present in the HIV-positive partner.

A less frequently studied issue is the effect of HIV on the incidence of STIs. There is evidence to suggest that the incidence of genital ulcer disease and genital warts is increased in individuals with weakened immune systems. Women who are immunocompromised are also more likely to experience candidiasis, a reproductive tract infection that is not usually sexually transmitted.

A related question is whether HIV infection alters the natural history of STIs, and whether STI infection alters the natural history of HIV. In individuals with herpes, the incidence of HSV-2 viral shedding and the frequency of symptomatic reactivation both increase significantly in the presence of HIV infection. It has also been found that the duration of episodes of bacterial vaginosis is longer in HIV-positive women than in HIV-negative women, and that pelvic inflammatory disease is more severe in women who are HIV-infected.

There is no consistent evidence to suggest that HIV affects the efficacy of treatment for other STIs, although many early studies suggest that single dose treatment for chancroid is less effective in the presence of HIV infection. There is some early evidence to suggest that serologic tests for syphilis become less accurate in individuals who are HIV-positive, but there is no other evidence that diagnostic techniques are less accurate in the presence of HIV infection.

The prevalence of classical STIs in South Africa

Epidemiologic monitoring of classical STIs in South Africa is not complete. Surveys of the general population are rare, and the vast majority of STI surveillance data in South Africa are obtained from health facilities. Most common among these are surveys of women attending antenatal clinics and family planning clinics.

The high prevalence of STIs in the general population in South Africa is demonstrated in TABLE 12.1 below. The prevalence of syphilis, gonorrhoea and chlamydia from two South African household surveys are compared with prevalence levels observed in household surveys in four other African countries. In most cases, the prevalence is highest in South Africa. STI prevalence in Africa is, in turn, substantially higher than in the developed world.

TABLE 12.1 Prevalence of STIs from household surveys in six African populations
Source: Buvé et al. (2001), Williams et al. (2000), Colvin et al. (1998)

	Kisumu (Kenya)	Ndola (Zambia)	Cotonou (Benin)	Yaounde (Cameroon)	Carletonville (South Africa)	Hlabisa (SA)
Syphilis						
Men	3.1%	11.3%	1.8%	6.0%	6.1%	9.3%
Women	3.9%	14.0%	1.2%	5.6%	9.7%	8.5%
Gonorrhoea						
Men	0%	0.6%	1.1%	1.6%	3.4%	2.3%
Women	0.9%	2.3%	0.9%	2.7%	6.9%	5.8%
Chlamydia						
Men	2.6%	2.1%	2.3%	5.9%	5.2%	5.6%
Women	4.5%	2.9%	1.3%	9.4%	8.1%	6.4%

Cross-sectional studies from family planning and antenatal services show different results. FIGURE 12.1 shows the weighted average prevalence levels from nine different surveys of women attending antenatal clinics or family planning clinics over the past 20 years. The average prevalence observed is 5% for gonorrhoea, 7% for syphilis, 11% for chlamydia, 26% for candidiasis, 30% for trichomoniasis, and 31% for bacterial vaginosis. However, many of these studies have been conducted in KwaZulu-Natal, and they might therefore not be representative of prevalence in the rest of South Africa. In addition, the studies are not representative of women at older ages, and women using private-sector health facilities. The studies therefore probably over-estimate STI prevalence in the adult female population.

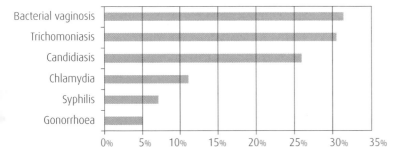

FIGURE 12.1 STI prevalence in women attending antenatal and family planning clinics

Public STI clinics are a further source of surveillance data, and provide most information on the prevalence of chancroid and herpes. Studies of men and women with genital ulcer disease (GUD) in the 1980s show a high proportion of GUD cases attributable to chancroid and syphilis, and the proportion attributable to herpes was 10% or less. More recent studies have shown a substantially higher proportion of GUD caused by herpes, though it is not clear whether this is associated with rising HSV-2 seroprevalence. A rise in the seroprevalence of HSV-2 might be expected, due to the strong epidemiologic interaction between herpes and HIV, which has only become highly prevalent in South Africa over the last decade. In addition, HSV seroprevalence is a marker of sexual activity, and internationally, prevalence of herpes has risen over the last few decades, and the locally observed increases may be associated with these international trends.

Although herpes and HIV are the most frequently studied viral STIs, there is also evidence that viral STIs such as hepatitis B and human papillomavirus are common. There has been little investigation into the relationship between *Lymphogranuloma venereum* and donovanosis and HIV. Although these bacterial STIs are believed to be fairly rare in South Africa, they appear to be common in certain regions, such as KwaZulu-Natal.

Although STI prevalence in South Africa has been extremely high over the last two decades, certain STIs are showing signs of significant declines in prevalence. For example, syphilis prevalence levels in the annual national antenatal clinic surveys have decreased steadily from 11.2% in 1997 to 2.8% in 2001. This decrease is partly the result of the syndromic management protocols that were introduced in the public sector in the mid-1990s, which had the effect of substantially improving the quality of treatment in the public health sector. Syndromic management is the provision of treatment for all the organisms that commonly cause STI symptoms such as discharges and ulcers. The decline may also be due, to some extent, to increased condom usage, in response to rising AIDS mortality and programmes that have promoted change in sexual behaviour. For other STIs, there is little evidence of significant changes in prevalence. Herpes, trichomoniasis, bacterial vaginosis and candidiasis are very prevalent, both in South Africa and other African countries, when compared with other 'traditional' STIs such as syphilis, gonorrhoea and chlamydia. However, the extent to which these infections are likely to present a significant obstacle to HIV prevention efforts is not known.

The treatment of STIs and the effect on HIV incidence

The World Health Organisation recommends that STIs be managed at the first point of contact with the health services, using the syndromic approach. Syndromic management is the provision of treatment for all the organisms that commonly cause the STI symptoms experienced by a patient in a particular area, eg treatment for syphilis and chancroid if the patient presents with an ulcer. The provision of information, education and counselling on the mode of transmission of STIs, as well as counselling on compliance and the treatment of partners, is recommended.

Three experimental studies have revealed conflicting results of the effect of the treatment of STIs on the incidence of HIV.

The Mwanza study, conducted from 1991 to 1994 in Mwanza district Tanzania, showed a decrease in the incidence of HIV following improved services for persons seeking treatment for STIs. Twelve villages were paired and an intervention was randomised to one of the villages in each pair. Health workers were trained in syndromic case management, a regular supply of effective medications was ensured, there were regular supervisory visits to health facilities and community-based campaigns were conducted to improve health seeking behaviour for STIs. A cohort of randomly selected HIV-negative adults was followed and the study showed a 38% reduction in HIV incidence in the villages where the intervention was conducted. There was also a 49% reduction in the prevalence of symptomatic urethritis in men, although this was not statistically significant.

The Rakai study, conducted from 1994 to 1998 in Rakai district, Uganda, showed no decrease in the incidence of HIV following mass treatment for STIs. Five of ten clusters (of 56 rural villages) were randomly selected to receive the intervention. This consisted of three rounds of single dose, directly-observed and effective treatment for STIs at ten month intervals for all adults. Surveys conducted among the entire adult population showed no decrease in HIV incidence in the intervention clusters. There was also no significant reduction in the prevalence of gonorrhoea or chlamydia.

The Masaka study was conducted between 1994 and 2000 in Masaka district, Uganda. It showed no decrease in HIV incidence following three interventions, one of which included improved services for persons seeking treatment for STIs. Eighteen communities were randomly allocated to one of three interventions. The first intervention involved the provision of information, education and communication according to a specific behaviour change model. The second involved training on syndromic management, the provision of a regular supply of effective medication and service supervision together with community-based STI health education. The third focused on community development, support and general health promotion. There was no significant difference in HIV incidence in the three different arms of the study.

There are a number of possible explanations for the different results in the three studies. First the trials tested different interventions in different HIV epidemic settings. A possible explanation is the difference in the stage of the HIV epidemic, which can influence exposure to HIV and the distribution of viral load in the infected population. The prevalence of HIV in Mwanza at the time of the study was much lower than when the studies were conducted in Rakai and Masaka. In addition, the prevalence of incurable STIs (such as genital herpes) was lower in Mwanza. In Mwanza and Masaka, STI services were improved whereas in Rakai intermittent mass STI treatment that would cover both symptomatic and asymptomatic STIs was provided to the community. Another possible explanation is the importance of asymptomatic STIs. The prevalence of asymptomatic STIs was not determined in Mwanza and Masaka but was shown to be high in Rakai. Fourthly it appears that the incidence of HIV was already decreasing in Uganda when the Masaka study was conducted due to other earlier behavioural interventions.

An observational study of the effect of periodic presumptive treatment of STIs in high risk 'core transmitters' of HIV such as sex workers on the overall prevalence of STIs in the community, has yielded positive results in a mining town in South Africa where there are large numbers of male migrant workers. A user-friendly service was initiated for women who had multiple partners and included good quality STI services with syndromic management, as well as monthly presumptive treatment of the STIs in asymptomatic women. In addition, STI services were improved for the miners. Although HIV incidence was not monitored the study showed a decrease in the prevalence of STIs in both the women and the miners.

The relative significance of various relationships in the interaction of HIV and STIs is the subject of much speculation, and several mathematical models have been created to simulate the complex interplay between HIV and other STIs.

These models have been used to demonstrate a number of important principles:

- The proportion of new HIV infections attributable to other STIs is likely to reduce as the HIV epidemic matures and HIV prevalence increases, and STI treatment programmes are therefore likely to be most effective when implemented in the early stages of an HIV epidemic.
- Management programmes that treat persons presenting with STIs are more likely to be effective in preventing the spread of HIV than mass treatment programmes.
- STI treatment programmes that target 'core transmitters' of classical STIs are likely to be more cost-effective than treatment programmes implemented in the general population.

The role of STIs in HIV transmission is well accepted. The challenge is to identify and conduct studies that test different combinations of interventions, including improved STI services with syndromic management, mass STI treatment and periodic presumptive STI treatment, in order to determine the most cost-effective way to conduct programmes that can play an important role in containing the HIV epidemic in South Africa.

Bibliography

BUVÉ A, WEISS H, LAGA M, VAN DYCK E, MUSONDA R, ZEKENG L ET AL. 'The epidemiology of gonorrhoea, chlamydial infection and syphilis in four African cities'. *AIDS* 2001; 15 (suppl 4): S79–S88.

COLVIN M, ABDOOL KARIM S, CONNOLLY C, HOOSEN AA, NTULI N. 'HIV infection and asymptomatic sexually transmitted infections in a rural South African community'. *International Journal of STD & AIDS* 1998; 9: 548–550.

DEPARTMENT OF HEALTH SOUTH AFRICA. '*National HIV and syphilis sero-prevalence survey in South Africa: 2001*'. Government Printers, Pretoria. 2002.

DESCHAMPS M, PAPE J, HAFNER A, JOHNSON W. 'Heterosexual transmission of HIV in Haiti'. *Annals of Internal Medicine* 1996; 275: 122–127.

DUERR A, SIERRA M, FELDMAN J, CLARKE LM, EHRLICH I, DEHOVITZ J. 'Immune compromise and prevalence of Candida vulvovaginitis in human immunodeficiency virus-infected women'. *Obstetrics and Gynecology* 1997; 90: 252–256.

FLEMING D, WASSERHEIT J. 'From epidemiological synergy to public health policy and practice: The contribution of other sexually transmitted diseases to sexual transmission of HIV infection'. *Sexually Transmitted Infections* 1999; 75: 3–17.

GHYS P, DIALLO M, ETTIÈGNE-TRAORÉ V, YEBOUE KM, GNAORE E, LOROUGNON F ET AL. 'Genital ulcers associated with human immunodeficiency virus-related immunosuppression in female sex workers in Abidjan, Ivory Coast'. *Journal of Infectious Diseases* 1995; 172: 1371–1374.

GRAY R, WAWER M, SEWANKAMBO N, SERWADDA D, LI C, MOULTON LH ET AL. 'Relative risks and population attributable fraction of incident HIV associated with symptoms of sexually transmitted diseases and treatable symptomatic sexually transmitted diseases in Rakai District, Uganda'. *AIDS 1999*; 13: 2113–2123.

GROSSKURTH H, HOSHA F, TODD J, MWIJARUBI E, KLOKKE A, SENKORO K ET AL. 'Impact of improved treatment of sexually transmitted diseases on HIV infection in rural Tanzania: Randomised control trial'. *Lancet* 1995; 346: 530–536.

JAMIESON D, DUERR A, KLEIN R, PARAMSOTHY P, BROWN W, CU-UVIN S ET AL. 'Longitudinal analysis of bacterial vaginosis: Findings from the HIV Epidemiology Research Study'. *Obstetrics and Gynecology* 2001; 98: 656–663.

KAMALI A, QUIGLEY M, NAKIYINGI J, KINSMAN J, KENGEYA-KAYONDO J, GOPAL R ET AL. 'Syndromic management of sexually-transmitted infections and behaviour change interventions on transmission of HIV-1 in rural Uganda: A community randomised trial'. *Lancet* 2003; 361: 645–652.

KORENROMP E, DE VLAS S, NAGELKERKE N, HABBEMA J. 'Estimating the magnitude of the STD cofactor effects on HIV transmission: How well can it be done?' *Sexually Transmitted Diseases* 2001; 28: 613–621.

KORENROMP E, VAN VLIET C, GROSSKURTH H, GAVYOLE A, VAN DER PLOEG CP, FRANSEN L, ET AL. 'Model-based evaluation of single-round mass treatment of sexually transmitted diseases for HIV control in a rural African population'. *AIDS* 2000; 14: 573–593.

O'FARRELL N, HOOSEN A, KHARSANY A, VAN DEN ENDE J. 'Sexually transmitted pathogens in pregnant women in a rural South African community'. *Genitourinary Medicine* 1989; 65: 276–280.

OVER M, PIOT P. 'Human immunodeficiency virus infection and other sexually transmitted diseases in developing countries: Public health importance and priorities for resource allocation'. *Journal of Infectious Diseases* 1996; 174 (suppl 2): S162–S175.

PAXTON L., SEWANKAMBO N., GRAY R., SERWADDA D., McNAIRN D., LI C, WAWER M. 'Asymptomatic non-ulcerative genital tract infections in a rural Ugandan population'. *Sexually Transmitted Infections* 1998; 74: 421-425.

PHAM-KANTER G, STEINBERG M, BALLARD R. 'Sexually transmitted diseases in South Africa'. *Genitourinary Medicine* 1996; 72: 160–171.

ROBINSON N, MULDER D, AUVERT B, HAYES R. 'Proportion of HIV infections attributable to sexually transmitted diseases in a rural Ugandan population: Simulation model estimates'. *International Journal of Epidemiology* 1997; 26: 180–189.

ROTCHFORD K, STRUM W, WILKINSON D. 'Effect of coinfection with STDs and of STD treatment on HIV shedding in genital-tract secretions: systematic review and data synthesis'. *Sexually Transmitted Diseases* 2000; 27: 243–248.

RØTTINGEN J, CAMERON D, GARNETT G. 'A systematic review of the epidemiological interactions between classic sexually transmitted diseases and HIV: How much is really known?' *Sexually Transmitted Diseases* 2001; 28: 579–597.

SCHACKER T, ZEH J, HU H, HILL E, COREY L. 'Frequency of symptomatic and asymptomatic herpes simplex virus type 2 reactivations among human immunodeficiency virus-infected men.' *Journal of Infectious Diseases* 1998; 178: 1616–1622.

WASSERHEIT J. 'Epidemiological synergy: Interrelationships between human immunodeficiency virus infection and other sexually transmitted diseases'. *Sexually Transmitted Diseases* 1992; 19: 61–77.

WAWER M, SEWANKAMBO N, SERWADDA D, QUINN TC, PAXTON LA, KIWANUKA N ET AL. 'Control of sexually transmitted diseases for AIDS prevention in Uganda: A randomised community trial'. *Lancet* 1999; 353: 525–535.

WEISS H, BUVÉ A, ROBINSON N, VAN DYCK E, KAHINDO M, ANAGONOU S ET AL. 'The epidemiology of HSV-2 infection and its association with HIV infection in four urban African populations'. *AIDS* 2001; 15 (suppl 4): S97–S108.

WILLIAMS B, GILGEN D, CAMPBELL C ET AL. 'The natural history of HIV/AIDS in South Africa: A biomedical and social survey in Carletonville'. Council for Scientific and Industrial Research. Johannesburg. 2000.

WINTER A, TAYLOR S, WORKMAN J, WHITE D, ROSS JD, SWAN AV ET AL. 'Asymptomatic urethritis and detection of HIV-1 RNA in seminal plasma'. *Sexually Transmitted Infections* 1999; 75: 261–263.

CHAPTER 13
Safe blood supplies

Anthon Heyns and Johanna P Swanevelder

SOUTH AFRICA HAS A blood service based on voluntary non-remunerated donors who have an HIV prevalence much lower than the general population. The Department of Health has delegated responsibility to autonomous, non-profit blood transfusion services and there will be a single blood transfusion service formed under the National Health Act.

The greatest risk of HIV infection from transfused blood arises from the window period of infectivity, although this has been significantly reduced by more sensitive HIV assays. However, the quality and safety of the blood supply ultimately depends on the donor population and their education is a key component in the provision of safe blood.

The policies and procedures in place to ensure a safe blood supply in South Africa have been successful and depend on actively selecting donors who are not at risk of infection with HIV or other infections transmitted by transfusion.

An effective blood transfusion service is an essential component of a successful health care system. South Africa is fortunate that it has a model blood service based on voluntary non-remunerated blood donors with an HIV prevalence much lower than that of the general population. The devastating impact that HIV/AIDS may have on blood safety is highlighted by the infection of haemophiliacs in the 1980s, before the cause of the disease was recognised and before blood donations were routinely screened for the presence of HIV antibodies.

The World Health Organisation (WHO) estimates that every year 80 000 to 160 000 cases of HIV are transmitted to patients by blood and blood products. About 20% of all blood donations are not screened for HIV, and hepatitis B and C (the transfusion transmissible diseases) and approximately 545 000 donations are not tested for the presence of HIV. The risk of acquiring HIV through a transfusion is particularly high in the developing world. The WHO has reported that 80% of the world population has access to 20% of the safe blood that is available.

The effect of the window period of infectivity and the steady increase of HIV-infection, even in the select population of blood donors, has necessitated the introduction of measures to minimise the impact of HIV and other transmissible diseases on the blood supply.

Governance of the blood service

It is universally recognised that a well-structured and well-governed, financially viable 'fee for service' organisation, supported by the government, is the foundation of a sustainable, effective and equit- able blood service. The value system and code of ethics of such a service must be above reproach if it is to retain the support of the community and credibility with the blood users and patients.

The Department of Health is ultimately responsible and account- able to the public for the provision of safe blood supplies to the country's patients. In South Africa this responsiblity has been delegated by the National Department of Health to autonomous, non-profit blood transfusion services. The National Health Act (2004) makes provision for a single national blood transfusion service licensed by the Department of Health. The intent of the minister is that the two existing services, the South African National Blood Service (SANBS) and the Western Province Blood Transfusion Service, should merge. The majority of members of the Boards of Directors of the blood transfusion services are blood donors who act as the custo- dians to protect the interests of the blood donors and the patients that they serve. The governance and operational activities of the national blood transfusion service are overseen by the Department of Health. The principles guiding the practice of blood transfusion, including the safety of the blood supply, are set out in the *Policy with regard to Blood Transfusion in South Africa* (1998) and the *Policy to Protect the Safety of the Blood Supply against the* HIV/AIDS *Pandemic* (2000). These high-level policies are expressed in the National Health Act (2004) and the Regulations regarding Blood and Blood Products scheduled by the Minister of Health. The National Health Act and the Regulations pertaining to the practice of blood transfusion are complemented by the *Standards for the Practice of Blood Transfusion in South Africa*, published by assent of the Minister of Health. SANBS has a Blood Safety Policy that addresses all procedures related to the safety of the blood supply. The blood transfusion services are accredited with the South African National Accreditation System.

This well-structured and controlled blood service is the foundation of the quality service delivered to patients. This is expressed in the mission statement of the SA National Blood Service (SANBS) to provide sufficient safe blood in an equitable manner to the patients of the country. This statement recognises that self-sufficiency is the primary goal, but the code of ethics of the organisation states that above all the patient will not be harmed. This approach includes observance of the 'precautionary principle' that calls for a blood service to introduce measures that may protect the patient even though there may be no unequivocal scientific evidence that such measures will be effective.

Sufficient safe blood and the window period of HIV infectivity

The major HIV risk to the safety of the blood supply is the so-called window period of infectivity, which limits the value of the available laboratory screening tests for HIV. Simply stated, this is the period between infection with HIV and detection by a laboratory test (for further details on HIV diagnostic testing see CHAPTER 6). Transfusion of such blood will result in the infection of the patient with the infective agent. The window period, which varies from test to test, makes it impossible to rule out the possibility of the transmission of the virus by the blood transfusion. The increased sensitivity of new generation laboratory tests has significantly decreased the residual risk of transmitting HIV (FIGURE 13.1). It should be noted that because of the large

FIGURE 13.1 Reduced risk of undetected HIV units/100 000 by consecutive generations of screening tests that shorten the window period – based on 1998 incidence levels

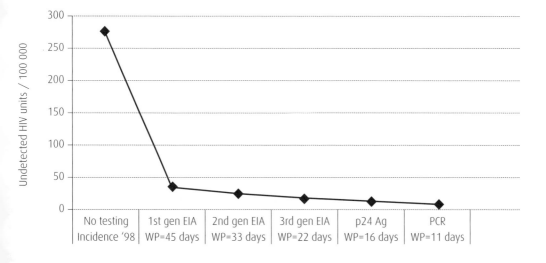

CHAPTER 13 SAFE BLOOD SUPPLIES

volume of blood given during a transfusion, 89 to 100% of those patients who receive HIV-positive blood will become infected.

In South Africa all blood donations are routinely screened for the presence of HIV-1/2 antibody and p24 HIV-1/2 antigen by sensitive and specific third generation enzyme-linked immuno-assays (EIA) test systems that conform to the highest international standards. Blood donations in South Africa are currently not screened for viral nucleic acid (nucleic acid testing; NAT). Taking into consideration the marginal reduction in residual risk and the expense of NAT, it is debatable whether it can be justified in a country with limited resources and other health priorities.

It is recognised that the quality and safety of the blood supply ultimately depends on the risk profile of the donor population and the lifestyle of the blood donor population. In the light of the risk associated with the window period, it is particularly important to identify those blood donors who have recently been infected by HIV. Thus, education of blood donors about HIV/AIDS and the exclusion of individuals who have participated in risk behaviour or who have been exposed to high risk incidents (TABLE 13.1) that will put the blood supply at risk, is the key to a safe blood supply.

Blood transfusion is regarded as a medical intervention. Therefore the well-being of the recipient of the blood product is the primary concern of the Service. Although blood donors, as the only source of blood, and their commitment to help their fellow citizens is vital, their interests are secondary to the needs of the patients. In the context of the diseases that may be transmitted by blood, the Blood Service thus does not procure blood from prospective blood donors who do not satisfy the rigid requirements of the Service. These criteria are universally accepted.

- Having more than one sex partner or engaging in casual sex in the preceding six months
- Sex with someone whose sexual behaviour is not known to the donor
- Men who have had sex with other men within the preceding five years
- Sex with a prostitute or sex in exchange for money, drugs, goods or favours
- Having had a sexually transmitted disease
- Accidental exposure to blood or body fluids (eg needle stick injury)
- Victim of sexual assault
- Intravenous injection with drugs or substances not prescribed by a doctor

---

TABLE 13.1 The activities and exposures that are included in the blood donor self-exclusion questionnaire. Prospective donors who participate in any of these activities or have been exposed to these events, are not accepted

It should, however, be kept in mind that the first priority of a blood service is to provide sufficient blood to all patients. The risk posed by undetected HIV to the blood supply is less than the dangers faced by a patient who needs blood if this is not available. The policies to ensure a safe and adequate blood supply therefore must be in balance.

These principles and issues are further developed in the Blood Safety Policy.

The Blood Safety Policy

The Blood Safety Policy of SANBS is based on the following key principles:
- a coordinated programme to procure sufficient blood from low-risk voluntary, non-remunerated blood donors
- a programme that aims to be nationally self-sufficient for low-risk blood products
- issuing blood according to a hierarchy of risk
- recognising the right to privacy of the individual donor
- protecting the health of blood donors, recipients of blood products and staff members
- educating blood donors, particularly learners, on the importance of donating blood, the spread and pathogenesis of HIV/AIDS, and the effect of a safe healthy lifestyle on the quality and safety of the blood supply.

The policy recognises that the voluntary non-remunerated donor, who donates regularly, is the safest donor. It is, however, also recognised that the demographic, social, economic and cultural characteristics of a community determine its safety as a source of blood donors. It is therefore important to take the diversity of communities into account when recruiting new blood donors and promoting blood procurement programmes. It is also acknowledged that a structured educational programme is a powerful tool to change attitudes on blood donation and to induce an ethos of serving the community by the 'gift of life'. This is particularly important in the young.

The Blood Safety Policy therefore is supported by procedures that:
- develop donor recruitment and selection programmes that minimise the effects of the epidemiological and demographic factors that determine the risk of transmitting HIV by transfusion
- use information on epidemiology and risk behaviour to develop criteria to recognise donors who are unlikely to be infected with HIV
- develop programmes of sensitive, culturally appropriate forms of communication with donors
- develop a process whereby donors will not present themselves for donating blood if they regard themselves as participants in risky

activities or behaviour, or in certain cases will inform the blood service that the blood that they have donated should not be used

- minimise the danger that the public may use the blood transfusion service as a testing facility for HIV
- ensure that the blood system supports, cares for and counsels donors where necessary
- maintain links with the national HIV/AIDS programme and brings our education programme in harmony with those of others

Outcome of the Blood Safety Policy

The policy and the procedures to maintain the safety of the blood supply have been successful. Although it is not possible to accurately compare the rates of HIV in the population donating and not donating blood, a persuasive indication of the impact on the donor recruitment policy is the very significant difference in the prevalences between the attendees at antenatal clinics in South Africa and the population donating blood for SANBS (FIGURE 13.2). Noteworthy is the decrease in HIV rates in the blood collections after implementation of the Blood Safety Policy.

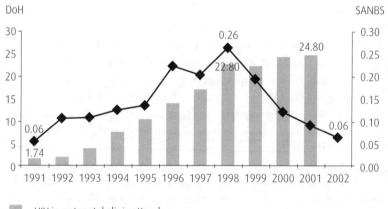

FIGURE 13.2 The rate of HIV infection in attendees of antenatal clinics has increased significantly since 1991 (scale on left). In contrast, the HIV rate in blood collections (scale on right) has always been much lower although showing the same rate of increase. Since the introduction of the Blood Safety Policy in 1999 this rate has decreased significantly and in 2002 was at the same level as 1991

The policy focuses on actively selecting donors not at increased risk for HIV infection. The procedure is based on demonstrating, by multivariate regression analysis of blood donations collected in 1996 and 1997, that the significant determinants of HIV seropositivity in blood donations are whether the donor is donating for the first time or is a regular donor, the time lapse since the previous donation, the ethnic status and gender of the donor and the location of the clinic where the blood is collected.

It is possible to stratify the blood donations according to these determinants into categories based on observed HIV prevalence levels (FIGURE 13.3). Four such risk categories (RCs) have been defined. The HIV prevalence rates of the cohorts that constitute the RCs are:

- RC I " 0.0099%;
- RC II 0.0100 – 0.0999%;
- RC III 0.10 – 0.99% and
- RC IV ≥ 1.0%.

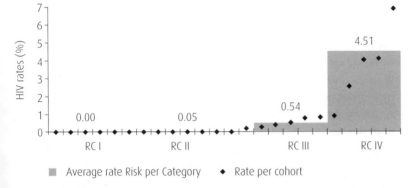

FIGURE 13.3 The blood donation cohorts have been stratified into four risk categories. These risk categories include cohorts of blood donations with HIV prevalence rates falling into the Risk Category limits. The HIV rate of Risk Category I donations is significantly lower than that of Risk Category IV. The residual risk of transmitting HIV inherent in the window period risk, is related to these Risk Categories. (RC = Risk Category)

It is evident from FIGURE 13.3 that there is a major difference in the HIV rates between the low-risk RCs I and II, the relatively high-risk RC III, and the high-risk RC IV. The prevalence of HIV in the cohorts constituting RC IV is particularly high.

The implementation of this policy has not created a shortfall in blood supply from the low-risk categories I and II. This has been avoided by instituting a recruitment programme that focuses on increasing the number of donations from repeat donors at the same time as closing clinics with high observed HIV prevalence.

The self-exclusion and health questionnaire has been refined, and an outcome of the education initiative has been the Club 25 programme aimed at recruiting learners to become regular blood donors. These young donors commit themselves to maintain a safe and healthy lifestyle and to donate at least 20 units of blood before they reach the age of 25. This programme aims to foster a lifelong commitment to regular donation, thus ensuring a source of safe blood for the future.

The Safe Blood Policy was implemented in the Inland Region of SANBS, servicing Gauteng, Mpumalanga, Limpopo, North West, Northern Cape and Free State in 1999. As a result, the rate of HIV positivity in donations decreased from 0.26% before the programme was instituted in 1998 to 0.06% in 2002. This decrease is mirrored by a five-fold decrease in the estimated incidence of HIV in all blood collected from 275 per 100 000 in 1998 to 57 per 100 000 in 2002.

As additional safety measures, blood platelet concentrates and blood components for paediatric use are prepared from Risk Category I donations. Fresh frozen plasma is quarantined for at least 56 days and only released for transfusion if the donor donates again and is shown to be free of infection with transmissible disease. Unfortunately the retest procedure cannot be undertaken with red cells and platelets because the shelf-life of these components is less than the minimum period of 56 days between donations. These procedures restrict the risk of transmitting HIV from one undetected infected donation to more than one recipient, and enhance the safety of plasma products by further reducing the risk of the window period.

The combined effect of all the activities of the Blood Safety Policy has been to change the donor profile. Low-risk blood donations now constitute 96% of the blood collections compared with 91% in 1998 (TABLE 13.2). It is also noteworthy that 86% of blood is procured from repeat donors. Low-risk donations now satisfy the demand for blood products.

	1998				2002			
	Donations	Donors	HIV rate (%) Donations	HIV rate (%) Donors	Donations	Donors	HIV rate (%) Donations	HIV rate (%) Donors
Risk Category I	73.07%	51.67%	0.01%	0.02%	79.37%	59.37%	0.01(%)	0.02(%)
Risk Category II	17.88%	34.68%	0.09%	0.09%	16.27%	33.94%	0.05(%)	0.06(%)
Risk Category III	5.42%	6.03%	0.63%	1.19%	2.96%	3.75%	0.32(%)	0.57(%)
Risk Category IV	3.63%	7.61%	5.74%	5.74%	1.40%	3.18%	3.07(%)	3.06(%)

TABLE 13.2 The implementation of the Blood Safety Policy in 1998 has resulted in procuring more blood from low-risk donors and a decrease in the rate of HIV in all the cohorts that comprise the four donor risk categories. The safety of the blood supply is ultimately dependent on the proportion of low and high-risk blood donations and whether the need for blood and blood products can be fulfilled from low risk blood. In 1998 a total of 588 547 units of blood was collected; of these 73% was from RC I; 18% RC II, 5% RC III; and 4% RC IV. In 2002 there were 523 562 donations, 79% RC I; 16% RC II; 3% RC III; and 1% RC IV

Although it is recognised that a blood transfusion is a medical intervention that will expose the patient to some risk, this risk has to be acceptable both to the patient and the health care provider. This raises the question of what acceptable risk is.

Risk is commonly defined as the combination of the likelihood and the impact of any adverse reaction. This simplistic view does not, however, take into account the perception of risk. For instance, the public and health workers view the risk of being infected by HIV through a blood transfusion as disproportionately high because of the perceived dreadfulness of the disease.

The ALARP principle (as low as reasonably possible) attempts to define a level of risk that is negligible and tries to identify that level of risk that is not acceptable to society. Assessment of acceptability of such risk must, however, be related to the potential benefit of the intervention, in this case the blood transfusion. In this context, it has been suggested that acceptable risk is more or less proportional to the third power of the benefits.

It should also be noted that people are more willing to accept the risk that they are exposed to from voluntary activities (such as driving a motor vehicle or smoking cigarettes) than from involuntary activities. Blood transfusion is viewed as an involuntary risk.

Although there have been many studies of risk, risk-benefit, risk and cost-benefit and acceptable risk, it is clear that there are no universally acceptable options. The acceptance or rejection of risk associated with an event therefore depends on the consequences, available choice, perceptions and facts that are examined in the process of deciding on the risk involved.

Although the transfusion of blood products is generally regarded as one of the most effective medical interventions available, its benefit cannot be quantified and it is thus not possible to express the risk of transfusion in absolute terms. As a consequence, both the public and health care providers tend to have an exaggerated fear of the possibility of the transmission of HIV by a transfusion.

Transfusion-associated HIV infection was first recognised in 1982. Once the relationship between the disease and high-risk behaviour was perceived, persons at increased risk for HIV were asked not to donate blood. The introduction of the self-exclusion questionnaire giving the donors the opportunity to indicate that their blood should not be used for transfusion, decreased the risk of transmitting HIV *before* the introduction in 1985 of screening tests for the presence of HIV antibodies. The development of more sensitive tests for HIV, tests for HIV type 2 and the HIV type 1 group O serotypes, together with the introduction in South Africa in 1996 of routine screening of all blood donations for HIV p24 antigen, decreased the risk further.

The residual risk of transmitting HIV by a blood transfusion is potentially related to errors in testing for transmissible agents, issuing contaminated blood to a patient because of mismanagement of the inventory, and administrative errors that link a blood donation to the wrong donor. These human errors have been minimised by instituting a quality management system encompassing all procedures of the Service.

The window period of infectivity is thus left as the most common cause of the residual HIV risk. This residual risk can be estimated in three ways.

First, by mathematical modelling (the incidence/window period model): such a model is based on knowledge of the incidence of HIV in the donor population and the length of the window period between exposure to infection and antibody detection according to the laboratory test or tests used. The likelihood of laboratory errors with the laboratory test system can be included.

Secondly, the residual risk can be determined from donor repository prevalence/transmission studies using 'look backs'. In this method, which is only possible with repeat donors who have seroconverted, it is ascertained whether a recipient had been infected by the blood product/s of a previous negative donation.

Thirdly, prospective controlled studies of transfusion recipients can be used to establish the risk of transfusion-transmitted infection. Recipients are followed-up after transfusion and if it can be demonstrated that an HIV positive patient has similar genotypes to the donor who has seroconverted, HIV transmission can be verified.

The residual risk given in TABLE 13.3 was estimated using the incidence/window period model. Note that in this model the residual risk of blood obtained from a high-risk donor population group is orders of magnitude higher than that of the low-risk donor population.

It is clear that the Safe Blood Policy has had a major impact on the safety of the blood supply. It is estimated that if only RC I and II blood is used for transfusion, seven patients will be infected per year. However, the risk using the mathematical model is considerably higher than the observed risk from retrospective analyses. In the period January 1992 to December 2002 a total of 21 cases of transmission of HIV was reported. This is approximately two per year with a residual risk of about 1 : 400 000. This discrepancy may be ascribed to several factors: the high prevalence of HIV/AIDS in patients who receive blood products, the high mortality of patients who receive blood because of their underlying disease, and the difficulties

	1998			2002		
	Incidence /100 000	Residual Risk /100 000	Estimated infected units in blood collected	Incidence	Residual Risk /100 000	Estimated infected units in blood collected
All	275.14	12.06	70.98	63.84	2.80	14.65
Risk Category I	26.72	1.17	5.04	19.43	0.85	3.54
Risk Category II	76.30	3.34	3.52	41.46	1.82	1.55
Risk Category III	1865.28	81.77	26.06	710.97	31.17	4.83
Risk Category IV	3879.24	170.05	36.38	1473.32	64.58	4.74
Low Risk	36.47	1.60	8.56	23.18	1.02	5.09
High Risk	2673.97	117.22	62.43	955.64	41.89	9.57

TABLE 13.3 The residual risk, related to the window period, has decreased significantly since the implementation of the Blood Safety Policy. There is a relationship between risk category (RC) and residual risk. If all blood collected in 2002 was available for transfusion, 15 undetected HIV-infected units would have been included in the blood supply. Restricting the blood supply for transfusion to 96% Risk Category I and II blood, 5 window period donations were probably included in the blood supply

sometimes encountered in tracing patients once they have left the health care facilities where they have received blood products.

Informed consent and other legal aspects of blood transfusion

The *Policy with regard to Blood Transfusion in South Africa* and the *Policy to Protect the Safety of the Blood Supply against the* HIV/AIDS *Pandemic* states that the blood service must not collect blood in communities where the prevalence of diseases that may be transmitted by blood is high. The *Standards of Practice of Blood Transfusion in South Africa* and the *Regulations regarding Blood and Blood Products* also prescribe the tests that must be performed on all donations, the criteria for the deferral of prospective blood donors, and the procedures to be followed to ensure positive identification of the blood unit, the patient and the donor.

So-called product liability, or strict liability for harm caused to a consumer by a defective product, is not part of South African law. Accordingly, if it is proved that a patient has been infected with HIV as the result of a transfusion with HIV positive blood, this will not necessarily be taken to indicate that the Blood Service or the doctor of the patient acted negligently.

The patient will only be successful in a claim for damages if it can be proved that a wrongful act or omission on the part of the blood service or the doctor caused the damage to the plaintiff. Furthermore, it will have to be proved that there was negligence on the part of the Service or the attending doctor. In this regard, such a fault or negligence implies that a legal norm has been violated. Negligence in this context is present if 'the reasonable man' would have foreseen harm to the patient and would have taken steps to avoid such damage.

The Blood Services go to great lengths to ensure that blood products comply with the requirements as stated in the Standards for Practice. It will therefore be very difficult indeed to prove that the Blood Service or doctor acted negligently if they adhered to the legislation, regulations and minimum requirements stated in the Standards.

However, legal opinion is that if it could be proved that the Standards themselves are inadequate to safeguard the safety of the blood supply, the Blood Service, the Board of Directors of the Service (who compiled the Standards) and the Department of Health (who sanctioned the Standards) could be held liable.

The important issue is that according to considered legal opinion the Service and the Department of Health may be held accountable if blood is collected from known high-risk donor groups and if donor clinics are established in areas with an unacceptably high prevalence of HIV infection. This is particularly important if the needs of the community for blood products can be satisfied by procuring blood from low-risk donors. In the light of this, it is important for the Blood Service to have a clear-cut policy with procedures underpinning it to ensure that these requirements are satisfied and that 'reasonable' steps are taken to maintain the safety of the blood supply.

An important legal issue is liability due to lack of informed consent. Although this also applies to the blood donor, it is particularly relevant to the patient. From a legal standpoint, the question is whether the attendant doctor could be held liable if he/she had not warned the patient that blood, although tested for HIV, may still be infected with the virus.

The legal position is that informed consent is always required if a patient is subjected to a medical intervention, including a blood transfusion. This informed consent is only waived under exceptional circumstances such as when the patient is unconscious or unable to give consent.

In relation to the issue of the risk of transmitting HIV by a transfusion, it needs to be considered what information should be given to a patient to enable him or her to make an informed judgement. Legally, the judgement will depend on the assessment of whether a 'reasonable' person in this position, if warned of the risk of a transfusion, would have attached significance to it. This would apply to both the patient and his or her doctor. Notably, in South Africa the court has adopted a patient-oriented standard. The importance of this is that the patient, rather than the doctor, should be the one to make the decision. Doctors should therefore take into account that a reasonable person who is a patient due to receive a blood transfusion certainly will attach significance to the fact that there is a risk that the blood product may be infected with HIV.

The Blood Service supports the right of a patient to freedom of choice. Patients should be fully informed of the potential benefits and risks of a transfusion, and the alternative forms of treatment that are available, such as the option of autologous transfusion where medically feasible. Failure to do so could be interpreted as failure to obtain informed consent, and this may make the doctor legally liable.

Withdrawing blood from a blood donor is also a medical intervention. The Blood Service must adhere to the prescribed requirements for the procedure as outlined in the Standards for Practice. The donor should, however, give informed consent for the intervention. The donor also has to be informed of the nature and the consequences of the withdrawal of the blood and that a sample of the blood is to be tested for HIV and other diseases that may be transmitted by transfusion. Regarding HIV, it is accepted in South African law that the patient or, in this case blood donor, must be informed specifically that his or her blood will be tested for HIV and that the donor must give consent for this. The donor has to be informed of the serious medical, legal, ethical and psychological implications of a positive HIV test result. Clearly a 'reasonable' person who is tested for HIV, will regard such a test and the result of the test as significant.

It is also required that the donor be informed of the risks inherent in the withdrawal of the blood. If the donor is not warned of the potential side-effects of the withdrawal of a unit of blood, this may be regarded as a failure to obtain the donor's informed consent for the intervention.

An extension of informed consent and the involvement of the patient in the decision-making process is that it is incumbent on the health care provider to use blood only when necessary and appropriate. This ensures that the patient will be exposed to the minimum risk. The Blood Services facilitate the process by publishing the *Clinical Guidelines on the appropriate Use of Blood*. These guidelines are updated regularly, are widely distributed and form the basis for structured educational programmes to blood users and health care providers.

The future

There has been some progress in the manufacture of blood substitutes and artificial oxygen carriers. These products have, at best, limited clinical use and remain unproven as viable alternatives to blood and blood components. Also, some of these products are manufactured from bovine haemoglobin and thus have their own inherent and unique risks. There are promising results with techniques to virus-inactivate cellular and fresh blood products such as platelets, red cells and fresh frozen plasma. These techniques have not been validated and, if introduced, are likely to be expensive.

It should be noted that the use of such products will add considerably to the cost of blood products and thus possibly compromise the delivery of other, perhaps more important, health services. The decision to use or not use such technology is not just a scientific issue, but also a sociopolitical one, closely related to the risk that a society is willing to accept, their health priorities, and how society wants to spend the money that is available for health care.

These questions should be carefully considered when evaluating the risk that HIV poses to the blood supply and the very high costs that must be incurred to make a blood product safer, often only marginally so. There is little doubt that the most cost-effective approach is to focus on the blood donor, recognising that the risk profile of the donor determines the quality of the blood supply. We are indeed fortunate to have a high-quality blood donor population in South Africa. This has enabled us to maintain a blood supply as safe as that of most industrial countries. The challenge is to maintain such a low-risk donor base and a safe blood supply in the face of an escalating HIV/AIDS epidemic.

Bibliography

BUSCH MP, YOUNG MJ, SAMSON SM, MOSLEY JW, WARD JW, PERKINS HA AND THE SAFETY STUDY GROUP. 'Risk of human immunodeficiency virus (HIV) transmission by blood transfusions before the implementation of HIV-1 antibody screening'. *Transfusion* 1991; 31: 4–11.

DEPARTMENT OF HEALTH SOUTH AFRICA. *'Annual national HIV surveys in women attending antenatal surveys. 1990 to 2001.'* Government Printer. Pretoria 2002.

HEYNS A DU P. 'Risk of transmitting HIV and other diseases with a blood transfusion in South Africa'. *CME* 1999; 17: 854–861.

KLEINMAN SH, BUSCH MP. 'The risks of transfusion-transmitted infections – direct estimation and mathematical modelling'. *Baillière's Clinical Haematology.* 2000; 13: 631–649.

VAN WYK C. Liability for the transfusion of blood in South Africa'. *CME* 1999; 17: 867–874.

WINSLOW R.M. 'New Transfusion Strategies: Red Cell substitutes'. *Annual Review of Medicine* 1999; 50: 337–353.

CHAPTER 14

Intravenous drug use in South Africa

Ted Leggett

SHARING NEEDLES FOR INJECTING drugs is a potent vector for
the transmission of blood-borne diseases because infected blood is
injected directly into the user's system. The more damaging trends in
global drug abuse did not emerge in South Africa until the mid-1990s
because of apartheid isolation.

Now, intravenous drug use is a small, but growing trend, particularly among white youth in Cape Town and Gauteng.

Heroin is the drug most commonly associated with injection, but,
until recently, has been little used in South Africa. However, there has
been an escalation in arrests for heroin since 1997 and demand for
heroin is known to be rising. Most current South African heroin users
'chase' their drug: vaporising it and then inhaling. But variations in
quality of heroin, an emerging problem in South Africa, may result in
increased injection use of the drug.

The relationship between sex workers, intravenous drug use and
HIV infection is a potentially potent one in increasing drug-related
infections.

The possibility of needle exchange programmes to mitigate this
effect in South Africa is explored.

The sharing of needles for intravenous drug use is one of the most
potent vectors for the transmission of HIV and other blood-borne
diseases, because infected blood is injected directly into the user's
system. The Ukraine is often cited as an alarming example of how
quickly the virus can spread through an injecting population: the
number of diagnosed HIV infections in that country rose from
virtually zero in 1995 to 20 000 a year from 1996 onwards, and 80%
of these new cases are injecting drug users. Since drug users also
have sex with non-users, and these couples give birth to children,

epidemiologists have begun tracking 'injection-related transmissions', which include the partners and offspring of the injector. With this expanded definition, injection emerges as the major driver of the epidemic in many parts of the world, particularly in Asia and the former Soviet Block countries but also in many Western cities.

Because of its isolation during the apartheid era, South Africa was for many years spared the more damaging global trends in substance abuse. The South African Police seized their first rocks of crack cocaine in 1995, more than a full decade behind the peak of the crack epidemic in America. Likewise, heroin was relatively rare before the transition to democracy. But things have changed, and today intravenous drug use is a small but growing trend, especially among white youths in Gauteng and Cape Town. There is a risk that drugs could become a potent adjunct to sexual transmission and aggravate an already dire situation.

This chapter first reviews South Africa's unusual injection drug history, looking at how the market evolved to its present state. It then looks at the present state of affairs and assesses the extent of injection use of heroin, with an eye to predicting future developments. Finally, it considers the possibilities of needle exchange programmes and whether they would have any impact on the risks of transmission.

A brief history of South African injection drug use

In the past, injection drug use has not been much of an issue in South Africa. Known locally as 'spiking', there has been very little reporting of injected cocaine, amphetamines, or other non-narcotic drugs. Indeed, there have been relatively few seizures of pure amphetamines until recent years, when methcathinone and methamphetamine emerged as issues. In 2003, the police seized 33 local methcathinone labs, and sentinel surveillance of rehabilitation admissions in the Western Cape where methamphetamine was mentioned as a primary or secondary drug of abuse grew from less than 1% in the first half of 2002 to 18% in the first half of 2004. South Africa's drug markets are in a state of flux, and it is essential that interested parties keep abreast of potential new developments.

Prior to 1994, the primary drug injected in South Africa was a synthetic opiate called Wellconal® (dipipanone), known on the street as 'pinks' and sold abroad under the trade name Diconal®. A prescription painkiller in tablet form, the drug is still used medically in cases of severe pain. Street supplies are diverted via theft and fraud: pharmaceutical stores are burgled, stolen prescription pads are used, and terminal patients are paid to gather multiple scripts for sale. While the drug is designed to be taken orally, street users dissolve the tablets in water before injecting. Wellconal® contains silicon (which damages veins) and cyclizine (an antihistamine/anti-emetic). Most pinks addicts die within a few years from complications related to injection or an overdose. As a result, this drug, and injection in general, has never been widespread in South Africa.

Internationally, heroin is the drug most commonly associated with injection, but very little heroin use was reported in South Africa until recent years. While law enforcement data show a clear trend with a number of drug types from 1990, heroin arrests were inconsistent until a pronounced escalation occurred after 1997 (FIGURE 14.1).

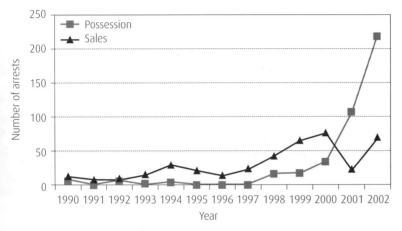

FIGURE 14.1 Heroin arrests started increasing after 1997. Note that the acute dip in enforcement seen in 1996 was a result of changes in police organisation that impacted across drug types
Source: SANAB

According to one sentinel-site monitoring network, national treatment demand for heroin has escalated consistently in recent years, and the drug has emerged in centres where no demand existed previously. For example, the share of heroin admissions to treatment in Gauteng province grew from nothing in the first half of 1998 to 8% in the second half of 2003. The great majority of patients were young and white, but black patients increased from 1% of heroin admissions in Cape Town and Gauteng in 2001 to 5% and 7% respectively in the first half of 2003. In Cape Town, 32% of heroin admissions were of 'coloured' people in the second half of 2003, compared with 2% in the first half of 2001. And heroin has emerged for the first time in Mpumalanga, a largely rural province situated along trafficking routes between Mozambique and the major urban centres. The heroin share of admissions to treatment grew from nothing in the second half of 1999 to 7% in the second half of 2003.

Why is heroin emerging only now? While apartheid isolation did limit South Africa's exposure to the global drugs market, it did not render the country impenetrable to contraband. Indeed, both state and liberation forces smuggled all manner of material across the borders, including vast quantities of Mandrax (methaqualone), another street drug. If there had been a local market for heroin, supplies would surely have found their way into the country.

The reasons for heroin's late arrival may have more to do with the lack of a pusher community than with barriers to import. The fall of apartheid opened South Africa to a rush of immigrants from other parts of the continent. Nigerian nationals, credited with supplying 40% of America's heroin, were among these migrants. In addition, East Africans arrived with connections to traditional sea transport routes from Central Asia. Enforcement data and qualitative research suggest that these two groupings are disproportionately involved in heroin trafficking and sales.

The drug first emerged as a problem in central Johannesburg, where Nigerian nationals and sex workers are concentrated. This area, specifically the residential hotels of Hillbrow and Berea, remains a major source of supply to the region and country as a whole, but areas such as Sunnyside in Pretoria and Seapoint in Cape Town have become equally problematic. As with drugs such as cocaine and ecstasy, heroin has impacted on the white community first and most powerfully, but, as the sentinel site data cited above show, it is rapidly expanding among other ethnic groups.

The present

There are currently two main types of heroin in South Africa: brown heroin (called 'brown sugar' or simply 'heroin') and white heroin ('Thai white'). The brown was introduced first, with white heroin making a more recent appearance. In keeping with international trends, the white was initially seen as a far better grade of heroin. The difference in colour is due to the refining process, but may also be associated, as the name suggests, with country of origin.

While members of all ethnic and national groups are involved in the market, foreign nationals are particularly prominent. Nigerians, especially those of the Igbo language group from the southeast corner of the country, import the drug and market it in inner-city areas, such as Hillbrow in Johannesburg and Seapoint in Cape Town, where sex workers form a major pillar of their consumer base. They have connections to other expatriate communities of Igbo in supplier cities such as Bangkok. East Africans, especially Tanzanians and Burundians, market the drug in the suburbs of Cape Town and Pretoria.

The sex worker/Nigerian interface is particularly worrying from an epidemiological perspective, because widespread injection could facilitate the transmission of HIV among the sex workers and through them to their clients. While little research has been done on the topic, the few studies that have been published indicate a sero-prevalance level of about 50% among street sex workers, with significant differences between ethnic groups within the profession. White sex workers, who have relatively low levels of HIV, are most likely to be heroin users, according to both qualitative research and arrestee testing. Sharing of needles between ethnic groups could dramatically impact overall infection rates. In addition, street sex workers who use drugs have a strong incentive to introduce their clients to substance use, in the hopes that the client will pay for mutual consumption.

The presence of heroin does not automatically result in an injection problem, because heroin can be ingested in a number of ways. At present, most heroin users in this country 'chase' their drugs: they vaporise the powder on aluminium foil using a lighter and draw the fumes into their lungs with a straw. In addition, heroin can be snorted or mixed with cannabis or tobacco and smoked.

International experience shows, however, that variations in the quality of heroin, and in particular a decline in purity, can create pressures toward injection. Once markets become established, wholesalers can control for variations in supply by 'cutting' the drug with various inert and psychoactive substances. As market chains become more protracted, intermediaries maximise profits by additional cutting. In South Africa, heroin (especially the brown grade in Cape Town) has been found to be cut with a range of substances, including caffeine, benzodiazepines and barbiturates.

Non-injection users can become just as addicted as injection users, and when purity levels decline, the need for a more direct method of ingestion increases. In addition, experienced users develop a tolerance. Desire to recapture the intensity of earlier experiences, as well as financial pressures, can push users toward injection. One study found that more than 15% of heroin snorters monitored moved to drug injection during an average period of a little more than a year.

While there have been variations in quality and availability, South African heroin remained quite pure for some time. This allowed users to continue to receive a satisfactory experience from chasing. Once injection is tried, it presents attractions not seen in other methods of ingestion. Intravenous use is accompanied by a 'rush' – a short period of intense sensation – in addition to the longer lasting sense of euphoria found in less direct routes. For some users, this sensation is enough to overcome initial reservations around needle use.

There is evidence that this transition has already started to take place. In Johannesburg and Cape Town at the end of 2003, just under half of all of those admitted for heroin treatment reported some injection use (TABLE 14.1), and 38% of heroin patients in Cape Town reported injection as their primary means of using heroin. Thus, of those who said they had tried injecting, 87% considered it their primary method of ingestion. This is up from 56% in the first half of 2000, so a growing share of those who have experimented with needles have come to prefer injection.

	Jul–Dec 1999	Jan–Jun 2000	Jul–Dec 2000	Jan–Jun 2001	Jul–Dec 2001	Jan–Jun 2002	Jul–Dec 2002	Jan–Jun 2003	Jul–Dec 2003
Cape Town									
Number of heroin users	49	63	88	105	90	103	94	111	117
% injecting	29%	49%	47%	47%	51%	45%	34%	38%	44%
Gauteng									
Number of heroin users				172	191	202	145	196	165
% injecting	n/a	n/a	n/a	31%	36%	42%	48%	49%	49%

TABLE 14.1 Proportion of heroin users reporting some injection use
Source: SACENDU

Data on needle sharing are lacking for South Africa. Anecdotal reports suggest accessibility of pharmaceutical sources varies quite a bit by location, with retailers in areas better known for drug consumption being more reluctant to supply needles. Many heroin addicts are under constant financial pressure due to the cost of their habit, and even the small cost involved in procuring a new needle can be a disincentive. In addition, the distance of amenable suppliers from consumption sites can make the choice to share needles more attractive.

Needle exchange programmes

'Needle exchange' or 'syringe exchange' programmes are a harm-reduction technique in which users are encouraged to turn in used needles in exchange for new ones at no cost. The idea is that fewer users will share needles as old ones grow dull or break. A number of nations with heroin problems considerably more advanced than South Africa's have successfully employed needle exchange pro-grammes as a means of reducing the risks of drug-using behaviour associated with the transmission of HIV and other blood-borne diseases, such as hepatitis. In addition, needle exchanges can provide a gateway to methadone programmes or other forms of treatment. The costs of such programmes need to be weighed against the costs of providing lifetime treatment to those infected with the virus.

Despite their efficacy, these programmes have encountered resist-ance from those who feel abstinence is the answer and allege that these programmes encourage use. There has been little research to support this position, however. Those interested in taking heroin intravenously are usually operating under conditions where the availability of a clean needle is an afterthought. It is for precisely this reason that needle exchanges need to be made as accessible as possible. Resistance from community groups to an apparent suborning of drug use can be addressed by consultation in the creation of such programmes. In the United States, needle exchanges are problematic because possession of drug paraphernalia is criminalised in most states, and many active needle exchanges are technically illegal. Fortunately, South Africa has no such legislation.

Several important lessons emerge from the international experience:

- In addition to formal needle exchanges, the rate of new needle use can be augmented by encouraging 'no questions asked' sale by local pharmacies.
- It is important that the needles be brought to the location where the drugs are used, and that they be available during the hours of usage. This may involve none-state actors, such as pharmacies, as well as impersonal methods of distribution, such as vending machines. It may even involve use of 'runners' employed to deliver clean needles to the primary injection sites.
- It is important that needle exchange be teamed with information about the risks of borrowing and lending needles, but excessive 'education' can become a deterrent to users taking up the service. Information should not be limited to HIV, but should also include other blood-borne diseases as well as hazards specific to injection, such as circulatory and clotting issues. Information should also be given on how to sterilise needles with bleach when new needles are not available.
- It is important that users be alerted to the dangers of sharing all injection equipment, including cooking spoons and filtering devices, as these can also become vectors for infection.

The potential for South Africa

At present, South Africa does not appear to have a major intravenous drug use problem, so it is easy to become complacent about issues such as needle exchange. Unfortunately, history has shown that levels of infection among injecting drug users can skyrocket overnight where needle sharing is common. The fact that half of all heroin users in treatment are experimenting with injection should ring alarm bells, especially given the levels of infection among the general population in this country, and the fact that many users are also sex workers. The growing number of users from highly infected communities means that injection drug use could become a bridge between population groups in a way that, for historical reasons, sexual contact is unlikely to become.

Due to limited resources, it is likely that needle exchanges and other interventions focused on the drugs – HIV link will be sidelined in favour of efforts aimed at reducing sexual transmission. This would be a mistake. The fact that the problem is at present small means that the time is ripe for intervention. A relatively low-cost, carefully targeted programme could plug this particular hole in the lifeboat, before it becomes a major hazard. This is possible in part because the problem is still limited, for the most part, to a minority community in a few well-known geographic areas. Indeed, a half-dozen well-selected and well-publicised sites could conceivably capture the majority of those at risk today.

If even this minor effort is considered too much, a lot could be achieved by simply making the state's position on the issue clear. The national government is good at making ground-breaking policy statements, and this talent should be put to work here. The Central Drug Authority should formally adopt a harm reduction stance in this area. This should be communicated to retail pharmacies and other sites where needles might be purchased, particularly those in high-risk areas. In other words, if the state is not willing to pay for needles, at least it can encourage retailers to sell to addicts, no questions asked.

In the end, successful intervention in this area will produce no great fanfare. Making the lives of junkies safer has never been high up on the list of public priorities. It will never be clear whether efforts actually saved lives. But if done properly, South Africa can rest confident in the knowledge that it drew on the best in international experience and took sound measures to reduce the risk of infection for all of its people.

Bibliography

CENTRAL DRUG AUTHORITY. 2001.'Heroin Use in South Africa'. Cape Town and Pretoria: Medical Research Council and the United Nations Office for Drug Control and Crime Prevention.

LEGGETT T. 2001.'Rainbow Vice: The drugs and sex industries in the new South Africa'. Cape Town: David Phillip Publishers and London: Zed Books.

LEGGETT T, PARRY CDH, PLÜDDEMANN A. 'Illicit drug-using offenders and dealers in South Africa: A profile for law enforcement.' Acta Criminologica 2004; 17: 155–167.

LEGGETT T. 'Drugs, sex work, and HIV in three South African cities'. Society in Transition 2001; 32: 101–109.

LEGGETT T OP CIT. 2001; TED LEGGETT (ED). 2002. 'Drugs and crime in South Africa: A study in three cities'. ISS Monograph Series No. 69. Pretoria, Institute for Security Studies.

Liu M. 'The curse of 'China White'. *Newsweek,* October 14, 1991.

Mathias R. 'Heroin snorters risk transition to injection drug use and infectious disease'. *NIDA Notes* 1999; 14(2). Rockville: National Institute on Drug Abuse, National Institutes of Health, December 1999.

Parry C, Pluddemann A, Bhana A, Harker N, Potgieter H, Gerber W. 2003. *'SACENDU Update'.* Cape Town: Medical Research Council.

Pluddemann A, Hon S, Bhana A, Harker N, Potgieter H, Gerber W, Parry C. 2002. *'Proceedings of the South African Community Epidemiological Network on Drug Use Report Back Meetings, Phase 12'.* Cape Town: Medical Research Council.

UNAIDS. *'Report on the Global HIV/AIDS Epidemic June 2000'.* Geneva. 2002

United States Drug Enforcement Administration. *'Country Profile: Nigeria.'* Unpublished report. 1992.

CHAPTER 15

New prevention strategies under development and investigation

Salim Abdool Karim and Cheryl Baxter

INTERVENTIONS FOR PROTECTION FROM HIV infection beyond behaviour modification and barrier methods are urgently required if we are to alter the course of the epidemic. This chapter discusses important prevention strategies that are under development. Besides vaccines and microbicides, the use of antiretroviral therapy, male circumcision, and the treatment and prevention of Herpes Simplex Virus Type 2 (HSV-2) as yet unproven HIV prevention modalities, are discussed.

An AIDS vaccine remains an important hope for the control of HIV/AIDS. Despite significant advances in AIDS vaccine research, including new vaccine constructs, new vectors and prime-boost strategies, its realisation is still several years away. The significant challenge of a lack of correlates of protection remain and further phase III efficacy trials are required. Microbicides provide real potential to influence the course of the HIV epidemic as a woman-controlled prevention method. There has been substantial progress in microbicide development with several potential products entering phase III trials this year.

The use of antiretroviral therapy to reduce viral load and thus the probability of transmission of HIV is one prevention strategy for HIV positive persons and studies to evaluate the efficacy of such a strategy are currently underway. The presence of HSV-2 has been shown to greatly increase the transmission probability of HIV and thus prevention and treatment of HSV-2 infection is a promising new prevention strategy under investigation.

Although some studies suggest that circumcised men are less likely to become infected with HIV, the current evidence is insufficient to consider male circumcision as a public health intervention.

Randomised controlled trials are currently underway to assess the feasibility, acceptability and efficacy of such an intervention.

The results from current trials of HSV-2 treatment, male circumcision and antiretroviral therapy for HIV prevention should become available in the next two to four years and may provide valuable additional options to curb the spread of HIV.

Vaccines

It is now widely accepted that an effective, preventive HIV vaccine would provide the best method for controlling the catastrophic HIV/AIDS pandemic, especially in less developed countries.

Clinical trials of HIV vaccines have been underway for more than 15 years but the first phase III efficacy trial was completed only recently. Vaccine development and assessment has primarily taken place in developed, western countries and most early phase human clinical trials have been done in the USA and Europe. Globally, there have been more than 80 phase I and II trials but only one product – a bivalent, recombinant gp120 vaccine, AIDSVAX, has reached large-scale phase III efficacy testing in North America, the Netherlands and Thailand. Despite many years of research, most of the experimental vaccines are still limited to testing in animal models and no efficacious HIV vaccine for humans has yet been identified.

A wide variety of vaccine approaches are currently being pursued. For many years the vaccine pipeline was limited to monomeric gp120 or gp160 proteins based on laboratory strains of the virus, different synthetic peptides, and simple poxvirus-HIV-1 recombinant vectors. The pipeline has recently expanded to include gp120 constructs based on clinical isolates of HIV-1, conformational envelope antigens, complex canarypox vectors expressing multiple HIV-1 genes, different constructs of naked DNA vaccines, new live vectors, including the modified vaccinia Ankara (MVA), and the Venezuelan Equine Encephalitis virus replicon. The most promising candidates are attenuated live vectors containing HIV genes. Examples of such vectors include Sindbis, adenovirus, associated adenovirus, and Venezuelan Equine Encaphalitis virus. These vectors have been attenuated so that no infection by the vector can take place after administering the vaccine formulation. In addition to these vectors, a host of recombinant DNA constructs are available using HIV genes from various subtypes. Vaccine classes and types are summarised in TABLE 15.1.

The ability of a vaccine or a component of a microorganism to stimulate an immune response is key to memory in the immune response for future protection. Designing a successful vaccine against HIV has been hampered by the lack of an immune correlate of

HIV VACCINE CLASSES AND TYPES

	Class	Product Name	Producer
1.	Canarypox vectors	ALVAC vCP 1452	Aventis Pasteur
2.	DNA Plasmid vaccines	TBD -Clade C Gag-Env plasmids	Chiron
		EP HIV-1090	Epimmune
		pGA2/JS2 DNA	Emory
		Gag and Env DNA/PLG microparticles	Chiron
		VRC-HIVDNA-009	NIH VRC
		WLV003	Wyeth
3.	Fowlpox vectors	TBC-F357; TBC-F349	Therion
4.	Lipopeptides	LIPO-5	Aventis Pasteur/ ANRS
5.	Modified Vaccinia Ankara vectors	MVA pGA/JS2	NIAID-LVD
		TBC-M358	Therion
		TBC-M335	Therion
6.	Non-Replicating Adenovirus vectors	MRKAd5 HIV-1 Gag	Merck
		VRC-HIVDNA-010	NIH VRC
7.	Peptides	Wyeth me CTL peptide vaccine	Wyeth
8.	Proteins	AIDSVAX B/B	VaxGen
		Gp120 MN	VaxGen
		TBD - Clade C Env subunit	Chiron
		gp140 SF-162 – oligomeric V2-deleted	Chiron
		NefTat + gp120W61D	GlaxoSmithKline
9.	VEE vectors	AVX-101	AlphaVax
10.	Yeast vectors	HIVAX-GS	GlobeImmune
11.	Live attenuated vector	VSV	Wyeth

TABLE 15.1 HIV Vaccine classes and types
Source: The Pipeline Project HIV vaccines in development
http://chi.ucsf.edu/ vaccines

protection, ie it is not clear which type of immune response is needed to provide protection against HIV. Unfortunately, animal protection experiments and natural history studies have failed to produce conclusive results and no animal model proposed so far can adequately mimic human disease infection and disease progression.

Cellular immune responses

Cytotoxic T lymphocytes (CTL) are part of the cellular immune response and are associated with control of viral replication. CTLs are capable of directly destroying HIV-infected cells and thus vaccines designed to stimulate CTL responses are more likely to lead to control of viral replication and therefore viral load as opposed to creating sterilising immunity which would prevent primary HIV infection. A subset of T lymphocytes (CD8+ T-cells) have CD8 receptors on their surfaces and are the dominant effector cells responsible for defending the host against cellular level viral infections. Other CD8+ T-cells are capable of suppressing HIV replication without necessarily killing the infected cell. CD8+ T-cells may be critical to resisting HIV infection. (For a more detailed description on immune responses refer to CHAPTER 8).

A further component of cellular immunity includes the regulatory T-cells, which are capable of directing antibody- and cell-mediated immune responses. The main regulatory T-cell, the helper T-cell or CD4+ T-cell, is also HIV's main target.

CD4+ T helper function is typically measured by measuring T-cell proliferation following incubation with viral antigens. Most HIV-infected subjects have weak or undetectable proliferative responses to HIV antigens. Monitoring of cellular immune response to vaccination has advanced significantly in the last few years; the more complex chromium release assay has been superseded by new assays that allow a rapid identification of T-cell responses. Specifically, the gamma-interferon enzyme linked immunospot (Elispot) assay and the intra-cytoplasmic cytokine (ICC) assay are now being commonly utilised worldwide to measure T-cell functional response to HIV.

The failure of vaccinated or infected subjects to develop virus-specific proliferative responses is common and may result from infection and subsequent death of HIV-specific CD4+ T-cells when they encounter an HIV-infected antigen-presenting cell. Relatively vigorous HIV-1-specific CD4+ T helper responses have been reported in HIV-infected long-term nonprogressors and patients who received potent antiretroviral therapy early in the course of primary infection. Induction of strong HIV-specific proliferative responses may therefore be an important goal for candidate vaccines, although there is at present no definitive evidence for this conclusion.

Humoral immune responses

Humoral (antibody-mediated) immunity refers to protection provided by antibodies, the secreted products of B lymphocytes. Antibodies are important because they are the immune system's first line of defence and are thought to be the key to preventing viruses from ever contacting the cells they infect.

Antibodies function either by binding to part of the virus that may or may not have antiviral effects (binding antibodies) or by inactivating or preventing the virus from infecting cells (neutralising antibodies). By virtue of their ability to prevent viral entry and infection, neutralising antibodies represent the best possibility of inducing sterilising immunity, ie prevention of infection. Thus the ability to stimulate a neutralising antibody response remains a desirable endpoint of vaccination. However, this has been exceedingly difficult to attain. These difficulties have arisen because HIV has the ability to mutate at a rapid rate and several subtypes of the virus exist.

Gp160, a protein located in the outer envelope of HIV, has been identified as important for stimulating neutralising antibodies. However, several features, eg glycosylation and the oligomeric form of the HIV envelope limit its ability to be neutralised by antibodies. Initial candidate vaccines were recombinant antigens of HIV envelope proteins that stimulated neutralising antibody responses to laboratory-adapted viruses but were unable to neutralise primary viruses. This is because these vaccines comprised monomeric gp120 or gp160 and thus did not present the correct conformational epitopes to the immune system. In addition, it has become clear than laboratory-adapted viruses are relatively easy to neutralise compared with primary viruses. This resulted in a rethinking of the immunogens used to stimulate neutralising antibodies and a new phase in the approach to envelope vaccine design. Basic research is ongoing into the use of modified *Env* proteins from primary isolates that can either retain the trimeric structure or mimic a conformational form that exposes neutralisation-sensitive determinants.

A variety of different assays have been used to characterise humoral responses against HIV, including binding to viral proteins (as assessed by either ELISA or Western blot), inhibition of syncytia formation, complement fixation, ability to mediate antibody-dependent cell-mediated cytotoxicity (ADCC), ability to neutralise infectivity or cell fusion, and ability to block CD4-gp120 interactions. At present, whether any of these assays are more likely than another to measure antibody responses relevant to protective immunity is unknown.

Current HIV candidates elicit reasonably potent cellular immune responses, but only low levels of neutralising antibodies. Such CTL-based vaccines (eg DNA vaccines) do not prevent infection, but can have a beneficial effect on disease course. A combination of both humoral and cell-mediated immune responses may be needed for effective protection.

Mucosal immune responses

In addition to cellular and humoral immunity responses, the stimulation of mucosal immunity may also be necessary to achieve protection against HIV. The majority of HIV infections occur via mucosal routes and stimulating the mucous membranes that line the rectal and genital tract to induce mucosal immunity may be an essential requirement of an effective HIV vaccine.

Induction of protective immunity against mucosal challenge with SIV or SHIV has been reported in several macaque models. Although these animal model results cannot be assumed to hold true for humans exposed to HIV, there is evidence from studies on highly exposed persistently seronegative (HEPS) individuals that mucosal immune responses are possible.

The prime-boost strategy

One way currently in vogue to enhance immune responses to HIV is the combination approach called prime-boost strategy. This strategy endeavours to get the immune system both to make neutralising antibodies and to launch a strong cell-mediated response. The immune system is first primed with one vaccine, eg naked DNA, and then boosted with a different vaccine, eg live vector/protein. The boosting strategy serves to focus CD8+ T-cells to recognise an array of epitopes.

By itself, a naked DNA vaccine stimulates production of memory T-cells but few antibodies. The prime-boost combination, however, can stimulate a strong cellular immune response, including persistent killer CD8+ T-cells as well as antibodies that neutralise the virus. Several methods to measure CD8+ T-cell responses in vaccine recipients have been developed and are discussed further in CHAPTER 8. The prime-boost method has shown promise in animal models and better protection has been achieved using this method than any other HIV vaccine strategy to date. This strategy has also been tested in human clinical phase I and II trials, where it has been found to be safe and effective.

Implications of the VaxGen trial results

The results of the first phase III AIDS vaccine (AIDSVAX B/B) trial were announced in February 2003. Although safe, the vaccine did not show an overall reduction of HIV infection in the vaccination arm of the entire study population. These results suggest that narrowly defined antibodies are not effective in providing protection against HIV infection.

Protein-based vaccines, such as AIDSVAX B/B, generally elicit only a humoral response, without significant stimulation of the cellular arm of the immune system. The vaccine may not have succeeded either because the antibodies generated by the vaccine did not coincide with the antigens on the viruses, which led to infection in the study population, or because the antibodies on their own were not sufficient to protect HIV infection. More phase III trials are needed to understand this better.

South Africa's contribution to the AIDS vaccine

The uncertainty over whether a vaccine effective for one subtype will be effective for another has encouraged researchers in developing countries to develop vaccines for strains of HIV-1 that are dominant in their own countries. South African researchers have taken the responsibility for vaccine work aimed at the subtype C strain of HIV, the dominant form in South Africa. The South African AIDS Vaccine Initiative (SAAVI) was established in 1999 to coordinate the local research, development and testing of HIV/AIDS vaccine for subtype C strains. Most HIV vaccines that have been tested in clinical trials to date have been developed for the subtype B virus. The overall mission of this initiative is to develop a safe, effective, affordable and accessible HIV vaccine for South Africa. SAAVI is a national project that is sanctioned by the South African Government and is coordinated by the Medical Research Council of South Africa.

SAAVI consists of a coordinated network of researchers who are currently working on making novel HIV vaccines; developing clinical trial sites of the SAAVI vaccines and other vaccines from international groups; performing laboratory immunology assessments of these vaccines; developing locally relevant ethical frameworks for these investigations, and providing community education, mobilisation, legal and human rights, advocacy and communications.

Making candidate vaccines

The two main institutions involved in developing candidate HIV vaccines for the subtype C HIV virus in South Africa are the Universities of Cape Town and Stellenbosch.

The University of Cape Town is generating candidate HIV vaccines, using DNA, modified vaccinia Ankara (MVA), Bacille-Calmette-Guérin (BCG), salmonella, and virus-like particles (VLPs), and testing these in animal models. This centre was instrumental in selecting and patenting HIV isolates for SAAVI candidate vaccines at the University of Cape Town and abroad. The other international initiatives using these genes include the Venezuelan Equine Encephalitis – VEE (Alphavax), adeno-associated virus and oligomeric gp140 vaccines. The VEE was one of the first vaccine candidates approved for phase I testing by South Africa's Medicines Control Council in 2003.

An immunology and testing laboratory in the Department of Virology, University of Stellenbosch, is generating candidate HIV vaccines in collaboration with Chiron, using a DNA construct, as well as mammalian and fungal cell expression systems, and testing these in animal models. This laboratory serves primarily as a facility for monitoring the immunogenetic potential and overall efficacy of vaccine constructs generated in the US. At present the main focus is on the first primate vaccination study – a DNA prime (cordon-optimised, *Gag, Pol, Env*), protein boost (modified *Env*) vaccination protocol, which is being assessed in baboons.

What are microbicides and why is their development important?

Microbicides are substances that are able to kill bacteria, viruses and parasites. A microbicide is any substance that can substantially reduce transmission of sexually transmitted diseases, including HIV, when applied to either the vagina or rectum. The development of microbicides as a women-controlled mechanism is particularly important given that almost six out of ten new HIV infections occur in women. Microbicides would fill an important gap for women who are unable to successfully negotiate mutual monogamy or male condom use. Gender and power issues, especially in the South African setting, also strongly influence the ability of women to negotiate safe sexual practices with their partners (discussed further in CHAPTER 16). Microbicides are not yet available, but as many as 60 products, including 11 that have proven safe and effective in animals, are currently being tested in many countries, including South Africa.

Mechanisms of action

Several microbicides are under development and are designed to target different points in the HIV infection process. Microbicides can use one or more of the following mechanisms of action to combat infection. They can support normal vaginal defences, destroy surface active pathogens by disrupting membranes, inhibit pathogen entry into mucosal cells by creating a barrier between the pathogen and the vagina, prevent fusion between the membranes of the pathogen and mucosal cells and inhibit a virus from replicating once it has infected the cells that line the vaginal wall. Examples of microbicides capable of these actions are presented in TABLE 15.2 A successful microbicide product will probably include a combined strategy that targets multiple components of HIV infection to maximise its effectiveness.

Microbicide studies in South Africa

Several microbicide studies have been conducted in South Africa. Completed phase I trials include: a randomised cross-over double blinded study which was conducted with 20 sex workers in 1999 to establish the acceptability of Nonoxynol-9 film. This study showed that Nonoxynol-9 was an acceptable product for use in this population of sex workers. Some side-effects occurred, such as genital lesions, with increased viral loads associated with the lesions. The placebo provided less protection against sexually transmitted infections. A phase I study of PRO 2000/5 (P) gel which was conducted among HIV-uninfected and abstinent HIV-infected women and

Action	Microbicide examples
Maintenance or mobilisation of normal vaginal defences	· Buffer Gel · Engineered lactobacillus · Hydrogen peroxide/peroxidases
Destroying surface active pathogens by disrupting membranes	· Nonoxynol-9 / Octoxynol-9 · Benzalkonium chloride · C31G – Savvy · Chlorhexidine zinc gel
Inhibiting pathogen entry into mucosal cells	· Carraguard® / PC-515 · PRO2000 gel · Emmelle / Dextrin-2–Sulfate
Preventing fusion between the membranes of the pathogen and mucosal cells	· CCR5 inhibitors · Soluble CD4
Inhibiting post-fusion replication (poorly absorbed ARVs)	· Nucleoside reverse transcriptase inhibitors (PMPA) · NNRTIs (UC-781) · Protease inhibitors (WHI-07)

TABLE 15.2 Mechanism of action of microbicides

assessed the acceptability of once or twice daily exposure to two different concentrations of the gel. The results indicated that the product was well tolerated and no serious adverse events were evident. Another phase I study of PRO 2000/5 (P) Gel was conducted among healthy sexually inactive women and the gel was well tolerated. Phase I study of COL-1492 established that the multiple daily use of COL-1492 by female sex workers did not show an increase of local toxicity over that of a placebo.

A Phase II study was undertaken by the Population Council of its lead candidate microbicide, Carraguard®, in two sites in South Africa. This randomised placebo-controlled trial evaluated 150 woman-years of exposure to the council-developed product and a placebo. Women in both groups overwhelmingly found the gel and the applicator to be acceptable and they are proceeding with phase III studies of this product.

A phase II/III randomised, placebo-controlled, triple-blinded study with COL-1492, a nonoxynol-9 (N-9) vaginal gel, was conducted in 2002 in a cohort of 892 female sex workers. This study showed that the product did not have a protective effect on HIV transmission in high-risk women. Low frequency use of nonoxynol-9 causes neither harm nor benefit, but frequent use increases a women's risk of HIV infection. Multiple use of N-9 has been shown to irritate the lining of the vagina which may facilitate HIV infection. This drug can no longer be deemed a potential HIV-prevention method. A number of phase II and III trials of several products, eg PRO 2000, PMPA, Buffer Gel, Cellulose Sulphate and Carraguard®, are currently underway in South Africa and results from these trials will become available in the next three to five years.

Current state of clinical development of microbicides

Effective vaginal microbicides will probably be delivered in many forms, such as gels, creams, suppositories, films, sponges and vaginal rings. Many microbicidal products are in various stages of development but testing the efficacy and safety of microbicides takes many years and involves a number of carefully phased stages. A safe and effective microbicide is scientifically possible within the next five to seven years.

The current state of clinical development of microbicides includes several new generation products such as PRO 2000, Buffer Gel and Carraguard®, which are in advanced stages of testing. Several products are likely to enter phase III trials in 2004, with more in phase II and entering phase III in the near future. The pipeline of new products is growing rapidly and more than 20 products are progressing to human safety trials. Microbicides currently in development are summarised in TABLE 15.3.

Phase	Microbicide	
Phase I	UC-781	Human Monoclonal antibodies
	SPL7013 / Viva gel	Emmelle / dextrin-2-sulfate
	Pro 2000	Cellulose sulfate
	Polystyrene sulofonate	Cellulose acetate phthlalte (CAP)
	PMPA – topical formulation	Carraguard®
	PMPA – oral formulation	Buffer Gel
	Acidform	Benzalkonium Chloride (BZK)
	Lactin vaginal capsule	
Phase I / II	Invisible condom	
Phase II	Praneen Polyherbal formulations	Cellulose sulphate
	Lactocacillus suppository	Carraguard®
	Emmelle dextrin-2 sulphate	
Phase II / IIb	Pro 2000/5	
Phase II/III	C3IG / SAVVY	Buffer Gel
Phase III	Cellulose sulfate	C3IG/SAVVY
	Carraguard®	

TABLE 15.3 Microbicides under development *(Adapted from the Alliance for Microbicide development document on Protocol Summaries of Clinical Trials of topical microbicides – www.microbicide.org)*

Obstacles to microbicide development

Several obstacles have slowed the development of a safe and effective microbicide. The first obstacle centres on financial commitments. An estimated $775 million in product development costs are required over the next five years to develop safe and effective microbicide products, but only about $230 million has been committed thus far. A successful product will require extensive and sustained investment in research and development, access and advocacy.

To show safety and efficacy, the product must be tested on large numbers of sexually active people. Trials also need to be conducted among selected populations that are likely to be at high risk of acquiring HIV infection. Clinical trials are thus often carried out in developing countries that have high levels of infection or among sex workers. Counselling on use and provision of condoms as a proven HIV prevention method in addition to the experimental product is ethically required in all HIV prevention trials, including microbicide trials. Under these conditions the trial can only measure whether microbicides improve on the protection afforded by condom use. Other practical, ethical and scientific challenges include behaviours such as anal sex, and use of other intravaginal substances (see CHAPTER 16) and the lack of a true placebo.

Microbicide research and development has also been more challenging than vaccines as it has been difficult to mobilise pharmaceutical industry support. Without a proof of concept (that other vaginal products prevent STIs), investor concern is created about risks of investing in a product without evidence of its success. Other concerns surrounding the development of microbicide include the potential hazards related to reproductive toxicity and the increased risk of local toxicity from applying a product repeatedly to the same tissue that may enhance risk of infection. The threshold of acceptability and toxicity will differ between countries, and those with an aggressive spreading disease, such as developing countries, will be more likely to accept a partially effective product.

The future for microbicides

Acceptability studies among men and women in South Africa suggested that microbicides would be acceptable, and both men and women would be happy to use the product if it was available on the market. The first vaginal microbicides developed are not expected to provide complete protection against STIs and HIV. However, a microbicide even with 30 or 40% efficacy would have an enormous public health benefit.

A combination of microbicides, targeting multiple components of HIV infection, are more likely to prove effective than interventions that disrupt only a single step or target a single gene process. The development of a protection mechanism for women remains hopeful and provides real potential to influence the course of the HIV epidemic.

The rationale for the use of antiretroviral prophylaxis to prevent sexual HIV transmission comes from a Ugandan discordant couple study that demonstrates a strong relationship between how much virus is present and the probability of HIV transmission. Given that high viral load has a higher risk of transmission than low viral load, it begs the question whether interventions that can reduce viral load will consequentially reduce the probability of transmission of HIV. Several mathematical models estimate up to 80% HIV reduction with antiretroviral use. There are several studies underway that seek to evaluate the effectiveness of antiretrovirals to prevent heterosexual transmission of HIV in sero-discordant couples. The scale-up and increasing access to voluntary counselling and testing (VCT) and highly active antiretroviral therapy (HAART) creates a new opportunity to integrate prevention and care. The impact of HAART on reducing viral load presents an opportunity to assess whether HAART in HIV-positive people can reduce new infections thereby extending prevention strategies available to HIV-positive persons.

In South Africa, major companies and industries in the private sector including the mines, utility companies and clothing manufacturers are beginning to provide antiretroviral therapy to their employees. Until recently, antiretroviral drugs in the public sector were only available through pharmaceutical company sponsored clinical trials, and occupational post-exposure and perinatal transmission prophylaxis.

The recent decision of the South African government to make antiretroviral therapy available in the public sector has changed this. There is therefore an urgent need to develop simple and sustainable strategies for delivery of HIV care to large numbers of patients in the context of the existing under-developed health care delivery systems. The scale of the growing morbidity coupled with ongoing high HIV incidence rates demand an approach that addresses both treatment and prevention in an integrated manner. Access to antiretroviral therapy must be integrated into a comprehensive programme that includes VCT for HIV infection, the diagnosis, prevention and treatment of the major opportunistic infections (mainly TB, candida and other fungal infections) and screening for TB, cervical carcinoma and Kaposi's sarcoma.

Should the roll-out of antiretroviral therapy in South Africa fail to integrate treatment and prevention, the epidemic is likely to continue to rise. It is therefore essential for treatment to be accompanied by improved prevention so that both AIDS deaths and new HIV infections decrease, leading to a declining epidemic. The use of anti-retrovirals for treatment is discussed in greater detail in CHAPTER 33.

Herpes simplex virus (HSV) treatment as a prevention strategy

Herpes simplex virus type 2 (HSV-2) infection is sexually transmitted and causes genital ulceration. The development of accurate and sensitive laboratory tests to study HSV-2 over the last decade has contributed to our understanding of HSV infection and its role as a cofactor in the sexual transmission of HIV. In many sub-Saharan African countries, the HSV-2 epidemic has spread in parallel with the HIV epidemic. Although the link between genital ulcers and HIV-1 has been noted by epidemiologists for many years, only recently has HSV been recognised as a major factor behind this association.

Prevention and treatment of HSV-2 is a new HIV prevention strategy being studied. The rationale for this intervention is based on data demonstrating that clinically undetectable infection with HSV-2 increases the amount of HIV in the blood and thereby could lead to HSV-2 increasing the risk of transmitting HIV. Additionally, genital ulcer disease (GUD) causes a 4-fold greater chance of transmitting HIV, and thus, HSV-2 as the most common cause of GUD, may increase the risk of acquiring HIV.

Further, daily use of valcyclovir can reduce HSV-2 transmission among HSV-2 discordant heterosexual couples, supporting the notion that antivirals could reduce HSV-2 transmission. An HSV-2 vaccine which is currently under study may prevent HSV-2 infection or prevent shedding – this may be another future mechanism to reduce transmission. Preliminary data from Tanzania show HIV incidence rates about 13 times higher in men with newly acquired HSV-2 compared with about six times higher in men with existing infection. Similar findings were observed among sex workers and their clients in Pune, India. Whilst these data illustrate a strong relationship between HSV-2 and HIV, they are inadequate at this point to support any specific public health intervention. A randomised control trial to prove that suppressing HSV-2 infection can reduce HIV infection is needed and such a trial is currently underway.

Controlling STIs should be an integral part of HIV prevention and is one of the most fundamental issues that needs to be addressed if we are to limit further devastation caused by AIDS. Offering HSV-2 serologic counselling and testing at HIV counselling and testing sites might help prevent the spread of both infectious diseases. The treatment of STIs to reduce the risk of HIV is discussed in further detail in CHAPTER 12.

An analysis of several studies suggests a protective benefit of male circumcision in a range of high-risk groups. However, there are several important factors that also need to be considered such as sexual behaviour, religion, penile hygiene, viral load and immune status. Recent evidence from a large cohort study of discordant couples in Uganda revealed that there were no new HIV infections in HIV-negative circumcised men compared with 16.7% in uncircumcised men. Not all effects of circumcision are necessarily beneficial. In studies undertaken in the general population, there was a lack of association with HIV and male circumcision. Therefore, current evidence is insufficient to consider male circumcision as a public health intervention. Several randomised controlled trials are currently underway in Kenya, Uganda and South Africa. Results from these trials together with assessments of the feasibility and acceptability of widespread male circumcision will need to be carefully considered prior to any public health policy decision.

Bibliography

BERTLEY FMN, WANG SW, KOZLOWSKI P ET AL. *'Effective induction of virus-specific immunity induced by rectal or nasal dna-mva vaccination and its effects on SHIV challenge'.* 10th Conference on retroviruses and opportunistic infections, February 10–14th, 2003. Hynes Convention Center Boston, Massachusetts, USA (abstract 453).

BIASIN M, LO CAPUTO S, SPECIALE L, COLOMBO F, RACIOPPI L, ZAGLIANI A ET AL. 'Mucosal and systemic immune activation is present in human immunodeficiency virus-exposed seronegative women'. *Journal of Infectious Diseases* 2001; 182: 1365–1374.

BURTON DR. 'A vaccine for HIV type 1: The antibody perspective'. *Proceedings of the National Academy of Sciences of the United States of America* 1997; 94: 10018–10023.

CROTTY S, MILLER CJ, LOHMAN BL, NEAGU MR, COMPTON L, LU D ET AL. 'Protection against simian immunodeficiency virus vaginal challenge by using Sabin poliovirus vectors'. *Journal of Virology* 2001; 75: 7435–7452

ESPARZA J, BHAMARAPRAVATI N. 'Accelerating the development and future availability of HIV-1 vaccines: why, when, where, and how?' *Lancet* 2000; 355: 2061–2066.

GRAY RH, WAWER MJ, BROOKMEYER R, SEWANKAMBO NK, SERWADDA D, WABWIRE-MANGEN F ET AL. 'Probability of HIV-1 transmission per coital act in monogamous heterosexual, HIV-1 discordant couples in Rakai, Uganda'. *Lancet* 2001; 357: 1149–1153.

MAZZOLI S, TRABATTONI D, LO CAPUTO S, PICONI S, BLE C, MEACCI F ET AL. 'HIV-specific mucosal and cellular immunity in HIV-seronegative partners of HIV-seropositive individuals'. *Nature Medicine* 1997; 3: 1250–1257.

MBOPI-KEOU FX; ROBINSON NJ; MAYAUD P, BELEC L, BROWN DWG. 'Herpes simplex virus type 2 and heterosexual spread of human immunodeficiency virus infection in developing countries: Hypotheses and research priorities'. *Clinical Microbiology and Infection* 2003; 9: 161–171.

MCCUTCHAN FE, SALMINEN MO, CARR JK, BURKE DS. 'HIV-1 genetic diversity'. *AIDS* 1996; 10(suppl 3): S13–S20.

Perelson AS, Neumann AU, Markowitz M, Leonard JM, Ho DD. 'HIV-1 dynamics in vivo: Virion clearance rate, infected cell life-span, and viral generation time'. *Science* 1996; 271: 1582–1586.

Quinn TC, Wawer MJ, Sewankambo N, Serwadda D, Li C, Wabwire-Mangen F et al. 'Viral load and heterosexual transmission of human immunodeficiency virus type 1'. *New England Journal of Medicine* 2000; 342: 921–929.

Rosenberg ES, Billingsley JM, Caliendo AM, Boswell SL, Sax PE, Kalams SA et al. 'Vigorous HIV-1-specific CD4+ T-cell responses associated with control of viremia'. *Science* 1997; 78: 1447–1450.

Rustomjee R, Abdool Karim Q, Abdool Karim SS, Laga M, Stein Z. 'Phase I trial of nonoxynol-9 film among sex workers in South Africa'. *AIDS* 1999; 13: 1511–1515.

Schoub BD. 'Vaccination as an intervention against viral diseases: Will this work for HIV?' *CME* 2002; 20: 561–566.

Schrier RD, Gnann Jr JW, Landes R, Lockshin C, Richman D, McCutchan A et al. 'T-cell recognition of HIV synthetic peptides in a natural infection'. *Journal of Immunology* 1989; 142: 1166–1176.

Stone A. 'Microbicides: A new approach to preventing HIV and other sexually transmitted infections'. *Nature Reviews* 2002; 1: 977–985.

UNAIDS/WHO. *'Report on the global HIV/AIDS epidemic.'* 2002.

Van Rensburg EJ. 'Vaccine design and making vaccines for Africa'. *CME* 2002; 20: 577–580.

van Damme L, Ramjee G, Alary M, Vuylsteke B, Chandeying V, Rees H et al. 'Effectiveness of COL-1492, a nonoxynol-9 vaginal gel, on HIV transmission in female sex workers: a randomised controlled trial'. *Lancet* 2002; 360: 971–977.

SECTION 4
Focal groups for understanding the HIV epidemic

CHAPTER 16

Heterosexual transmission of HIV – the importance of a gendered perspective in HIV prevention

Quarraisha Abdool Karim

THIS CHAPTER PROVIDES A brief overview of the global burden of heterosexually transmitted HIV, the role of age, gender, migration and sexually transmitted infections as key factors driving the epidemiology of HIV transmission and some of the underlying biological mechanisms for the heterosexual transmission of HIV. Specific societal and economic factors that shape masculine and feminine identities, and contribute to differences in the risk of acquiring infection heterosexually between men and women, are presented. Within this context the limitations of the current paradigm of HIV prevention, namely abstinence, behaviour modification and use of male condoms are also considered. These data show that acquisition and prevention of sexual transmission of HIV is a multi-factorial and complex social and biological challenge. If we are to make an impact on the current trajectory of this epidemic we will need to adopt more gender-sensitive approaches in all aspects of our response to the HIV epidemic. In conclusion, the approaches for achieving this are highlighted.

Heterosexual transmission of HIV

Some indication of the importance of the heterosexual component of the global burden of HIV infection is shown by the UNAIDS estimates at the end of 2003. Of the estimated 37.8 million prevalent infections, about 87% were acquired through heterosexual transmission. Further, of the 4.8 million new infections and 2.9 million AIDS deaths in 2003, over 85% were in people who acquired HIV infection hetero-sexually. These data underscore the importance of this mode of trans-mission.

FIGURE 16.1 further highlights the centrality of reducing hetero-sexual transmission of HIV to achieve control of this epidemic in

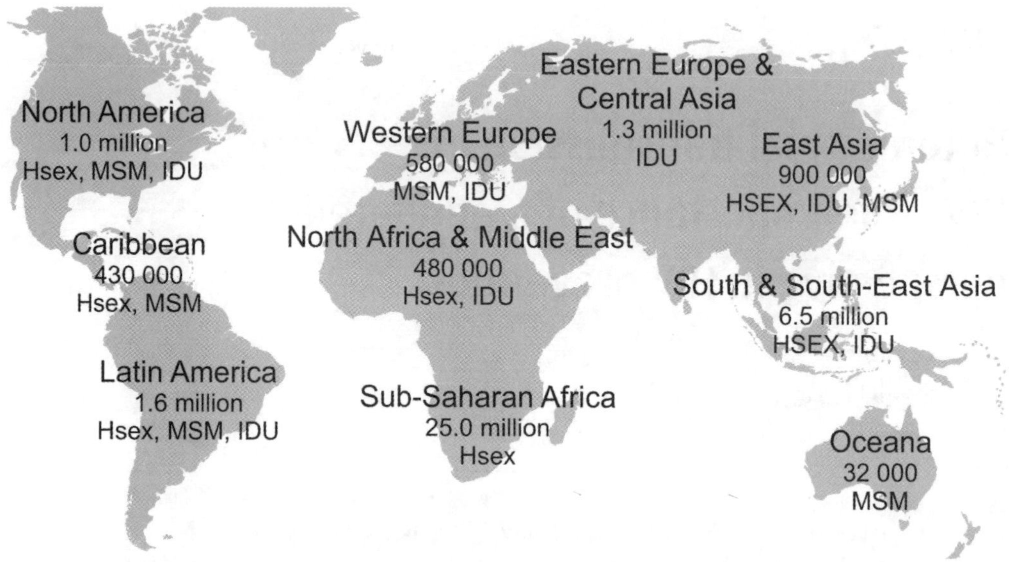

North America
1.0 million
Hsex, MSM, IDU

Western Europe
580 000
MSM, IDU

Eastern Europe &
Central Asia
1.3 million
IDU

East Asia
900 000
HSEX, IDU, MSM

Caribbean
430 000
Hsex, MSM

North Africa & Middle East
480 000
Hsex, IDU

South & South-East Asia
6.5 million
HSEX, IDU

Latin America
1.6 million
Hsex, MSM, IDU

Sub-Saharan Africa
25.0 million
Hsex

Oceana
32 000
MSM

FIGURE 16.1 Global burden: modes of transmission in 2003 *Source: Adapted from UNAIDS 2004 report on the global HIV/AIDS epidemic: 4th global report. Geneva Switzerland*

many parts of the world. The geographical distribution of the modes of HIV transmission indicate that heterosexual transmission of HIV is an important mechanism of transmission beyond sub-Saharan Africa to most countries around the world and particularly in south and south-east Asia, where a quarter of the new infections in 2003 occurred. Not only is heterosexual transmission important in driving the current major epidemic in sub-Saharan Africa but it is also a major factor driving the emerging epidemics in India and China. It is noteworthy that most of the epidemics in China and eastern Europe are being fuelled principally by injecting drug use, with sexual transmission as a secondary mode of spread by these individuals. The emerging patterns of injecting drug use in South Africa and its implications for HIV transmission are described and discussed in CHAPTER 14.

Epidemiological factors influencing heterosexual spread of HIV

Heterosexual transmission of HIV is shaped by several key epidemiological factors, which are discussed in this chapter.

Sex and age

The intersection of gender with age is an important determinant in the distribution of power in any society; younger members of society typically have less power than older members and younger women have less power than younger boys, while the overall power imbalances between men and women, at both societal and individual relationship levels, have their roots in adolescence.

Not surprisingly, a striking characteristic of heterosexual transmission is the disproportionate burden of HIV infection in young women compared with men. FIGURE 16.2 graphically illustrates the age-specific prevalence of HIV infection for men and women in rural South Africa. As can be observed from this diagram, not only are there more than twice as many infections in women compared with men, but women acquire HIV infection at least five to ten years earlier than men. While teenage girls are already close to peak prevalence by age 15 to 19 years, young boys aged 15 to 19 have little or no HIV infection.

In most African countries where heterosexual transmission is the major mode of transmission, a key factor in the epidemic is the high incidence rates in young women between the ages of 14 and 24 years. About a quarter of all new infections that occurred globally in 2003 were in people under the age of 25, highlighting the importance of youth in the pandemic and in South Africa.

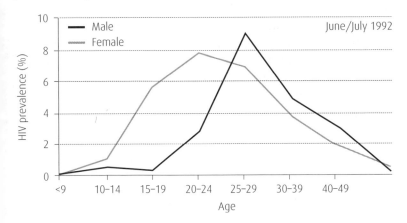

FIGURE 16.2 Age and gender specific prevalence of HIV infection in rural South Africa

The relationship between sex and HIV risk is a well-established fact demonstrated through several epidemiological studies conducted in the 1980s. The more efficient transmission of HIV from men to women compared with that from women to men (estimated to be seven times greater) is attributable to anatomical and physiological differences between men and women.

It is only more recently that there has been growing recognition and appreciation of the critical importance of gender in influencing the risk of acquisition of infection with HIV. This also affects a woman's access to services and social support when infected or affected by HIV/AIDS and single-handedly compounds the effects of biological risk.

Notwithstanding context-specific differences, there is consistency in role differences between men and women, particularly in access to resources and in decision-making authority, that create and sustain an unequal balance of power. Typically men are expected to be bread-winners and to generate income through economic activities outside the home, while women are expected to be responsible for maintaining the home through nurturing and rearing, but also through subsistence farming. Almost uniformly across the world, women have less access to and control of productive resources outside the home. Evidence for this imbalance in power includes the gender gaps in literacy levels, employment patterns, access to credit, land ownership and school enrolment rates. This imbalance in access to, and control of, productive forces and resources translates into an unequal balance in sexual relations in favour of men.

Some indication of the unfolding catastrophe for women is shown by the temporal trends in age-specific HIV prevalence in pregnant women in rural South Africa in Table 16.1. These data are presented in three-year intervals starting with 1992 through to 2001. In 1992, the peak prevalence of HIV infection was 6.9% in women aged between 20–24 compared with the lower prevalence observed in older women. While women in the 20- to 24-year-age group continue to experience high rates of HIV infection, the magnitude of that risk has grown substantially with time. HIV infection in 20 to 24-year-old women increased from 6.9% in 1992, to 21.1% in 1995, to 39.3% in 1998, and against all odds reached 50.8% in 2001.

TABLE 16.1 Temporal trends in the age-specific HIV prevalence (%) in ANC attendees in rural South Africa

Age Group	1992	1995	1998	2001
20–24	6.9	21.1	39.3	50.8
25–29	2.7	18.8	36.4	47.2
30–34	1.4	15.0	23.4	38.4
35–39	0.0	3.4	23.0	36.4

However, the real picture of the devastation in this community is best illustrated by the experience of a birth cohort of 1972 who were 20 to 24 years old in 1992. In TABLE 16.1 again, but this time focusing not on row one but on the diagonal which illustrates the HIV prevalence in this cohort of women aged 20 to 24 years in 1992, we see that the prevalence of HIV infection increased from 6.9% in 1992, to almost one in five infected by 1995, growing to almost one in four of those infected in 1998, until by 2001 almost one in three are infected with HIV.

Migration and HIV

While at a global level the economic divides between North and South have grown substantially in the past five years, the challenges in terms of unemployment, wage gaps, literacy levels and occupational segregation are greatest for poor, indigenous women. There is growing evidence of the link between women's low economic status and increased risk of acquiring infection with HIV. Immediate survival is a more pressing need than reducing HIV risk, which is perceived as a threat several years away. Specific ways that women's economic status influences their HIV risk relates to exchange of sex for survival, dependency on sexual partners for accommodation and security, access to information and services and the impact of migration.

Poverty is emerging consistently as the root cause of women using sex as a commodity. The definition of sex work is complex and ranges from the simple exchange of money for sex to a variety of other ways in which women use sex to make ends meet: sex to buy food or school uniforms, to pay school fees, to secure accommodation. Where marriage is rare, women enter into a series of monogamous relationships to ensure their and their children's survival. Often these women have a child to ensure continued financial support from the father, and in the course of a lifetime may end up having several children with different biological fathers. Pre-occupied with survival, and with limited access to information and health services, the risk of infection and options to reduce risk are not priorities for these women.

Poverty and lack of economic opportunities are more pronounced in rural and geographically isolated areas and influence both men and women to migrate in search of employment and income. In some settings it is more likely that men leave their families in rural areas to seek employment in cities. Where men are away from home for prolonged periods or seasonally, conjugal stability and social cohesion are disrupted and this increases the risk of HIV and other sexually transmitted infections. Men and women away from home are likely to establish new sexual networks that present a greater risk of HIV acquisition; on their return home, gendered role expectations and dominant ideologies around marriage and procreation make it unlikely they will use barrier methods.

While overall poverty increases HIV risk in both men and women, gender-related factors increase women's economic vulnerability and their dependency on men, and in turn their HIV risk. In contrast, gender-related norms and economic need force men to migrate without their families in search of work, fostering conditions for multiple sexual relationships and increasing HIV risk. Restricted access to information and services limit an individual's ability both to prevent infection and to cope when infected with HIV.

In South Africa, an important factor contributing to the high prevalence of HIV among women is the wide-spread 'circular migration' of men who work in the cities where they have 'town wives' while maintaining their spouses and children in rural areas. These circumstances place young women in rural areas in a uniquely vulnerable situation for acquiring HIV. In one rural survey the prevalence of HIV infection in women who saw their partners less than ten days a months was 15% compared with 0% in women who saw their partners more frequently. HIV infection in mobile couples is two to three times higher than that of more stable couples.

Other sexually transmitted infections

The sexual transmission of HIV is also influenced by the presence of other sexually transmitted infections (STIs). A Cochran analysis of eight studies show that STIs increase the risk of HIV transmission on average about fourfold, as shown by the position of the diamond on the bottom line in FIGURE 16.3. The size of the effect, as an odds ratio or a relative risk, is shown by the position of the squares on each line, and the size of the square indicates the relative sample size of each study. The burden of untreated STIs is high in many developing countries and this exacerbates and accelerates the spread of HIV.

FIGURE 16.3 Sexually transmitted diseases and HIV infection
Source: Adapted from Røttingen JA, Cameron WD, Geoffrey GP. A systematic review of the epidemiologic interactions between classic sexually transmitted diseases and HIV: how much really is known? Sexually Transmitted Diseases 2001; 28: 579–597

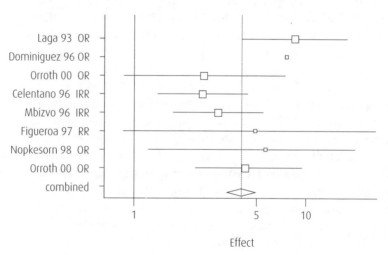

Gender norms define and determine access to health services. Many health services are not designed to reach men or meet men's needs, being modelled around societal norms that place the responsibility of nurturing, parenting and caring in the hands of women. Yet in allocation of household resources, particularly in poor communities, it is male members of the household who get priority. It is not uncommon to find women sacrificing their own health for that of their children and husbands. Two additional considerations are the judgemental attitudes of health care workers towards women seeking treatment for STIs and substantial asymptomatic presentation of STIs in women.

In South Africa, the prevalence of other STIs in pregnant women and family planning clients is high. One survey of antenatal and family planning clients using public sector primary care facilities in rural KwaZulu-Natal showed that 60% of the attendees had one or more STIs. The presence of other STIs substantially increases the risk of acquiring infection with HIV. In women, infection with other STIs is more likely to be asymptomatic and access to services may be limited.

HIV transmission – biological mechanisms

Our understanding of the underlying biological mechanisms of HIV transmission is incomplete. Studies have shown that semen and vaginal secretions have both cell-free virus and T-cells and macrophages which contain HIV. HIV shedding is not reduced by vasectomy suggesting that spermatozoa and other components of semen emanating from the testis are not the sole source of HIV in semen. While it is clear that both semen and vaginal secretions are able to transmit infection, the relative importance of cell-associated and cell-free viruses as the source of infectious virus is not known. Further, it is unclear whether epithelial cells play any role as targets of infectious virus. CD4-positive cells are present both in the male urethra and female vagina – but it remains unclear whether CD4 cells in the lumen or in the mucosa are both involved in the infectious process. If mucosal CD4 cells such as dendritic cells and macrophages are the primary focus of genital infection, it is unclear whether the conventional wisdom that breaks in the genital epithelium are absolutely necessary for infection to occur is true.

Some important epidemiological observations provide clues: immune status, that is, CD4 cell count, independent of blood viral load, correlates closely with the presence of HIV in semen and in the vagina; and HIV is most often detected during advanced stages of the disease.

These factors in combination result in a risk of HIV infection of three per 10 000 contacts for the male partner and a risk of 20 per 10 000 contacts for the female partner in peno-vaginal sex. Hence, on average, women are seven times more likely to become infected. This ratio rises in peno-anal sex, where the gender ratio exceeds 20:1, marking the importance of anal sex as an important factor not only for men but for women as well. Given that prevention messages seldom mention anal sex in women, this form of sex is increasing in several settings both to avoid pregnancy but also because of the seriously misguided notion that this may be safer. Comparing the risk of heterosexual transmission to other modes of transmission, needle sharing was associated with a risk of 60 per 10 000 and receptive anal sex with a risk of 80 per 10 000 contacts (TABLE 16.2).

HIV ESTIMATES FOR SOUTH AFRICA FOR 2000	
Exposure	**Risk per 10 000 contacts**
Needle sharing	
Source: Kaplan & Heimer 1992	60
Occupational needle stick	
Source: Gerberding 1995	33
Receptive anal	
Source: DeGruttola 1989	80
Receptive vaginal	
Source: Peterman 1996; Padian 1991	20
Insertive anal and vaginal	
Source: Padian 1991; Downs 1996	3
Receptive vs Insertive vaginal sex	± 7:1

TABLE 16.2 Estimates of per-contact HIV risk

Source: Kaplan EH, Heimer R. HIV prevalence among intravenous drug users: model-based estimates from New Haven's legal needle exchange. Journal of Acquired Immune Deficiency Syndrome. 1992; 5: 163–9. Gerberding JL, Lewis FR Jr, Schecter WP. Are universal precautions realistic? The Surgical Clinics of North America. 1995 Dec; 75: 1091–104. DeGruttola V, Seage GR 3rd, Mayer KH, Horsburgh CR Jr. Infectiousness of HIV between male homosexual partners. Journal of Clinical Epidemiology. 1989; 42: 849–56. Padian NS, Shiboski SC, Jewell NP. Female-to-male transmission of human immunodeficiency virus. JAMA. 1991 Sep 25; 266: 1664–7. Downs AM, de Vincenzi I. Probability of heterosexual transmission of HIV: Relationship to the number of unprotected sexual contacts. European Study Group in Heterosexual transmission of HIV. Journal of Acquired Immune Deficiency Syndrome Human Retrovirology 1996; 11: 388–395

Preventing sexual transmission of HIV

The epidemiological and biological data described above guide the prevention goal, which has two components: firstly, reduction in the number of discordant sexual acts; secondly, reduction of the risk of HIV transmission in discordant sexual acts.

The first can be achieved through: abstinence, sex between concordantly negative individuals with 'zero-grazing', and sex between concordantly positive individuals

At a programme level, the 'ABC' approach, which entails the promotion of abstinence, behaviour change and promotion of male condoms has been most widely promoted in HIV prevention.

Abstinence and behaviour change

Abstinence and lifelong mutually faithful monogamous relationships are critical to reduce the number of discordant sexual acts, and should be promoted as part of any comprehensive prevention strategy. However, they should not be promoted to the exclusion of all else as abstinence and monogamy may not be an option for many, such as migrants, who are at risk of acquiring infection with HIV.

Hence for those who are unable to, or fail to, reduce their number of discordant sexual acts, the prevention goal is to reduce the probability of transmission in discordant sexual acts. In this context, male and female condoms provide a proven prevention option. Microbicides, vaccines, antiretroviral prophylaxis, control and prevention of herpes simplex virus-2 infection and male circumcision are unproven prevention options which may have great potential in the future.

Male condoms

There is convincing data from several studies collated in a Cochran review that consistent condom use reduces HIV incidence by at least 80%, within the context of the varying levels of effectiveness described in different studies. To highlight just one study in discordant couples, there were no new infections in those who used condoms consistently, while the HIV incidence was 4.8% in those who used condoms inconsistently. For protection against unintended pregnancy, condoms are 86% to 97% effective. Hence, there is compelling evidence that condoms are effective if used consistently. CHAPTER 10 highlights the challenges to consistent and correct use of male condoms.

In the past decade female condoms have become available as an additional barrier method. *In vitro* data support their impermeability to HIV. Several studies demonstrate that they are as effective as male condoms in preventing STIs and pregnancy. Some concern has been expressed that the promotion of the female condom will reduce male condom use such that female condoms will merely displace male condoms and not really increase overall condom use. Data from the the female condom programme in Brazil, however, which used community-based and health care settings, consistently showed that there was a substantial increase in the number of protected coital acts with the introduction of the female condom, regardless of the way in which they are introduced. In other words, the overall number of sex acts protected by a condom rose substantially, showing the beneficial effect of introducing the female condom.

HIV prevention beyond the research setting

While there is compelling evidence for success in reducing sexual transmission of HIV in a research context, another important consideration is how successful the intervention is in real life. In other words, can implementation of interventions for heterosexual transmission that show efficacy in research settings lead to reduction of HIV transmission and control of HIV at country level?

Evidence from Uganda demonstrates that a range of social, political and biological interventions can, used together, reduce HIV incidence rates. In contrast, HIV continues to spread at alarmingly high rates in Uganda's neighbours and in most other countries in sub-Saharan Africa. While postponement of sexual debut played a key role in Uganda, the increase in condom uptake and campaigns to promote knowledge of one's HIV status, also played a prominent role in their successful HIV control efforts.

Evidence from the Thai 100% condom promotion programme in sex workers, introduced in 1993, indicates that this initiative has had a major impact on HIV incidence rates in Thailand and substantially altered the projected trajectory of HIV infections in Thailand, averting an estimated six million infections. The promotion of male condoms to reduce HIV is effective in both research and in the real world and it can play a critical role in preventing heterosexual HIV transmission in developing countries; this has been clearly demonstrated both in Thailand and Uganda. The introduction and promotion of female condoms, in addition to male condoms, can increase overall condom use and hence increase the number of protected coital acts – thereby reducing HIV transmission. It is critically important to appreciate that we can control and prevent the spread of HIV with proven, currently used tools and interventions. The new technologies and new interventions being developed will be useful additions to our existing and growing armoury of options to reduce heterosexual transmission of HIV.

In South Africa, whilst some successes have been noted in the implementation of life skills programmes for those at school, distribution of male condoms, mass communication strategies, increasing access to VCT and syndromic management of STIs, have not been sufficient to have an impact on the continued spread of HIV infection.

Social and cultural factors influencing HIV risk reduction

Cultural prescriptions of masculinity and femininity – when they control and determine what men and women know, how they communicate with each other and how they behave within their relationships – significantly affect not only men's and women's sexual behaviours and attitudes but also their respective access to services and information and their ability to cope when ill. These norms are enforced by societal institutions such as schools, work-places, communities and health systems.

For example, in most societies women are cast in a subordinate, dependent and passive role where the ideal virtues include virginity, motherhood, obedience, and ignorance – particularly about their bodies. In contradistinction, masculinity is cast in terms of aggression, dominance, independence and invincibility, where the key virtues are strength, courage and virility. Yet both between and within socie-ties, through social interactions, and simply in the course of the inevitable vicissitudes of an individual's life, there are all sorts of variations and modulations in the force of these norms. This diversity and dynamism implies that there is space in most societies for modifications of harmful dominant ideologies of masculinity and femininity.

'Good women' in most societies are expected to be ignorant about sex and passive in sexual interactions. Numerous surveys consistently demonstrate higher levels of correct knowledge about HIV/AIDS in men compared with women. This imbalance in knowledge is a major obstacle to women's ability to assess their risk and take steps to reduce it; ignorance fosters myths and fears about both risk and prevention options and makes it very difficult for women to be pro-active in negotiating safer sex.

These dominant ideologies also define for women that sexual practices linked to reproduction are moral and those linked to pleasure are immoral; and for men they endorse variety in numbers of sexual partners. This double standard for men and women in acceptable sexual behaviour seriously challenges HIV prevention efforts targeted at promoting monogamy and fidelity.

In many cultures, children define a woman's social identity and they guarantee her status in her community and in some instances also her very survival through financial support from the child's father. In these circumstances the promotion of condoms and other barrier methods pose significant hurdles for women. Given the risk of transmission from infected mother to infant, it also has implica-tions for the decisions that she makes governing her own and her child's well-being. In many instances prevention of mother-to-child transmission (PMTCT) programmes disregard this reality for women and reinforce gender stereotypes. Sole responsibility for whether or not to test, whether or not to breastfeed, the chosen mode of delivery, whether or not to terminate her pregnancy, not to mention the initial responsibility of taking home positive test results, is placed on the mother.

While in most societies women are expected to be dependent on men to make decisions and access resources, men are socialised to be self-reliant, which has concomitant implications for the control of the epidemic. The expectation of invulnerability associated with being a man encourages denial of risk from HIV risk-taking behaviours such as lack of condom use and/or multiple partner relationships and it influences health-seeking behaviours.

The social milieu for the majority of black women in South Africa is riddled with the disadvantage of having little power, knowledge, skills or support. In a study of rural and peri-urban women in KwaZulu-Natal, knowledge of HIV/AIDS was high, yet women under-estimated their personal risk of acquiring HIV/AIDS. In this study, despite the high likelihood of their partners being HIV positive, unprotected sexual intercourse was still the norm. A key reason for the women not acting or being able to act on their knowledge and perception of HIV risk was that most did not believe they had a right to refuse sex or to insist on condom use; this belief was present whether the partner was a husband or a boyfriend. Additionally, most women thought that their male partner had a right to have multiple partners. Further, women did not perceive abstinence or non-penetrative alternatives such as thigh sex or masturbation as viable options, nor were they preferred. Only the male condom was perceived as a potential protective option, but use was limited because it required that the man approve its use. Many of these women indicated that they knew that their partners were not monogamous. Women stayed in these relationships mainly through fear of violence and because of financial dependence on their partners. This was exacerbated by the fact that many of the women were unemployed, and few had skills that would make them employable. Sexist customs and practices such as the payment of *lobola* (bride wealth) and *inhlawulo* (a custom where-by a man who makes an unmarried women pregnant is required by the traditional leader to pay a certain amount of money to compensate her family) were dominant themes in the interviews.

The findings of this study illustrate how prevailing cultural norms place South African women at risk for HIV; they also make it clear that, in some settings in South Africa, sex is viewed as a conjugal right and a male prerogative. As in other parts of Africa and the developing world, simply being married is one of the biggest risk factors for acquiring infection with HIV.

Ethnicity, caste, race and HIV risk

Social and economic marginalisation based on ethnicity, race and/or prolonged discrimination creates serious deficiencies in schooling, employment, health-seeking behaviours and access to services. When there are few opportunities for development and little hope for the future, not surprisingly, risk behaviour that increases the possibility of HIV infection is more common. Pre-existing prejudices based on race and ethnicity fuel the stigma, discrimination and ostracisation commonly associated with being HIV infected and, whilst both men and women in marginalised communities are vulnerable, women are more vulnerable than men. It is also the case that issues of race and ethnicity tend to be sensitive and highly politicised, which often restricts the availability of data that could improve understanding and help target interventions and resources.

In the evolution of the HIV epidemic in South Africa an over-arching factor has been the intersection of gender with race in the historical legacy of apartheid: huge inequalities in schooling, employment opportunities, land ownership, and access to health services and information rendered all African communities, men, women and youth disproportionately vulnerable to HIV infection and AIDS. But black women, and young black women in particular, had the least access, in the time of apartheid, to social, economic or political power and they bore a double burden of race and gender. In the current era, they bear the additional burden of HIV, creating what is sometimes referred to as the 'triple jeopardy' faced by African women. In the Constitution of democratic South Africa there are indeed numerous laudable provisions to redress the historical imbalances that patriarchy and white supremacy so disproportionately imposed upon African women, but these legal provisions have yet to be translated into meaningful action at a grassroots level where the need is greatest.

Sexual behaviours and practices and HIV risk

Age of sexual debut

Early sexual initiation has been found to be associated with subsequent sexual behavior and risk of STIs in several studies in Africa and elsewhere. Women who became sexually active between the ages of ten and 14 years were more likely to have had sex with men who were at increased risk for HIV and STDs. They are also more likely to have a greater number of partners than those who become sexually active at a later age.

Several studies in South Africa have found a similar age of sexual debut for both genders. Younger age of first sexual intercourse is associated with increased risk of infection. In a population-based study in an urban South African township outside the mining town of Carletonville, the mean age at first sex was 15.9 years for men and

16.3 for women, suggesting that age of sexual debut is not sufficient to explain the gender difference in age-prevalence of infection.

Age difference between partners

There is some data to suggest that very young girls are perceived as an 'HIV-free' group and are preferred as sexual partners by older men. Several studies have demonstrated that some young women often form partnerships with older men who have some source of income and who are able to provide them with personal gifts and favours as well as money for household necessities and school fees.

In a statistical simulation it was shown that the sex ratio of HIV prevalence increases as a function of the percentage of women who have male partners five to ten years older than themselves, holding constant the ratio of male-to-female versus female-to-male transmission probabilities. These model predictions have been confirmed using data from a population-based seroprevalence survey in rural Zimbabwe. Among sexually active respondents aged 17 to 24 years, older age of partner was a significant correlate of HIV infection. Among women, the median age difference with partners was six years older, whereas among men it was three years younger.

A study of HIV risk behaviours among black adolescent females in the USA concluded that the relationship dynamics between adolescents and sexual partners who are at least two years older does not favour the adoption of HIV risk-reduction behaviours.

There is little behavioural data from South Africa to assess the role of sexual coupling patterns and specifically the role of age difference in partners as a risk factor for HIV acquisition in young women and as a possible explanation of the observed epidemiological differences.

Teenage pregnancy

Studies conducted in the early 1980s demonstrate high rates of teenage pregnancies. These rates have been steadily increasing. The most recent South African Demographic and Health Survey showed that by age 19. 35% had been pregnant. While many young women are in consensual sexual relationships, large numbers of young women are coerced into being sexually active. A case control study comparing women under the age of 19 years attending prenatal services in South Africa to age-matched school or neighbourhood controls who had never been pregnant, demonstrated that cases were more likely where the household was more materially stressed, where there was a greater mean age difference between the woman and both her current and her first sexual partner and where the relationship with the current sexual partner was relatively new. Among young women who described their sexual initiation as forced or rape, the risk of pregnancy was higher. Young women who engaged in sex out of fear had an increased risk of pregnancy and experienced a higher frequency of beatings.

Anal sex and HIV

It is a common misconception that anal intercourse is an exclusively homosexual male practice. Recently, an increasing number of publications indicate that heterosexual anal intercourse is far more common than generally acknowledged. These surveys indicate that an estimated 10 to 30% of women and their male consorts engage in anal sex with some regularity. It has been suggested that the risk of contracting HIV through anal intercourse is far higher than for vaginal coitus.

Several studies elsewhere demonstrate that women practising anal intercourse are less likely to use condoms and more likely to engage in risky behaviours. The most commonly cited reason for lack of condom use during anal intercourse was that pregnancy was not then an issue. In some settings, anal intercourse is viewed as an alternative to vaginal sex to preserve virginity. In countries in Africa where female circumcision is practised, anal intercourse is often experimented with during the weeks and months before vaginal penetration can be achieved.

The risk for sexual transmission of HIV is heightened in women who experience violence and threats of violence. A study investigating the trends between violence and HIV sexual risk behaviours showed that women who are raped, physically assaulted or threatened with assault were more likely to have multiple sex partners and engage in unprotected anal intercourse. A survey of adolescent risk behaviours in low-income African-Americans established that 39% had engaged in anal intercourse and that youth who had engaged in anal intercourse were significantly more likely to report having being sexually molested.

Data on anal sex practices or its role in HIV transmission in Africa is almost non-existent. One of the very few sources is research that the South African Medical Research Council has been undertaking for almost a decade on female sex workers at truck-stops in KwaZulu-Natal. Of note is the increase in the practice of anal sex in this cohort over time – in 1992 the practice of anal sex was rare but by 1996 had increased to 42.8%. Based on self-reported anal sex, the researchers established an HIV prevalence of 61.3% among sex workers who practised anal sex compared with 42.7% in those who did not. Anal sex was associated with a higher risk of HIV infection in a multiple logistic regression model controlling for age, condom use, number of clients per week and duration of sex work.

As elsewhere in Africa, no data exist on the role of anal sex in HIV acquisition in women in the general population in South Africa and this information is urgently needed.

Violence

The most disturbing and alarming outcome of the expectation of physical and sexual domination in men is violence against women. There is growing evidence of the nexus between violence, risky behaviour and reproductive health. Several studies have established a strong association between experience, or fear, of violence and HIV risk. Fear of violence prevents women even from discussing HIV risk with their partners, let alone requesting condom use. In some countries there has been a shift from intimate/domestic violence to more random acts of violence against young women in particular. In some countries with high HIV prevalence there is evidence suggesting that the increase in rape of young women could be related to a perception of sexually active women being vectors of HIV infection and of virgins being 'disease-free'. In some settings, HIV-infected women using health services are about ten times more likely to report violence compared with similar aged HIV-negative women. Gender violence is a recurrent theme in South African life, with 13% of women in the last national Demographic and Health Survey reporting being beaten by a partner. Several studies have uncovered high levels of violence and coercion to obtain sex among urban teens, but this issue has not been systematically examined in relation to sexual coupling patterns, sexual practices, or HIV infection in heterosexual relationships. One qualitative study found that the conditions under which young girls have sex were determined by their male partners' use of violence and gender-role expectations about love, sex, and compliance with male partners' desires. The changing patterns in adolescent sexual practices and the age differential between girls and first-sex male partner (men on average five years older than women) could further contribute to young girls' risk of HIV/STIs. The power and maturity advantage that these males hold over young girls suggests that sex may sometimes be coerced.

The recent promotion of virginity testing for young women in KwaZulu-Natal, in part as a response to high rates of teenage pregnancy and HIV/STDs, may reinforce gender inequality by placing the burden of responsibility on females. This practice may also increase their vulnerability to disease, as girls identified as virgins become prey for sexual assault.

Opportunities for reducing the sexual risk of acquiring infection with HIV

While in any given society there are many different kinds of masculinity and femininity that vary by age, ethnicity, social class and sexuality it is the dominant ideology that influences women's and men's attitudes and behaviours, making both vulnerable in the context of the HIV epidemic. On the other hand, the diversity and dynamism of masculine and feminine identities imply that it may be possible, over time, to modify gender identity in the direction of more equitable relationships that promote safer sex.

The past decade has resulted in an enormous growth in our knowledge about the gender-related determinants of risk and vulnerability to HIV and the consequences of AIDS. However, translating this knowledge into action at a policy and programme level has remained a major challenge. Attempts to integrate gender into AIDS programmes have resulted in a range of outcomes from harmful, through perpetuation of sexual stereotypes, to empowering, through addressing the root causes of gender imbalances in society. To fill this gap Gupta et al have developed a framework to categorise the different approaches to integrating gender into HIV/AIDS programmes. The first step in their four-step continuum is about **minimising harm** potentially arising from interventions that reinforce the damaging gender and sexual stereotypes that emanate from dominating ideologies: stereotypes that determine, for example, what men and women should or should not know, what sexual behaviours are sanctioned, or which services can be accessed by men and which by women. The next step in this continuum is the establishment of **gender-sensitive** programmes that recognise that the needs of men and women differ and explore ways of meeting these needs. The next level introduces a more complex set of approaches targeted at **gender transformation** through creating conditions where men and women can examine damaging aspects of gender norms and experiment with new behaviours to create more equitable roles and relationships. The final step in this continuum is structural interventions that **empower** women and girls by increasing their access to the social and economic resources that in the long term protect women, men and their families in the HIV epidemic, thereby also altering the economic and social dynamic of gender roles and responsibilities.

Challenges in reducing HIV infection in women

Clearly, there are many factors that could be contributing to the excess risk of HIV infection in women, and young women in particular. It is unlikely that the observed age and gender differences can be attributed to a single factor but it is likely that some of the factors outlined above could be playing a greater role than others. There is an urgent need to elucidate the attributable risk from each of these factors in order to develop a more nuanced understanding of HIV risk in relation to gender and age, along with appropriate and targeted interventions to alter this risk profile.

Current safer sex options need to be refined to convey to married women the risk they face if their partners are not in mutually monogamous relationships with them. In addition, there is a need for more investment to develop biomedical interventions such as vaccines and microbicides that will reduce HIV risk in women.

The challenge in reducing HIV risk in women cannot be divorced from efforts to reduce risk in men and women jointly. Given the greater power and control men have compared with women, all interventions ultimately hinge on men taking greater responsibility and being more actively involved in efforts to reduce women's HIV risk both at an individual and societal level.

The Gupta model provides a practical gender-sensitive approach for reducing HIV risk along a continuum: from simply doing no harm, to addressing specific needs of men and women, to the creation of an enabling environment for risk reduction, and ultimately to redressing the power imbalances that make women disproportionately vulnerable.

Bibliography

ABDOOL KARIM Q, FROHLICH J. 2000 'Women try to protect themselves from HIV/AIDS in KwaZulu-Natal, South Africa'. In: Turshen M (Ed). *Women's Health in Africa*. Africa World Press, Lawrenceville, NJ.

ABDOOL KARIM Q, STEIN Z. 2000. 'Women and HIV/AIDS: A global perspective'. In: Goldman M, Hatch M (Eds). *Women and Health*. Academic Press.

ALAN GUTTMACHER INSTITUTE. 1998. *Into a New World: Young Women's Sexual and Reproductive Lives*. New York, Alan Guttmacher Institute.

ALDERMAN H, GERTLER P. 1997. *'Family resources and gender differences in human capital investments: The demand for children's medical care in Pakistan. Intrahousehold Resource Allocation: Methods, Application, and Policy'*. L Haddad, J Hoddinott and H Alderman. Baltimore, Johns Hopkins University Press.

BARKER G, LOWENSTEIN I. 'Where the boys are: Attitudes related to masculinity, fatherhood, and violence toward women among low-income adolescent and young adult males in Rio de Janeiro, Brazil'. *Youth and Society* 1997; 29: 166–196.

BASSETT M, MHLOYI M. 'Woman and AIDS in Zimbabwe: The making of an epidemic'. *International Journal of Health Services* 1991; 21: 143–156.

DIXON-MUELLER R. 'The Sexuality Connection in Reproductive Health'. *Studies in Family Planning* 1993; 24: 269–282.

DOWSETT GW, AGGLETON P ET AL. 'Challenging gender relations among young people: the global challenge for HIV/AIDS prevention'. *Critical Public Health* 1998; 8: 291–309.

GUPTA GR, WHELAN D, ALLENDORF K. 2003. *Integrating gender into HIV/AIDS Programmes.* WHO, Geneva

GUPTA GR. 'The Best of times and the worst of times: Implications of scientific advances in HIV prevention in the developing world'. *Annals of the New York Academy of Sciences* 2000; 918: 16–21.

GUPTA GR. *'Gender, Sexuality, and HIV/AIDS: The What, the Why and the How.'* (Plenary address). XIII Conference on HIV/AIDS, Durban, South Africa, 2000.

GUPTA GR, WEISS E. 1993. *Women and AIDS: Developing a New Health Strategy.* Washington DC, International Center for Research on Women.

HEISE L, ELIAS C. 'Transforming AIDS prevention to meet women's needs: A focus on developing countries'. *Social Science and Medicine* 1995; 40: 933–943.

HEISE L, ELLSBERG M ET AL. *'Ending Violence against Women'.* (Population Reports, Series L, No. 11). Baltimore, Johns Hopkins University School of Public Health, Population Information Programme, 1999.

INTERNATIONAL CENTER FOR RESEARCH ON WOMEN. 1989. *'Strengthening Women: Health Research Priorities for Women in Developing Countries'.* Washington DC, ICRW.

JEWKES R. 'Violence against women: An emerging health problem'. *International Clinical Psychopharmacology* 2000; Suppl 3: S37–45.

ORUBULOYE, IO, CALDWELL JC ET AL. 'African Women's Control over their Sexuality in an era of AIDS: A study of the Yoruba of Nigeria'. *Social Science and Medicine* 1993; 37: 859–872.

PARKER, R, AGGLETON P. 1999. *Culture, Society and Sexuality: A reader.* London: UCL Press.

PURNIMA M, AGGLETON P. 'Gender and HIV/AIDS: What Do Men Have to Do With It?' *Current Sociology* 2001; 49: 23–37.

SANDERS D, SAMBO A. 'AIDS in Africa: The implications of economic recession and structural adjustment'. *Health Policy and Planning* 1991; 6: 157–165.

SUZANNE M, CAMPBELL J ET AL. 'The Intersections of HIV and Violence: Directions for Future Research and Interventions'. *Social Science and Medicine* 2000; 50: 459–487.

TALLIS V ET AL. *Agenda special issue on Women and AIDS.* Ed: Tallis V. Durban, 2000.

UNAIDS. *Gender and HIV/AIDS: Taking stock of research and programmes.* UNAIDS. Geneva 1999.

UNAIDS. *Working with men in HIV prevention and care.* UNAIDS. Geneva 2001.

WEISS E, GEETA RG. *Bridging the gap: Addressing gender and sexuality in HIV prevention.* International Centre for Research on women, Washington 1998.

WINGOOD G, DiCLEMENTE RJ. 'Application of the theory of gender and power to examine HIV related exposures, risk factors, and effective interventions for women'. *Health Education and Behaviour* 2000; 27: 539–565

WORLD HEALTH ORGANISATION. *Integrating gender into HIV/AIDS national programmes.* WHO. Geneva 2003.

CHAPTER 17

Young people and HIV/AIDS in South Africa: Prevalence of infection, risk factors and social context

Abigail Harrison

AMONG YOUNG PEOPLE IN sub-Saharan Africa, the HIV epidemic is super-imposed on already poor sexual health outcomes, including high levels of unintended pregnancy. Young people, particularly women, are disproportionately represented in the epidemic, with high prevalence in the age group 15–24. In South Africa, one-quarter of young adult women aged 20–24 are now HIV infected.

Adolescence is a time of exploration and experimentation that can enhance sexual risk. Young girls face particular risks. Biological immaturity of the genital tract increases a young woman's chance of sexually transmitted infection and gender inequality decreases her negotiating power in sexual matters. Young girls are likely to be sexually active with older boys and men, who, in turn, may have multiple sexual partners. There is increasing recognition that awareness and prevention campaigns that promote abstinence, monogomy and condom use without addressing wider societal changes are not effective because they ignore existing gender inequalities that young women find it difficult to overcome.

Certain social and structural factors are most commonly associated with HIV infection in young South Africans. Evidence points to associations between HIV infection and partner's age, school attendance and completion, parental absence, participation in community and sports organisations, and other measures of social capital.

Interventions in the early teen years and beyond need to address both individual and structural causes of infection. Interventions that emphasise negotiation skills, assertiveness training and self-esteem can enhance young people's ability to protect themselves. Interventions with potential to reduce the number of new HIV infections in youth include 100% condom promotion, youth-friendly services,

voluntary counselling and testing, income generation, keeping
young people in school, and protecting sexual and human rights.

In sub-Saharan Africa, HIV/AIDS is an epidemic of young people,
especially women. UNAIDS estimates show that between 10 and 15% of
the 15–24 age group are HIV infected in this region. The HIV epidemic
has been superimposed on already poor sexual health outcomes in
young people, most notably high levels of unintended teen pregnancy.
In many ways, high levels of HIV infection among young people are
not surprising. Adolescence is a time of exploration and experimentation, with sexuality a major area of development and change. Also,
since levels of infection are so high in the general population, simply
being sexually active places young people at high risk. Further, unique
characteristics of sexual partnerships for many South African youth
predispose them to acquisition of HIV. For young women, the main
risk factor for HIV infection is the tendency to have partners on
average three to five years older than themselves. For young men, the
widespread practice of maintaining multiple partnerships puts both
themselves and their partners at high risk. Other risk factors for HIV
infection in young people include infrequent or inconsistent condom
use, as well as high levels of fluidity and mobility in relationships and
high levels of sexual coercion, particularly around sexual initiation.

   This chapter explores these issues in relation to young people in
South Africa today, presenting an overview of the HIV epidemic and
its impact on young people. First, HIV prevalence, sexual risk behaviours and the proximate determinants of HIV infection in young
people are examined, followed by a discussion of youth-focused
prevention strategies. The chapter concludes with a discussion of the
challenges inherent in preventing HIV infection among young South
Africans.

Who are 'young people'?

Who is included in the definition of young people? In this chapter,
both the terms 'adolescent' and 'young people' are used. Adolescent
refers to a specific developmental stage that spans the period from
puberty into young adulthood, and which is characterised by transition, physical and emotional development, and change. Youth generally refers to the ages ten to 24, while young people comprises a
broader category that can include men and women into their early
thirties. The standard definition preferred by the World Health
Organisation (WHO) for young people is ten to 24 years of age. In this
chapter the term 'young people' generally refers to those aged 15 and
older, because few data exist to document the experiences of younger

adolescents in the ten to 14 age range. Most standardised surveys, for instance, collect data on persons of reproductive age, generally defined as 15 to 49 years of age. Many behavioural studies have focused specifically on adolescents, usually including a sample from 14 to 19 years of age. However, behaviours and life experience may differ greatly between younger and older adolescents, as well as between teenagers and those in their early twenties. Where possible, such contrasts and distinctions are discussed throughout this chapter.

In many ways, young people represent a difficult population group to study. Adolescence is a powerfully formative stage of life, in most societies encompassing the transition to adulthood. In recent decades, global trends toward rising ages at marriage and expanded opportunities for young people in terms of education and employment have created an expanded period of adolescence. With more young people leaving home and living for extended periods on their own prior to entering adulthood, the needs for youth-focused programmes have become more apparent. By definition, adolescence is a time of transition, and a high level of mobility, instability and change are characteristic of young people's lives during this phase.

Adolescence is a time of experimentation and risk, often leading to heightened vulnerability, as young people make the transition to greater social and psychological independence. Peer pressure, socio-cultural norms, and expectations are social factors that influence the process of adolescence enormously. Sexuality is a typical area of experimentation and exploration during the teen years and beyond. Other developmental factors that influence adolescent sexual risk are the advent of puberty and associated physiological changes, coupled with the emergence of sexual expression and the desire to experiment. During this transitional period, young people are vulnerable for multiple reasons, including emotional and physical development, age, inexperience and financial dependence.

Importantly, sexual risk is influenced by multiple social, behavioural and situational factors, making adolescents hugely vulnerable to HIV/AIDS. In particular, young people often do not perceive themselves to be at risk, preventing them from accessing or using prevention when needed. Age puts young people at risk, in terms of inexperience and inability to negotiate the terms of relationships. Certain biological or developmental factors also confer risk, as does the broader social context, which for many young people includes poverty and related issues such as access to education or employment.

Gender and the heightened vulnerability of young women

The importance of gender as a dominant force in young people's relationships has been shown through research in a number of settings. Adolescence can be a particularly important time with regard to gender roles. In many societies, differentiation of gender roles heightens after puberty, with the world expanding for boys while girls often face new restrictions. Adolescence may thus be a time when boys gain autonomy, mobility, opportunity and power, including in the sexual and reproductive realm, while girls are deprived of the same privileges. Young women are also biologically vulnerable, with the immature genital tract and cervix providing increased opportunity for the transmission of infection. In general, while both young men and women are vulnerable, adolescent women represent one of the most vulnerable population groups in relation to HIV/AIDS. Women represent the majority of those living with HIV/AIDS in sub-Saharan Africa. Further, women are generally infected at younger ages than men, making adolescence a particularly vulnerable time period for women and HIV risk.

In South Africa, gender role norms contribute to the pronounced gap between HIV awareness and practices and the social processes that influence young women's disproportionate risk for HIV. There is increasing recognition that public health approaches that promote abstinence, fidelity, and condom use in the absence of wider societal changes are not effective because they ignore existing gender inequalities that young women have difficulty overcoming. However, a better understanding of these dynamics and how they serve as prevention barriers is needed. Sociocultural norms about sexual expression within the confines of accepted masculine and feminine behaviour limit choices of protection from pregnancy and disease and increase the vulnerability of South African youth to HIV and other sexually transmitted infections (STIs). Often, these norms are manifested in young women's lessened ability to negotiate the terms of their relationships and sexual activity, discussed below.

Less has been written about men and their social roles in the context of sexual health, but these issues are equally important when discussing young men's risks. While men may control decision-making and hold power within relationships, poor self-image may contribute to sexual aggression and related behaviours. Also, peer group influences, socialisation within a dominant male culture, and a lack of 'affective' sexual and social experiences in childhood and adolescence may contribute. In South Africa, this may be exacerbated by a social situation characterised by poverty, lack of opportunity and general social disempowerment. Also, the position of young men in a world characterised by failure and hopelessness strongly influences masculinity, sexuality and attendant decisions in the realm of relationships.

Profile of risk among young people

Each year, more than half of all new HIV infections globally are in young people aged 15–24, and over two million people aged 10–24 become infected each year. At the end of 2001, 11.8-million young people globally were infected, most of them young women. More than eight million of these HIV-infected young people are in sub-Saharan Africa, where two-thirds of infected youth are women.

The epidemic in southern Africa is particularly severe. More than 20% of youth aged 15–24 are infected in South Africa and the neighbouring countries of Botswana, Lesotho, Zimbabwe and Namibia. In South Africa, it is estimated that as many as 40% of the current generation of young men will die of AIDS in adulthood, assuming no change in the risk of becoming HIV infected. However, young women are typically at higher risk than men of the same age. Studies of HIV infection in adolescents throughout Africa generally show sharply increasing prevalence in women during the teen years, with large sex-disaggregated differences in infection levels. Teenage women often experience prevalence levels as much as four to five times higher than men of the same age. Further, young women's risk of infection per partnership is substantially higher than their male peers, largely because women have partners on average five years older than themselves and these partners are more likely to be already HIV infected.

HIV and STI prevalence

South Africa's HIV epidemic is severe, disproportionately affecting teenage women and men slightly older than that. Patterns of prevalence – measured through pregnant women attending antenatal clinics – are similar to other high prevalence areas in Africa. Of the more than five million South Africans now infected with HIV, over half are young people aged 15–24. A recent nationally representative survey of youth found that HIV prevalence was 15.5% in women aged 15–24, compared with 4.8% among men. Among women aged 20–24, prevalence was 24.5%.

The national antenatal surveys conducted annually in public clinics show a steady rise in the epidemic during the 1990s. About one-quarter of all pregnant women attending antenatal services nationally are HIV infected, with young women under age 25 forming a high-risk group. HIV prevalence in teenage women, those aged 15–19, has declined from the mid 1990s (FIGURE 17.1). In 1999, prevalence was measured at 16.5% in this age group, compared with 15.4% in 2001. However, in the next age group – those aged 20–24 – such declines have not been observed. Prevalence now stands at 28.4% in this age group, a slight increase from 25.6% in 1999. Considerable provincial variation in the epidemic exists, with the highest prevalence among antenatal women, 33.5%, found in KwaZulu-Natal.

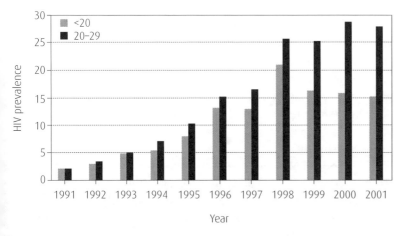

FIGURE 17.1 HIV prevalence in young South African women attending antenatal clinics: 1991–2001

Discrepancies between data from household surveys and antenatal data are to be expected. Use of antenatal data to estimate prevalence in young women is likely to overestimate levels of infection. Models of the HIV epidemic using age- and sex-specific prevalence data indicate that both young men and young women face a heightened risk of HIV infection, with prevalence peaking for women by the mid-twenties, but for men not until the early thirties. Yet even if prevalence for younger age groups is overestimated from antenatal data, these age and gender patterns are likely to be valid.

Links between pregnancy and HIV/AIDS

Levels of pregnancy are very high among teenage and young adult women in South Africa. This occurs in spite of a low overall total fertility rate (total number of births per woman), in fact one of the lowest in sub-Saharan Africa, and a high use of contraceptives. Use of contraception, particularly modern hormonal methods, is often delayed until after the birth of a first child, meaning that many adolescent women do not experience the benefits of prevention. Such high levels of unprotected sexual activity underscore the high level of sexual risk faced by young South African women. Also, non-use of contraception by those who have recently become sexually active means that opportunities for counselling regarding condom use and dual protection against HIV and pregnancy are missed, leaving young women vulnerable to both HIV and pregnancy.

Knowledge and attitudes about HIV/AIDS

In South Africa, adolescent sexuality in the context of the HIV epidemic is characterised by high knowledge and awareness. However, while most studies have noted high levels of knowledge about HIV/AIDS transmission and methods of prevention, particularly among school-going youth, they have also noted the presence of numerous myths related to HIV/AIDS and sexuality more broadly. Further, many adolescents possess a poor understanding of the physical changes of adolescence and reproductive biology. Information and education about sexuality comes mainly from peers. In addition, widespread education and associated high levels of knowledge have done little so far to contribute to a decline in HIV prevalence.

Sexual behaviour

For young South Africans, sexual activity is the predominant mode of HIV transmission. Sexual behaviour describes the set of behaviours and practices that define sexual risk for HIV, typically including partnership characteristics, sexual networking and the timing and experience of sexual initiation. Understanding adolescent sexual behaviour is important, since people in this stage of life face high risk coupled with unique developmental issues. Also, as the period between puberty and marriage has lengthened in recent decades, creating an expanded adolescence, the likelihood of premarital sexual relationships and unintended pregnancy has increased in this age group. And where young people are at risk for pregnancy, they are also at risk for HIV and other STIs.

Cross-national studies of sexual behaviour across age groups have shown that marital status, gender, and age are the strongest determinants of sexual networking patterns. In South Africa, the availability of nationally representative data on sexual behaviour was limited until recently. In the mid 1990s, two national surveys of youth knowledge, attitudes and practices were conducted (TABLE 17.1). A growing literature exists on the sexual behaviour of young South Africans, although most studies to date have focused on individual parameters of risk, such as knowledge, attitudes and condom use.

Sexual debut

Initiation of sexual intercourse places young people in a high risk group for HIV, other STIs, and unplanned pregnancy. In the context of HIV/AIDS, age at sexual debut is an important marker of risk as it

	Ever Used Condom		Frequency of Use		Used at Last Intercourse	
	Male	Female	Male	Female	Male	Female
National Surveys						
Pettifor et al., 2004	Not measured		39% always used w/most recent partner	28% always used w/most recent partner	57%	48%
Human Sciences Research Council, 2002			33.9% said always (15–24 years)		57.1 (those aged 15–24, sexually active)	46.1
Demographic and Health Survey, 1998		28.4% teen women (15–19 years)		4% aged 15–19 use as current contraceptive		19.5%
Kaiser Family Foundation, 1998	53%	55% said always				
Richter et al., 1996	20%	4%				
Research Studies						
Abdool Karim et al., 1992	47%		None said 'always'			
Kelly, 2000	70% men and women aged 15–30 nationally		60% men and women are frequent users		52% men and women aged 15–30 nationally	
Williams et al., 2003	63.2%	59.3%				
Jewkes, 2003*	*In 31.2% of relationships, women suggested condom use. 44% of men agreed.					
Kaufman, 2002					49%	46%
Reddy et al., 2003			28.8% consistent users (male and female)			
Harrison, 2003	39.5% aged 15–19, sexually active	29.6% aged 15–19, sexually active	25.1% used frequently (15–19 years)	37.1% used frequently (15–19 years)		

determines length of exposure to infection. Those who begin sexual activity in the early teen years are likely to have a higher chance of infection than those who delay, although risk is also highly dependent on choice of partner. Historically, sexual initiation was linked to marriage and subsequent childbearing, and remains a key marker of the transition from adolescence to adulthood.

Throughout sub-Saharan Africa, the average age of sexual initiation falls between 15 and 17 for both young men and women. A substantial proportion of both men and women initiate sex in the early to

TABLE 17.1 Condom use among South African youth: summary findings

mid-teens, often with a higher proportion of young men sexually active in the early teen years.

In South Africa, findings from various studies indicate a range in age at sexual initiation from 14 to 17 for both young men and women. In the 1998 South African Demographic and Health Survey (DHS), median age at first intercourse for women was approximately 18 years.

However, a recent review of the South African literature on adolescent sexual behaviour estimated that more than half of young men and women are sexually active by age 16, although the studies reviewed were older and mainly school-based. Reporting of data on sexual behaviour is subject to bias due to the highly sensitive nature of the topic, and may also vary widely in different regions of the country, and also between urban and rural areas. For instance, a study among urban youth in KwaZulu-Natal found a mean age at sexual initiation of 16.5 years, and first sex was more likely to be protected among young women who initiated sex later. In contrast, studies in rural KwaZulu-Natal have found an older age at sexual initiation, ranging from 16 to 18 (TABLE 17.2).

A younger age at sexual initiation has also been associated with greater sexual risk. Younger adolescents may be less likely to use condoms, because of limited knowledge, fear, uncertainty or lack of negotiating ability. Importantly, those who initiate sex at younger ages may be less likely to protect themselves at sexual initiation than older persons who are better prepared for this event.

Some studies also indicate that a younger age of sexual initiation is associated with greater sexual risk later in life. Some evidence suggests, for instance, that young men who start sex younger establish patterns of sexual networking that continue into adulthood. Involvement in multiple partnerships as a teen may thus continue as a risk behaviour later in life.

Partnership characteristics and patterns of sexual networking

Patterns of sexual networking, including type of partner, age differences between partners, numbers of partners and a partner's broader sexual contacts, are among the main determinants of risk for HIV infection. In particular, the typical pattern of sexual partnerships in which young women have partners on average three to five years older than themselves is a major risk factor for HIV infection. Similarly, young men's propensity to engage in multiple partnerships, sometimes concurrently, underlies their risk for HIV infection. Further, men are more likely than women to have casual partnerships. Casual partnerships, however, are the situations in which condoms are often used, and therefore men may be more protected within

	Age at first sex		% Young people sexually active		More than one partner in last year	
	Male	Female	Male	Female	Male	Female
National Surveys						
Pettifor et al., 2004	16.4 years (mean)	17 years (mean)	67%	68%	24% had >5 lifetime partners	6% had >5 lifetime partners
HSRC, 2002	Median Age: 17 (25–34 age group)		55.6%	57.9%	23%	8.8%
Demographic & Health Survey, 1998		Median: 18		40% (had sex in year prior to survey)		2.9 % (teen women aged 15–19)
Kaiser Family Foundation, 1998			54% (16–17 year olds) 60% teens overall			
Richter et al., 1996	Median Age: 16		70% (16–20 yrs)	66% (16–20 yrs)		
Research Studies						
Abdool Karim et al., 1992			57.7	8.3		
Kelly, 2000	15.7	17	78%	68%	42% (> 1 partner now)	18% (> 1 partner now)
Williams et al., 2003			82% aged 15–24	87.6% aged 15–24	71.7% ongoing casual p'ship	69.7% ongoing casual p'ship
Jewkes, 2003		14.2				1.8 = mean number boyfriends
Kaufman, 2002			49%	46%	18%	2%
Reddy et al., 2003	25.4% < 14 years	5.6% < 14 years	50.1%	34.1%	66.4% (lifetime)	38.1% (lifetime)
Harrison, 2003	17.1	17.3	52.3% (15–19 yrs)	43.5% (15–19 yrs)	61.8% (w/in last 3 years)	7.3% (w/in last 3 years)

such relationships. Numerous studies in South Africa have shown that most young men and women who are sexually active report that they have a regular boyfriend or girlfriend. Within such relationships, condoms may not be used because they are perceived to be a violation of trust. Both men and women report encountering resistance when trying to negotiate condom use, as a partner will often view this as a suggestion that he or she is thought to be untrustworthy or unclean (see CHAPTER 9 for more details on the lack of condom use).

TABLE 17.2 Sexual behaviour and HIV risk among South African youth: summary findings

Reporting of sexual contact and partners is subject to certain biases. In the 1998 DHS, most teenage women reported no sexual partner in the previous year. Only about 20% indicated they were sexually active in the month prior to the survey. Most studies have found that women report only one or two lifetime partners. For instance, the 1998 DHS found that multiple partnerships among women were rare. At the same time, men may sometimes exaggerate the number of sexual partners they report, out of a desire to prove virility or conformity with accepted norms for young men.

Some studies have found a low frequency of sexual activity among young people, in spite of the participation of many sexually active young people in regular partnerships. In the recent HSRC survey, 29% of youth aged 15 to 24 reported having no sexual activity in the past month. Frequency of sexual activity is even lower for women: another recent study found that more than half of teen women reported the last sexual activity with their current partner was more than one month ago. Low sexual frequency among young people may relate to opportunity, mobility, distance and migration, to difficulties in spending time with partners, especially for younger women and also to an idea among young people that they may prevent HIV by having sexual intercourse less often.

Prevention of HIV/AIDS

Condom use
Studies have shown increased acceptability of condom use, especially among young people, where consistent messages are promoted and support for continued use is provided. For instance, in the United States, condom use among unmarried and adolescent women has increased in recent years following almost two decades of concerted efforts to prevent HIV infection. In some studies among specialised populations, such as sex workers or factory workers, increased condom use has been associated with changes in sexual risk behaviour. Among youth, perceived self-efficacy, or the belief that one knows how to use a condom correctly, may also be closely linked to successful condom use. Refer also to CHAPTER 10 for further details on condom use.

Use of other contraceptives
In South Africa, studies generally document low levels of contraceptive use, including condoms, among young people. However, the DHS indicates high contraceptive use among young women, with two-thirds of sexually active 15–19 year olds reporting current use of a modern contraceptive, and injectable contraceptive use is high. Among teenage women only 4% report condoms as the contraceptive

method they currently use. In many instances the condom may not even be promoted within family planning services as a regular contraceptive method. Social barriers to contraceptive use also exist, particularly among young people, often including communication difficulties between adolescents and parents and avoidance of responsibility for contraception by male partners.

Abstinence or delayed onset of sexual activity

Abstinence, or refraining from sexual activity, is an often-cited prevention strategy among young people, especially women. Abstaining from sex is an important prevention strategy, as it prevents any chance of infection. In reality, however, abstinence often refers to a strategy of delaying sexual initiation for a limited period of time, as sexual activity increases steadily from about age 15 onwards for both young men and women.

A number of South African studies, including national surveys, have found that just about half of teenage men and women report being sexually active. However, when disaggregated by age and examined by single-year intervals, data from most sources demonstrate steadily increasing levels of sexual activity throughout the teen years. As data from one recent survey indicate, although 20% or fewer of both young men and women report being sexually active by age 15, this proportion has increased to more than 75% by the end of the teen years (FIGURE 17.2).

An increase in age at first sex is now commonly cited as a contributing factor in the decline in HIV infection in Uganda, where increased abstinence among the young is cited as one of the factors that has led to lower overall HIV prevalence. Similar trends have not, however, been observed in South Africa, where recent studies have noted a decline in the age at first sex. This is most probably due to a general trend toward the liberalisation of society and to overall societal changes that affect this generation of youth.

'Secondary abstinence' refers to a prolonged period without sexual activity among those who have already been sexually active. The recent HSRC/Nelson Mandela Children's Fund survey noted that almost 20% of men aged 15 to 24 and 13.9% of women in the same age group reported having no sexual intercourse in the last twelve months although they had previously been sexually active. An increase in secondary abstinence would suggest behavioural change in response to HIV prevention messages, although such change is impossible to measure until more than cross-sectional data are available.

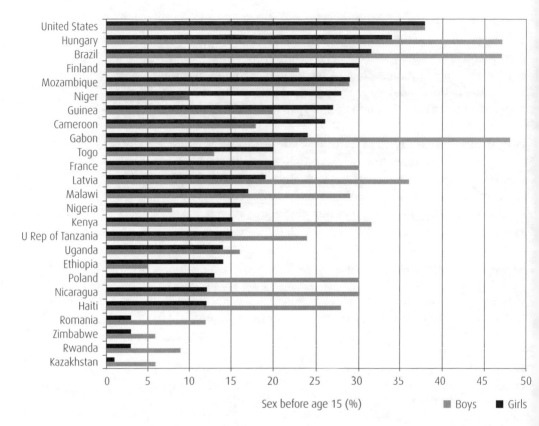

FIGURE 17.2 Sexual initiation prior to age 15 among young people in selected countries
Source: Demographic and Health Surveys (DHS) 1998–2001. Health Behaviour in school-aged children survey 1998.

Power and decision-making in sexual relationships

Negotiation and communication

Findings from a wide range of settings indicate that young women are especially vulnerable within relationships, due to power imbalances largely determined by prevailing gender norms. Even where awareness and knowledge of reproductive health are high, and the risks of HIV and pregnancy are understood, decision-making and negotiation of safer sexual practices remains difficult. In many societies, men are socialised to exert authority in all matters, including reproductive decision-making, and the concepts of sexual 'decision-making' and 'negotiation' may not be relevant for many women.

Different issues may prevail when discussing negotiation within adolescent relationships. Sexual decision-making for adolescents is a distinct process and a combination of factors, including the physiological changes of adolescence, the importance of peer influences, and a different understanding of risks and their consequences, make adolescent relationships unique. Further, adolescence is a possible time for intervention to improve young people's capabilities in this area.

In South Africa, gender imbalances are so entrenched that in some cases the male partner's domination of all aspects of decision-making, including the timing of sex, may be viewed as acceptable or normative by their female partners. Absence of any formal decision-making process or communication between partners, characterised by 'non-negotiation', is common. Also, a number of studies have identified a link between constraints to decision-making and gender-based violence. Poor inter-generational communication often compounds these problems.

Sexual coercion and gender-based violence

Sexual coercion within relationships, whether emotional, financial or physical, compounds women's inability to protect themselves. Gender-based violence may be an independent risk factor for HIV infection. One study found that the conditions under which young women have sex were determined by their male partners' use of violence and gender-role expectations about love, sex and compliance with male partners' desires. Because male partners are usually older, the power and maturity advantage that they hold creates an environment conducive to sexual coercion. Older partners may also provide financial or material benefits, and thus young women's power to negotiate safe sex is often inversely related to the age of their partner. In fact, young women are vulnerable at multiple levels, because of their age and inexperience, as well as gender, which effectively cedes control within relationships to the male partner. These pressures further contribute to their inability to engage in protected sex. Violence in the sexual arena may also be a negative response to the HIV epidemic, with some young people seeking to spread infection, or seeking virgin partners whom they believe to be safe. Few data exist to document men's perceptions of sexual violence, nor to complement findings on sexual violence from research with women.

Structural factors: The social context of risk

A growing body of research addresses the multifactorial ways in which societal or contextual factors shape adolescent sexuality and risk.

Access to services

Globally, access to services and accurate information about prevention and reproductive health for young people is problematic. In South

Africa, a number of reports have documented the poor quality of care that young people receive in the public health services. Throughout southern Africa, this poor quality of care for young people encompasses limited access to services, poor reception and treatment from service providers, and non-availability of preventive methods that young people need, most notably condoms. Some have suggested the need for separate youth services, in response to problems encountered by young people in accessing family planning or other prevention services.

Lack of access for South African adolescents is not limited to physical constraints, but is also characterised by social inaccessibility. Service providers are often overtly hostile to serving young clients, particularly for their reproductive health needs. In fact, clinics are often conveniently located near schools and so could play an important role in meeting the prevention needs of young clients. Anecdotal accounts of young clients being chased from clinics abound and research data support this.

Community participation and social capital

More recently, research has begun to examine community factors, encompassed in the concepts of community participation and social capital and their impact on sexual risk. How young people use their time may strongly influence their sexual risk-taking behaviours. For instance, work and employment may occupy young people's time and reduce their ability to participate in sexual risk activities. Also, some evidence suggests that young people who belong to community organisations may experience protective effects from doing so. These effects may be different for young men and women, with young women appearing to benefit most from membership in various organisations. For men, membership in sports organisations is most common, but the effect of participation on HIV risk is ambiguous, with some studies indicating that men who participate in sports are actually at increased risk. Use of community organisations for structural HIV prevention interventions should be further explored.

Schooling and educational achievement

Links between education and improved sexual health outcomes, such as a reduced incidence of teen pregnancy, have been observed in South Africa and globally. Few such analyses have been extended to the realm of HIV/AIDS. Available evidence does suggest that school enrolment or attendance lowers sexual risk for young people. Intuitively, this makes sense: those in school may be less likely to be involved in relationships, more positively engaged in other activities and thus less likely to be sexually active. However, the causal mechanisms of this lowered risk are difficult to understand. Young women, for instance, may leave school because they are pregnant, thus making it appear as if those remaining in school are at lower risk. How these mechanisms operate in terms of HIV risk is an important area for further study.

Sociocultural norms and values

Social and community norms remain important to young people, such as conflict between social norms and sexual feelings, gendered power imbalances within young people's relationships, aspects of male sexuality, and peer norms and values. A number of studies have examined how gender, operating at a contextual level, determines the conduct of relationships at an interpersonal level. Strong sociocultural norms that are firmly adhered to in many communities influence gender relations and perpetuate longstanding gender inequalities.

Only a few studies, however, have looked in any detail at the role of societal norms and culture in influencing adolescent sexual risk. Conservative social norms remain dominant in many South African settings, making the acknowledgement of relationships and sexuality by young people difficult. Some young people, particularly women, may hide relationships for fear of sanction by the larger community, thus limiting their ability to access prevention or guidance. High levels of participation in religious institutions that promote conservative viewpoints such as abstinence and the value of virginity may also limit young people's prevention options. Further, cultural sanctions against discussion of sexuality limit the opportunity for inter-generational education or guidance.

Some aspects of cultural practices related to sexuality, such as non-penetrative sex, or the instruction of young people in sexual matters by their elders, could have positive implications for HIV prevention if adapted to the needs of contemporary youth. Further study of such issues is needed. Too often, practices that may be harmful to young people, such as virginity testing or initiation ceremonies, are promoted as having value in terms of safe sex or HIV prevention. An emphasis on virginity may be detrimental for young women, for instance, if they feel pressure to 'prove their virginity' through sexual intercourse with a male partner or be pressured to practise anal sex to preserve their virginity. Further education about positive and negative aspects of cultural practices are needed for young people, many of whom are strongly influenced by the societal values that promote them.

Youth-focused prevention strategies

As the severity of South Africa's HIV epidemic has heightened among South Africa's youth and the general population, intervention efforts have increased in number. However, the number of interventions evaluated for efficacy – or their ability to achieve the desired outcomes – remains few. In this chapter, a distinction is made between *programmes*, which are broad-based efforts designed to reach a large population, and *interventions*, which are more narrowly focused efforts designed to be evaluated for efficacy. If successful, interventions may be scaled up for programme implementation to reach a larger audience. In South Africa as elsewhere, school-based efforts are a predominant method of delivering programmes to young people, because of the greater ease in reaching the target population. High levels of school enrolment throughout the country mean that such efforts may reach most young people. However, the fact that out-of-school youths may represent a small but important risk group should not be overlooked.

Intervention design

Reviews of interventions in other settings suggest the importance of including certain components in youth-oriented interventions in order to ensure success (TABLE 17.3).

Outcomes: Aim for effect on timing and frequency of sexual intercourse, numbers of partners, use of condoms or other contraceptives
Objectives: Include a narrow focus with few behavioural goals
Content: Give clear, consistent messages; focus on reducing sexual behaviours that lead to unintended pregnancy and HIV/STIs; include basic, accurate information and repeat essential messages; be specific to age and culture; use a theoretical framework
Skill-based focus: Include experiential activities, especially modelling and practise; training on coping skills; interpersonal negotiation and communication
Participation: Involve students, address social pressures, motivate teachers and parents to participate
Community: Acknowledge the importance of young people's community norms; use appropriate language and cultural references; situate AIDS interventions in broader contexts, acknowledge structural factors
Evaluate: Measure impact in relation to stated goals and outcome measures, disseminate findings, replicate

TABLE 17.3 Components of successful interventions

In addition to the points detailed in TABLE 17.3, UNAIDS provides ten steps for promoting behaviour change among young people, developed from global experience working with young people. These include:
- addressing stigma
- providing young people with adequate knowledge and information
- equipping young people with life skills
- providing youth-friendly health services

- promoting voluntary counselling and testing
- working with young people and encouraging their participation
- engaging young people living with HIV/AIDS
- creating safe and supportive environments
- reaching out to young people most at risk
- strengthening partnerships and monitoring progress.

These and related points will be discussed in relation to existing interventions in South Africa.

Whether in South Africa or elsewhere, interventions aimed at HIV prevention in youth should emphasise the points outlined below.

Provide accurate factual information

Provision of accurate and specific factual information is an important primary goal for intervention programmes. Even with the high levels of knowledge about transmission of the virus and the HIV epidemic, many myths remain. It is important to ensure a common basis of factual knowledge and understanding as a foundation for intervention programmes. Information provided in HIV prevention programmes needs to extend beyond HIV transmission and prevention to include basic facts about reproductive biology, pregnancy and contraception. Often, failure to practise safe sex behaviour is related to myths about how young people cannot become pregnant at first sex, or that there are certain times when young women cannot become pregnant. Since preventive behaviour is often motivated by a desire to prevent pregnancy, addressing these issues along with HIV prevention is important.

Promote clear and informed choices

Second, promoting informed choices such as condom use and delay in the onset of sexual activity are critical. The very high levels of infection make evident the fact that young people do not easily translate information into action when it comes to HIV prevention. Providing concrete options and strategies to implement them is a key second step for interventions.

Develop communication and negotiation skills

Even where informed choices exist, the ability to negotiate their use is often absent for young people. Because of this, providing information and education to young people is not enough. Interventions need to acknowledge the difficulties in communication and negotiation for young people within relationships, identify steps to address these difficulties and then emphasise skills building to achieve this. Such interventions operate at the interpersonal level, rather than relying on individuals to make changes on their own. Communication, deci-sion-making and negotiation are extremely difficult for young people in the South African context given the prevailing gender inequities in many young people's relationships. Discussion of gender role norms and how these need to change also needs to be a part of skills develop-ment around negotiation and decision-making.

Participation of youth in intervention design and implementation

Participatory involvement of youth in intervention design and imple-mentation, in contrast to being involved only as participants, has become an increasingly important part of standard youth-focused intervention design. Many interventions now begin with formative research among the target population, to develop an understanding of their needs and the most appropriate methods of addressing them.

One way to involve youth in interventions is through the use of peer education, which has become an important component of many youth-oriented interventions. Peer education refers to the use of trained individuals from a particular target group to educate their peers, particularly as these programmes are generally aimed at empowering as well as educating participants. A number of South African interventions have used peer education, with some documen-tation of the strengths and weaknesses of this approach.

Some programmes have gone one step further, to involve youth in the actual design of the interventions themselves. Such efforts typically begin with formative research, but continue to include the target population in analysis and interpretation of the data, as well as actual intervention design. Such programmes then become youth-designed and executed.

Recently, the idea of social franchising of youth interventions has gained recognition. In this process, successful interventions are taken and adapted widely through a process of replication, often using NGOs and sometimes with broad-based participation.

Interventions for South African youth

In recent years, a number of large-scale programmes have been devel-oped to address the HIV prevention needs of South Africa's youth. The national campaign LoveLife has promoted safer sexual relationships through mass media and prominent messages on billboards, buses and taxis. These have been supplemented by peer education efforts and youth-friendly clinics.

The national Life Skills programme targets youth in schools, and has become a part of the secondary school curriculum in many locations. This programme aims to increase knowledge and offer skills-based solutions to behavioural change. Implementation of the programme varies according to province, with some very strong programmes,including peer education and other methods designed to involve youth in a participatory manner.

An evaluation of the DramAidE programme in KwaZulu-Natal, using a randomised controlled trial design, found increased condom use after exposure to the school-based drama education programme. Smaller interventions evaluated for efficacy remain relatively few, however. Interventions in the early stages of the epidemic focused primarily on raising knowledge and awareness of HIV/AIDS, with the further aim of promoting condom use as a prevention strategy. In Cape Town, secondary school youth exposed to an intervention in schools experienced increased knowledge of HIV transmission and prevention and greater acceptance of people with AIDS, as well as some behavioural effects.

A number of interventions have begun to address the issue of gender and gender inequity which many consider to be the most important factor underlying young people's risk for HIV/AIDS. Stepping Stones, which uses participatory methods to address issues of gender and relationships in relation to HIV prevention, has been adapted for use in South Africa and will soon be formally evaluated. Other interventions, such as Men as Partners and Teaching Men to Care, employ similar approaches. In northern KwaZulu-Natal, the Mpondombili Project is a school-based programme that addresses gender through skills-based and factual learning, while incorporating the perspectives of youth peer educators and adult role models in the design. In addition to increasing knowledge and changing attitudes, the majority of interventions have focused on condom distribution and promotion, and the promotion of youth-friendly services.

Where are the gaps?

Increasingly, there is a call to target interventions at the structural causes of HIV/AIDS, rather than assuming that individual behaviour change will follow from educational programmes. Structural interventions include improving access to prevention technologies for young people, or addressing some of the underlying causes of the HIV epidemic, such as poverty and gender inequality.

Condom promotion

Although condoms have become the ubiquitous symbol of AIDS prevention in South Africa as well as globally, young people often face significant barriers to condom use. First, although condom access is generally thought to be good in most of the country, young people's access may be limited by a number of factors. Having to access condoms in public places, such as clinics, may make obtaining them difficult, especially for girls. And even where access is not a problem, the social barriers to using condoms remain significant. Negative images of condoms prevail among young people, and negotiation of their use may be difficult in many situations. This is compounded by fear and hesitation in accessing condoms publicly.

Youth-friendly services

Problems with young people accessing high-quality preventive and reproductive health care are well documented in South Africa. While a number of interventions, including LoveLife, have begun to tackle the issue of youth-friendly services, attitudes toward young people in the public sector remain an important gap. There is a need to focus on services that young people receive as well as young people themselves, on the training and sensitisation of providers, and possibly on dedicated youth services that can address prevention in the context of youth's broader needs. LoveLife's efforts to combine youth centres that offer recreation and other services along with health and prevention needs are important, but an evaluation of their success and popularity among youth has not yet been conducted.

Voluntary HIV testing and counselling services

With the advent of expanded treatment options, voluntary counselling and testing will become an increasingly important need for young people. Access is an even more important issue for young people than for other population groups, and the special needs of youth should be kept in mind while planning.

Keeping young people in school

Keeping young people in school represents an indirect but important intervention to prevent HIV/AIDS. With evidence beginning to accumulate regarding the risks to young people of not being in school, efforts to keep young people in school should be enhanced. Further, specialised HIV interventions for out-of-school youth, who are likely at highest risk, should be considered.

Protecting sexual and human rights

Because of South Africa's high levels of sexual coercion and violence, young people need to be made aware of their rights and to learn to assert themselves. Young people need to know that sexual coercion and discrimination based on HIV status are not acceptable, and that they are protected by law. Such intervention efforts can help to increase young people's ability to protect themselves.

Some of the challenges inherent in providing interventions to prevent HIV/AIDS in young people are evident from the discussion above. Young people are a difficult group in which to intervene because of developmental issues such as a sense of invulnerability, other priorities, little direct evidence among peers of the need to change, and other related concerns. While there is some evidence that having experienced the death of a close associate may contribute to increased sense of risk and decreased vulnerability, youth are likely to remain the most vulnerable group with the most need to change. On the positive side, change is probably easiest to promote in youth, although better ways to sustain and encourage behavioural change in the long term need to be defined. Some intervention efforts do show promise and these should be expanded to enhance young people's ability to protect themselves. Preparing for a future when young people will receive treatment and move beyond behavioural interventions alone is an important goal. Also, expanding interventions to focus on structural issues related to risk is important, including poverty, stigma and discrimination, gender inequality and sexual rights. Structural interventions could include vocational training, employment transition and assistance, income generation and other strategies to address the underlying causes of risk for HIV/AIDS.

Bibliography

ABDOOL KARIM Q, ABDOOL KARIM SS, NKOMAKAZI J. 'Sexual behaviour and knowledge among urban black mothers. Implications for AIDS prevention programmes'. *South African Medical Journal* 1991; 80: 340–343.

ABDOOL KARIM Q, PRESTON-WHYTE E, ABDOOL KARIM SS. 'Teenagers seeking condoms at family planning services. Part I. A user's perspective'. *South African Medical Journal* 1992; 82: 356–359.

BLANC AK, WAY AA. 'Sexual behaviour and contraceptive knowledge and use among adolescents in developing countries'. *Studies in Family Planning* 1998; 29: 106–116.

BRADSHAW D, PETTIFOR AE, MACPHAIL C, DORRINGTON R. Trends in Youth Risk for HIV, Chapter 10 in Health Systems Trust, *South African Health Review* 2004, Durban, 2004.

CAMPBELL C, MACPHAIL C. 'Peer education, gender and the development of critical consciousness: Participatory HIV prevention by South African youth'. *Socical Science and Medicine* 2002; 55: 331–345.

DEPARTMENT OF HEALTH, REPUBLIC OF SOUTH AFRICA, MEDICAL RESEARCH COUNCIL, AND MACRO INTERNATIONAL. *South African Demographic and Health Survey 1998: Preliminary Report.* Pretoria: Department of Health, 1999.

EATON L, FLISHER AJ, AARO LE. 'Unsafe sexual behaviour in South African youth'. *Social Science Medicine* 2003; 56: 149–165.

HARRISON A, XABA, N, KUNENE P. 'Understanding safe sex: Gender narratives of HIV and pregnancy prevention by rural South African school-going youth'. *Reproductive Health Matters* 2001; 9: 63–71.

Harrison A, Xaba, N, Kunene P, Ntuli N. 'Understanding young women's risk for HIV/AIDS: Adolescent sexuality and vulnerability in rural KwaZulu/Natal'. *Society in Transition* 2001; 32: 69–78.

Jewkes RK, Levin JB, Penn-Kekana LA. 'Gender inequalities, intimate partner violence and HIV preventive practices: Findings of a South African cross-sectional study'. *Social Science and Medicine* 2003; 56: 125–134.

Jewkes R, Vundule C, Maforah F, Jordaan E. 'Relationship dynamics and teenage pregnancy in South Africa'. *Social Science and Medicine* 2001; 52: 733–744.

Kaiser Family Foundation/LoveLife. *'Hot Prospects, Cold Facts: National Survey of South African Youth'.* Johannesburg: LoveLife and Kaiser Family Foundation, 2000.

Kaufman CE, Clark S, Manzini N, May J. *'How community structures of time and opportunity shape adolescent sexual behavior in South Africa'.* New York: Population Council Working Paper No. 159, 2002.

Kaufman CE, DeWet T, Stadler J. 'Adolescent pregnancy and parenthood in South Africa'. *Studies in Family Planning* 2001; 32: 147–160.

Kelly K. *'Communicating for Action: A Contextual Analysis of Youth Responses to HIV/AIDS'.* Pretoria: Department of Health, Beyond Awareness Campaign and Action Research Connection, February 2002.

Leclerc-Madlala S. 'Infect one, infect all: Zulu youth response to the AIDS epidemic in South Africa'. *Medical Anthropology* 1997; 17: 363–380.

MacPhail C, Campbell C. '"I think condoms are good but, aai, I hate those things": Condom use among adolescents and young people in a Southern African township'. *Social Science and Medicine* 2001; 52: 1613–1627.

MacPhail C, Williams B, Campbell C. 'Relative risk of HIV infection among young men and women in a southern African township'. *International Journal of STD and AIDS* 2002; 13: 331–342.

Manzini N. 'Sexual initiation and childbearing among adolescent girls in KwaZulu/Natal, South Africa'. *Reproductive Health Matters* 2001; 9: 44–52.

Mensch BS, Bruce J, Greene M. *'The uncharted passage: Girls' adolescence in the developing world'.* New York: The Population Council, 1998.

Pettifor AE et al. HIV and sexual behaviour among young South Africans: A national survey of 15–24 year olds. Johannesburg: Reproductive Health Research Unit, University of the Witwatersrand, 2004.

Preston-Whyte E. 'Gender and the lost generation: The dynamics of HIV transmission among black South African teenagers in KwaZulu/Natal'. *Health Transition Review* 1994; 4(Suppl): 241–255.

Reddy P et al. 'Umthente Uhlaba Usamila – The South African Youth Risk Behaviour Survey 2002'. Cape Town: South African Medical Research Council, 2003.

Richter L. *'A Survey of Reproductive Health Issues among Urban Youth in South Africa'.* Pretoria: Society for Family Health, 1996.

Shisana O, Bezuidenhout F, Brookes HJ, Chauveau J, Colvin M, Connolly C, Ditlopo P, Kelly K, Moatti JP, Loundou DA, Parker W, Richter L, Schwabe C, Simbayi LC, David Stoker D, Toefy Y, van Zyl J. *Nelson Mandela/HSRC Study on HIV/AIDS.* Human Sciences Research Council. Cape Town 2002.

Varga C. 'Sexual decision-making and negotiation in the midst of AIDS: Youth in KwaZulu/Natal, South Africa'. *Health Transition Review* 1997; 7(Suppl 3): 45–67.

Williams G, Taaljard D, Campbell C et al. 'Changing patterns of knowledge, reported behaviour and sexually transmitted infections in a South African gold mining community'. *AIDS* 2003; 17: 2099–2107.

Wood K, Maforah F and Jewkes R. '"He forced me to love him": Putting violence on adolescent sexual health agendas'. *Social Science and Medicine* 1998; 47: 233–242.

UNAIDS. Young People and HIV/AIDS: Opportunity in Crisis. Geneva: UNICEF/UNAIDS/WHO. 2002.

CHAPTER 18

Female sex workers

Gita Ramjee

THE COMPLEXITY OF SEX work in South Africa makes it a challenging task to regulate the sex work industry in order to implement effective HIV prevention programmes. Effective programmes of peer education and behaviour change can be implemented through targeted interventions and have been successful elsewhere in the world. However, since sex work is a criminal offence in this country, identifying sex workers for targeted interventions could result in further violence, stigma and social ostracism of these women.

However, the fact that sex work is illegal in no way limits the occupation. Sex has become a commodity to ensure survival and may be exchanged for food and shelter as well as money. This chapter concentrates on the more traditional female sex workers who exchange sex for money. Most come from stable working class families.

Income among sex workers is racially skewed, with white women receiving the highest fees per coital act. The prevalence of HIV among sex workers also reflects racial differences, with the highest prevalence seen among black women.

The mining industry and truck stops are important working areas and several studies have focused on the incidence of sexually transmitted infections (STIs), including HIV, among these sex worker populations and their clients.

Condom use is an economic issue, with penetrative sex (vaginal or anal) attracting higher fees if no condom is used.

Successful HIV and STI prevention programmes would require the government to recognise and accept the sex worker industry in the country by decriminalising sex work and promoting health-seeking behaviour among sex workers and their clients.

In countries where HIV transmission is predominantly through sexual contact, having multiple sexual partners is a key risk behaviour. Sex workers, by virtue of the nature of their work, which is characterised by multiple sex partners and frequent coitus, have a higher risk of acquiring and transmitting HIV than the general population. The high prevalence of HIV observed in sex workers in several countries in Africa and Asia is attributable not only to high-risk sexual behaviour but also to common background characteristics, such as poor social conditions, limited knowledge of HIV/AIDS and a high prevalence of other sexually transmitted infections (STIs). Sex workers and their clients are therefore seen as important 'core transmitter groups/bridging populations' for the spread of HIV to the general population. The success of interventions targeted at sex workers and their clients depends on an understanding of the social context within which behaviour changes must occur. In settings where negotiation of safer sex methods is difficult, the social, economic and medical needs of sex workers needs to be well defined and understood. A deeper understanding of sex work and sex worker networks is critically important in terms of targeting HIV prevention interventions country-wide, especially during the early stages of the HIV epidemic.

Sociodemographic characteristics

With the social and economic constraints that limit women's access to resources in so many developing countries, sex becomes a commodity to ensure survival. In such a context, the definition of sex work is complex as there are many transactions that it can encompass in a scale extending from serial monogamous relationships, sporadic or occasional exchange of sex for transport, school uniforms and fees, food, accommodation, all the way through to more conventionally identified formal occupation as a sex worker. This chapter focuses on formal sex work and only on the female sex worker industry. The fact that sex work is illegal in South Africa in no way diminishes its ubiquity.

The sex work industry in South Africa includes men and women in a range of settings such as escort agencies, massage parlours, street workers, and truck stops. Race, the male:female ratio in terms of clients:sex workers, who controls where sex work takes place, and the financial cost of the sexual transaction are all important determinants for HIV risk. Sex workers based at escort agencies and massage parlours are more likely to be white and regulated by employers in terms of condom use and regular HIV and STI screening, and therefore also more likely to be at the lower end of HIV risk. In contrast, street sex workers, sex workers at truck stops and around male migrant workplaces, are more likely to be black, working independently or in small, closed groups, with limited access to HIV testing, condoms and reproductive health services, and therefore at higher risk of acquiring infection with HIV. Although sex workers have been broadly grouped by the setting within which they work, there is some movement between the groups. The socio-demographic characteristics of sex workers in several settings in South Africa are described below.

Year of Study	Carletonville	3 Cities in South Africa	Truck Stops	Johannesburg
	1998	1999–2000	1996–2000	1996–1998
Condom Use (Casual Partner)				
Never (<25%)	58.5 (n=94)	NA	41	8
Sometimes (%)	15.9	NA	11	51
Most of the time (%)	25.5	NA	0	30
Anal Sex (%)	NA	<3%	41	7
No. of Clients (Range) (Week)	NA	5 to 30	5 to 30	5 or less
Use of Drying Agents for 'Dry Sex' (%)	9.1	NA	94 (n=142)	NA
Cost of Sex (Street workers)	R20	>R90	R70	–
STI				
Syphilis (%)	23.3	NA	30	28
N Gonorrhoeae (%)	5.7	NA	10	30
C Trachomatis (%)	9.1	NA	12	10
T Vaginalis (%)	NA	NA	36	NA
HIV Prevalence (%)	68.6 (n = 100)	78 (n = 175)	50 (n = 416)	45 (n = 247)
Substance Abuse				
Crack/Madrax (High income sex workers)	NA	High	NA	High
Dagga	NA	Yes	Yes	Yes
Alcohol consumption	High	High	High	High

TABLE 18.1 HIV/STI prevalence among sex workers from various studies

NA = not available * Williams B G, Macphail C, Campbell C, Taljaard D, Gouws E, Moema S, Mzaidume Z, Rasego B. The Carletonville-Mothusimpilo Project: Limiting transmission of HIV through community-based interventions. South African Journal of Science, 2000; 96: 351–359.

Leggett T. Drugs, sex work, and HIV in three South African cities. Society in Transition 2001; 32: 101–109.

Legget T. Poverty and sex work in Durban, South Africa. Society in Transition 1999; 30: 157–167.

Ramjee G, Gouws E. Prevalence of HIV among truck drivers visiting sex workers in KwaZulu-Natal, South Africa. Sexually Transmitted Diseases 2002; 29: 44–49.

Rees H, Beksinska M E, Dickson-Tetteh K, Ballard R C, Htun Y. Commercial sex workers in Johannesburg: Risk behaviour and HIV status. South African Journal of Science. 2000; 96: 283–284.

Dorothy Nairne. 'Please help me cleanse my womb' A hotel-based STD programme in a violent neighbourhood in Johannesburg. Research for Sex Work 2, 1999

The illegal status of sex work in South Africa has limited the feasibility of undertaking research and/or interventions in this group. The few studies that have been conducted have largely been cross-sectional, collecting socio-behavioural data. There is little data on the prevalence or incidence of HIV and other STIs or on links with behavioural risk factors. TABLE 18.1 presents data from sex workers on HIV risk behaviours from a variety of settings and cities in South Africa. A cross-sectional study among sex workers in massage parlours, escort agencies and on the street in the central business district of Durban in 1998 demonstrated that the majority came from working class families. Family structures were stable with both mother and father present.

Sex workers based at escort agencies have a fixed hourly rate determined by the agency which also takes a fixed percentage of the income generated. Although injecting recreational drug use is limited, there is extensive use of non-injecting recreational drugs and alcohol. Some respondents claimed that this helps them to be sex workers, but as it also consumes a large proportion of their income it creates a vicious cycle of dependency and further impoverishment. See CHAPTER 14 for a more detailed description of sex workers and substance abuse.

A survey conducted in 2000 of HIV risk in sex workers from three South African cities, Durban, Johannesburg and Cape Town, confirmed that income is racially skewed with white women earning the highest and black women the lowest. The majority of white women are urban based and earn at least R90 per coital act, with occasional coital encounters where condoms are not used.

In contrast, black sex workers tended to be at a substantially lower socioeconomic level and based in mining towns such as Carletonville, along major trucking routes across southern Africa, or on the streets in high-density urban areas. TABLE 18.1 describes the available data we have from various studies in terms of condom use, sexual practices, substance use, number of clients, and HIV and STI prevalence. Condom use is very low with the majority of coital acts unprotected. The number of clients per sex workers ranges from five to 30. Cost of sex differs between the sex worker groups, with sex workers in Carletonville charging a lower fee compared with women in the cities.

Recreational substance use, especially drugs such as Mandrax or Crack, has been reported mainly among women in the cities, and is especially prevalent among women with a higher income. Alcohol consumption is high with many women reporting alcohol consumption prior to sex.

Reports on anal sex practice are varied. It is possible that women may not have been comfortable in divulging this information as anal sex is generally regarded as 'taboo' in many heterosexual relationships. Of concern, though, is the likelihood that men and women are equally unaware that receptive anal sex is a significant risk factor for HIV infection (see also CHAPTER 16).

Carletonville sex workers

The mining industry employs several hundreds of thousands of black men in the economically active age group. They are recruited from various rural areas in South Africa as well as neighbouring countries in the southern African region. These migrants leave their wives and families in their rural areas of origin and spend about 11 months of the year housed in single-sex dormitory accommodation at the mines. CHAPTER 19 provides a more detailed description of this phenomenon and its relationship with HIV rate. Not surprisingly, a sex industry has developed at the periphery of these mines that is utilised extensively by the mineworkers. High levels of alcohol consumption by clients mitigate against the use of condoms in these coital encounters. Whilst the miners have good access to health care, the sex workers, because of their isolation, have limited access to reproductive and other health services.

Sex workers in Hillbrow, Johannesburg

It is estimated that there are between 5000 and 10 000 female sex workers living and working in Hillbrow, central Johannesburg. These women operate through hotels and flats, and many of these establishments have been transformed into brothels where sex workers both live and see their clients.

In a cross-sectional study of 278 women, the women reported soliciting clients from streets (53%), bars (29%) and hotels (8%). Only 30% of the women used condoms consistently (70% of sexual acts). The women, on average, saw five or fewer clients on a working day. A small percentage of women practised anal sex at least once a week.

Sex workers at truck stops

The South African Medical Research Council has been undertaking research on sex workers based at truck stops along the national road between Johannesburg and Durban. In 1996, as part of a phase III microbicide trial, a cohort of 470 female sex workers, also refered to as the Du Cohort, was established at five truck stops in the KwaZulu-Natal midlands. During the three year follow-up period HIV and STI prevalence and incidence rates were established. Data from sex workers who seroconverted during the trial have generated valuable data on the natural history of early HIV infection in a HIV subtype C population.

Clients included truck drivers and men from neighbouring towns. Preliminary research among 12 sex workers at one truck stop in 1992 indicated that limited employment opportunities, lack of access to health services including condoms, limited skills to negotiate condom use, loss of income if they insisted on condom use and experience of violence increase their risk of acquiring infection with HIV.

At each stop there are usually about 15 to 20 sex workers. The most senior sex worker in terms of age and/or length of stay at the truck stop – also referred to as the 'Boss' – determines who works at the stop, the number of sex workers at the truck stop at any given time, and the price of the sex. She also takes a fixed percentage of the income earned by the sex workers. The 'Boss' also actively recruits new, young sex workers to attract more clients.

Most of the women sex workers are migrant workers from other rural areas or cities. Lack of employment opportunities and a high number of dependants often lead them to prostitution. Many also have intimate relationships outside of sex work. Some women work as sex workers during the day and go home to their partners and families at the end of the day. While some sex workers are able to get their clients to use condoms, in their personal relationships they face similar challenges to women in the general population in trying to practise safe sex.

Some sex workers sell beer and dagga (marijuana) to their clients to supplement their income from sex work.

Sex work was categorised as 'short-jobs' which usually involves a single coital act or 'long-jobs' which may involve several coital acts over several hours. The cost of a coital act was dependent on whether a condom is used or not and type of sexual practice. Condom use resulted in a loss of income. For example, peno-vaginal sex with a condom is about R60 compared with R120 without a condom. Anal sex without a condom fetched the highest price.

Of the 416 sex workers screened in 1996, 41% never used condoms, while 11% indicated 100% condom use during peno-vaginal intercourse, while 41% reported the practice of anal sex with their clients, which is usually unprotected. At the end of the three year follow-up period, unprotected anal sex was reported by 75% of the sex workers in this cohort. Notwithstanding the limitations of self-reported sexual behaviours and practices, there is clearly an increase in reported unprotected anal sex that is also associated with a higher risk of infection with HIV.

The prevalence of HIV infection in 145 sex workers screened in 1995 as part of a phase I microbicide trial was 61.3% among those who also practised anal sex as compared with 42.7% among sex workers who did not practise anal sex. Anal sex was associated with a higher risk of HIV infection in a multiple logistic regression model controlling for age, condom use, number of clients per week, and duration of sex work. Stratifying for these variables demonstrated that anal sex was consistently associated with a higher risk of HIV infection.

Douching, intravaginal substance use and dry sex practices

There have increasingly been reports of douching, intra-vaginal substance use and dry sex practices by women for reasons of hygiene and/or for sexual enhancement in both sex- and non-sex worker populations in sub-Saharan Africa. While concerns about its implications for HIV transmission have been raised, the relationship of these practices to HIV acquisition has not been established.

Sex workers at the truck stops reported the use of a variety of herbs and chemicals for either contraceptive or hygienic reasons, as well as for 'dry sex'. Products range from household cleaning agents to over-the-counter sexual enhancers to traditional medication. Although 33% of the women interviewed did not enjoy 'dry sex' as they found it painful, they continued with the practice to attract male clients.

Prevalence of HIV and sexually transmitted infections

HIV prevalence in groups of sex workers studied in South Africa is alarmingly high and ranges from 17 to 66%. Black sex workers showed substantially higher infection rates compared with other race groups. In the three cities study, over 66% of black sex workers in the sample of 249 were HIV positive compared with 18% of whites and 17% of coloureds. The HIV prevalence among Carletonville sex workers is significantly higher than that at truck stops. Given that the clients of these Carletonville sex workers are mainly migrants, the probability of transmission of viruses from these clients to their sexual partners in rural areas is high and is discussed in greater detail in CHAPTER 19.

The prevalence of sexually transmitted infections (STIs) in the truck-stop sex worker population is relatively high (TABLE 18.2) compared with other sex worker cohort studies conducted elsewhere in Africa.

The relationship between HIV and STI was first recognised in epidemiological studies that showed a high prevalence of HIV among individuals with a history of STI. (See CHAPTER 12 for a more detailed assessment of STIs and the associated risk of acquiring HIV.) Ulcerative infections such as syphilis and gonorrhoea have been reported to increase the rate of HIV transmission, and given the low rate of condom use, it is likely to have an enormous impact on the risk of STI infection.

Data on the prevalence and incidence of sexually transmitted infections including HIV among sex workers at the truck stops between 1996–2000 are presented in TABLE 18.2. The high HIV and STI incidence rates despite intensive and ongoing counselling provide some indication of the challenges faced by these sex workers in implementing condom use.

TABLE 18.2 Baseline prevalences and incidence rates of STIs and HIV among sex workers at truck stops between 1996–1999

STI	Prevalence (95% CI) (N = 472)	Incidence Rate (% per person years of follow-up) (95% CI) (N = 198)
T vaginalis	36.1% (31.6–40.6)	114.0% (102–126)
N gonorrhoea	11.3% (8.4–14.3)	42.0% (34.8–49.2)
C trachomatis	12.7% (9.4–15.9)	43.2% (34.8–50.4)
Syphilis	31.9% (27.6–36.2)	–
HIV	51.3% (46.7–55.8)	18.2% (13.0–23.0)
HPV	18.4%	–
HSV-2	84%	38%

The overall prevalence of human papillomavirus (HPV) was high among both HIV-positive and HIV-negative sex workers.

Prevalence of herpes simplex virus type 2 (HSV-2) was high in this cohort. At baseline, 84% of the sex workers screened were already HSV-2 positive. Infection with HSV-2 was predictive of HIV seroconversion.

HIV seropositivity and safe sex practices

The impact of knowledge of HIV-positive status on safer sex practices was assessed in a group of 77 HIV-positive sex workers at the KwaZulu-Natal midlands truck stops. This cohort of sex workers was followed up for a period of one year and the incidence of STIs ascertained as a proxy marker for risky sex practices. The incidence rate per 100 women-years of follow-up was 150 for *Trichomonas vaginalis* infection; for *Neisseria gonorrhoea* infection; *Chlamydia trachomatis* infection; and 244 for any STI. TABLE 18.3 indicates the number of STI infections among the women. Some women had no infections, whilst others came with multiple infections (TABLE 18.3). Despite their participation in the HIV prevention programme where HIV prevention education, safe sex counselling and intensive condom promotion was offered, the incidence remained high. Behavioural and counselling data showed that women who were positive were not willing to give up sex work as they had no other options for employment. Given that HIV-positive women are having unprotected sex during the course of their infection, it is highly likely that STIs including HIV will be transmitted to their sexual partners and clients. There is also the added risk of acquisition of infection with new strains of HIV leading to super-infection.

# of infections	T. vaginalis		N. gonorrhoea		C. trachomatis	
	Max	Min	Max	Min	Max	Min
None	30	30	57	58	64	64
1	21	24	11	10	10	12
2	15	17	3	6	2	1
3 or 4	11	6	6	3	1	0
Total	89	76	37	32	17	14

TABLE 18.3 Incidence rate of bacterial STIs in HIV-positive sex workers in 1999

Prevalence of HIV among clients of sex workers

Although the role of mobile populations in the spread of HIV has been well documented, there are few data comparing HIV prevalence among truck drivers in South Africa to that of the sex workers they frequent. A cross-sectional study conducted among 320 truck drivers frequenting sex workers at five truck stops in the KwaZulu-Natal midlands showed that the HIV prevalence among truck drivers was 56%. Sixty-six percent of these truck drivers reported having an STI in the past six months. Condom use varied, with 20% never using condoms and 47% reporting condom use for all coital acts. The truck drivers travelled to three or more provinces in South Africa and 65% also travelled to neighbouring countries where they had sex with other sex workers. While 42% of the men reported practising anal sex, only 23% of these acts were protected. The HIV prevalence among truck drivers and sex workers at each truck stop is presented in TABLE 18.4. Overall HIV prevalence in both sex workers and their clients is alarmingly high. At one truck stop, 95% of the men tested were

Truck Stop	Truck Drivers		Sex Workers		RR
	N	Prevalence (%)	N	Prevalence (%)	
A	75	37	29	38	0.97
B	44	57	55	44	1.30
C	48	52	24	42	1.24
D	32	50	13	62	0.81
E	56	52	31	74	0.70
F	55	95	52	64	1.48
Total	310	56	204	56	1.00

TABLE 18.4 HIV prevalence among truck drivers and sex workers at truck stops

already HIV infected. The study further illustrates the high-risk behaviour of mobile populations and their role in the spread of HIV in southern Africa.

Preventing HIV infection in sex workers

The general ability of women to negotiate safer sex practices within the current paradigm of HIV risk reduction strategies is low. The ability of sex workers to negotiate in sexual contacts is expected to be lower, especially where sex work is illegal and carries with it few social or legal rights. The sex workers, especially those at truck stops and gold mines, already carry a substantial burden of HIV infection or are at high risk of heterosexually transmitted HIV but they have little power to negotiate safer sexual practices both in their commercial and intimate sexual relationships. Violence, or the threat of it, plays an important role in their disempowerment.

For these sex workers, living in poverty and overcrowded conditions and with several dependants, the risk of infection that may not materialise for many years is perhaps not so alarming a spectre. HIV infection is one more consequence of their lack of social and economic power.

Sex with condoms brings a lower price. Hence sustaining earnings while using condoms requires more clients. Time constraints and competition for clients limits the feasibility of this option. Thus to maintain prices while insisting on condom use would require a co-operative approach, with the sex workers standing together as suppliers in the market place.

To address the issues central to the disempowerment of sex workers, long-term programmes that redress the worker's lack of social and legal rights are required. In the shorter term enabling sex workers to get their clients to use condoms and expanding the availability of methods that women can initiate and control will increase their options to protect themselves from HIV infection. To empower these sex workers in their relationships with their clients would be a step toward developing their ability to reduce the threats to their health that might have far-reaching effects on the reduction of HIV incidence rates. Negotiation and communication skills, information and access to health care services are a start to this process.

Successful experiences from select South African sites in 100% condom use, peer education programmes and decriminalisation of sex work are presented in the following case studies.

Case study

The first cases of AIDS in Thailand were described in the early 1980s, initially among injecting drug users and soon afterwards among sex workers and their clients. Infection in the wives and/or sexual partners of the clients of sex workers highlighted how HIV infection was being introduced into the general population. The Thai Government acted early and decisively by launching its 100% Condom Programme, a nationwide campaign to reduce HIV infection by promoting universal and consistent condom use among commercial sex workers located in brothels and other settings. See CHAPTER 9 for a more detailed description of this programme.

Given the diversity of the sex worker population in South Africa, the fact that sex work is largely unregulated, and the already high rates of HIV among sex workers, the introduction of a 100% condom use programme may have little impact on the epidemic in South Africa but could have enormous benefits for new sex workers entering the industry. The development and promotion of chemical and non-chemical barrier methods are discussed more fully in CHAPTER 15.

Case study

The Sex Worker Education and Advocacy Task Group (SWEAT) has been playing an important role in mobilising sex workers, especially those working in escort agencies and massage parlours, around their rights, access to health services and techniques for erotocising condom use to encourage acceptance by clients.

The peer-education programme in Carletonville encouraged sex workers to identify and seek medical attention during the early stages of infection with STIs. The programme also aimed to increase the sex workers' self-esteem and recognise personal vulnerability to HIV as a way of promoting condom use. The programme had a tremendous impact on the confidence of the peer educators and this sense of pride and achievement spread to the community beyond the peer education team. It was also successful in resolving community divisions so as to initiate discussions around issues of sexual health and condom use.

Prevention of sexually transmitted infections

Globally, female sex workers are a stigmatised group, but all the more so with the advent of the HIV epidemic in which they are targeted as vectors of HIV transmission. The ambivalence of their position in the epidemic (vectors or victims) makes it difficult to prioritise intervention projects.

Regular STI treatment in core groups such as sex workers has proved both to be cost effective, and to reduce the spread of the infection in the general population. Unfortunately, provision of quality service to high-risk groups also results in stigma and may not be acceptable. Many countries in Africa and elsewhere have introduced STI services to sex workers through channels such as government clinics, private practitioners and brothel-based delivery that ensure privacy, confidentiality and convenience.

A study currently undertaken by the Reproductive Health Research Unit aims to assess the cost-effectiveness of brothel-based STI treatment for sex workers in Hillbrow, Johannesburg. Preliminary results indicate that 252 HIV infections and 6273 cervical infections were averted in a sample of 1431 women with 2523 visits.

Promoting behavioural change

Efforts to promote behavioural change have been coupled with biological interventions for preventing the spread of HIV infection. Strategies aimed at this, which include raising HIV awareness, promotion of male and female condoms and reducing multiple partners among high-risk groups, have proved effective among some sex workers – although it is also the case that while they and their clients may be motivated to use condoms in sex-work encounters, a majority of sex workers fail to use protection with their regular partners. Even so, a recent study suggests that while researchers focus on mobile populations as bridges to the spread of the virus, the same population may also be bridges to the spread of positive attitudes about condom use and HIV education.

Bibliography

ABDOOL KARIM Q, ABDOOL KARIM SS, SOLDAN K, ZONDI M. 'Reducing risk of HIV infection among South African Sex Workers: Socioeconomic and gender barriers'. *American Journal of Public Health* 1995; 85: 1521–1525.

CONNOLLY C, RAMJEE G, STRUM AW, ABDOOL KARIM SS. 'Incidence of sexually transmitted infections among HIV-positive sex workers in KwaZulu-Natal, South Africa'. *Sexually Transmitted Diseases* 2002; 29: 721–724.

CORBETT E L, STEKETEE R W, TER KUILE F O, LATIF A S, KAMALI A, HAYES R J. 'HIV-1/AIDS and the control of other infectious diseases in Africa'. *Lancet* 2002; 359: 2177–2187.

MASTRO TD, LIMPAKARNJANARAT K. 'Condom use in Thailand: How much is it slowing the HIV/AIDS epidemic?' *AIDS* 1995; 9: 523–525.

MORRIS M, WAWER MJ, MAKUMBI F, ZAVISCA JR, SEWANKAMBO N. 'Condom acceptance is higher among travellers in Uganda'. *AIDS* 2000; 14: 733–741.

Moses S, Plummer FA, Ngugi EN, Nagelkerke NJD, Anzala AO, Ndinya-Achola JO. 'Controlling HIV in Africa: Effectiveness and cost of an intervention in a high-frequency STD transmitter core group'. *AIDS* 1995; 5: 407–411.

Nairne D. '"Please help me cleanse my womb" A hotel-based STD programme in a violent neighbourhood in Johannesburg'. *Research for Sex Work* 1999; 2: 18–20.

Plummer FA, Simonsen JN, Cameron DW et al. 'Cofactors in male to female transmission of HIV-1'. *Journal of Infectious Diseases* 1991; 163: 233–239.

Ramjee G, Abdool Karim SS, Morar N, Gwamanda Z, Xulu G, Ximba T, Gouws E. 'Acceptability of a vaginal microbicide among female sex workers'. *South African Medical Journal* 1999; 89: 673–676.

Ramjee G, Gouws E. 'Prevalence of HIV among truck drivers visiting sex workers in KwaZulu-Natal, South Africa'. *Sexually Transmitted Diseases* 2002; 29: 44–49.

Rosenburg MJ, Gollub EL. 'Commentary: Methods women can use that may prevent sexually transmitted disease, including HIV'. *American Journal of Public Health* 1992; 82: 1473–1478.

Stigum H, Magnus P, Bakketeig LS. 'Effect of changing partnership formation rates on the spread of sexually transmitted diseases and Human Immunodeficiency Virus'. *American Journal of Epidemiolology* 1997; 145: 644–652.

Stover J, Walker N, Garnett GP, Salomon JA, Stanecki KA, Ghys PD, Grassly NC, Anderson RM, Schwartländer. 'Can we reverse the HIV/AIDS pandemic with an expanded response?' *Lancet* 2002; 360: 73–77.

Varga CA. 'Coping with HIV/AIDS in Durban's commercial sex industry'. *AIDS Care* 2001; 13: 351–365.

Van Damme L, Ramjee G, Alary M, Vuylsteke B, Chandeying V, Rees H, Sirivongrangson P, Mukenge-Tshibaka L, Ettiègne-Traoré V, Uaheowitchai C, Abdool Karim SS, Mâsse B, Perriëns J, Laga M. 'Effectiveness of Col-1492, a Nonoxynol-9 vaginal gel, on HIV transmission in female sex workers'. *Lancet Infectious Diseases* 2002; 360: 971–977.

Wawer MJ, Serwadda D, Gray RH, Sewankambo NK, Li C, Nalugoda F, Lutalo T, Knode-Lule JK. 'Trends in HIV-1 prevalence may not reflect trends in incidence in mature epidemics: Data from the Rakai population-based cohort, Uganda'. *AIDS* 1997; 11: 1023–1030.

World Health Organisation/Global Programme on AIDS: *Global prevalence and incidence of selected curable STDs: Overview and estimates.* Geneva: World Health Organisation (WHO/GPA/STD95.1). 1995.

CHAPTER 19

Population movement and the spread of HIV in southern Africa

Mark Lurie

MIGRATION, OR POPULATION MOVEMENT, has played a critical role in the spread of HIV throughout southern Africa, but relatively few studies have attempted to understand the underlying processes in detail or to develop ways to reduce the spread of infection among migrants and their partners.

For many years, even with limited empirical evidence, the central assumption in migration research has been that of the unidirectionality of spread: it has long been assumed that the predominant patterns of spread have been from returning migrants who became infected while away to their rural partners who they infected when they returned home.

There is now increasing evidence that the unidirectionality of spread was very much true early in the epidemic and was likely a major factor in the spread of HIV from urban to rural areas during the early 1990s. However, in the mature epidemic that southern Africa now faces, with high rates of infection both in urban and rural areas, the patterns of spread have changed and there is now evidence for a significant amount of HIV transmission occurring locally in rural areas. This does not absolve migration as being an important risk factor for HIV transmission – indeed it continues to be a critical factor – but instead it further illustrates the complex relationship between population movement and the spread of disease during a mature epidemic.

The epidemiological and social evidence argues strongly for the need for intervention programmes aimed specifically at migrants and their partners.

The spread of disease in societies is shaped, at least in part, by the political, social and economic environment in which people live. In sub-Saharan Africa, where 'circular' migration is fundamental to the way in which society is ordered, migration has been an important determinant of the spread of infectious diseases, and has contributed to the extraordinarily rapid spread of HIV.

It is generally assumed that when young men leave their rural homes in search of work in urban areas they may engage in sex with women at high risk, and are themselves at high risk of infection (FIGURE 19.1). When they return to their rural homes, they may carry the virus with them and infect their rural partners. This circular migration typifies the pattern of movement of many young men throughout southern Africa.

However, the role of migration in the spread of HIV and other sexually transmitted infections (STIs) is not well understood. Studies of migration tend to concentrate on the urban, or 'receiving' areas with little attention being paid to people living in the rural or 'sending' areas. Furthermore, there have been few well-designed epidemiological studies documenting the relationship between migration and infectious diseases. Even more importantly at this late stage of the southern African HIV epidemic, there have been few intervention programmes, even on a small scale, which attempt to reduce transmission among migrants and their rural or urban partners. Finally, no attempt has been made to address the structural factors that force people to migrate in the first place.

To develop a better understanding of the role that migration plays in the spread of HIV in the region, prospective studies are needed. Inevitably, however, prospective studies are difficult to implement among migrant people given the logistical difficulties and financial costs that arise when trying to keep track of people who are 'on the move'.

FIGURE 19.1 Conceptual framework for the role of migration in the spread of HIV/STI. Main decision points are shown in blocks; main risk factors are shown in circles
Source: Lourie M. Migration and the spread of HIV in South Africa. Doctoral Dissertation, John Hopkins University School of Hygiene and Public Health, 2001

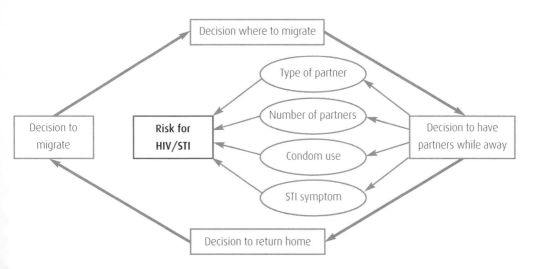

This chapter begins with a brief examination of the origin and extent of population movement in southern Africa, reviews the literature on the role of migration in the spread of HIV and STIs, identifies current intervention needs among migrants and concludes by discussing some areas in which further research is needed.

The history and extent of migration in southern Africa

The migrant labour system was central to the way in which the political economy of South Africa was ordered in the last century and was intimately bound up with the structure and functioning of the system of apartheid. Current estimates are that more than 2.5 million legal, and many more illegal, migrants are drawn to work in South Africa's mines, factories and farms from rural areas within South Africa and from neighbouring countries. Estimates of the prevalence of migration should, however, be interpreted cautiously as they are likely to underestimate the true extent of migration since illegal and undocumented migration is notoriously difficult to quantify and is reported to be increasing. While many migrants are employed in the formal economic sector, many more find employment in the informal sector and the latter are unlikely to be counted in the official statistics. What is clear, however, is that large-scale migration is not just an issue for South Africa; it is a regional issue with far-reaching consequences.

One way to begin to quantify the extent of migration in South Africa is by examining census data, either local or national. FIGURE 19.2 shows the distribution of men and women by age-group in KwaZulu-Natal and Gauteng. It is clear that in both provinces the ratio of men to women under the age of 15 is essentially one, but that by age 20 the proportion of men in KwaZulu-Natal begins to decline. At the same time there is a subsequent increase in the proportion of men at migration destinations such as Gauteng. As these data are from the 1996 census, it is unlikely that they reflect significant AIDS mortality; instead these patterns are mainly the result of large-scale population movements; outmigration of young men from KwaZulu-Natal and inmigration to Gauteng.

The extent of migration is also clearly seen in a demographic profile of men and women from one rural district in KwaZulu-Natal (FIGURE 19.3). The number of women falls rapidly after the age of 17 years, but the number of men falls even more rapidly, leading to a distorted sex ratio. By age 32, the proportion of men falls to about 35% and then increases again as migrant workers return home, often with severe and debilitating disease.

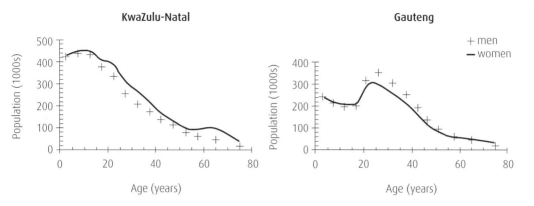

FIGURE 19.2 Number of people (in thousands) by one year age groups, Gauteng and KwaZulu-Natal, South Africa, 1996
Source: Udjo E and Hirschowitz R (Eds.) The People of South Africa Population Census 1996: Summary Report. Statistics South Africa, Pretoria 2000.

Migration patterns in South Africa were an integral part of the way in which government, with the support of industry and in particular the mining industry, structured South African society from early in the twentieth century culminating in the system of apartheid. During the early decades of the twentieth century the movement of labour was strictly controlled to ensure a continuing supply of cheap black workers for agriculture, industry and commerce while simultaneously protecting the relative privilege of white workers. The demise

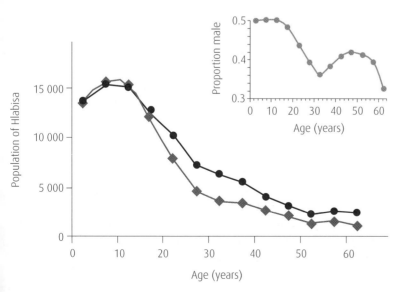

FIGURE 19.3 Demographic Profile of Men and Women in Hlabisa District, South Africa: The number of men (squares) and women (circles) in Hlabisa in five year age bands and the proportion that are male (inset)
Source: Williams BG, Gouws E, Lurie M, Crush J. Spaces of Vulnerability: Migration and HIV/AIDS in South Africa. Cape Town – IDASA, 2002

of apartheid and the rise of democracy will change the pressures and demands for labour, but it is still not clear how this will affect the form and patterns of labour migration in the new South Africa.

The changing and dynamic nature of migration in southern Africa can best be understood by examining the way in which sources of rural livelihoods changed over the course of the last century. In the mid-1930s between 40 and 50% of rural subsistence food requirements were still met by rural production. Over the next 40 years, however, remittances from family members working in urban areas increased in importance and by 1970, agricultural production in these rural areas had declined to the point where only 10% of the total income for most rural households came from agriculture, with the balance of household incomes coming from remittances by family members employed as migrant labourers. In KwaZulu-Natal, for example, by the late 1980s remittances from migrant workers made up over three-quarters of rural household income.

The patterns of migration in South Africa have changed considerably over the last three decades and the political changes in South Africa that have taken place since the democratic election of 1994 ensure that dramatic changes will occur in the near future. In the early decades of the last century, migrant workers tended to work in the mines or other sectors of the economy for a few years after which time they would return permanently to their rural places of origin. In 1936, for example, there was a greater than 75% chance that by the time a migrant was 45 years old, he would have ceased to engage in migrant labour.

Today, migrant labour tends to be more long-term, with more frequent returns home. Several factors have combined in recent years to encourage easy and rapid movement of people in southern Africa. These include the lifting of apartheid laws that restricted the movement of the majority of the population, the development of a significant transportation infrastructure and as a result of strengthening trade unions, the negotiation of more flexible work contracts. All of these events have made it easier for migrants to return home more frequently than they could in the past.

Migration to the gold mines

Much of the published research on migrant labour in South Africa has focused on the gold mines which have drawn large numbers of workers from all over the sub-continent; by the end of the 1980s, for example, more than 800 000 men were employed on the gold mines. Because these men live almost exclusively in single-sex hostels, without their wives or families, they are inevitably at high risk of contracting STIs including HIV.

The pattern of migration to the gold mines has changed considerably over the last two decades. In the early 1970s, almost 80% of the workforce came from outside South Africa; today less than 40% of gold miners come from outside South Africa's borders. In addition, large-scale retrenchment over the last decade has come about as a result of falling levels of production, a dramatic drop in the international price of gold and the historical marginality of South Africa's gold mines. For example, in 1992 the gold mines employed 32% fewer workers than they did in 1986, and retrenchments have continued since 1992.

Despite these changes, important aspects of mine migration have persisted: over 90% of the industry's black employees are migrants. The vast majority live in single-sex hostels and visit their rural families only occasionally. Foreign workers on the mines are generally able to return home less frequently than their South African counterparts and their partners are less likely to be able to visit them on the mines.

The number of men living in single-sex hostels is slowly declining as the mining industry experiments with the introduction of married housing. But in 1993, 89% of miners still lived in single-sex hostels and only 2.1% lived in married housing. The rest opted for their own accommodation, separate from that provided by mining companies.

Other types of migration

When one speaks of migration in South Africa, one tends to think mostly about young rural men working on the gold mines, but in fact population movement in the southern Africa region takes many forms. Indeed there are many different 'types' of migration (FIGURE 19.4) and each may carry with it different levels of risk for the acquisition and spread of HIV and other STIs.

→ Long-term/short-term
    – seasonal
→ Across the border
     – legal
     – Illegal
→ With family; without
→ Refugees, other forced removals
→ Rural ⇒ Urban/Urban ⇒ Rural/Urban ⇒ Urban/Rural ⇒ Rural
→ Males/Females/Children/Adults
Most prevalent type of migration in SA:
→ Circular/oscillating migration, both across international borders and within countries, predominantly but not exclusively male

FIGURE 19.4 Different types of migration in southern Africa

In spite of the attention paid to the gold mines, the majority of migrant workers are employed in other sectors or are in the process of seeking work and large gaps exist in our knowledge of other forms of migration in South and southern Africa, particularly for those engaged in the informal sector. Indeed, while single-sex hostels are discussed almost exclusively in relation to gold mines, they are common outside of the mining industry as well. Within a 12 kilo-metre radius of Durban, for example, there are at least seven men's hostels with an excess of 43 000 officially registered beds, one women's hostel with over 1000 beds and one mixed hostel with 11 000 beds.

Women in particular are increasingly mobile, with one survey in KwaZulu-Natal finding that about one-third of women between the ages of 19 and 49 were migrant (defined as spending most nights away from home). Unlike their male counterparts, female migrants tended to stay closer to home and were therefore able to return home more frequently.

Forced migration, usually as a result of political conflict, has produced large numbers of refugees in southern Africa. Although little work has been done among these populations the dynamics of HIV/STI spread among refugees is likely to be quite different from that of urban male migrants living in single-sex hostels. It is therefore important to recognise that migration takes many different forms in southern Africa and that each of these different forms may be associated with different risk factors for the spread of HIV/STI and that each may require slightly different intervention strategies.

Migration and HIV/STIs

In several parts of the world, geographic mobility, migration and widespread population displacement have been identified as significant risk factors in the transmission of HIV and migration has become an important theme in the discussion of AIDS. A number of studies have shown that migrants are at greater risk of infection with HIV and other STIs than are non-migrants, both in South Africa and elsewhere, but few of these studies have been able to measure biological outcomes such as HIV or STI prevalence or incidence. A summary of the major African studies on migration and HIV is presented in TABLE 19.1.

The association between migration and HIV is more likely to be related to the conditions and structure of the migration process than to the actual dissemination of the virus along corridors of migration. Despite this fact, much research has focused along these corridors and on people who move along them. Studies along trucking routes and major highways are examples of this research (Refer to CHAPTER 18).

Location, year (authors)	Population	Main findings
South Africa, 2003 (Lurie et al.)	Migrant men and their partners; and non-migrant men and their partners	Migrant men 2.4 times more likely to be infected with HIV than non-migrant men; high rates of HIV discordance among couples; women the infected partner in 30% of discordant couples
South Africa, 2003 (Zuma et al.)	Migrant & non-migrant women near a South African mining town	HIV prevalence among migrant women was 46%; migrant women were 1.6 times more likely to be HIV-infected than non-migrant women
Uganda, 1995 (Nunn et al.)	Rural Ugandan residents & migrants	People who moved within last 3 years were 3 times more likely to be infected with HIV than those who had stable residence for 10 yrs
Senegal, 1993 (Pison et al.)	Seasonal migrants in rural areas	HIV spread mostly first to men who became infected during seasonal migration, then to their rural partners when they returned
South Africa, 1992 (Abdool Karim et al.)	Rural KwaZulu-Natal residents & migrants	HIV 3 times more likely among those who had recently changed their place of residence
South Africa, 1991 (Jochelson et al.)	Urban male mine workers	Migration disrupts family life and creates a market for prostitution in mining towns
Zimbabwe, 1990 (Bassett et al.)	Urban male factory workers	HIV+ men more likely to live apart from their wives and to have multiple sex partners

A study in Uganda showed a strong correlation between HIV infection and migration status. People who had moved within the last five years were three times more likely to be infected with HIV than those whose residence had been stable for more than ten years. The lowest infection rates were among those who had been living for the longest time in the same place. Also, individuals who migrated reported more sexual partners than their non-migrant counterparts.

TABLE 19.1 Summary of the major African studies on migration and HIV/AIDS

In rural Senegal, a study of seasonal migration and HIV found that HIV was transmitted first to adult men through sexual contacts with infected women they met during their seasonal migration and then to their wives or regular partners once they are back home. Since this study concentrates on seasonal migration – where men spend on average half a year or more away from their rural homes – the implications for South Africa may be important as the migration patterns in the two countries appear to be similar.

In a study of male factory workers in Zimbabwe, HIV-positive men were more likely to live apart from their wives and to have multiple sexual partners than HIV-negative men. This is supported by a study in Ghana where Anarfi has argued that migration acts to increase the extent of sexual networking.

In South Africa high rates of STIs have been found in gold miners although there have been no studies on the prevalence of HIV or other STIs among returning migrants. Nevertheless, it has been argued – with little empirical evidence – that the rate of HIV infection among migrants is 50% higher than among their non-migrant counterparts. In a study of HIV seroprevalence in a rural KwaZulu-Natal community, people who had recently changed their place of residence were three times as likely to be HIV infected as those who had not.

While the link between migrant labour and high-risk sexual behaviour has not been explored in detail in South Africa, it is clear that migrants' frequent and lengthy absences from home are likely to disrupt their familial and stable sexual relationships. It has also been argued that the migrant labour system created a market for commercial sex in mining towns and recent work from the Carletonville gold mines has confirmed this. This argument is not new. As early as 1949 it was noted that the widespread prevalence of gonorrhoea and syphilis in both urban and rural areas of South Africa was due to the migrant labour system and that prostitution resulted from the separation of husbands from their wives and families.

Another South African study has provided insight into the link between migration and HIV. The study found HIV prevalence among migrant men to be 25.9% compared with 12.7% among non-migrant men, so that migrant men were 2.4 times more likely to be HIV infected than non-migrant men (FIGURE 19.5). In multivariate analysis,

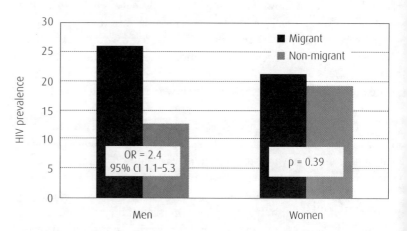

FIGURE 19.5 HIV prevalence among migrant and non-migrant men, and women whose partners were migrant or not
Source: Lurie M, Williams B, Zuma K, Mkaya-Mwamburi D, Garnett GP, Sturm AW, Sweat MD, Gittelsohn J, Abdool Karim SS. The impact of migration on HIV-1 transmission: A study of migrant and non-migrant men, and their partners. Sexually Transmitted Diseases 2003; 40: 149–156

the main risk factors for HIV infection among men were being a migrant, ever having used a condom and having lived in four or more places during the course of a lifetime. The study also found very high rates of HIV among women. Overall 17.5% of women were HIV infected; however, women whose partners were migrants were as likely to be HIV infected as women whose partners were not migrants.

The study further examined patterns of HIV concordance and discordance among migrant and non-migrant couples. These patterns shed light on the directionality of spread of the epidemic. The study found that migrant couples were more likely than non-migrant couples to have one or both partners infected (35% versus 19%) and to be HIV discordant (27% versus 15%).

It has long been assumed that in the context of migration, HIV transmission is unidirectional from returning migrant men – who themselves became infected while away – to their rural partners when they return home. But if this were the case, it would be the man who was the infected partner in all migrant HIV-discordant couples. However, in this study the woman was the infected partner in 29% of discordant couples; this did not differ by migration status. Clearly a woman who is HIV infected – and whose primary partner is not HIV infected – could not have been infected by her partner. The study raises questions about the sexual networks of rural women and challenges the common assumption of directionality of HIV transmission in the context of large-scale population mobility. This finding highlights the importance of understanding the rural, as well as the urban, dynamics of the epidemic and implies that successful prevention efforts should concentrate not only on the urban 'receiving' areas but on the rural 'sending' areas as well.

These findings are particularly interesting given the maturity of the South African epidemic. It is likely that early in the epidemic the role of migration was critical in dissemination of the virus from urban to rural areas and relatively more important than in the later stages of the epidemic. Isolating a single causal factor – when background prevalence is already high – is likely to be difficult. The fact that, even against the background of extremely high HIV prevalence, migration is an independent risk factor for men highlights the importance of migration as one explanation for the size and rapidity of spread of the southern African AIDS epidemic.

Research gaps

While much is known about the role of migration in the spread of HIV in southern Africa, important gaps remain. Southern Africa's circular migration patterns put people at risk for HIV and other STIs at both ends of the migration spectrum. However, migration studies have concentrated largely on the *determinants* of migration and most studies have been concerned with migration to the gold mines, so that little work has been done to document the effects of circular migration on South Africa's rural areas. While there is some understanding of the relationship between migration and susceptibility to HIV, little is known about how migration affects the risk of HIV and STIs in partners of migrants. Some of the areas in which further research is needed are discussed below.

Population-based studies

There have been very few population-based studies of HIV and STI prevalence and incidence in sub-Saharan Africa. The studies carried out in Rakai, Uganda and Mwanza, Tanzania are exceptions, as is a series of studies conducted on the Carletonville gold mines and their surrounding communities, but apart from these there have been almost no community-based studies. Prevalence estimates of HIV in southern Africa, therefore, tend to rely heavily on antenatal clinic data, which may or may not give a reasonable estimate of overall prevalence among women. Furthermore, there are surprisingly few studies that measure the age-specific HIV prevalence among men.

Migration and AIDS

The work that has been done generally on migration, and on migration and AIDS more specifically, has focused almost exclusively on migrants at their place of work. This is reflected in the abundant literature, both contemporary and historic, on migration to the gold mines and to a lesser extent on migration to other urban destinations. Reasons for this include the cost and logistical difficulties in identifying and tracing migrants. A lesser focus of migration research in southern Africa has been on rural sending areas. The few studies that have researched rural issues have provided important insight from the perspective of a migration sending area, some even following communities over time. However, studies on HIV and migration in rural areas are few and far between.

Understanding both sides of the migration spectrum

While understanding the context of migration both from the perspective of sending and receiving areas is clearly important, it is equally important to study both sides of the migration spectrum at the same time; no studies were found that looked concurrently at migrants at work and their partners at home. This weakness is particularly important in the study of HIV and STIs, where understanding both sides of the spectrum is particularly important if successful intervention programmes are to be implemented. The circular migration patterns in South Africa put people at risk for HIV and other STIs at both ends of the migratory movement and it is important to know how these combine to determine the direction and the extent of the flow of infection.

Interventions

Given the speed with which HIV has spread both in space and in time in South Africa, interventions aimed at migrants and their partners are needed as a matter of urgency. Sadly, though, interventions on a regional or national scale have been almost non-existent; also absent has been rigorous evaluation of the few programmes that do exist. Instead, the few interventions that are active tend to be isolated and sometimes unsustainable, aimed mainly at migrants at their work places and occasionally at migrants at transition points like border crossings.

Effective interventions to limit the spread of HIV and STIs among migrants and their partners are urgently needed. Peer education and condom distribution programmes among people in this high-risk group would be a good start and should be combined with efforts to improve access to services and to upgrade the quality of the services, for the treatment and management of STIs. Clearly, any effective intervention must cover people both in the labour sending and receiving areas if the chain of transmission is to be broken.

Mining communities have been the focus of interventions aimed at migrants, in part because industry has finally begun to realise the impact that HIV will have on their workforce. These interventions have tended to include improving STI services, training peer educators, promoting condom use, providing voluntary counselling and testing, and education. While these interventions appear to be fairly widespread in the mining community, the degree to which they have been adopted among other industries is unclear. Furthermore, well-designed evaluations aimed at measuring the impact of such workplace programmes have been few and far between. Recently mining companies have announced, then rescinded, then re-announced that they will start to provide antiretroviral therapy to miners infected with HIV, although the scope and scale of antiretroviral provision has not yet been determined.

An intervention study in one mining community (Welkom) was able to substantially reduce the prevalence of STIs among gold mine workers through an intervention aimed solely at commercial sex workers, who received monthly presumptive STI treatment with azithromycin. Although the study did not evaluate the impact of presumptive treatment on HIV prevalence or incidence, it highlights the critical role of sex workers operating near mining communities. Based on these results, the intervention has been implemented in several other mining communities.

In addition, similar intervention studies in the Carletonville community should yield valuable lessons for the control of HIV/STI in an urban setting with a very large number of migrant mine workers and high rates of in-migration.

In addition to the Carletonville and Welkom interventions, there have been some modest efforts made to intersect migrants, particularly at border posts, where free condoms and occasionally education are provided. But these interventions are patchy at best, and no thorough evaluations have been published.

Mining companies could move more quickly towards providing more family-friendly housing. Mathematical models have shown that eliminating single-sex hostels on the mines could have a substantial impact on HIV transmission and would be cost-effective. While some companies have begun to move away from single-sex hostels in favour of family-friendly accommodation, this movement has been frustratingly slow and today more than 90% of mine workers still live in single-sex hotels.

These kinds of structural interventions – which alter the environment and conditions that foster the spread of HIV/STI are critically needed. While most interventions have been aimed at altering individual behaviour, also needed are interventions that address the larger contextual factors that put individuals at risk. Structural interventions would include changing single-sex housing to more family-friendly environments, investing in rural development and creating jobs in rural areas to minimise the need to migrate in the first place. These sorts of structural interventions, while long-term and complex, are more likely to have a much greater overall impact on HIV transmission than interventions aimed at improving individual behaviour. And given that the migrant labour system was so central to the establishment and maintenance of apartheid, one would hope that this issue would be addressed in the post-apartheid democratic South Africa.

Acknowledgements

The author would like to thank all members of the Migration Project Team, as well as Brian Williams, Geoff Garnett, Ari Johnson and Chitra Akileswaran for their input into this chapter.

Bibliography

ABDOOL KARIM Q, ABDOOL KARIM SS, SINGH B, SHORT R, NGXONGO S. 'Seroprevalence of HIV Infection in Rural South Africa'. *AIDS* 1992; 6: 1535–1539.

ANARFI J. 'Sexuality, Migration and AIDS in Ghana – A Socio-Behavioural Study'. *Health Transition Review* 1993; 3: 45–67.

BASSETT M, EMMANUEL J, KATZENSTEIN J ET AL. *'HIV Infection in Urban Males in Zimbabwe'*. VI International Conference on AIDS, San Francisco (Abstract ThC581) 1990.

CAMPBELL C. 'Selling sex in the time of AIDS: The psycho-social context of condom use by sex workers on a Southern African mine'. *Social Science and Medicine* 2000; 50: 479–494.

COFFEE M, GARNETT G, LURIE M. 'Modelling the impact of circular migration on the rate of spread and the eventual scale of the HIV epidemic in South Africa'. Poster presented at the XIII International AIDS Conference, Durban South Africa. 2000.

CRUSH J. 'Mine migrancy in the contemporary era'. In *Crossing Boundaries: Mine Migrancy in a Democratic South Africa* (Eds.) J. Crush and W. James. Cape Town: IDASA/IDRC. 1995.

DAVIES RH. 1979. *'Capital, State and White Labour in South Africa 1900–1960'*. New Jersey: Humanities Press.

DE BEER C. 1984. *'The South African Disease: Apartheid Health and Health Services'*. Trenton, New Jersey: Africa World Press.

DECOSAS J, ADRIEN A. 'Migration and HIV'. *AIDS* 1997; 11(Suppl. A): S77–S84.

DECOSAS J, KANE F, ANARFI J ET AL. 1995. 'Migration and AIDS'. *Lancet* 1995; 346: 826–828.

EVIAN C. 'AIDS and Social Security'. *AIDS Scan* 1995; 7: 8–11.

GEBREKRISTOS H, LURIE M. *'The impact of family housing on the HIV/AIDS epidemic among mine migrants in South Africa'*. Poster presented at the XIV International AIDS Conference, Barcelona Spain. 2002.

HUNT C. 'Migrant Labor and Sexually Transmitted Disease: AIDS In Africa'. *'Journal of Health and Social Behavior'* 1989; 30: 353–373.

IJSSELMUIDEN C, PADAYACHEE W, MASHABALA W. 'Knowledge, beliefs and practices among black goldminers relating to the transmission of human immunodeficiency virus and other sexually transmitted diseases'. *South African Medical Journal* 1990; 78: 520–523.

JOCHELSON K, MOTHIBELI M, LEGER J. 'Human Immunodeficiency Virus and Migrant Labor in South Africa'. *International Journal of Health Services* 1991; 21: 157–173.

KARK S. 'The Social Pathology of Syphilis in Africans'. *South African Medical Journal* 1949; 23: 77–84.

LURIE M. *'Preserving White Privilege: Industrial Unrest on the Witwatersrand, 1913'*. Unpublished Masters Thesis, University of Florida. 1992.

LURIE M, HARRISON A, WILKINSON D, ABDOOL KARIM SS. 'Circular migration and sexual networking in rural KwaZulu/Natal: Implications for the spread of HIV and other sexually transmitted diseases'. *Health Transition Review* 1997; 7(Suppl. 3): 15–24.

LURIE M, WILLIAMS B, ZUMA K, MKAYA-MWAMBURI D, GARNETT GP, SWEAT MD, GITTELSOHN J, ABDOOL KARIM SS. 'Who infects whom? HIV concordance and discordance among migrant and non-migrant couples in South Africa'. *AIDS* 2003; 17: 2245–2252.

LURIE M, WILLIAMS B, ZUMA K, MKAYA-MWAMBURI D, GARNETT GP, STURM AW, SWEAT MD, GITTELSOHN J, ABDOOL KARIM SS. 'The impact of migration on HIV-1 transmission: A study of migrant and non-migrant men, and their partners'. *Sexually Transmitted Diseases* 2003; 40: 149–156.

LURIE P, HINTZEN P, LOWE R. 'Socioeconomic Obstacles to HIV Prevention and Treatment in Developing Countries'. *AIDS* 1995; 9: 539–546.

Mabey D, Mayaud P. 'Sexually transmitted diseases in mobile populations'. *Genitourinary Medicine* 1997; 73: 18–22.

May J. 1990. 'The Migrant Labour System: Changing Dynamics in Rural Survival'. In *The Political Economy of South Africa.* Cape Town: Oxford University Press.

Murray C. 1981. *'Families Divided: The Impact of Migrant Labour in Lesotho'.* Cambridge: Cambridge University Press.

Natrass J. *'The Migrant Labour System and South Africa's Economic Development, 1936–1970'.* 1976. Unpublished Ph.D Thesis, University of Natal.

Nunn A, Wagner H, Kamali A, et al. 'Migration and HIV-1 Seroprevalence in a Rural Ugandan Population'. *AIDS* 1995; 9: 503–506.

Packard R. 1989. *'White Plague, Black Labor: Tuberculosis and the Political Economy of Health and Disease in South Africa'.* Berkeley: University of California Press.

Pison G, Le Guenno B, Lagarde E, et.al. 'Seasonal Migration: A Risk Factor for HIV in Rural Senegal'. *Journal of Acquired Immune Deficiency Syndrome* 1993; 6: 196–200.

Platzky L and Walker C. 1985. *'The Surplus People: Forced Removals in South Africa.'* Johannesburg. Ravan Press.

Quinn T. 'Population Migration and the Spread of Types 1 and 2 Human Immunodeficiency Virus'. *Proceedings of the National Academy of Sciences.* 1994; 91: 2407–2414.

Steen R, Vuylsteke B, DeCoito T, Ralepeli S, Fehler G, Conley J, Bruckers L, Dallabetta G, Ballard R. 'Evidence of declining STD prevalence in a South African mining community following a core-group intervention'. *Sexually Transmitted Diseases* 2000; 1: 1–8.

Wilson F. 1972. *'Labour in the South African Gold Mines 1911–1969'.* Cambridge: The University Press.

Williams BG, Gouws E, Lurie M, Crush J. 2002. *'Spaces of Vulnerability: Migration and HIV/AIDS in South Africa'.* Cape Town: IDASA.

Williams M. 'Hostel leaders vow to fight violence in run-up to elections'. *The Natal Mercury* 1998; Sept 25: 1.

Zwi A and Bachmayer D. 'HIV and AIDS in South Africa: What is an Appropriate Public Health Response?' *Health Policy and Planning* 1990; 5: 316–326.

Zuma K, Gouws E, Williams BG, Lurie M. 'Risk factors for HIV infection among women in Carletonville, South Africa: migration, demography and sexually transmitted diseases'. *International Journal of STD and AIDS* 2003; 14: 814–817.

CHAPTER 20

Young men

Gethwana Makahye

GENDER IS A SOCIETAL CONSTRUCT that encompasses widely
shared expectations, norms, customs, beliefs and practices within a
particular society. Gender is about roles and responsibilities as determined by different societies. Society expects men and women to
behave in a particular manner based on the prevalent beliefs, practices
and norms of that society. These expectations are learnt in families,
workplace, schools and other institutions. They define appropriate but
different behaviour for both men and women. Men are expected to be
more powerful than women in all respects and are expected to be
providers by bringing food, money and other commodities for their
families. Gender inequality has contributed to the spread of HIV in
many ways. As discussed more fully in CHAPTER 16 it is women who are
disproportionately affected by HIV/AIDS and bear the burden of responsibility for HIV/AIDS by persuading their partners to practise safe sex, to
care for HIV-positive and terminally ill family members and for orphans.
As a consequence, much of the work on HIV/AIDS prevention has been
directed at women. Ironically, the very behavioural strategies that are
likely to be most effective for reducing the spread of HIV, ie condom
use and faithfulness to one partner, are the strategies that are the least
in the control of women.

While there has been a growing realisation of the importance of
gender at the centre of the HIV pandemic, gender issues have often
been interpreted as women's issues and many HIV interventions have
placed an even greater burden of responsibility on women, with a
tendency to overlook the constructive engagement of men. There is a
general unwillingness on the part of men to regard HIV/AIDS as a
problem that concerns them and there is a general paucity of
HIV/AIDS research and intervention programmes for men. Numerous
recent documents from organisations such as UNAIDS and the

Voluntary Services Overseas Organisation (VSO) have highlighted the importance of the constructive engagement of men in HIV prevention and intervention programmes. While men hold a position of power in social interactions, training them to use their power creatively will allow men to protect themselves and thus their female partners. If there is to be a major change in the current HIV/AID pandemic, it is primarily the behaviour of men that must undergo dramatic change.

Introduction

This chapter discusses the two main intervention programmes that have been implemented in South Africa by the Targeted AIDS Intervention (TAI). TAI targets young men and boys as people at risk of HIV in an attempt to involve them in protecting themselves and their loved ones from sexually transmitted infections (STIs) and HIV/AIDS.

The Targeted AIDS Intervention

The Targeted AIDS Intervention is a non-governmental organisation that initially began by focusing on women, educating them on HIV/AIDS and its modes of transmission. It soon became evident that when women tried to implement the lessons they had learned, they were met with resistance and often abuse, negating their attempts to make any significant change in their HIV risk. Recognising that the beliefs and practices around masculinity play a major role in generating and maintaining HIV risk, the organisation shifted its focus to men. In South Africa the TAI is one of the best examples of a non-governmental organisation-based response to involving men in prevention programmes. Through its peer education activities developed in local soccer leagues and in schools across KwaZulu-Natal, creative possibilities for gender-based HIV interventions have been implemented.

Much of the TAI's intervention with boys has involved examining how they see men and masculinity. Interestingly, when asked what the desired characteristics of a man are, the boys often initially give negative responses. Their experiences of older men, including their fathers, have shown them what they do not like in men and therefore what they would like to avoid in themselves. Many of the young men included in these projects are born to unmarried women and have no male role model at home or no contact with their fathers.

There is an apparent ignorance of HIV among men. Further, men do not see it as their responsibility to protect themselves or their children from HIV. Infected men often hold their wives responsible for HIV infection in their children. Generally, boys see men as legitimately in control of sexual relations. One of the marks of a successful man is sexual prowess and performance and the ability to have and satisfy multiple girlfriends. Boys appear to think that multiple partners are sanctioned for men but not for women. Furthermore, women are seen as vectors of disease.

Intervention projects

In establishing a network of men, the TAI targeted the amateur football league in KwaZulu-Natal. The 'Shosholoza' Project began in 1998 as an HIV/AIDS education campaign operating through a network of soccer players, attempting to use the sport's language, beliefs and behaviour as a creative medium for facilitating change in the risk behaviours leading to HIV.

Through this project it became apparent that men between the ages of 16 and 24 had been sexually active for some time, with most boys reporting their sexual debut between 14 and 15 years. These data are consistent with other studies on high school students in KwaZulu-Natal, which showed that the average age of sexual debut for girls was 15 and that 76% of girls and 90% of boys were sexually active. Of those who were sexually active, 95% had never used condoms; all those who were sexually active had more than one sexual partner and only 3% said that a woman has a right to say 'no' to sex.

This led TAI to establish another project: 'Inkunzi Isematholeni'. This focused on HIV/AIDS education among younger boys still at school. Since youth is the generation highly at risk, schools offer a good opportunity to address both gender inequality and HIV/AIDS. Those at school are still negotiating their gender identities and exploring their sexuality. These institutions can be used to campaign for the promotion of gender equity. The aim of the 'Inkunzi Isematholeni' project is to influence younger boys through education and role modelling before they become sexually active and influenced by older boys with higher levels of HIV risk behaviour.

Since this is a project for soccer players, the province of KwaZulu-Natal was demarcated according to the South African Football Association (SAFA) regions (FIGURE 20.1) SAFA KZN Midlands, SAFA Eastern KZN, SAFA Northern KZN for the intervention. Twenty schools from these three regions were targeted and soccer players between 11 and 18 years were included in the project.

Both interventions use a peer-educator model where groups of young boys are recruited and offered training in HIV/AIDS and are then encouraged to share their information and skills with their peers. This is encouraged through focus group discussions, workshops and debates, drama, role plays, simulations and message development.

The focus groups discuss risky behaviours, including early sexual debut, unprotected penetrative sex including anal sex, multiple sexual relations, sex in the presence of STIs and under the influence of drugs and alcohol, casual sex and sex with multiple partners. Condoms are distributed through peer educators and the South African Football Association offices.

These projects have received great support from local communities and football associations for their focus on men's sexual behaviour and attitudes. Other football clubs and schools in KwaZulu-Natal have expressed interest in becoming involved. Representatives from all regions were involved in decision making, ensuring that the project was owned and supported by the clubs and so was sustainable.

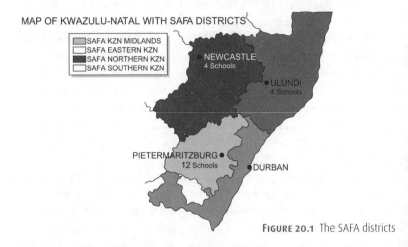

FIGURE 20.1 The SAFA districts

Men as victims of the gendered system

The findings of the TAI reveal that boys and men are commonly victims of the gendered system, despite the many advantages that society offers them. Sociocultural norms prevent men from participating in reproductive responsibilities, which include family planning; antenatal services and child health services. An important assumption about masculinity that in fact victimises men is the idea that 'men know everything', preventing them from seeking advice, or using appropriate sources of information. One example is the common assumption that the onset of wet dreams indicates that boys should become sexually active, creating considerable, but unquestioned, pressure on adolescent boys to actually become sexually active.

Young men are under pressure to conform to rigid gender expectations and often lie about their sexual experience to their peers. This meant that there was often a discrepancy between what the boys said in the company of their peers and when they were interviewed alone. In this study, one of the most fascinating findings is the way in which boys are trapped in a cycle of deception, which arises from the pressure on them by their peers to conform to gender expectations, influencing young men to become sexually active. Some young men explained how their sexuality is questioned if they have never been seen with girls. Others explained that they lie and say they are having sex with girls who are not in the same school for fear that the questioner may want to check with the girl concerned. However, as the young men attended more counselling sessions in the programme they gained confidence and became more comfortable about not being sexually active.

Competition and change in gender construction

The work by the TAI has revealed a growing awareness among boys of the unacceptability of certain patterns of behaviour, such as the abuse of women and children or the phenomenon of 'sugar daddies' and older men attracting younger girls with money and gifts.

Attitudes to girl's behaviour is revealing. 'Isigcebe' or girls' wearing of short skirts is an interesting example. Some of the boys see this as an invitation to abuse and rape; others not. Social group discussions show the gradual emergence of 'caring' as an acceptable and appropriate performance of masculinity. However, caring is still shown in very instrumental and paternalistic ways, eg fathers providing money for children's education.

In some groups, there is evidence that boys are choosing to behave differently for reasons related to HIV risk. The way some boys view the women in their lives is also changing and many have expressed a desire to be more helpful at home to show their gratitude. However, many of the traditional masculine behaviours of boys are expected by girls, reinforcing them. Failure to conform to these particular patterns of masculine behaviour leaves these boys unsuccessful in their relationships with girls, presenting a particular challenge to the intervention programmes. Women and girls make an important contribution to the maintenance of the gendered system, often because of their economic vulnerability and need. One of the major challenges is the development of strategies that can foster gender change without undermining a sense of masculine security and identity.

Conclusion

Young men represent an important focal group who have an impact on the HIV/AIDS pandemic. Work by the TAI demonstrates that it is possible to effectively and creatively intervene among young men, regarding both HIV risk and gender. The exploratory work on masculinity initiated by the TAI has produced both valuable data on local constructions of masculinity and offered a forum for young men and boys to begin examining beliefs and attitudes about what masculinity is. Interventions that target young boys can facilitate the development of a culture of self-respect and respect for others. These interventions are a good opportunity to interact with the boys in an attempt to bring about changes in their lives with the aim of reducing their vulnerability to STIs, unwanted pregnancies and HIV/AIDS. They also teach young boys to be responsible partners and fathers of the future. Once men get enough information and skills to change their patriarchal attitude towards sex and women, they can play a meaningful role in the mitigation of HIV/AIDS.

Bibliography

ABDOOL KARIM Q, ABDOOL KARIM SS. 'South Africa: Host to new and emerging epidemics'. *Sexually Transmitted Infections* 1999; 75: 139–147.

ABDOOL KARIM Q AND ABDOOL KARIM SS. 'The evolving HIV epidemic in South Africa'. *International Journal of Epidemiology*. 2002. 31: 37–40.

AKANDE A. 'Risky Business: South African youths and HIV/AIDS Prevention'. *Educational Studies*. 2001; 27: 237–256.

CATANIA J, KEGELES SM, COATES T. 'Towards an understanding of risk behaviour: An AIDS Risk Reduction Model (ARRM)' *Health Education Quarterly* 1990; 17: 53–72.

DEPARTMENT OF HEALTH SOUTH AFRICA. 2002. *Overview of Youth Programmes (Lifeskills Programme)*.Government printer. Pretoria.

KELLY JA. 'Community-level interventions are needed to prevent new infections'. *American Journal of Public Health* 1999; 89: 299–301.

LINDEGGER G, DURRHEIM K. 2001. 'Men and AIDS'. In: Stones CR (ed). *Socio-Political and psychological perspectives on South Africa*. New York. Nova Publishers.

MADLALA LS. 'Infect one, infect all: Zulu youth response to the AIDS epidemic in South Africa'. *Medical Anthropology* 1997; 17: 363–380.

MAKHAYE G. 'Shosholoza's goal: Educate men in soccer'. *Agenda* 1998; 39: 93–96.

MORRELL R. 2001. *'Changing men in South Africa'*. Pietermaritzburg and London: University of Natal Press and Zed Books Ltd.

MOORE SM, ROSENTHAL D. 'The adolescents' perception of friends and parents' attitudes to sex and sexual risk taking'. *Journal of Community and Applied Social Psychology* 1991; 1: 189–200.

TALLIS V. 'Gendering the response to HIV/AIDS: Challenging gender inequality'. *Agenda* 2001; 44: 58–66

WEISS E, WHELAN D. 'Gender, Sexuality and HIV: Making a difference in the lives of young women in developing countries'. *Sexual Relationship Therapy* 2001; 15: 233–245.

SECTION 5
The impact of AIDS

CHAPTER 21

Shattering the silence – an auto-biographic, reflective narrative on living with HIV/AIDS

Lilian Benita Mboyi

I AM A 37-YEAR-OLD black woman, a mother of two boys, a lover, a partner, and a researcher living with HIV/AIDS trying to uncover the circumstances that brought me here. Understanding how and why I got here will, I hope, give me, and more importantly others, a clearer understanding of this epidemic and the painful silences that have come with it. This is my way of shattering the silences both within me, and externally in the world that I work and live in.

My story

I am privileged to have been born into a black middle class family, which meant that I had access to good education early in life. It is this privilege that spared me the many childhood diseases of poverty that afflict many African children of my age group, and somewhat guaranteed a future free of economic struggle. With this in mind I have wondered if the best outcome of my upbringing was to delay the onset of an HIV infection by a few years? These thoughts are based on the close encounters I have had with AIDS; with Bill, for example, who with his girlfriend and child were lost to AIDS in 1996–1997. With the fact that in Zimbabwe, where I was born and raised, one in four people between the ages of 15 and 49 are HIV positive and more than 3000 people die every week due to AIDS-related causes.

Loving Mr Solomon

My divorce in 1997 at the age of thirty opened a new chapter in my life, establishing new relationships with men. I first met Mr. Mzamo Solomon (I have given my lover's name in full because I had permission to do so given by him before he died). Mr Solomon was murdered on the 20th May 2002. However I will refer to him as Mr S because that was the pet name I used with him on the 5th September 1998 in a church at Bloubergstrand, Cape Town, the day of his cousin's wedding. I was in the process of putting the shame and dramatic events of my divorce behind me and I was tired of dating married men. I knew that he would feature in my life, with his shy smile, strong body and air of sophistication. My best friend Nandipha's younger brother, he was years younger than me. However, that was not reason enough to stop me from pursuing what I wanted. After three weeks of courting him into my world, dancing and sightseeing, I invited him to my 32nd birthday party on the 28th of September and by the end of that evening our fate was sealed. Having fallen deeply in love with each other we both knew what we wanted. The following day we made love, knowing the rules of engagement; I arrived armed with a variety of condoms for our pleasure. This was the most beautiful experience I had had in a long time, and was the beginning of a relationship that would change the course of my life forever.

October was a month of passion, I was happy and blossoming; we were inseparable, a beautiful couple drawing attention wherever we went. On the 6th November 1998 my flight of fancy was brought to a rude and abrupt halt just five weeks into our relationship when he indicated he wanted to end the relationship. I was shattered, robbed of a wonderful chance at happiness and feeling I could not take such blatant rejection. Refusing to accept the truth and trying to convince him to see reason I pleaded with him to allow me to visit him in the evening so that we could finish our discussion. With the wisdom of hindsight, I should have just swallowed my pride and let it go.

Demons visit in the night

The night of the 6th November 1998 stands alone as the most significant night of my life, the night the demons took over and madness reigned. Driving back to Mr S, charged with rejection, I had no real plan, other than finding a way to keep my new found love. At the back of my mind, perhaps, I was hoping that new tricks in bed would make him want to hang around longer and not put me through this shame of rejection. Against all reason, and in an act of passion, I abandoned all the rules of sexual engagement that had almost become my 'ten commandments' of sexual encounters; two crucial words were uttered at the beginning of our Russian roulette game, 'condoms' and 'AIDS', but neither made any difference. Now, with hindsight, I can say that there is a worst kind of rejection and stigmatisation that makes child's play of being a divorcee. If only I had contended with the reality of the stigma and discrimination that would come with an HIV-positive status. Many tears have been wept and many sleepless nights have been spent because of that reckless behaviour. Perhaps that was the night that I was actually infected with the virus, I don't know. What it did do was open an outlet for reckless loving punctuated by sporadic safe sex. I will always consider the 6th of November as the day I was infected with HIV.

A downward spiral begins

Mid-December 1998 I had an unexplained but desperate urge to send my two children home to my mother in Zimbabwe for the school holidays. I did not have any leave due to me, but I managed to fly them to Bulawayo via Harare so that I could be back at work on the Monday. Nandipha fetched me on my return from the airport on the Sunday night and took me to my house around 22h00. I got into the house and put down my bags and lay on the couch to rest in front of the television. That couch was to cushion my painful body for the next five weeks. The following morning my body was screaming in pain, I could hardly lift my arms, let alone stand up from the couch. I was battling to breath and I had to crawl on all fours to get myself to the toilet which was about ten metres away. I was scared, alone and very confused. My condition deteriorated as the day progressed, and got worse as the days came and went. Mr S volunteered to come and look after me during this time. I could hardly keep my food down and I would throw up at the most unexpected of times. Mr S cleaned up after me and carried me around in his arms if I needed to go to the toilet or to go into the tub for a bath. I have a vivid memory of him holding a bucket and a rag wiping off vomit from the corridor wall that I had splashed when I had tried to walk unaided to the toilet. That image shall remain with me for the rest of my life because it was so compassionate and brings to light the devastation caused by AIDS. Mr S' role shifted from that of a caring lover to a caregiver. Yet at the time neither of us was aware of the seriousness of what we were dealing with. All I felt was that I was dying and I watched myself become a shadow of the person that I had been. The vibrancy was gone and so was the energy. When I eventually felt strong enough to leave the house and seek medical attention and venture back to work it was with calculated slow steps and an effort that took all the inner strength that I could master. I would experience blackouts while I was behind the steering wheel to and from work, and trying to type a document would leave me so exhausted my wrists would ache and I would be left short of breath.

My visits to the doctor or rather the referrals to consult with specialists did not yield much. Blood tests carried out in the first week in January showed that I was very anaemic and very low on iron, but the HIV test was negative. The doctor suspected that I had probably picked some viral infection in Zimbabwe and referred me to a specialist to do further checks. I was put on two weeks bed rest and waited for my appointment with the senior specialist at the City Park Clinic in Cape Town. The iron deficiency explained the blackouts that I had been experiencing and the bed rest took care of that.

Unfortunately life was not waiting for me. Mr S had to go back to his sister's place where he was helping her run the house. My responsibilities beckoned. Schools opened and I requested that my mother send my older son Ndumiso back to Cape Town so that he could go to school and I asked her to look after Njabulo in the meantime, while I recovered. Ndumiso is my first born son now aged 17; it took a disclosure of my status on a television programme for me to finally tell him just before his 16th birthday in September 2003. Njabulo is my second son aged nine, I only disclosed my HIV-positive status to him in March 2004 and I disclosed to him because I felt that the net was closing in on my silence and I also needed him to understand my bouts of fatigue and get his support. The disclosure was largely more a need to protect him from being teased by school mates as a result of my public disclosure. It was not a planned disclosure and it took fours years to do. Ndumiso's return highlighted just how sick I was. I could not be a mother to him in the way that he was used to. It literally took me three quarters of an hour to wash his white school shirt. I would start with the collar and rub it with soap while I leaned against the bath tub; I would then have to gasp for breath and rest my wrists before proceeding. Halfway through the task, I would lie down on the bathroom floor to rest for about ten minutes before proceeding to complete washing the shirt. Food preparation was done with me lying on the couch and through the hatch that separated the kitchen from the lounge I would instruct Ndumiso on what to do. At best it was heart-breaking; at its worst it brought me very close to the painful realities of millions of mothers in sub-Saharan Africa who succumb to AIDS. I was scared and did not understand what was happening to me.

Everything that could have gone wrong in my body did go wrong. I started snoring in my sleep because I had developed sinusitis. My body ached in places I did not even remember I had. For the first time I came face to face with the thick yoghurt-like fungus called candida in my genitals. I started nose-bleeding which is something I had last experienced in my childhood. I was so sick I felt like a wet dog. I lived from moment to moment, I just was not sure if I could live through to see the next day. The thought of dying and leaving my children so young also scared the hell out of me.

The specialist at the City Park Clinic gave me a thorough consultation and took his time asking questions to try and understand how I had arrived at this almost vegetable state. We discussed HIV and he wanted to know if I practised safe sex with my boyfriend. He said seeing that I was HIV negative, but not strictly adhering to safe sex practices, I could be placing myself at a high risk for AIDS especially considering that my boyfriend was from Zimbabwe. Unbeknownst to both of us he was trying to lock the stable door and the horse had already bolted. The 6th of November 1998 had come and gone and I was already reaping the harvest of that reckless night of passion. The verdict of my visit to the specialist was that my problems were related to the central nervous system. He explained that he would put me on a course of fluoxetine which is an antidepressant that works by inhibiting the neuronal uptake of serotonin in the central nervous system. He recommended that I have a further three weeks bed rest until the medication started working in my system. He advised that I take the antidepressants for at least six months.

It was with a sense of relief that I walked away from his rooms R275 poorer, but freed from the fear of some terrible viral infection possibly picked up from Zimbabwe. I was just relieved to know that I was not dying of some mysterious disease and that if all went well I would be back on my feet in just a few weeks time. I started on my medication straight away. As the weeks went by, strength slowly flowed back into my limbs and the black-outs receded into memory. It was quite convenient to forget the pain and the hardship that came with it and that being sick and feeling close to death had been a terrible shock that was best left in the past. Towards the end of my bed rest, I attended an alternative healing course that I had registered for some time back. It was the Indian head massage course run by Dr Iqbal Badat. By the end of the course I felt much stronger and on the road to wellness. This course was not only to benefit me in my healing process, but also to put food on the table when I lost my job.

In April Mr S moved in with me because his sister was relocating to the United Kingdom. We became the cosy happy couple, and he focused his full attention on me. Our relationship was quite developed then and somehow we had totally stopped using condoms. In July I took a holiday to Zimbabwe and when I returned from my holiday mid-July, the atmosphere had not only changed on the home front, but was also different at work. I could not place my finger on it, but something was wrong. My manager called me into her office one afternoon and told me that there was to be a re-structuring in our division and my job was under review; I was being side-lined. On reflection I realise that I was paying for my sickness earlier in the year. I was too shocked to fight; losing my job was the last thing I expected; I was broken.

It was only many months later as I wallowed in depression that I pinned the pieces of the puzzle together. I suspect that I was fired from my job for a suspected HIV sero-conversion. Initially my manager had been quite concerned when I became ill at the beginning of the year; she had arranged for me to see the medical staff at the clinic in case I needed support to cope with my illness. Innocently I had kept her informed about my illness and that my HIV test had been negative, although I was not obliged to show her my test results. I suspect that since the organisation in question did not have an AIDS policy at the time, it was easier to terminate my employment contract with them, rather than be burdened with expensive claims in the case of me getting fullblown AIDS and dying. To date I still wrestle with the pain and humiliation of my job loss because it was immediately followed by a positive HIV diagnosis.

Death in spring

'An unannounced pregnancy shattered the peace with the ring of the phone on a beautiful September day. The gestation had been too long – November, 6 1998 to September 3 1999. The baby chose to announce its presence way past its due date.' Lilian Mboyi, Date unknown.

One Friday evening as I discussed my future plans with Mr S the phone rang to intervene in my preparations for the life that lay ahead. Having decided to have a medical check up a few weeks back to take advantage of my medical aid, I had also done a routine HIV test in the process. HIV, I felt, was the least of my worries because I had had a negative result earlier in the year. The test was done because someone was paying for it and because I had been in the habit of having one regularly. No comebacks were expected and hence very little pre-test counselling took place.

The unexpected call from the doctor's rooms was, therefore, a total shock to my system. It really felt like someone had told me that I had been mysteriously pregnant and was just about to deliver. The doctor indicated that I should come and see her on Monday because she would need to re-do the HIV test; this without saying that the result had been positive. I felt scared and angry. Deep inside I felt the significance of what she was saying. Within the space of a few hours my thoughts had done so many somersaults, although I wanted to run into the street and scream and pull my hair out; I did not. I wanted to ask Mr S why he had done this to me. In the end I could not and I did not; I simply informed him that my HIV test was positive and that since we had occasionally indulged in unprotected sex, he should also go and be tested. When my little boy, not even five years old yet, walked into the room I looked at him with sadness as potentially he would be an orphan by the age of ten. My heart was broken and I hated myself for bringing this on my children. I spent the whole weekend in a daze, except for the first shared shock hug, Mr S and I barely touched each other the whole weekend. The thought of having sex with him revolted me, and, in a way I think he had similar thoughts. Thoughts of that significant day, the 6th November 1998 constantly filled my mind. On the designated Monday I went to see the doctor in Mr S' company, wanting information about our options as neither of us were on medical aid. I did another test to confirm the result. The doctor advised us both to go to the public Day Hospital in Woodstock where Mr S could be tested and we could both get assistance. Unfortunately in South Africa in 1999, not many physicians were interested in or very informed about HIV/AIDS. The doctor proceeded to give us advice that in retrospect was really dangerous for our health, for example, that we should guard against infecting other people but that we could engage in unprotected sex. This in ignorance of the fact that we could re-infect each other and further compromise our immune systems. The following week we picked up Mr S' HIV test result. As expected, he was HIV positive with a CD4 count below 200 and a viral load in the hundred thousands. The reality of my situation hit me hard when we walked into that waiting room. There was just a multitude of sick people sitting on rows of benches patiently waiting to be seen by the Polish doctor who was the AIDS expert. I had also taken my results along and went in to be seen. The sister-in-charge was very kind, understanding and very empathetic. She gave us some sachets of vitamins and another batch of tablets called bactrim which she explained were antibiotics. Taking antibiotics when I was not sick did not seem right to me; the little I had learnt through alternative therapies had informed me that antibiotics weakened the system and were not to be taken in vain. I took advantage of her kindly nature and bombarded her with questions. I asked her about clinical trials and if she knew if there were any taking place at the hospital. Something told me that if I was to survive and not end up like the people I had seen sitting on the benches I had to equip myself with information. She immediately referred me to an old colleague of hers by the name Ashraf Grimwood who was interested in the field of HIV/AIDS. Calling him there and then, he said we should see him in his consulting rooms on Saturday the 18th September. That is one phone call that I will always be grateful for.

At our consultation on Saturday morning he explained in easy terms that we were facing a disease that had the ability to consume its victims at great pace and that we needed to get help as quickly as possible. To illustrate his point he compared my initial negative blood test carried out in January which showed a CD4 count of 700, with the second test taken barely eight months later with a CD4 count of about 350. I believe I owe my life to this early intervention, otherwise I would have succumbed to the devastation of AIDS long ago. Dr Grimwood explained about the clinical trials he was recruiting for and said if we were interested he would take both our bloods to assess if we met the study criteria. Confident that Mr S would get in since his CD4 count was around 200, he indicated that I might be excluded because my CD4 count was slightly higher than the study requirements. I was more concerned about Mr S getting help because he seemed to be fading in front of my eyes.

After an anxious week of waiting I was accepted to participate in the study, and Mr S was not. I felt relieved for my sake, but at the same time very sad for him as I thought he had a greater need to be in the clinical trial than I did. On the 29th September, instead of celebrating the first anniversary of our affair, I was reading study consent forms and bombarding the doctor with questions motivated by fear of being a guinea-pig. As much as I had wanted to participate in clinical trial to save my life, the reality of signing into one was scary. I started thinking about the way AIDS drugs were represented in the media and the fact that many were new drugs that had not been used elsewhere. Through experimenting on us, the drugs might be passed as safe and effective. I lost lots of sleep on this. Even worse was the fact that I could not discuss any of this with Mr S as he was depressed at not having been enrolled onto the study.

I took my study medicines religiously and my adherence was more than 95%. The study staff liked me since I never missed any visits. I valued the R50 transport money that I got on my visits once a month. It contributed a lot towards the food I needed to eat. I made an effort to follow a healthy diet whenever I could afford to, but it was not always possible. Close friends of mine kept me supplied with fruits, vegetables and some basic groceries. A good balanced diet and peace of mind do go a long way towards the health of an HIV-positive person.

I kept listening out for other clinical trials that Mr S could enroll on. At the end of February 2000 he began falling ill on and off, and missing work. The more he missed work the more the rumours flew that he had AIDS, which depressed him even further and he would numb his sorrow in liquor. In March he became very sick and it was as if overnight he lost a great deal of weight. He could not walk to the toilet barely two metres from the corner where we slept, he shivered and sweated and the bed linen would become soaking wet; he complained of his feet being cold and very painful. Barely a year later our roles had reversed. I had become the caregiver and he was the patient. I nursed him fearing that at anytime he would die. Taking him to Dr Grimwood's rooms we were both seen by another wonderful doctor, Douglas Wilson. He was concerned about my fatigue, depression and the sinus problem and took time to explain the different conditions, how they related to HIV, and smoothed over any stigmas that were attached to taking antidepressants. An invitation to come to Somerset hospital where he was running an HIV research clinic was aimed at trying to get Mr S into one of the clinical trials that came up every now and then. A recommendation that I start managing my depression and sinus medically has, with time, taught me to manage both my depression and fatigue by accepting my limitations, resting often and not taking on too many responsibilities. However, by openly living with my HIV-positive status, I do at times get overwhelmed with the emotional demands of the support I have to give to other people.

Having received medical attention, Mr S eventually got back to his feet and went back to work. Unfortunately for him, getting back onto his feet also meant finding his way to the pub. Looking after him throughout his illness had left me very drained and I knew that if I hoped to survive I could not afford to nurse him through another episode like the previous one. Ending my relationship with him was the most painful decision that I had to make because I loved him, and when he was available, his company was great for my dark days.

I continued utilising the private clinic for my study drugs and any opportunistic infections that had an impact on the research. I went to the public hospital research facility run by Dr Wilson for my antidepressants and my sinus medicine; additionally I had to go for my antidepressants once a month since they were controlled drugs and the doctor had to examine me with every visit. Dr Wilson was interested in my total well-being and I thrived under his care. He cared about my diet, how I lived and was interested in my business and job-hunting prospects. When he realised that I had been hibernating in my flat and not going out at all, he encouraged me to venture out and meet people. He so much wanted me to find the joy in life again. Dr Wilson had a way of making one feel normal again. The specialised care I received taught me the importance of love and nurturing in medicine where no one has answers and fear reigns. In June I consulted a psychic, Kalinka who told me things about my health taking a turn for the better and that I would be able to take something that would allow me to have a baby. The upswing in my health was confirmed by Dr Wilson when I consulted with him on the 29th July for my monthly study visit. My CD4 count was up to 700 and my viral load was undetectable. Nothing can rival the feeling of hope, life and elation that I felt on that day. I can still hear his laughter of joy and excitement when he shared the news.

Re-negotiating sexual relations

Under treatment, good diet, lots of rest and spiritual well-being, I thrived and blossomed and eventually even got some of my old confidence back. It took me a year after breaking off with Mr S to think beyond the four walls of my flat besides the odd casual job and the hospital and doctor's visits. In March 2001, I slowly ventured into the outside world. My first sexual encounter after a year of celibacy was very important because it helped to re-establish myself as an attractive woman who had sexual needs and not a diseased woman. I had other casual sexual encounters after that. It was not always easy because I also found out that while I was deeply immersed in the world of HIV/AIDS and safe sex, other people were still in a world where those things were remote from their lives. Many people, especially in the crowd that I was inclined to hang out with, saw AIDS as something that happened to other people. I have found that AIDS statistics mean nothing for many people. The statistics represent other people out there who have nothing to do with them. I suppose 'othering' and placing distance between oneself and HIV/AIDS makes it easier to deal with a disease that is very complex.

In my time of isolation I had worked hard on my spiritual development. Part of my strength outside the medical interventions I believed came from the long hours of meditation that I put in. This also meant that I began to be attracted to and hang out with similar minded people. One of the people that I met through my spiritual interests was a guy I will call Peter. Peter was a very earthy and grounded guy, and a dedicated karate practitioner, with whom I shared a love of meditation, spiritual chants, the dance floor and classy restaurants. When we found ourselves alone one evening Peter introduced me to the sexual world of oral sex. As this was a significantly positive experience, I feebly protested that it was not safe to do so. I consoled myself with the fact that I could not possible infect him seeing that my viral load was undetectable. We did discuss the importance of safe sex afterwards though. This is one sexual encounter I still feel guilty about because there is a part of me that knows I behaved recklessly and placed another person at risk for my own pleasure. May it be noted, however, that when the other person breaks the rules of safe sex it is not always easy to disclose one's HIV/AIDS status.

Discordant couples

In September 2001 I met a guy who fell head over heels in love with me. After telling him about my HIV status he was stressed for some hours mulling over the facts and then seemed to accept it. Since he lived in Johannesburg and I was based in Cape Town, we did not have that much of a sex life. It is only when he visited me in Cape Town six months into the relationship that I realised that his acceptance was largely based on ignorance and a whole lot of other things that I don't think I fully comprehend.

In spite of the fact that I had taken my time to explain my circumstances to him, he seemed to keep forgetting that we needed to use condoms and I had to keep reminding him. I was given a glimpse into his ignorance and the stigmatisation of HIV-positive people when I had to stop at my friend Nandi's place and we found Mr S there. My new friend could not hide his disgust at the sight of Mr S and one would have thought afterwards that he was talking about a corpse. We went away for the weekend and for much of the time, without saying so, he was abusive and angry with me about my HIV status. Raising different issues it sounded as though I had forced him into a relationship with me. His obsession about a skeletal death did not stop him from having forced anal sex without a condom, as in his mind, he could not contract HIV that way. I felt violated and abused and at the same time powerless because I had disclosed my status in what I thought was a safe environment. This experience was significant as it showed me the personal vulnerability that comes from selective disclosure. When we drove back from what was supposed to be a romantic weekend I made a vow that I would never again be in such an abusive relationship no matter how desperate I was for love. I ended that relationship soon after that trip and never found out what that person's HIV status was.

At a time when I was experiencing both an air of despondency and renewed confidence regarding long-term relationships, I met Pone. We spent many weekends caught up in long discussions and establishing a friendship before we even ventured into any intimacy. Though we shared a lot, I never discussed my HIV status with him and I felt justified in not doing so. It was not as if everybody else was discussing their HIV status with me and yet I was saddled with this burden to share my status with those who dared get close. I did not share my HIV status with him until our first sexual encounter, and he was not amused even though we had practised safe sex. He felt that it was unfair of me and that I needed to give him all the facts and let him make the choice based on those facts. After the abusive incident with my previous boyfriend I felt that I was the one who ended up telling people about my HIV-positive status thus opening myself to abuse, so my reasoning had become that we engage in safe sex and life goes on. Pone set a meeting to see me one lunch time and brought his HIV results which were negative and indicated that he wanted us to have a serious relationship. It has not all been all smooth sailing. The first few sexual encounters after my disclosure were very complicated involving safe sex taken to the extreme. Over and above using condoms, Pone would guard against any cuts and soon after intercourse would scrub his hands and genital area clean with disinfectant. It made me feel so dirty and diseased. Things got to a head when we had an incident with a burst condom. I cried when he looked terrified even after his scrubbing session. The incident opened up an opportunity to talk openly. Voicing my feelings to him, we discussed our differences, acknowledged each other's fears and feelings, and eventually found safety in one other. I greatly admire Pone for the love that he has for me. I always ask myself if I would have been able to handle it were the tables turned.

Pone has had to put up with a lot of challenges since we started going out. Early on in our relationship, he was roped into helping me care for my brother who was sick with AIDS. He did it with care and tenderness, from helping with the cooking to dressing his boil. A few weeks after my brother's arrival, Pone stood by my side when I buried Mr S and wordlessly grieved for him. There are times when I have felt that he does not fully understand what I am going through since he is not HIV positive. When I opted to seek solace in an HIV/AIDS support group, he felt that I was undermining his support and unnecessarily dragging my life and his into the public forum. At times I act on impulse and selfishly think of my own feelings and in the process forget that I have children and a man who loves me. In September 2003, when I consulted with a psychic on a national television programme to facilitate making contact with Mr. S after his death I publicly disclosed my HIV status without consulting Pone. He felt that he and the children stood to be harmed more by my public disclosure than I stood to benefit. We spent many hours discussing, arguing and fighting about this until he understood my need to break the silence and make peace with Mr S' death. I feel we emerged from that process stronger and freer as a couple. Pone is now very supportive of my disclosure as long as I remain cognisant of the impact on those close to me and I consult and share with them in my process.

We have been together for about three years now and are still deeply in love. We hope to get married and have a child or two together. I dream of having twin girls since I already have two boys. There is, however, debate in the public forum facilitated by those who see themselves as gatekeepers of what is moral and right, which questions an infected woman's right to bear children who could be infected. In answer to this, all I can say is that as a woman of childbearing age I cannot suppress my maternal instincts and my HIV-positive status has not taken away my desires to bring life into this world. I will take my chances like any other woman infected or not infected.

A few weeks after I started a very committed relationship with Pone, arrangements were made for my brother Hudzani, to travel to Cape Town to seek medical attention. I had seen him during the previous Christmas holidays in Zimbabwe and he had been quite sickly. Rumours had been flying in the family about his condition and the cause of it. Much grief and pain had already been caused with the unofficial pronouncement of an HIV/AIDS diagnosis by gossiping family members. The family had already endured the suffering of being stigmatised and discriminated against. It still shames me to think that in my family, one that I considered highly educated and informed, my own brother had to suffer the indignity of having his utensils and laundry separated from everyone else's. My experience of being infected and working among other infected people has taught me that HIV/AIDS stigma and discrimination has no educational or social status. Given this history, it was not surprising that I met a broken man at the airport on the evening of the 2nd of May 2002. His main message to me was to take care of his children was he to die, as he had lost all hope of living. After getting his HIV results and seeing that his CD4 count was 38, I realised that more than anything it was the desire to leave his two daughters in good hands that had kept him alive for the past few months.

Working closely with Hudzani and supporting him through his HIV tests and early days of taking antiretrovirals was both physically and emotionally draining. My first painful hurdle was actually sharing my HIV status with him. Although my relatively good health was meant as an encouragement to him, it devastated him as he had pinned his hopes on me raising his children were he to die. On another level, it empowered him because he could no longer hand over the baton of caring for his children to somebody else; he needed to get up from his sick bed and find strength to live for their sake. I had done it, and I had faith he could do it too. It devastated me, however, to care for Hudzani because it meant that to give him hope I had to share my own status with him. I had to invite him into my secret and ask him to perpetuate the silence around HIV/AIDS. My logic says I did not want him sharing this information with my mother who would be broken by news of having two children who could be dying, but somewhere I wonder if my reasoning was motivated by not wanting my mother to know that I had made a dreadful mistake.

It required a lot of physical effort on my part to make sure that my brother had eaten well and taken his medicines and to keep checking at night that he was warm and had not tossed the blankets away because of the sweating. I had a demanding job in the day and I had never fully recovered my physical strength since my bout of illness when I became infected with HIV. Emotionally it was hurting to see my baby brother so wasted and so close to death. I had to keep a brave front through it all and assure him that he would be fine.

With Pone's support, it was uplifting to see my brother gain his strength day by day. His appetite kept improving and he started gaining weight. It was with such joy that six weeks into his recovery process we went to a party together and I watched him dance with the energy of a man who had come too close to death and greatly valued the gift of just being alive. It was touching to see what a few weeks of love, care and medical intervention in non-judgemental circumstances could do for a human being. If only it had come sooner and saved him from the shame of being diseased. Although I knew that Hudzani had negotiated the first hurdle of living with HIV, which is moving beyond a sick body, I knew through my own experience that many challenges lay ahead. No challenge can compare, however, to living in a body that is daily being devoured by a living organism over which you have no control. My brother still needed to either face his family and disclose his status or come up with a lie to explain his long illness and sudden recovery in Cape Town. He still needed to go back and deal with those who had discriminated against him, and stigmatised and shamed him during the course of his illness. He was still to spend hours asking himself what had gone wrong, which sexual encounter had left him infected, and with whom? These are the questions that one is faced with now and then when one contemplates the past. When sick, the main prayer is for access to antiretroviral medicines, and once access is achieved the silent prayer is for a cure to be freed from the silence and shame of a devouring virus.

It still gives me great pleasure to look at the photos of that party and think of what was averted. I enjoy talking to Hudzani on the phone and hear that he is a well man, working hard for his children and living like a normal human being who does not have to suffer public scrutiny because of his skeletal looks.

Bibliography

PROFILE SOCIAL MARKETING AND COMMUNICATIONS SERVICE FOR HEALTH. Population Services International. August 2004 Harare, Zimbabwe

As I bask in the fortune of good health, and enjoy the benefits of being on antiretrovirals, I am continuously grateful. I am always reminded of my good fortune in the context of my work, because every day I have to meet people who are in different stages of their struggle with the disease. I hope that sharing my story will save at least one person from getting infected, and touch another who is already infected by making them realise that it is possible to thrive with HIV after all. That with love and care there is room to ease stigma and discrimination even though it is not possible to eradicate it. However, I question the seriousness of the scientific world for its failure to halt the continued existence and spread of a virus 25 years into its existence.

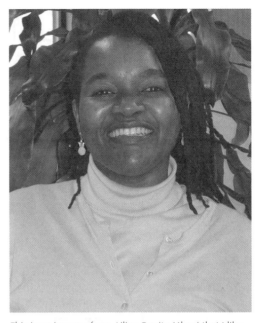

This is an image of me, Lilian Benita Mboyi that I like to hold close to my heart and as an example of a healthy 38 year old HIV+ woman who is on antiretrovirals

CHAPTER 22

Impact of AIDS – the health care burden

Mark Colvin

AS THE LEADING CAUSE of illness and death in sub-Saharan Africa, HIV and AIDS have become an added burden on already strained health care systems. The full extent is not yet apparent because of the latent period between infection and illness and death. Data on the effect of AIDS on health care systems are scarce, most studies being small and cross-sectional.

The main impact on adult health services appears to be increased hospital admissions, leading to ward overcrowding and possible exclusion of HIV-negative patients as a result. The increasing incidence of TB that accompanies HIV in southern Africa has also had an effect on hospital and other health care services. Increased mortality is seen in both patients infected with HIV and those who are not.

A disproportionate increase in the numbers of medical paediatric admissions against surgical admissions suggests that paediatric HIV is having an impact on paediatric health care services. Studies have found that HIV-positive children have more contact with health care services than those that are negative and mortality among those infected with HIV is consistently higher than among those who are not.

Treating intercurrent illness appears to be more costly among patients who are HIV positive than among those who are not infected. This was particularly the case for those co-infected with HIV and TB according to a study from Kenya.

It is unlikely that the public health sector is going to be able to sustain the increasing costs of treating HIV-positive patients, which means that some form of rationing is inevitable and is probably already happening.

It is likely that the marginal costs of HIV in the private health sector will not rise as much as this sector already spends more per patient than the public health sector. However, those private schemes that cater for the lower end of the market may be faced with escalating costs as this is the population with the highest HIV prevalence.

AIDS is now the leading cause of morbidity and death in sub-Saharan Africa including South Africa and the epidemic has therefore become an added burden on already strained health care systems. It is estimated that in 2002 there were between 4.5 million and 6.5 million people living with HIV and AIDS in South Africa and of this, about 25% (1.1 to 1.6 million people) were likely to be symptomatic including 7% (315 000 to 455 000 people) with full-blown AIDS. Because HIV infection affects predominantly young adults, among whom health status is usually good, the epidemic is changing the pattern of disease and placing an increased demand on health care services.

However, the full extent of the impact has not yet been felt because of the length of the latency period between acquiring HIV infection and the development of HIV-related illnesses. The individuals with AIDS who are now seeking health care are predominantly those infected more than seven years ago when the antenatal prevalence of HIV was 10%, substantially below the 24.8% estimate for 2001. Indeed, it is estimated that the number of AIDS cases is likely to climb sharply to 500 000 by 2005 and to 800 000, or double the current numbers, by 2010.

There is a scarcity of data on the impact of HIV on health care services with most of it coming from small, cross-sectional studies. Even the longitudinal data tends to be focused on specific wards and with no large-scale studies published, there are few data on the impact on health services more broadly. Nevertheless, there are trends and patterns that emerge from what data are available.

This chapter describes the impact on health services resulting from an increasing disease burden and a shifting in the patterns of disease. It also discusses the rising prevalence of HIV among health workers and the negative impacts of this overwhelming epidemic on their functioning.

Impact on adult health services

During the late 1980s and early 1990s reports from eastern African cities described HIV prevalence rates of up to 80% among hospitalised patients and hospital bed occupancy rates approaching 200%. The pattern was similar in other parts of Africa stretching from Guinea Bissau to Zambia. In Nairobi, Kenya, bed occupancy in the Infectious Diseases Hospital rose from 69% to 81% from 1985 to 1990 with an increase of 61% in the number of registered TB cases and a significant rise in TB-related mortality.

The HIV epidemic was established in South Africa later than in eastern and central Africa, but by the early 1990s HIV was beginning to have an impact on health care services. A study conducted in the rural district of Hlabisa on the eastern seaboard of South Africa tracked the impact of the epidemic on the district hospital from 1991 until 1998. During this time there was no increase in hospital beds but total hospital admissions increased by 81%. The most dramatic rise in adult patient numbers was because of a 360% increase in ward admissions for tuberculosis whilst the HIV prevalence among TB patients went from 35% in 1993 to 68% by 1997. Mortality among TB patients in the same district rose by 46% from 1991 until 1995. Over the same period the HIV prevalence among pregnant women went from 4% to 29%. This rise in TB case load in tandem with a rising HIV prevalence has been reported elsewhere.

Most other South African studies have been conducted in larger, city-based hospitals and available data on the HIV prevalence among hospital patients are presented in TABLE 22.1. During 1998 the prevalence of HIV among medical inpatients in a tertiary hospital in Durban was 54% with 84% of these patients having AIDS according to the WHO expanded case definition of AIDS. In comparison to HIV-negative patients, HIV-positive patients were significantly younger, were 2.4 times as likely to die whilst hospitalised and were more likely to be transferred. Mean length of hospital stay was similar for the two groups.

At the 2003 Durban AIDS conference the Human Sciences Research Council (HSRC) released preliminary results of a study on the prevalence of HIV among health care workers and patients in four provinces. Within the public sector, the overall prevalence of HIV among a combination of all patients was 28% with the prevalence being 26% among clinic attendees and 46% among inpatients (TABLE 21.1). More women (31%) than men patients (22%) were HIV positive but this was not statistically significant.

Reference	Study setting	Year	No tested	% HIV+	% HIV+ with AIDS	Mortality HIV+	Mortality HIV-
HSRC 2002	Patients from health facilities in 4 provinces	2002	581	28%			
Colvin 2001	Adult medical wards, tertiary hospital, KZN	1997	507	54%	84%	22%	9%
Wilkinson 1999	Gynaecology wards, district hospital, KZN	1997	196	42%		1%	1%
Hassig 1990	Medical wards, public hospital, Kinshasa Zaire	1988	251	50%	50%	50%	30%

TABLE 22.1 Summary results from HIV prevalence studies among adult users of health services in southern and East Africa

Unfortunately, there are little additional non-anecdotal data on the impact on health services but impressions are that the services are under strain. In KZN, arguably the province with the highest HIV prevalence rate, medical beds at hospitals such as Northdale and Edendale in Pietermaritzburg and in several rural hospitals are running at 120% over capacity because of AIDS, according to a report in the *South African Medical Journal* in 2001. The superintendent at Hlabisa, a rural district hospital, claimed that for three years his medical wards have run at 140% occupancy. The shortage of beds means that during inclement weather and overnight, each bed is occupied by one or two patients and sometimes there is another patient on the floor underneath.

Patterns of illness and disease

HIV/AIDS is also changing the way in which patients present and the pattern of diagnoses. In 1990, when the heterosexual HIV epidemic was beginning in South Africa, it was noted that the most common diseases presenting to the Baragwanath AIDS clinic in Soweto outside Johannesburg were tuberculosis followed by pneumonia, herpes zoster and 'slim' disease. Later in the 1990s a study was done on the distribution of presenting symptoms and initial diagnoses among HIV-infected and uninfected patients admitted to the adult medical wards of a large tertiary hospital in Durban (the results are given in TABLE 22.2). Another study conducted in an HIV clinic in a large Soweto hospital had similar findings with the most common presenting problems being lymphadenopathy, weight loss, TB and oral candidiasis.

Disease/clinical findings	% with disease among HIV infected (n=131)	% with disease among HIV uninfected (n=87)	RR of having disease if infected with HIV
Oral/oesophageal candidiasis	43% (56)	2% (2)	18.6 (4.7–74.2)
Generalised lymphadenopathy	49% (64)	7% (6)	7.1 (3.2–15.6)
Unexplained fever	48% (63)	7% (6)	7.0 (3.2–15.6)
Chronic diarrhoea	21% (28)	3% (3)	6.2 (1.9–19.8)
> 10% weight loss	41% (54)	9% (8)	.5 (2.2–8.9)
Pulmonary TB	56% (74)	7% (6)	3.1 (1.9–4.9)
Extra-pulmonary TB	6% (8)	0% (0)	not calculable

TABLE 22. 2 Risk of selected symptoms, signs and diseases among HIV infected compared with HIV uninfected patients for medical ward patients in a large, tertiary hospital in Durban, South Africa

This synergy between HIV and TB is posing a significant threat to TB control in sub-Saharan Africa, which has the greatest TB burden in the world and is growing at an annual rate of 6% (see CHAPTER 29 for a more detailed discussion of the association between HIV and TB).

In summary, there is evidence that over the last ten years total hospital admissions have been rising and an increasing proportion are due to people with HIV-related disease. The pattern of admissions is also changing with the average age of patients decreasing and HIV-related diseases such as tuberculosis, pneumonia, diarrhoea and disseminated fungal infections becoming more common. The overall mortality of hospitalised patients is increasing but this is largely due to the higher mortality rates among the HIV infected. The impact on HIV-negative patients is not clear although there must be some 'squeezing out' of these patients. The potential negative impacts on those uninfected with HIV, such as rising mortality or decreasing hospital stays, has not been demonstrated in South Africa, although it has been shown in some other African countries.

Impact on paediatric health care services

The prevalence of HIV among children in Africa and the morbidity and mortality rates among these children is likely to be more severe than experience from the industrialised countries may indicate. The reasons for this are listed in TABLE 22.3.

TABLE 22.3 Likely reasons for higher rates of morbidity and mortality in children born to HIV-positive mothers in Africa compared with experience in the industrialised countries

- *Higher rates of mother – to – child transmission*
- *Increased and variable risk of infection from the environment*
- *Poor nutrition*
- *Limited access to standard and specialist medical and social care*
- *Ill-health in the mother and other potential carers*
- *Stigmatisation of infants with real or presumed infection*

For South Africa, Dorrington and colleagues, using the ASSA model, predicted a total of just under 1.2 million births for the year 2002 with an estimated 89 000 (6.7%) children being HIV infected at birth and through breast feeding. In the absence of a national antiretroviral programme, it is expected that 50% of these children will die of AIDS-related disease within three years and 90% by nine years. Prior to death these children will be accessing health services for their pre-morbid illnesses.

Turning from modelled to measured data, TABLE 22.4 shows the results of studies in southern and eastern Africa that have estimated the proportion of HIV-positive children using health services.

Estimates vary from 8% to 63% of paediatric patients with the proportion who are HIV positive decreasing with age. The only longitudinal data published was a report from a rural district hospital in KZN that indicated that there was a 68% increase in medical paediatric admissions between 1991 to 1996 with only an 18% increase in surgical admissions. The disproportionate increase in medical patients was attributed to an increase in HIV-related medical illnesses. As with the adult studies, most of the published studies are cross-sectional and focus on specific hospital wards, which makes it difficult to assess the overall impact. Nevertheless, there are some consistent findings across the published literature.

Importantly, the mortality of HIV-positive children is consistently and substantially higher than among the HIV-negative.

Most studies found that length of hospital stay was not different between HIV-positive and negative children. However, one study in

Ref	Study setting	Year	No tested	% HIV+	Mortality HIV+	Mortality HIV-
Pillay 2001	Paediatric wards, tertiary hospital, KZN	1997	160	63%	20%	12%
Meyers 2000	Paediatric wards, tertiary hospital, Gau	1996	507	29%	17%	5%
Johnson 2000	Paediatric wards, tertiary hospital, Gau	1998	176	18%	NA	NA
Yeung 2000	Paediatric wards, rural hospital, KZN	1996/7	281	26%	21%	7%
Roux 2000	Paediatric wards, 18 hospitals in Cape Town	1999	1264	8.3%	NA	NA
Kawo 2000	Paediatric wards, Dar es Salaam	1995/6	2015	19.2%	21.4%	8.4%

TABLE 22.4 Summary results from HIV-prevalence studies among paediatric users of health services in southern and East Africa

Soweto found that HIV-positive children stayed in for an average of eight days compared with an average of six days among the HIV-negative children. This lack of difference in hospital stay may be partly due to the fact that HIV-positive children have a higher mortality and higher referral rate. To clarify this point future studies should report the length of stay for only those who are discharged.

Most studies have also found evidence that HIV-positive paediatric patients have previously had more contact with the health care system than HIV-negative children. In the Durban study, HIV-positive patients were 2.7-times as likely to have been previously admitted and 2.3-times as likely to have had an outpatient consultation, whilst a study in a rural KZN district also reported that HIV-positive children were more likely to have been previously admitted. In a Soweto study 48% of HIV-positive children had previously been admitted compared with 20% of HIV-negative children.

The prevalence of HIV and HIV-related disease is increasing among paediatric patients using public sector health services. Whilst the spectrum of disease is not substantially different between the HIV – positive and HIV – negative cases, certain diseases such as pneumonia, diarrhoea, fungal infections and malnutrition are more common among the HIV positive and tend to have a higher mortality rate. HIV-positive children do respond to standard treatment protocols but clinicians need to be ready to change therapy should response be poor.

The increasing burden on health care facilities may have a negative impact on the care of the HIV-negative children and alternative care strategies, such as more rational use of clinics and home-based care, need to be developed. The impact of HIV among children could be substantially reduced if there was an effective, national mother-to-child transmission (MTCT) prevention programme and universal access to antiretrovirals.

Impact of HIV on other paediatric infectious diseases

From the beginning of the epidemic, there have been concerns that the immunosuppressive effect of HIV infection may affect the natural history or epidemiology of other infectious diseases including the vaccine preventable illnesses and traditional tropical diseases. HIV infection may make children more susceptible to other infections or make the infections more severe and could conceivably cause the population's herd immunity to fall making it susceptible to new epidemics. Although the number of clinical studies is limited there is evidence that HIV-infected children suffer a similar clinical spectrum but with more severe and recurrent forms of a number of infections, including bacterial infections, pneumonia, septicaemia, diarrhoeal diseases and measles.

In local studies of children attending health care facilities, infectious diseases were the most common reasons for admission, regardless of HIV status. However, certain diseases, including pneumonia and gastroenteritis, tended to occur more commonly among the HIV-positive patients. In a Soweto study, pneumonia and gastroenteritis occurred 1.7-times and 1.4-times as frequently among the HIV positive and in a study in Durban, HIV-positive children were three times as likely to have a diagnosis of pneumonia and 18 times as likely to have a diagnosis of oral candidiasis. A number of researchers have also found that malnutrition is significantly more prevalent among the HIV positive.

Whilst common pathogens are believed to be responsible for the bulk of cases of pneumonia and diarrhoea among children in sub-Saharan Africa, the significance of opportunistic infections such as *Pneumocystis carinii* pneumonia (PCP) and cytomegalovirus have been overlooked, mainly because of the lack of diagnostic facilities. In a study in Johannesburg among two- to 24-month-old HIV-infected children hospitalised with severe pneumonia, PCP was found in just under half of the 105 children and cytomegalovirus pneumonia was diagnosed histologically in 44% of 18 postmortem cases. In another local study, PCP was the AIDS-defining event in 20% of hospitalised children and was associated with a significantly higher mortality.

Several researchers have reported that HIV-positive children respond well to antibiotic therapy, but at least one local study found that a satisfactory response to initial antibiotic therapy was less frequent in the HIV positive (56%) than in the HIV negative (73%).

Health service utilisation and costs

Once the natural history of HIV infection became apparent in the mid 1980s, it was anticipated that this would be an expensive disease to manage and would substantially increase the burden on the health care system. International studies bore this out and found that health service utilisation and resulting costs increased with the severity of illness and were particularly high in the three months before death.

A few studies in Africa have attempted to determine the resource utilisation or cost of managing HIV-positive patients in comparison to HIV-negative patients. A study in Nairobi, Kenya found that treating TB in HIV-positive patients was, on average, 25% more costly than treating HIV-negative patients, mainly because of the costs of drugs for treating intercurrent infections in the former group. However, a study conducted in Kinshasa, Zaire (now Democratic Republic of the Congo) found that hospitalisation costs did not differ between HIV-positive and HIV-negative inpatients.

The escalating burden on the public health care system described above will require an increasing level of resources to care for individuals with AIDS. Whilst the costs of managing the HIV/AIDS epidemic are not routinely measured, ABT and Associates have used demographic projection models and data on currently observed HIV-associated health care costs to make ten-year forecasts. The model used assumed that levels of care offered in the mid-1990s and the associated costs would continue to be made available over the next ten years despite increasing levels of illness. The costs and potential cost savings of providing antiretroviral therapy were also not considered. FIGURE 22.1 shows the estimated costs until 2010 in constant 2000 terms for acute in- and outpatient care but excludes long stay, rehabilitation activities and administration and managerial costs. The figure shows that acute health care costs are likely to double in real terms in the public sector if current levels of care are maintained.

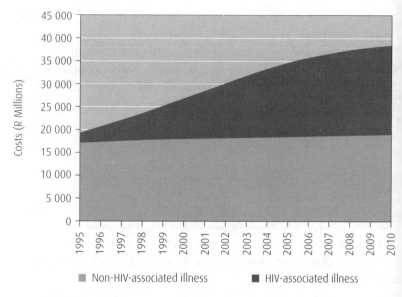

FIGURE 22.1 Cost of public sector health care by year – constant 2000 rands

Non-HIV-associated illness HIV-associated illness

Impacts of increased case load burden and escalating public sector health care costs

The estimated resources required to maintain current levels of health care, particularly for inpatients, are unlikely to be sustainable which means that some form of rationing will have to be implemented. While data demonstrating rationing are scarce, a few studies in East and southern Africa have found that a decreasing proportion of patients are HIV negative and that among these patients the absolute and relative mortality rates have increased. The rise in mortality of non-HIV-infected patients, which has increased in tandem with the overcrowding of hospitals, has been cited as evidence of declining health care standards. An increase in mortality from 13.9% to 23% among HIV-negative patients in a Nairobi hospital over a four year period was attributed to increasingly stringent hospital admission requirements and that this was favouring HIV-positive patients at the expense of HIV-negative patients.

There is now some evidence that rationing of health care may already be occurring in South Africa as demonstrated by FIGURE 22.2 which shows that HIV-infected children are staying in hospital for increasingly shorter periods.

In the rural district hospital of Hlabisa, the superintendent was reported as claiming that, 'Blood pressure readings and medications are missed, or are wrongly dispensed by inexperienced nurse-aides and that many diabetics and hypertensives, disenchanted with the levels of care, no longer bother to come in.' Dr Kimesh Naidoo of

Grey's Hospital says that at regional hospitals community service doctors are making life or death decisions simply because of the lack of consultants. 'They have to decide how far they must go, when to drop IV or antibiotics, should they ventilate this child? If the kids are HIV positive we don't ventilate and the kids die – that's become general practice'.

One strategy for reducing the impact of HIV/AIDS on the health services is to make more rational use of primary health care facilities and appropriate referral policies. Even before the HIV/AIDS epidemic it was clear that many patients were being treated in referral and specialist facilities when this was not necessary. In 1990 a study reported that 42.2% of attendees at a tertiary level hospital in Durban, KZN could have been medically managed in a primary care facility. A later study which considered only HIV-positive patients attending the HIV clinic of a teaching hospital found that 69.3% of all consultations were deemed suitable for treatment at the primary-care level. However, it was noted that as the severity of the disease increases (ie people move from WHO stage 1 to 3) there is a decrease in the proportion of patients that may be treated at this level.

Whether or not there has been a shift towards more rational use of health facilities or not is not clear but this strategy does need to be revisited.

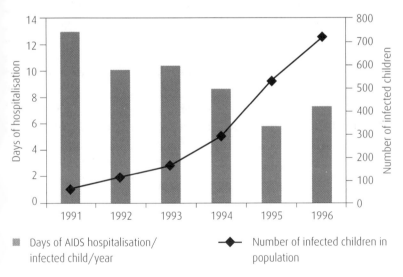

Days of AIDS hospitalisation/infected child/year

Number of infected children in population

FIGURE 22.2 Rationing of access to hospital care for children ill with AIDS with increasing levels of infection

Impact on the private health care sector

Approximately seven million people (15% of the population) in South Africa are not dependent on public health services but instead have access to private health care through membership of a medical insurance scheme. Membership of these schemes is usually linked to employment and so it is the relatively wealthier sectors of society that have access to private health care.

In the 1980s, the insurance and medical aid industries responded to the anticipated impact of the AIDS epidemic by attempting to contain the risk. They implemented an almost total, if ineffective, exclusion of HIV benefits. Annual benefits for HIV-related disease of R100 were the norm. Health care providers reacted by not disclosing the HIV status of patients whilst providing treatment for legitimately reimbursable illnesses such as pneumonia and chronic diarrhoea.

The largely futile response of the medical aid industry and objections to the discriminatory nature of their rules led to the implementation of the Medical Schemes Act in 1988, which banned previously widespread practices against people living with HIV/AIDS such as risk rating and excluding infected individuals from membership.

Another important development in HIV care within the private health sector has been the rise of managed care programmes. The primary aim of managed care is to contain costs and it has achieved mixed success. However, managed care has been more successful in the area of HIV/AIDS care because it is based on the premise that the major cost driver in managing HIV-related disease is hospitalisation and that antiretrovirals, although costly, are effective in reducing morbidity and improving survival. Managed care has also been able to address the underlying problems posed by the high cost of drugs, low benefits and the lack of expertise by most doctors in managing HIV/AIDS.

The largest managed care programme is AID *for* AIDS (AfA) which has 39 medical schemes contracted to it, covers two million beneficiaries, has 20 000 HIV-infected people registered and provides antiretroviral treatment to 12 000 persons. AfA claims to be a comprehensive and confidential disease programme that manages access to antiretrovirals and related drugs and disease monitoring, combined with a doctor and patient telephonic support system. AfA has also published data to support their claim to have reduced MTCT to 5.3%, improved virological and CD4 responses and stabilised hospitalisation costs. However, there are still no data published on the overall cost effectiveness of this programme.

Although there are few data on the prevalence of HIV among medical aid scheme members or on the impact of the epidemic on the schemes, it is likely that the private sector will be less affected than the public sector. This is in part because HIV prevalence is lower among medical aid scheme members because a higher proportion are of a higher socioeconomic status. Another reason is that the private sector already spends more than four times as much as the public sector per person covered and so the marginal impact of HIV/AIDS on overall costs will be relatively less. Nevertheless, there is some evidence that the schemes that cater for the lower end of the market, where there is a higher prevalence of HIV, are being threatened with runaway costs.

In spite of the changes in the legislation referred to above, businesses and industries in the private sector have more flexibility and scope to avoid the economic burden of AIDS than the government and there is evidence that the burden is being systematically transferred away from the private sector and private health care. Practices that shift the burden to households and government include reductions in employee benefits, restructured employment contracts, outsourcing of low-skilled jobs and selective retrenchments. Many firms have replaced defined-benefit retirement funds with defined-contribution funds, which eliminate risks to the firm but provide little for families of younger workers who become incapacitated or die of AIDS. Responsibility for the health care of these individuals and families falls back onto the households, NGOs and government. The widespread practice of contracting out previously permanent jobs also serves to protect companies from benefit and turnover costs. Whilst many of these changes are primarily responses to globalisation, they are potentially devastating for the households of employees with HIV/AIDS.

HIV/AIDS and health care workers

In addition to the risk of infection through the same routes as the general community, health care workers are at added risk through their exposure to HIV-contaminated blood and body fluids in the workplace. Risk of HIV infection is higher in Africa than elsewhere in the world because of the high prevalence of these diseases in the general population and because health care workers frequently lack the training and equipment to adequately protect themselves. A study conducted at Chris Hani Baragwanath hospital near Johannesburg found that 69% of interns reported one or more percutaneous exposures to blood during the intern year and 56% had suffered a penetrating injury during pre-clinical training and 18% recollected needlestick injuries involving HIV-positive patients. At Tygerberg Children's Hospital near Cape Town, it was recently reported that 91% of young doctors had suffered needlestick injuries and 55% had been exposed to HIV.

However, in spite of these occupational hazards, evidence suggests that the distribution of HIV and exposure to risk factors among health care workers are little different from the general community.

In the Human Sciences Research Council (HSRC) study of HIV in the health sector in four provinces, the HIV prevalence among public sector health care workers was 16%, which is lower than the Dorrington/Bradshaw estimate of 23.4% among 18 to 64 year olds but very similar to the Nelson Mandela/HSRC estimate of 15.6% among 15 to 49 year-old adults. A study in Zaire found that health care workers had a similar HIV seroprevalence to the general community and that neither injections nor the intensity of nosocomial exposure was related to risk of HIV infection. Several other studies in Africa conducted on indigenous health care workers and on expatriate medical workers point to similar conclusions, ie that the overwhelming majority of HIV infections among health workers are due to sexual exposure.

While the physical risks of acquiring HIV from workplace exposures may be small, the HIV/AIDS epidemic has had other, more subtle impacts on health care workers. The perceived threat posed by exposure to HIV-infected blood, body fluids and patients is a source of mental stress. A recent study in Kenya reported that the fear of contamination by HIV was having a negative effect on the motivation and aspirations to practise medicine for over 50% of young doctors interviewed. Even more of the doctors, 82%, stated that the overwhelming HIV/AIDS epidemic was having the same negative impacts. The study concludes that, among other reasons, the high number of AIDS patients has significantly affected the doctors' perceptions of themselves, their technical proficiency, their ability to care and feel for others and themselves and, for some, their entire sense of self. A 'roll on' negative effect on patients was also reported.

Nearer to home, in 2001 Dr Jim Muller, the Acting Head of Medicine for Edendale, Grey's and Northdale Hospitals, stated bluntly, 'People are dying prematurely because we are so stretched. Medical patients who don't have HIV/AIDS are being severely compromised because we have to discharge them prematurely – everybody is being compromised – the system just can't cope'.

BATEMAN C. 'Can KwaZulu Natal hospitals cope with the HIV/AIDS human tide?' *South African Medical Journal* 2001; 91: 364–368.

BUVE A. 'AIDS and hospital bed occupancy: An overview'. *Tropical Medicine and International Health* 1997; 2: 136–139.

COLVIN M, DAWOOD S, KLEINSCHMIDT I, MULLICK S, LALLOO U. 'Prevalence of HIV and HIV-related diseases on the adult medical wards of a tertiary hospital in Durban, South Africa'. *International Journal of STD and AIDS* 2001; 12: 386–389.

DORRINGTON RE, BRADSHAW D, BUDLENDER D. '*HIV/AIDS profile of the provinces of south Africa – Indicators for 2002*'. Centre for Actuarial Research, Medical Research Council and the Actuarial Society of South Africa. 2002.

FLOYD K, ALASDAIR REID R, WILKINSON D, GILKS CF. 'Admission trends in a rural South African Hospital during the early years of the HIV epidemic'. *Journal of the American Medical Association* 1999; 282: 1087–1091.

GILKS CF, FLOYD K, OTIENO LS, ADAM MA, BHATT SM, WARRELL DA. 'Some Effects of the Rising Case Load of Adult HIV-related Disease on a Hospital in Nairobi'. *Journal of Acquired Immune Deficiency Syndromes and Human Retrovirology* 1997; 18: 234–240.

HASSIG SE, PERRIENS J, BAENDE E, KAHOTWA M, BISHAGARA K, KINGELA N, AND KAPITA B. 'An analysis of the economic impact of HIV infection among patients at Mama Yemo Hospital, Kinshasa, Zaire'. *AIDS* 1990; 4: 883–887.

JOHNSON S, HENDSON W, CREWE-BROWN H, DINI L, FREAN J, PEROVIC O, VARDAS E. 'Effect of human immunodeficiency virus infection on episodes of diarrhea among children in South Africa'. *The Pediatric Infectious Disease Journal* 2000; 19: 972–979.

KARSTAEDT AS AND PANTANOWITZ L. 'Occupational exposure of interns to blood in an area of high HIV seroprevalence'. *South African Medical Journal* 2001; 91: 57–61.

KARSTAEDT AS. 'AIDS – the Baragwanath experience (Part III. HIV infection in adults at Baragwanath Hospital)'. *South African Medical Journal* 1992; 82: 95–97.

METRIKIN AS, ZWARENSTEIN M, STEINBERG MH, VAN DER VYVER E, MAARTENS G, WOOD R. 'Is HIV/AIDS a primary-care disease? Appropriate levels of outpatient care for patients with HIV/AIDS'. *AIDS* 1995; 9: 619–623.

MEYERS TM, PETTIFOR JM, GRAY GE, CREWE-BROWN H, GALPIN JS. 'Pediatric Admissions with Human Immunodeficiency Virus Infection at a Regional Hospital in Soweto, South Africa'. *Journal of Tropical Pediatrics* 2000; 46: 224–230.

PILLAY K, COLVIN M, WILLIAMS R, COOVADIA HM. 'Impact of HIV-1 infection in South Africa'. *Archives of Disease in Childhood* 2001; 85: 50–51.

RAVIOLA G, MACHOKI M, MWAIKAMBO E, DELVECCHIO GOOD MJ. 'HIV, Disease plague, Demoralization and "burnout": Resident experience of the Medical Profession in Nairobi, Kenya'. *Culture, Medicine and Psychiatry* 2002; 26: 55–86.

REGENSBERG L, HISLOP M. 'Aid for AIDS – A report back on more than four years of HIV/AIDS disease management in Southern Africa'. *Southern African Journal of HIV Medicine* 2003; February 7–10.

ROSEN S AND SIMON JL. 'Shifting the burden: The private sector's response to the AIDS epidemic in Africa'. *Bulletin of the World Health Organisation* 2003; 81: 131–137.

ROUX P, HENLWY L, COTTON M, ELEY B, AND THE PAEDIATRIC HIV CENSUS GROUP. 'Burden and cost of inpatient care for HIV-positive paediatric patients – status in the Cape Town Metropole during the second week of March 1999'. *South African Medical Journal* 2000; 90: 1008–1011.

RUTKOVE SB, ABDOOL KARIM SS, LOENING WEK. 'Patterns of care in an overburdened tertiary hospital outpatients department'. *South African Medical Journal* 1999; 77: 476–478.

SHISANA O, HALL E, MALULEKE KR, STOKER DJ, SCHWABE C, COLVIN M, CHAUVEAU J, ET AL. *The impact of HIV/AIDS on the health sector; National survey of health personnel, ambulatory and hospitalised patients and health facilities, 2002.* HSRC/Medunsa/MRC. National Department of Health, Pretoria, 2002.

STEINBERG M, KINGHORN AWA, SODERLUND N, SCHIERHOUT G, AND CONWAY S. 'HIV/AIDS – facts, figures and the future'. *South African Health Review* 2000: 301–326.

WALRAVEN G, NICOLL A, NJAU M, AND TIMAEUS I. 'The impact of HIV-1 infection on child health in sub-Saharan Africa: The burden on the health services'. *Tropical Medicine and International Health* 1996; 1: 3–14.

WILKINSON D AND DAVIES GR. 'The increasing burden of tuberculosis in rural South Africa – impact of the HIV epidemic'. *South African Medical Journal* 1997; 87: 447–450.

WILKINSON D, GILKS CF. 'Increasing frequency of tuberculosis among staff in a South African district hospital: Impact of the HIV epidemic on the supply side of health care'. *Transactions of the Royal Society of Tropical Medicine and Hygiene* 1998; 92: 500–502.

YEUNG S, WILKINSON D, ESCOTT S, GILKS CF. 'Pediatric HIV infection in a rural SA District Hospital'. *Journal of Tropical Pediatrics* 2000; 46: 107–110.

ZWI KJ, PETTIFOR JM AND SODERLUND N. 'Paediatric hospital admissions at a South-African urban regional hospital: The impact of HIV, 1992–1997'. *Annals of Tropical Paediatrics* 1999; 19: 135–142.

CHAPTER 23
The impact of AIDS on the community

Janet Frohlich

HIV IS HAVING A major impact on individuals and on community structures such as the family. Family has traditionally been the fundamental unit of any society but as the epidemic progresses this structure is being steadily eroded.

One of the most obvious changes has been in the increase in single-parent households. In South African society, women have previously often effectively been single parents as fathers have worked away from home. However, although this is still the case, 'skipped generation' households, headed by a grandmother, are increasingly common. The traditional absorption of orphans by the extended family is no longer possible as already strained communities struggle to cope with the increasing burdens of HIV and AIDS.

These burdens are made worse by the stigma attached to the disease, which among other effects, prevents those affected from being able to grieve openly. The traditional rituals associated with death are also often no longer followed as whole communities deny the existence of HIV as an illness. However, the numbers of orphans resulting from AIDS-related deaths in South Africa are predicted to rise to over five million by 2014, making effective community response to the epidemic essential.

Responses encompass different levels of care for orphans, community involvement in prevention and awareness efforts and continued advocacy and support for social change.

The state has a responsibility, underpinned by the Constitution, to provide assistance in the form of social grants for varying levels of need. However, these are often difficult to access.

As communities struggle to come to terms with the extent of the epidemic, psychosocial mechanisms such as ways of preserving memories and paying tribute to those who have died of AIDS (memory boxes and AIDS quilts) are becoming increasingly important in the response to the virus.

To address the social impact of HIV and AIDS on the family, children and orphans, there needs to be targeted advocacy and broad networks to mobilise and involve government, civil society, CBOs and NGOs in shared initiatives of community action.

Erosion of social structures

HIV and AIDS are now radically undermining the fundamental social fabric of affected countries such as those of southern Africa, with a relentless impact on the lives of individuals and on their family structures. What until the early 1990s was a 'silent' epidemic of HIV has now emerged as an inescapably visible AIDS epidemic with devastating effects on vulnerable communities. The sudden implosion of the epidemic in these communities was clearly manifest in the late 1990s in the bewilderment and concern of community members as they experienced ever more frequent funerals, a mounting population of orphaned children, withdrawal of children from school to care for ill family members and dwindling household incomes as the burden of the epidemic increasingly fell on the shoulders of older women.

Vulnerable communities and individuals become in turn increasingly at risk of HIV infection as their access to health services is more and more compromised by their deteriorating economic and social circumstances. And although the writing was on the wall for so many years, government and societal response has been desperately inadequate.

The breakdown of family structures

The impact of HIV and AIDS on society, family and community is complex. Traditionally, 'family' has been the fundamental institution of any society and, ideally, the primary point of provision to its members of care, nurturing and socialisation, affording them physical, economic, emotional, social, cultural and spiritual security. As the epidemic progresses, this nuclear 'family' unit is being drastically eroded – and the role of household head in particular is undergoing radical alteration. With the epidemic comes a very steep increase in single-parent households, in what have come to be known as 'skipped generation' households, headed by the elderly (by grandparents and very often by just one of these) and in a new pattern of child-headed households.

Households headed by a single woman are not uncommon in South Africa, particularly in the rural areas. This phenomenon has long established roots in the predominantly male migratory system and in a subsequent pattern of women seeking work in the cities for financial assistance and leaving their children with a grandmother or aunt. As the AIDS orphan population grows, child care has become even more the responsibility of single women – female grandparents and AIDS widows. And since in most rural communities it is women who also do the subsistence farming, the added burden of caring for AIDS orphans in turn exacerbates nutritional problems in these communities as it begins to have an impact on productive time for subsistence farming. Households like these are already vulnerable because of the limitation of economic opportunities for women, but the situation becomes even worse when traditional norms and customs so often see widows being severed from the extended family and denied access to land and housing.

'Skipped generation' households are likewise a long-established pattern, but these are both on the increase and taking on a new dimension as aging grandparents, usually the single grandmother, face the responsibility for dependent grandchildren orphaned by the HIV/AIDS epidemic. In the past children were frequently cared for by their grandparents because parents worked elsewhere and in certain cultures children born out of wedlock were customarily left with the maternal grandmother. The parent or parents nevertheless still retained contact with their child, but in the 'skipped generation' family unit of the HIV and AIDS epidemic this contact has gone.

For children who had lost both parents it was traditional for them to be absorbed by the extended family and cared for by aunts, uncles and grandparents – the general dictum was that there is no such thing as an orphan in Africa. But this is now also being eroded by the epidemic and relatives are unable, or no longer available, to cope with the rising number of AIDS orphans. And so a new type of 'family structure' emerges as an increasingly familiar pattern – the child-headed household where siblings are looked after by the eldest child.

The orphan challenge is an unfolding tragedy in which the erosion of family structures is set to continue for many years. Even if HIV infection rates drop, the number of orphans in southern Africa will continue to rise as parents and the heads of households continue to die of AIDS-related deaths. At the end of 1999 there were 14.6 million children globally under the age of 15 whose mothers had died of AIDS and of these children it is estimated that 1.5 million were HIV posi-tive. In South Africa the number of orphans under the age of 18 who have lost one or more parents is expected to peak around 2014 at an estimated level of 5.7 million. The extended families that would tradi-tionally have cared for these orphans are less and less able to do so as they are in turn financially and emotionally overburdened by the disease and so the traditions themselves break down and fade. In some situations orphans cared for by the extended family are treated as second-class family members, exploited by being given excessive household chores, forced to drop out of school to contribute to the added financial burden on the extended family, and subjected to physical and sexual abuse, with a string of knock-on consequences. The psychological impact of being abandoned increases the likelihood of these orphans ending up as school dropouts and street children, liable in turn to engage in antisocial behaviour and child prostitution with even greater risk to themselves of HIV infection and extended social instability over the long term.

The circle of silence, stigma, disenfranchised grief

By forcing the epidemic out of sight, HIV/AIDS-related stigma and discrimination obstruct disease prevention and treatment, and contaminate the resolution of personal grief.

> HIV/AIDS-related stigma comes from the powerful combination of shame and fear – shame because the sex or drug injecting that transmit HIV are surrounded by taboo and moral judgment, and fear because AIDS is relatively new, and considered deadly. Responding to AIDS with blame, or abuse towards people living with AIDS simply forces the epidemic underground, creating the ideal conditions for HIV to spread. The only way of making progress against the epidemic is to replace shame with solidarity, and fear with hope.
> *(Statement by Peter Piot, Executive Director UNAIDS, to Plenary of the World Conference against Racism, Racial Discrimination, Xenophobia and Related Intolerance, Durban, 5 September 2001.)*

Stigma has been a pervasive dimension of HIV/AIDS since the beginning of the pandemic. When first identified, HIV/AIDS was predominantly associated with socially ostracised groups such as male homosexuals and intravenous drug users. Though the disease has since infected individuals from all groups, the ostracism and stigma persists for those diagnosed with the disease. Stigma is an insidious, complicated phenomenon that feeds upon and reinforces and reproduces already present inequalities of class, race, gender and sexuality.

In South Africa, as elsewhere, stigma has gone hand in hand with discrimination. Discrimination against HIV-positive people hinges on a variety of perceptions and misconceptions of their gender, their race, their socioeconomic status, their HIV-positive status, and their sexuality. It has tangible consequences, such as segregation and denial of rights (to find or retain employment, to marry, to obtain life insurance), that may affect them at individual, community or societal level. Stigma induces discrimination, which induces violations of rights which in turn legitimise stigma and perpetuate the cycle.

Fear of stigma can produce extreme anxiety about sharing one's HIV status with others, and non-disclosure of HIV status is extremely common. People who do share their HIV or AIDS diagnosis with family or friends lay themselves open to stigmatisation (including reactions of fear, shock and blame), isolation (as a result of others' fears of casual transmission and the consequent likelihood of desertion), and potential loss of self-esteem. In South Africa, people who openly admit that they are HIV positive are often treated as outcasts, fired from their jobs, and sometimes even chased from their homes. In 1998, Gugu Dlamini, a woman in KwaZulu-Natal province, was beaten to death after she revealed her HIV status. Yet keeping the diagnosis of HIV a secret is very likely to hinder a person's ability to develop effective coping strategies, leaving them all the more vulnerable to fear, anger and depression. Nor will these problems fade for the infected individual as the progression of disease produces significant changes in behaviour, attitudes and physical appearance.

A crucial component of strategies to prevent new HIV infections is that persons at risk for HIV must have access to, and use, voluntary HIV counselling and testing. Care for HIV/AIDS cannot begin without the diagnosis of HIV infection and people who are infected and do not know it are more likely to engage in risky sexual practice and further spread the disease. Early diagnosis and induction into health care hold out obvious benefits to the individual and society – improved health and productivity, reduced hospitalisation costs, and decreased transmission from persons ignorant of their HIV status. And because most HIV-infected persons will probably adopt safer sexual behaviours after the diagnosis of HIV infection, raising the proportion of infected persons who know their serostatus is an important prevention goal. All of these objectives are compromised by the barriers of stigma and discrimination.

When people are afraid to speak openly about their HIV status there is, in effect, a climate of denial about the very existence of the epidemic. This discourages health-seeking behaviours among those who suspect they may already be infected with HIV and delayed health seeking after the onset of disease in turn increases debilitation and morbidity. Yet although the stigma of HIV/AIDS is tied to ignorance, informing people about the virus and the risk of HIV infection is not enough to eradicate it. Preventive education must also embrace serious education about discrimination, and at this level much still remains to be done. To challenge stigma and discrimination one must first understand the phenomenon, and reducing its influence entails wider confrontation with deep-seated cultural values and social attitudes. For communities to resist and take charge requires awareness raising, empowerment and community mobilisation that will give them the capacity to confront stigma and discrimination in relation not only to AIDS, but potentially also to other inequalities. Community awareness is fundamental to creating a climate that will foster self-understanding and encourage both individuals and groups to confront and process stigma. On the other hand, stigma is not a new problem in public health, nor is it unique to HIV/AIDS, but it does need to be addressed openly and measures that encourage general access to HIV testing will, by dissipating or diluting stigma, significantly strengthen HIV-prevention efforts.

To combat stigma and discrimination in the epidemic, community-based organisations (CBOs), NGOs, health service providers, community health workers and social services all need to work towards sensitising local communities to the needs of those affected by HIV/AIDS. Community mobilisation, advocacy and social change must go hand in hand with integrated interventions that make an impact on the broader context of people's lives. The greatest headway in addressing stigma and discrimination has always been made through the power and action of the community when people take ownership of the challenges that HIV/AIDS brings at a community level. UNAIDS lists a number of multi-pronged interventions to address stigma and discrimination for a more effective response to the HIV/AIDS epidemic:

- Community mobilisation and continuing advocacy with the support for social change of political and religious leaders in response to HIV/AIDS-related stigma and discrimination.
- Broad-based action to counteract gender, racial and sexual inequalities and stereotypes on which HIV/AIDS-related stigma and discrimination often feed.
- Promotion of life-skills education, risk-reduction counselling and support groups to help HIV-infected and affected individuals cope with stigmatisation in the home, school and community.
- Training and support for workplace initiatives, practical HIV-related training for health care workers and pre- and in-service training for teachers and religious leaders to promote better understanding and confidentiality and reduce unfound anxiety.
- Ensuring that comprehensive care services with community partnerships and advocacy are available to:
  - provide voluntary counselling and testing (VCT) with follow-up care that gives support to individuals when they learn their serostatus and enables them to disclose their status to important persons in their life

- raise awareness so that communities and women can access prevention of mother-to-child transmission care and support services and can hold government to account if these services are not available
- ensure there is concrete action for greater access to, and uptake of, treatment and drugs
- help people to understand that it is possible to live with HIV/AIDS and that treatment and wellness management promises real hope for the future; an important step in dissipating fear and anxiety about HIV/AIDS
- expand access to antiretrovirals – treatment itself significantly reduces stigma and discrimination; community fears lessen as HIV/AIDS increasingly comes to be seen both by health service providers and by the community as a manageable disease; and there is also a greater impact on prevention strategies and condom uptake when there is hope for a longer life.

Stigma and discrimination cruelly warp the lives of those infected with HIV/AIDS and their immediate caregivers, but death brings no further clarity to the widespread distortions of understanding. Most directly this is to be seen in the way that grief itself is perverted or suspended for those who survive – complexities that can best be described as the 'disenfranchisement' of grief.

Even in death communities remain locked in denial with all sorts of euphemisms being used to refer to an AIDS-related death: *'intsho-longwane'* (virus); *'hlengiwe ivy vilakazi'* (HIV); *'ugcunsula'* (sexually transmitted infections (STIs)); *'ubhubhane'* (the destroyer). It is also common for people to refer to AIDS deaths as the consequence of tuberculosis (TB), of 'being weak', of 'losing strength' and of bewitchment. Many factors complicate and compound the grief process among those who lose a significant other to an AIDS-associated death. In schools, teachers frequently encounter bereaved children, as well as having to cope with grief of their own at the death of a colleague, friend or family member. When, as often happens, they have neither the skills, nor the emotional or material resources to deal with these situations the processes of grief are simply disregarded. The aura of secrecy, stigma and social ambiguity that surrounds AIDS deaths leaves no pathway for the grieving process to follow. The immediate bereaved are left unsupported to confront a bewilderment of pain, sadness and fear, shunned, very often, by family and friends and by community or social networks because of the generalised uncertainty and fear that veil an AIDS-related death.

Disenfranchised grief can be said to occur when the loss is not socially recognised because of certain dimensions of that loss – for the griever, stigma and isolation intensify when they block public recognition of an AIDS-related death and consequently, too, the traditional practices and customs, the mourning rituals, which would normally channel the expression of sorrow and communal solidarity and foster the restorative process of grieving. With deaths from AIDS not socially sanctioned, they are left cloaked in a kind of 'invisibility' and the unrecognised 'hidden grief' can paradoxically intensify the loss and subvert the grieving process. Grief is in effect displaced by embarrassment and shame, and the closed circle of silence, stigma and disenfranchised loss is perpetuated and intensified.

In the context of AIDS, grief can be disenfranchised when:

- The elderly, children or young adults are socially defined as incapable of grieving. These grievers are not socially recognised.
- The cause of death is hidden or denied from others for fear of rejection or discrimination.
- The relationship is not be publicly recognised or socially sanctioned such as the partnership in a gay relationship, an extramarital partnership, a common law partnership, or in polygamous relationships.
- Caregivers hide their grief or disassociate themselves from the AIDS sufferer because of their own fear of rejection or discrimination and the stigma that extends to caring for those dying of AIDS.

Reducing the erosion

First impact

The impact on the family and community starts either when the parent and/or head of the household, or the child, is diagnosed with HIV or when that person becomes obviously ill with advancing disease. Either way, this is a juncture at which the psychosocial needs of the family too often go unrecognised. Parents, siblings and family members need support and advice in discussing difficult issues. Community volunteers, teachers and faith-based leaders can give them that support if they are trained in communication about the complex issues that embrace the HIV/AIDS epidemic. Community care and support services need to be provided for the ill parent or child and for the primary caregiver and future guardian.

Reinforcing support networks: Family, school, society

Older children can benefit from disclosure and honesty about parental illness and a top priority should be to prolong the child – parent relationship for as long as possible. The eldest child is usually most affected as the one who assumes the parental role when the parent becomes sick; their education invariably suffers as they stay away from school to do household chores and care for the sickly parent and siblings. In these situations it is imperative to link the parents and children to a PLHA (persons living with HIV and AIDS) support group as early as possible in the process.

The morale of children affected by HIV and AIDS can be raised through the provision of recreational activities and most especially by keeping them in school. Consistent schooling supports children's morale and preserves a degree of equilibrium in their lives during difficult transition periods; recreational activities integrate children with their peers and enhance their general wellbeing. On a policy level there is a strong case for reconsidering primary and secondary school fees for the children of AIDS-affected families and for subsidisation of uniforms, text books and school materials to mitigate the psychosocial and financial impact on them. Schools also have to be recognised as having a very important role in combating stigma and discrimination by preserving the peer integration of AIDS orphans and children living with HIV and AIDS.

Life prolonging care and support services (eg antiretrovirals and home-based community care) for the sick adult can minimise the effect on children living in the household, improving their access to school and delaying their orphanhood. Such services need to include assessment of the children's material needs for daily living and education and assistance in getting access to relevant social grants and support facilities. This also means embracing proactive succession planning – community workers and social services have an important role to play in engaging future guardians in family planning and dialogue in ways that give the children opportunities to acclimatise to the new circumstances of guardianship that lie ahead for them.

Local social and community networks invariably provide the greatest proportion of day-to-day care for vulnerable families and children. But as the epidemic escalates the burden of care grows ever heavier and local efforts by local CBOs, NGOs and community care workers will need to be reinforced by continued capacity building and support from more broadly established social services, faith-based organisations and the like. Community development that extends access to clean and safe water, food, health care, legal advice and psychosocial support needs to be integrated into all HIV/AIDS care and support initiatives. Lawyers, for example, with paralegals and trained volunteers, can run workshops to teach both men and women to write effective wills. And there will need to be mobilisation of communities and community leaders to uphold the property rights of women and children.

Rebuilding the social fabric 1: AIDS orphans and custodians of care

Many children affected by AIDS are left abandoned and vulnerable and in need of intervention for care and support. The possible sources of intervention will be the local community, civil society, and government. The fundamental objective for intervention will be to mobilise community-based responses that create an enabling environment for affected children and their caregivers; strengthening the capacity of the extended family, of child-headed households and of social networks and ensuring the provision of social services, social security and grants by government. In setting priorities for the care of orphaned children, interventions should take their lead in the first instance from the immediate community, but guidelines consolidated from a wide range of international sources emphasise the need for proactive community interventions including succession planning to lessen the social impact on the family at the time of death. The 1997 and 2000 editions of *Children on the Brink* include five basic strategies to care for children affected by HIV/AIDS. They have policy and programme implications for governments, faith-based organisations, NGOs, CBOs and communities:

- strengthen the capacity of families, extended family and community to cope with the increasing number of orphans
- strengthen and mobilise community-based responses
- increase the capacity of children and young people to care for themselves by meeting their own needs through access to quality education, and protection from exploitation and excessive labour
- create an enabling environment for children and families by ensuring their basic legal protection through laws and policies, decreasing stigma and discrimination, and increasing behaviour change interventions
- extend child protective services.

In South Africa the responsibility of state agencies is underlined by the Constitution; this lays specific obligations on government to secure to every child the right to family, parental care, or to appropriate alternative care when the child is removed from the family or no longer has a family environment and the right to basic nutrition, shelter, health care services, social development and education. It makes the best interests of the child paramount in every matter that affects and concerns that child.

Models of care

Radical thinking is needed when seeking to ensure care for children orphaned and abandoned by the AIDS epidemic, and there are various models of care:

Orphanages/residential care

Orphanages/residential care are generally not considered as the first line of response to the crisis as they have limited capacity and are difficult to sustain and they cost considerably more per child than good community-based support. Long-term institutionalised care separates children from family and social networks and is not in general conducive to healthy childhood development. It can exacerbate stigma and discrimination and is liable to encourage dependency and impede socialisation. Nevertheless these homes are needed in certain instances to serve as an interim respite or while alternative arrangements are being sought.

Child-headed households

The AIDS epidemic forces many young adolescents into drastically premature parenting roles, depriving them of their own childhood and thrusting upon them the responsibilities of caregiver and guardian. Struggling as they often do to keep their families intact, there are likely to be life skills that they urgently need to be taught. Siblings left to depend on one another for support may experience intensified feelings of family unity and loyalty to family roots, but equally the resolution of grief can be critical for children who head households while still overwhelmed and angry. They are consequently prone to transfer their anger to their younger siblings. The difficulties that the eldest sibling can encounter, and the inevitable sacrifices, are liable to be considerable and they need to be acknowledged. It is very important for child-headed households to be identified for sound community and social support.

The extended family

Here a family member is identified to care for the children after the death of the parents. Often this will be a grandparent who was previously dependent on the financial support of the deceased, but the model nevertheless lends itself to creative initiatives. One such is the initiative dubbed 'Go-go grannies' (*ugogo*: 'grandmother' in Zulu) which is part of the Alexandra AIDS Orphan Project in Alexandra Township north of Johannesburg. This project provides psychosocial, financial and material support to thirty grandmothers and includes one-off building grants to ensure that the 'expanded' family has adequate shelter, and also seeds and fertiliser so that they can generate both food and income from their nutritional garden.

The surrogate parent

The surrogate parent model places an adult/adults in the home of orphaned children. This model can benefit both the children and the adult if, for instance, the adult has previously been living in the poorest of housing (mud or shack) and now moves in with children who have better quality accommodation.

Foster care

In South Africa child fostering is culturally well sanctioned and a long-established practice, with biological parents (one or both) allowing the child to be raised by another adult, usually a grandparent. This was a recourse forced upon many black families by the conditions of racial segregation and migrant labour where parents living in rural and underdeveloped communities were (and still are) forced by financial exigency to move to the cities to seek employment. Rural parents may also place their children in the home of an urban family member where educational opportunities appear greater. For young children, the strength of the kinship structure that develops is likely to matter more than the location of the foster parent. Fostered children are socialised and integrated into society more readily than children who are in orphanages/residential care as family integration promotes psychological and social development.

Cluster foster care

Here a surrogate mother is hired to care for up to six orphans in the community. If possible, housing is provided and they live together as a family unit. Foster grants are accessed and the mother may receive a small stipend. The cluster foster care replaces the traditional orphanage.

Child care committees/community care committees – the collective approach

Where possible the priority should be to keep siblings together. Child care committees overseeing a clearly defined geographical area give support to orphaned siblings so that they can be left in their own home with a sibling old enough to provide supervision. In this way the expertise of different community-based organisations and individuals is pooled for a collective response to orphan care. These committees provide a supportive network that keeps check on school attendance, oversees the children's homework, makes sure they have a nutritional meal each day and monitors their health and their recreational activities. The child care committee also accesses and administers the child support grant. Strict monitoring and external auditing of these committees are critical to protect the children's interest.

The possibilities here can be illustrated in the example of the Community Child Care Committees, supported by the Thandanani Children's Foundation's Development Programme, which operates in seven areas of the Msunduzi Municipality (Pietermaritzburg). The interventions engaged in by the 80 community volunteers who serve on these committees include daily home visits of children in distress to provide nurturing, love, guidance and supervision with the primary goal being to keep siblings together.

Adoption

Formal adoption is intended to provide the child with new parents and an opportunity to be integrated into a family unit. Adopted children gain the security of having the same rights and privileges as other children in the adoptive family, with the adoptive parent bearing equal responsibility for both their biological and their adoptive children. But this is not a familiar concept in cultures where the care of orphaned children has been accommodated naturally through customary practices. For formal adoption to be accepted as a care option communities will need to be educated to modify traditional mechanisms. The stigma attached to HIV/AIDS presents a major deterrent to adoption.

Rebuilding the social fabric 2: Structural interventions

Many of those affected by HIV/AIDS, both children and adults, will become dependent on the state to provide them with shelter, care and support. The South African Constitution guarantees the right to social assistance to vulnerable groups in society, or those unable to take care of their own or their families' basic needs. The Department of Social Development is constitutionally responsible for the financial, emotional and psychosocial care of those made vulnerable by HIV/AIDS and currently provides social services to alleviate the impact of the disease through three main delivery channels. **Social assistance and social welfare** services provide financial assistance to public and private sector institutions such as homes for orphaned children. **The social development or poverty relief programme** facilitates social change based on community initiatives. This programme (still often referred to in rural communities as 'RDP', although the original government Reconstruction and Development Programme of the mid-nineties has now fallen away) seeks to provide income support through income-generating projects to those groups of vulnerable populations not covered by the security net. **Social security** cash grants include pensions for the aged and the severely disabled and child support for poor and orphaned children.

Additional state policy will still need to be implemented to protect the most vulnerable and ensure provision of essential services. Considerations that need to be taken into account in implementation programme design include the following:

- **Strengthening the care and coping capacities of families and communities:** The first line of response to meet the needs of children affected by HIV/AIDS comes from extended families. When these cannot cope, the task is to strengthen the capacity of communities to fill the gaps in the safety net traditionally provided by the extended family. Cluster fostering, surrogate caring and adoption may be the most efficient, cost-effective and sustainable ways of assisting orphans and other vulnerable children. Families and communities also play a crucial role in identifying children who are most in need, both those affected by HIV/AIDS and other vulnerable children.

- **Children and youth as part of the solution, not the problem:** Children themselves are an important resource in mobilising a community response: actively involving children in care initiatives can build their sense of self-esteem and efficacy and cultivate skills they can use in the future.

- **Building collaboration and advocacy into community initiatives:** To meet the needs of children affected by HIV/AIDS, there need to be broad networks and targeted advocacy to involve government, civil society, and NGOs in shared initiatives of community action for orphans and other vulnerable children.

- **Long-term perspective:** Children in South Africa will continue to be affected by AIDS for decades to come. The scale of the epidemic demands that programmes be sustainable and replicable. Although material and financial assistance are important, it is equally necessary to ensure that community projects are driven by community ownership and responsibility.

- **Integration with other services:** Care for children affected by HIV/AIDS should start at the earliest possible moment as their problems begin well before the death of their parents. These children are themselves at high risk of HIV infection due to economic hardship and the absence of parental care, support and protection. Services for vulnerable children should be integrated into a comprehensive package that includes voluntary counselling and testing for HIV, prevention interventions and care for those living with HIV/AIDS along with corresponding support delivered through the Department of Social Development and Department of Education.

Legal assistance

Legal mechanisms such as wills, foster care and social grants are foreign concepts for many communities, particularly those in rural areas. Ill parents often do not know that they can name guardians for their children prior to death. Education programmes can do much to inform communities about the legal implications of death – such as how to write a will – and as part of all post VCT services, counsellors should be trained to guide and assist their clients in handling these matters. In particular there is still widespread ignorance of the financial support available to communities, families and individuals affected by HIV/AIDS and education programmes are urgently needed to make people aware of the grants that they may be legally eligible for (and also of hurdles that can confront them in accessing these entitlements): See FIGURE 23.1.

- **Foster care grant.**
  Children who have been placed in the care of foster parents, through the courts, can access the Foster Care Grant. While the financial assistance from this grant can ease the burden on the foster parent to qualify, the child needs to be placed in foster care through the Children's Court, which can be a very lengthy process.
- **Child(minder) support grant**
  Children who pass the means test in terms of income can access the child support grant though their caregiver.
- **Care dependency grant**
  Adults and children so sick from HIV/AIDS that they are looked after full time at home are eligible for the care dependency grant. Persons with full-blown AIDS whose CD4 count falls below 200 qualify for this grant. However, they have to be declared 'in need' by a medical doctor and then apply to the nearest social development office. Many individuals do not have easy access to a doctor or to the Social Development Office and may not have the money for transport.
- **Disability grant**
  Adults diagnosed with WHO Stage 4 AIDS are entitled to a disability grant. The roll-out of antiretrovirals complicates access to this grant as once the condition of the individual improves and the CD4 count rises, the individual no longer qualifies for a disability grant.

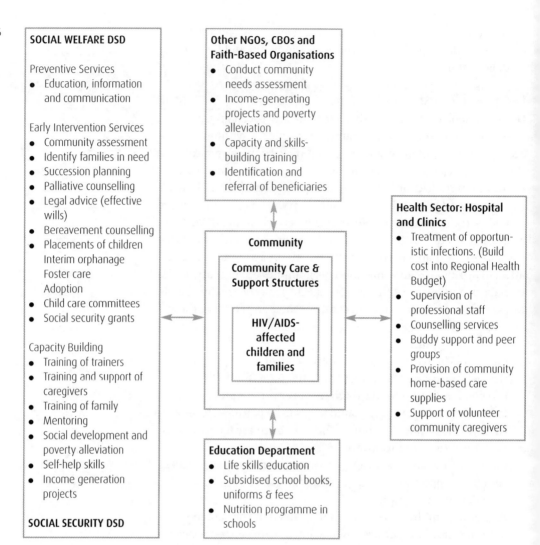

FIGURE 23.1 Community-Driven Model for integrated support of those families and children affected by HIV and AIDS. *Department of Social Development Community Driven Model. As adapted 2002*

A number of difficulties remain to be resolved in providing satisfactory access to these grants. There can be long delays before grants are approved, which seriously erodes the maximisation of benefit for the applicant. Many child-headed households struggle to access grants because they are headed by a minor.

Psychosocial resolution

The stigma attached to HIV and AIDS is a major barrier to families, friends and communities being able to speak freely about the multitude of feelings, fears and concerns the disease provokes. For this reason there is much to be said for promoting activities and projects

explicitly designed to stimulate and support emotional or psychological resolution.

Family memorabilia and shared anecdotes can be valuable starting
points for stimulating open discussion and disclosure and focused
planning for the future. One successful device for generating and
encouraging these has been the Memory Box Project, the central
theme of which is living positively with HIV/AIDS. Although the
Memory Box idea started as a bereavement-counselling tool it now
also includes focusing on the lives and stories of those currently living
with HIV or AIDS. Through facilitated workshops and group work the
heroic struggles of HIV-positive people are illustrated through words,
pictures, compiling a story book or creating a box container that
reflects their story. Memory 'boxes' or 'books' reflect different aspects
of the PLHA's family history, lifestyle, culture and beliefs. The project
may include skills-building workshops in creative writing techniques
to capture the description of the life of the PLHA. Videos can also be
created that capture singing, dancing and voices with messages that
can be reflected on in the future. Facing the possibility of death,
workshops can also focus on the practicalities of writing a will and
detailing ones hopes and wishes for children who are likely to be
orphaned. Memory boxes capture the personal and private journeys
both of the PLHA and of his or her family and assist all of them in
planning and shaping the future. Constructing and assembling a
memory box stimulates the kind of interaction among families,
communities and individuals through which stigma and discrimination can be most productively addressed and it also creates suitable
opportunities for realistic discussion and planning of future support.
Strong bonds with the deceased and the conscious decision to hold
on to their memory gives support to the grieving process and can do
much to ameliorate the disenfranchisement of grief that so often
threatens the bereaved in the bigotry that surrounds the AIDS
epidemic.

Another means to rebuilding the social fabric of traumatised
families and communities has been through making banners or
quilts. When family members, friends and community gather to sew
a banner or quilt they simultaneously weave a tapestry of stories and
recollections of courage, fear and anger of those who have struggled
against HIV and AIDS and whose memory is now enshrined. The AIDS
memorial quilt is a living memorial to those who have died of AIDS.
The South African contribution to this international project was
initiated in Cape Town in September 1989 by the NAMES Project
Foundation and continues to be promoted through organisations
such as DramAidE in KwaZulu-Natal (www.und.ac.za/und/dramaide/
aidsquilt.htm).

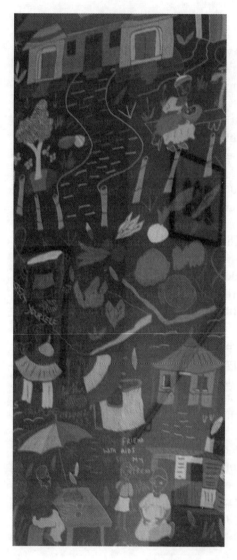

The goals of the AIDS memorial quilt project are:

- to provide a creative visual symbol of remembrance and healing for those whose lives have been affected by HIV/AIDS
- to illustrate the enormity of the AIDS epidemic
- to increase public awareness of AIDS and promote a greater understanding of the impact and effect that HIV/AIDS has on our lives
- to assist with HIV prevention and education and provide a starting point for action
- to acknowledge the lives that have lived behind the statistics
- to honour those who have died of AIDS and remember their dreams
- to reduce hostility and discrimination against people living with HIV/AIDS.

The importance of communities

From an early stage of the HIV/AIDS epidemic there has been recognition of the central role of community interventions in providing education, care, counselling and support. A mass, concerted response to the epidemic has to be driven through collaborative interaction between local community-based organisations, and larger public and private sector partnerships. Community care-driven intervention, taking the form of volunteer or community driven home and community-based support services represents the most fundamental of those integrated partnerships. The challenge will be to sustain the continuous nurture, renewal and innovation it needs to serve a complex and evolving epidemic environment.

Time to curb the untold suffering

AIDS is accomplishing a sweeping undoing of the liberation of the South African people in their new democracy and the advances made in the social upliftment and development of the country. Access to health services and care, as well as education are once again being undermined and the fabric of society is being threatened as a future generation of AIDS orphans mature in the absence of parents and family support structures. To address the social impact of HIV and

AIDS on the family, children and orphans there needs to be targeted advocacy and broad networks to mobilise and involve government, civil society, CBOs and NGOs in shared initiatives of community action. While the epidemic has been unfolding, the fight against AIDS has been substantially underresourced and financed by government at both national and provincial level, as well as by the donor community. Humanity demands an expanded effort in addressing the social implications of the epidemic and provide opportunities for new forms of solidarity.

More than ten years ago in 1990 Chris Hani who was tragically assassinated shortly before democracy was achieved said, 'We cannot afford to allow the AIDS epidemic to ruin the realisation of our dreams. Existing statistics indicate that we are still at the beginning of the AIDS epidemic in our country. Unattended, however, this will result in untold damage and suffering by the end of the century.' As a country, as communities and as individuals we are now experiencing the suffering. It is vital that the public sector, private sector and civil society act as one voice in directing their attentions to creating capacity that intervenes on the social impact of HIV and AIDS to curb the untold suffering of the South African people.

Bibliography

ABDOOL KARIM Q ABDOOL KARIM SS. 'The evolving HIV epidemic in South Africa'. *International Journal of Epidemiology* 2002; 31: 37–40.

ADAMS J, CLAASENS M, DIKWENI L, STREAK J. *Responding to the HIV/AIDS Pandemic in the Department of Social Development.* IDASA. Johannesburg. 1–34. www.welfare.gov.za. 2001

ASPAAS HR. 'AIDS and orphans in Uganda. Geographical and gender interpretations of household resources'. *Social Science Journal* 1999; 36: 201–206.

ATTARAN A, SACHS J. 'Defining and refining international donor support for combating the AIDS epidemic'. *Lancet* 2001; 357: 57–61.

BUSZA, JR. 'Promoting the positive: Responses to stigma and discrimination in Southeast Asia'. *AIDS Care* 2001; 13: 441–456.

CDC. 'HIV-Related Knowledge and Stigma – United States, 2000'. *Morbidity and Mortality Weekly Report* 2000; 49: 1062–1065.

FESKO L. 'Disclosure of HIV Status in the Workplace'. *Health and Social Work* 2001; 26: 235–245.

FOSTER G. 'Supporting community efforts to assist orphans in Africa'. *New England Journal of Medicicine* 2002; 346: 1907–1910.

GILBORN LZ, NYONYINTONO R, KABUMBULI R, JAGWE-WADDA. *'Making a difference for children affected by AIDS'.* Baseline findings from operations in Uganda. Populations Council. 2001. 1–33.

GOVERNMENT OF SOUTH AFRICA. 1996. *The Constitution of South Africa.* Pretoria. Government Printer.

HUNTER S, WILLIAMSON J. *Children on the brink: Strategies to support children isolated by HIV and AIDS.* USAID. Washington D.C. 1997.

HUNTER S, WILLIAMSON J. *'Children on the brink.'* USAID. Washington D.C. 2000.

JOHNSON L, DORRINGTON R. *'The impact of AIDS on Orphanhood in South Africa: A Quantitative Analysis'.* Centre for Actuarial Research. University of Cape Town. Care Monograph No. 4. 2001.

MARCUS T. 2002. *'Wo! Zaphela Izingane. Living and dying with AIDS'.* Johannesburg: Blesston Printing.

PARKER R, AGGLETON P. 'HIV and AIDS-related stigma and discrimination: A conceptual framework and implications for action'. *Social Science and Medicine* 2003; 57: 13–24.

RUSSEL M, SCHNEIDER H. Models of community-based HIV/AIDS care and support'. In Ntulia et al (Eds), South Africa. Durban Health Systems Trust. *Health Review* 2000; 327–333.

STRODE A, NONKOSI DEVELOPMENT SERVICES. 2003. *'The Nature and Extent of Problems Facing Child Headed Households within the Thandani Programme'.* Thandanani Childrens Foundation. Pietermaritzburg.

THOMAS K. 'Memory box project'. *AIDS Bulletin* 2001; 10: 17–20.

UNAIDS. *AIDS Epidemic update.* Geneva. UNAIDS, December 2002

UNAIDS. *A conceptual framework and basis for action. HIV/AIDS stigma and discrimination.* World aids Campaign 2002–2003. Geneva. 2003.

UNAIDS. *Report of the global AIDS epidemic: 4th Global Report.* Geneva. UNAIDS. 2004.

CHAPTER 24

The achilles heel? The impact of HIV/AIDS on democracy in South Africa

Mark Heywood

THE POLITICAL HISTORY OF HIV/AIDS in South Africa is one of controversy and denial. General opinion is that while the South African government has acknowledged that control and treatment of HIV is a national priority, they have been slow to put in place the programmes required to implement this. In the late 1980s and early 1990s several seroprevalence surveys showed that HIV had not yet established a firm hold in the country. HIV infection was detected among a relatively small number of people with identified high-risk behaviours, including men who have sex with men, and migrant workers. During this time, the ANC, COSATU and the UDF all realised the potential threat represented by HIV and took concrete steps to try to contain it. However, by the mid-1990s, HIV infection had begun to assume epidemic proportions, rising from a prevalence of 0.7% to 7.6%.

By 1999, the end of the first term of the newly elected democratic government, HIV prevalence had risen to 22.4%. There was little co-ordinated governmental effort to contain the epidemic prior to 1994. However, during Nelson Mandela's presidency, greater resources were made available for HIV and a new sexually transmitted infections unit was set up in the Department of Health. But, because this was still regarded as a health matter rather than a political priority, these measures did little to contain the spread of HIV.

The election of the second democratic government saw a shift in perspectives on HIV, both from government and within society. President Thabo Mbeki publicly questioned both the link between HIV and AIDS and the statistics showing rising morbidity and mortality resulting from the virus. The effects of this phase in South Africa's history of HIV/AIDS management are far reaching and have arguably had a negative impact on the development of the country's young democracy.

The prevention of HIV infection is one of the areas in which post-1994 South Africa has not succeeded. This is not sufficiently acknowledged by the South African government. Whilst there is some acknowledgement that control and treatment of HIV is a national priority, the government has not put in place the infrastructure, institutions or programmes with sufficient authority or reach to really make a dent on the incidence of new HIV infections or the overall growth of the epidemic.

Regrettably, this extends to the lack of proper acknowledgement of how the HIV epidemic will negatively impact on South Africa's ambitious programme of reconstruction and development and its quest for racial and social equity. This is amply evident in *Towards a 10-Year Review*, a document published in October 2003 by the Government Communication and Information Services (GCIS) assessing South Africa's progress after ten years. In the section dealing with health (pp 20–25) the Review admits that HIV prevalence increased from 0.7% in 1990 to 26.5% in 2002. But then optimistically, and without any supporting evidence, it claims that HIV prevalence rates 'seem to be stabilising between 1999 and 2002'. The Review also admits to 'about 400 000 people at an advanced stage of AIDS' (p 23), but does not discuss or give any further statistics on AIDS-related morbidity, mortality or the present or future impact of AIDS on development. This is not because there is no such evidence. Indeed, there is a wealth of analysis and evidence, including information generated by Statistics SA, the government's official body, which estimated accumulated AIDS deaths up to 2004 to be 1.49-million people.

The government's at times highly controversial response to HIV/AIDS in South Africa and its failure to act decisively and with conviction in implementing programmes that prevent or treat HIV infection by using antiretroviral drugs has drawn much national and international criticism. This chapter traces the outline of the political history of the response to HIV and AIDS in South Africa.

The beginnings of an epidemic

Several HIV seroprevalence studies undertaken in the late 1980s have demonstrated that the epidemic had not taken root and become established in the South African population generally. During this period, HIV infection was detected among small numbers of people but was confined to people with specific high-risk behaviours (such as men who have sex with men and sex workers) or immigrants from African countries where the HIV epidemic had already reached a more advanced stage. For example, in 1986, the largest HIV prevalence survey conducted up to that point found only 0.02% prevalence among South Africa mine workers, but a disproportionately higher prevalence (3.76%) in mine workers originating from Malawi. The same year, a survey of 1200 women, including 94 women believed to be sex workers, also demonstrated a 0% HIV prevalence. However, whilst HIV prevalence might have remained low throughout the 1980s, the social and political conditions that would facilitate the rapid growth of the epidemic in the 1990s were inherent to the political and economic system that was developed under apartheid. Some of the economic prerequisites for an explosive epidemic were the migrant labour system and the place of the mining industry generally in the economy. Thus in 1991, Jochelson et al warned with terrible prescience that:

> ... it appears that the migrant labour system has institution-alised a geographic network of relationships for spreading STDs. This network suggests that once HIV enters the hetero-sexual mining community it will spread into the immediate urban area, to surrounding urban areas, from urban to rural areas, within rural areas, and across national boundaries.

Political prerequisites for an explosive spread of HIV infection included the denial of access to health care services to millions of people on the basis of their race. In addition apartheid, and colonialism before it, had reinforced traditions of patriarchy and gender inequality. These systems facilitated the exploitation of African labour and rapid economic growth; they would also later facilitate the rapid transmission of HIV.

Thus, as predicted, between 1990 and 1994 (the first five years of annual antenatal surveillance), HIV entered and established a foothold in the population with prevalence beginning to rise from 0.7% to 7.6%. These years, between the release of Nelson Mandela in 1990 and South Africa's first democratic election in 1994, were politically charged and turbulent. However, despite the political volatility, it is significant that both the African National Congress (ANC) after its return from exile and the internal progressive movement that formed around the United Democratic Front (UDF) and the Congress of South African Trade Unions (COSATU) recognised the potential threat posed by HIV and proposed policies and actions to contain it. In its last years in exile, the ANC Health Department initiated a number of programmes on HIV, including the development of a video to alert its cadres to the threat of AIDS. In April 1990 a conference between the exiled ANC and internal progressive organisations to discuss this looming threat took place in Maputo. Upon their return to South Africa, the now unbanned ANC worked with health activists who had been aligned with the UDF, such as the South African Health Workers

Congress (SAHWCO) and the National medical and Dental Association (NAMDA), and with other parts of civil society, to develop a plan to contain the epidemic.

This is evident in the key policy documents of this period. The most advanced of these was the plan developed by the National AIDS Convention of South Africa (NACOSA), which was a multi-dimensional proposal that dealt with education, human rights and prevention and treatment. Importantly, in addition to AIDS-specific plans, HIV was listed as a priority in political programmes related to the post-apartheid period. On HIV/AIDS the *Reconstruction and Development Programme*, the ANC's main election policy document, promised:

> A programme to combat the spread of sexually transmitted diseases (STDS) and AIDS must include the active and early treatment of these diseases at all health facilities, plus mass education programmes which involve the mass media, schools and community organisations. The treatment of AIDS sufferers and those testing HIV positive must be with the utmost respect for their continuing contributions to society. Discrimination will not be tolerated. AIDS education for rural communities, and especially for women, is a priority. (Para 2.12.8)

Similarly the ANC's programme on health reform, *A National Plan for Health*, which was developed through a broad consultative process that included the World Health Organisation (WHO) made specific reference to the looming threat of HIV, stating:

> HIV/AIDS is emerging as a major public health problem, with over 2000 reported cases at the end of 1993, and 500 000 people infected with HIV. Forecasts to the year 2000 predict that there will be between four and seven million HIV-positive cases, with about 60% of total deaths due to AIDS, if HIV prevention and control measures remain unaddressed. Similarly, credible predictions indicate that by the year 2005, between 18% and 24% of the adult population will be infected with HIV, that the cumulative death toll will be 2.3 million, and that there will be 1.5 million AIDS orphans.

The envisaged response to HIV was set out in great detail in the Health Plan, (pp 27–29). Significantly, in view of the manner in which the ANC would later resist providing treatment to people with AIDS, the Plan was steadfast about the rights of people with HIV to medical treatment, when it declared that it was

> ... mandatory to define prevention and control interventions plus comprehensive care for those already infected, within the context of the Bill of Rights.

At this early point of the epidemic, the government-in-waiting had clearly articulated its conviction that HIV/AIDS was a human rights issue and not just a health issue; it had also recognised the social dimensions of the epidemic and the depth of stigma and discrimination that was associated with responses to people living with HIV. A 'Charter of Rights on HIV' which had been developed by the AIDS consortium, was supported by the major political parties and their leaders including Nelson Mandela, Mangosotho Buthelezi and the late Chris Hani. This charter became a road-map to the development of some of the world's most progressive legislation and jurisprudence on non-discrimination and HIV, being the foundation of two Constitutional Court judgments on the rights of people with HIV to non-discrimination in employment and of access to health care services. Support for integrating a human rights approach to HIV/AIDS was also supported by several other organisations. In 1992, at the instigation of Justice Edwin Cameron, the Centre for Applied Legal Studies established the AIDS Consortium, and later the AIDS Law Project, to tackle these issues. Further, the National Progressive Primary Health Care Network had established a national effort to involve communities in dealing with HIV/AIDS, and NACOSA had established itself as a loose coalition of organisations and individuals committed to tackling AIDS in a coordinated manner, thereby laying the foundations for the creation of a multi-sectoral national social movement against AIDS.

Thus, it seemed at this stage, that South Africa was well poised to tackle HIV/AIDS under a democratic government.

The response of the first democratic government

After South Africa's first democratic election in 1994, the ANC came to power as part of a coalition with the then National Party, known as the Government of National Unity (GNU). In 1994, with antenatal prevalence at 7.6%, it was clear that urgent and decisive action to translate statements of intention (described above) were needed to avert the epidemic from entering a phase of exponential growth that saw HIV prevalence rise to 22.4% by 1999, the end of the term of the first democratic government.

It is important to make it explicit here that the rapidly escalating HIV epidemic was not due to the onset of democracy or a change in government. In 2004, FW De Klerk, who was South African President from 1984 to 1994, told a conference in South Africa that before 1994 his health minister had already drawn up a detailed action plan on AIDS which was left to gather dust because 'anything from the apartheid era was somehow or other contaminated'. However, prior to 1994 the HIV prevention strategies of the National Party were at best half-hearted and at worst, overtly discriminatory.

By contrast, under the government of Nelson Mandela, greater resources were immediately made available for HIV prevention and a dedicated HIV/AIDS and sexually transmitted diseases unit was set up within the new Department of Health. Within months of the new government taking office the NACOSA plan was adopted as the official government plan. But despite these promising signs, in practice, the issue of HIV control was relegated to the status of a health matter rather than a political priority. Nelson Mandela himself, who became one of the world's most outspoken AIDS activists after he had stepped down as president, admitted much later that he had not wanted to discuss issues of sex and could have done more on HIV/AIDS during his presidency.

Unfortunately, however, this was not just a period of omission and an absence of political determination, but also one that saw the beginnings of conflict and confusion about the most appropriate response. In 1996, for example, there was a public and damaging controversy around the Department of Health's funding of the play 'Sarafina 2'. In addition to criticism of the play's flawed messaging and its cost, there were also allegations of unlawful tendering that led to an investigation by the Public Protector and the Parliamentary Portfolio Committee on Health.

This was followed by a damaging dispute over the substance virodene, which researchers from the University of Pretoria publicly claimed, with the support of the Cabinet of the South African government, to be a cure for AIDS. Sadly, this was not the case. But the political crisis around this quack cure was more damaging than the claim itself, after an investigation by the Department of Health and the University of Pretoria reported that the virodene researchers had violated basic ethical principles and government regulatory procedures governing clinical trials on human beings and had had privileged access to the Cabinet to present their 'research'.

These two major crises were followed by several smaller ones, including the public conflict over whether AIDS (not HIV) should be made a notifiable illness. The effect of these disputes was to detract attention and effort to secondary issues, whilst the crucial issues of HIV prevention and programmes to tackle the known social determinants of a growing HIV epidemic received insufficient attention.

The response of the second democratic government

Significantly, prior to 1999, there was no loud clamoring from civil society for a better response to the HIV/AIDS epidemic. Between 1994 and 1999, the HIV epidemic was growing exponentially but remained largely invisible because of the low levels of HIV-related mortality and high levels of stigma and discrimination. During the electioneering for the second democratic elections in 1999, the HIV/AIDS epidemic did not feature as one of the country's main priorities. This was in spite of a resolution of the ANC's 50th Congress in 1997, which had noted that 'the AIDS epidemic will massively impact on the economy, will impact socially with more orphans and the loss of breadwinners, and on the health service with additional new users.' The Congress had resolved:

> The message about AIDS awareness be included in political speeches of our entire leadership, with a pledge to fight the disease.

By 1999, South Africa was witnessing the growing reality of AIDS morbidity and mortality. As a result, civil society organisations such as faith-based and labour organisations became more vigourous in calling for more concerted action on AIDS, supported by the activism of groups such as the Treatment Action Campaign which had been launched in December 1998.

In 1999, Thabo Mbeki was elected President of South Africa. During the second ANC government, a significant shift in perspectives on HIV took place both in government and society. Whereas the first democratic government had effectively relegated HIV/AIDS to a matter for the Department of Health, the second democratic government inadvertently turned HIV/AIDS into a political issue.

When South Africa's national antenatal HIV prevalence was announced by government to be 22.4% in 1999, the HIV epidemic was – as is the routine course of epidemics of infectious diseases – coming out of its phase of exponential growth and demonstrating a continued rise in numbers of people infected but at a lower rate than was witnessed between 1994 and 1999. The response of the new government, however, was to question the accuracy of the statistics and for the first time, to justify inaction on key fronts of HIV prevention and treatment on a number of political and pseudo-scientific grounds.

By late 1999, a political debate was sparked over what should be an appropriate response to AIDS, as a direct result of growing demands for access to medical interventions that could either assist with HIV prevention, such as antiretroviral drugs that reduce the risk of mother-to-child transmission, or for access to treatment for people already infected with HIV. Ironically, at this point South Africa's government and civil society moved almost simultaneously onto two diametrically opposed paths.

In the years since 1999, the differences over AIDS policy have shifted, but the responses by government have shown thematic consistency. What has been common throughout all these responses has been an attempt to create a set of artificially juxtaposed positions between what government says it considers to be a priority and what it caricatures to be the demands of civil society, including the health professions. The most notable of these juxtapositions are:

- between HIV prevention (said to be government's priority) and treatment (said to be the priority of a range of others)
- between tackling poverty (government's priority) and tackling HIV (again the priority of a range of others)
- between providing poor people with basic nutrition (government's priority) and medicines (allegedly the priority of a range of others).

More recently, the President of South Africa and other officials have tried to insert further artificial juxtapositions into the debate, most notably between western medicines and traditional medicines; and between white people (who are allegedly using HIV as a convenient signifier to stereotype black people) and black people (who are resisting claims to be HIV infected because of being 'amoral, sexually depraved, animalistic, savage and rapist' as part of the global resistance against racism).

While the underpinnings of the political response to HIV are complex, it is arguable that the social consequence of the politicisation of AIDS sharpened the differences in a divided society instead of building unity of purpose in dealing with the crisis. This failure to confront the epidemic as a nation united in action, may have permitted a continued advance of the HIV epidemic. As a result, by 2003, antenatal prevalence had risen to 27.9% and surveillance studies showed higher that expected rates of infection among children aged two to 12; white people; youth and married women. In addition, the toll of AIDS-related mortality had begun to parallel the earlier exponential growth of the epidemic to the point where by late 2003, even the government was forced to admit to at least 500 000 people being clinically sick with AIDS and an uncertain number of people already having died.

The Presidential AIDS Panel

In early 2000, President Mbeki began a public debate over whether HIV causes AIDS. He established an international AIDS Advisory Panel, initially comprising 16 AIDS denialists and 16 'orthodox' scientists, where these two contending and allegedly equal sets of scientific positions were brought together with the mandate of advising him, and thus the country, on the most appropriate response to HIV. In his statement at the opening of the advisory panel, President Mbeki commented that:

> You have to respond to a catastrophe in a way that recognises
> that you are facing a catastrophe and here we are talking about
> people – it is not the death of animal stock or something like
> that, but people. Millions and millions of people.

Predictably the panel did not reach consensus and concluded its
work by presenting two sets of recommendations: one from the
denialists 'who did not support the causal link between HIV and AIDS'
and another from those who did. It is significant that, even though
one of the panel's experiments convincingly demonstrated the
'robustness of HIV ELISA tests' this did not cause the President to
correct a public statement made in 2000 questioning the value of
having an HIV test. In the face of this unbridgeable impasse, the work
of the panel ceased without any resolution or final report and no
heed seems to have been paid to either set of recommendations.

The panel left a vacuum and continued confusion over whether
the President supported the national imperative to deal with AIDS.
This was compounded by President Mbeki's opening speech at the
XIIIth International AIDS Conference held in Durban in 2000, where
he elaborated on a 1995 WHO report on mortality in order to dispute
claims that AIDS was the main cause of mortality. Later in 2000, to
overcome this void and prevent a policy crisis, the government
released a position statement that all government programmes and
activities in HIV/AIDS will be based on the premise of HIV as the cause
of AIDS and that the President will not comment further on the
matter.

Activism and antiretroviral drugs to reduce mother-to-child HIV transmission

The introduction of a national programme to prevent mother-to-child
HIV transmission (MTCT) is the best-known example of critically
important programmes becoming casualty to the politicisation of
AIDS. Clinical research had, in 1998, demonstrated the efficacy of a
short course of the antiretroviral drug AZT, in reducing the rate of
transmission of HIV from mother to child. At the time, this research
was welcomed by officials in South Africa's health department.
However, in the face of a contest over the aetiology of AIDS, and arguments by AIDS denialists that the drug AZT was the causative agent of
AIDS (not HIV), implementation of a programme to prevent MTCT was
delayed. Eventually, in 2001, the government opted to use a different
antiretroviral, nevirapine, but even then to limit its initial use for at
least a year to only 18 facilities throughout South Africa. This led to a
legal conflict between the government and doctors, children's rights
organisations and the TAC, which culminated in an order to the

Minister of Health from the Constitutional Court that a programme to prevent MTCT using nevirapine or any other effective drug, be implemented throughout the country. This conflict over a public health policy was unnecessary. Its needlessness is borne out by the 2004 Annual Report, of the South African Department of Health which highlighted that there are now 1600 facilities implementing the programme (up from 540 in 2002/2003), illustrating their strong commitment to the very goal they had earlier opposed at the Constitutional Court.

The result of conflict over AIDS policy has been that South Africa, which on a localised scale has pioneered and implemented some of the world's best clinical and social models in response to HIV, has acted in a fashion that has undermined public confidence. There is a direct causal relationship between this unfortunate situation and the growth of political activism around HIV led by, but not confined to, the Treatment Action Campaign. This political activism, which has often focused on what should have been non-contentious policies, has been a significant feature of the post-1999 non-governmental South African response to HIV/AIDS. It has focused on issues such as the need for national programmes on post-exposure prophylaxis (PEP) for rape survivors; prevention of mother-to-child transmission; and access to antiretroviral treatment for people with AIDS. Tragically, these programmes only came about after bitter legal and social disputes, which culminated in November 2003 with a government announcement adding a component of antiretroviral treatment to its strategic plan on HIV/AIDS. As a result, much now needs to be done to make this treatment programme a success. The Government Communication and Information Service *Review*, for example, points out that 'dedicated expenditure on HIV/AIDS programmes across national departments has increased from about R30 million in 1994 to R340 million in 2001/02' and that 'expenditure is further set to increase tenfold to R3.6-billion in 2005/06.' However, political leadership and better systems for monitoring implementation remain vital.

The poverty of the philosophy of poverty

Finally, it is worthwhile examining in greater detail the juxtaposition between the prioritisation of poverty alleviation versus HIV prevention and treatment. There is no disputing that the President and the government have been correct on insisting on the importance of confronting and gradually eliminating poverty in South Africa. Pervasive poverty is the most profound legacy of apartheid and manifests in high levels of adult illiteracy, homelessness and joblessness. Further, the demography of the apartheid economy, which deprived rural areas of income opportunity in order to facilitate the movement of labour to mines and manufacturing, makes rectifying poverty on a sustainable basis a great challenge.

The report of the WHO Commission on Macroeconomics and Health (2001) has described the links between health and development. Underdevelopment is a major cause of ill health and of the susceptibility of populations to a range of bacterial and virological pathogens. It is also a factor in higher than normal rates of non-communicable diseases. Investment in health is thus a form of direct investment in development.

However, whilst there is a general relationship between poverty and poor health, there is also a specific relationship between HIV and poverty. The post-apartheid legacy of socioeconomic displacement, high levels of adult illiteracy, lack of income opportunity outside of (and increasingly within) urban areas and of poor health care services, is a major factor that explains the difference between the epidemiology of HIV in a developing country, such as South Africa, versus a developed country, such as the United States. This is summed up in a recent article by Msimang and Ekambaram, a consultant with UNAIDS, who describes the failure of many HIV prevention programmes, as often 'exogenous to the programmes themselves.' Further, among poor people, HIV infection leads to more rapid deterioration in health, as well as greater social consequences for the family of an HIV-infected person.

However, a focus on poverty to the exclusion of HIV is as mistaken as a call for a focus on HIV to the exclusion of poverty. Unattended to, HIV will exacerbate poverty in ways that are already being documented in many southern African countries. Ironically, the response to HIV that is demanded of South Africa's government can be found in the words of President Mbeki. While electioneering in 2004 for the third democratic elections in South Africa, President Mbeki visited a rural area of KwaZulu-Natal and became embroiled in a dispute with a minister of an opposing political party, the Inkatha Freedom Party (IFP), who attacked the government policy of providing free food parcels, claiming people did not want food parcels but 'tractors so that they could produce their own food.' Mbeki's response was that while the government programmes are seeking sustainable solutions to poverty and hunger, 'you cannot really go to someone on Monday and say, "here is a tractor, go and farm and you will only have food in four months". When a person is hungry, he needs food immediately.'

Much the same might be said of access to life-saving HIV treatment. To tell people that poverty is the primary cause of AIDS but to do nothing about its immediate symptoms in millions of people, might have a theoretical foundation but is no relief to those people whose most immediate need is access to registered medicines that can stop the replication of HIV and its impact on the immune system, thereby preventing ongoing illness, restoring health and preventing premature death.

Conclusion

The growth of HIV/AIDS in South Africa between 1982 and 2004 is a matter of grave concern. Politics have made a deep imprint on the HIV epidemic in South Africa. Likewise, HIV/AIDS has made an impression on politics in South Africa. It remains a matter of debate among economists as to the extent to which HIV/AIDS may have an impact on key economic indicators such as gross domestic product or foreign direct investment. However, the social consequences of the HIV epidemic will be significant, particularly on health systems and the quality of life of South Africa's poor. Transforming and improving the public health system has been one of the priorities of the democratic government. But plans for health systems improvement were drawn up before the explosive epidemic of HIV, the concomitant epidemic of tuberculosis, and a growing burden of opportunistic infection and reduced capacity, due to HIV-related morbidity and mortality in its staff, of the health service itself. Tragically, the impact of HIV will thus fall most squarely on those who bore the brunt of apartheid; the urban and rural poor. The disruption of livelihoods, and the diversion of scarce resources to fill gaps left by those who have died, will rob the millions of poor people of prospects for income accumulation and social improvement. It is in this context that the next challenge of the AIDS epidemic must be viewed – expanding access to treatment is not only a moral, medical and legal necessity – it is also one of the critical ways of addressing the development goals of South Africa.

Bibliography

ABDOOL KARIM SS. 'Making AIDS a notifiable disease – is it an appropriate policy for South Africa'. *South African Medical Journal* 1999; 89: 609–611.

AIDS CONSORTIUM. *Charter of Rights on HIV/AIDS.* 1992.

AIDS LAW PROJECT. *The Implications of 'AIDS Notification' for Human Rights and HIV/AIDS Prevention in South Africa. An analysis of the proposed amendment to the Regulations Relating to Communicable Diseases and the Notification of Notifiable Medical Conditions. SA Government Gazette* R 485, 23 April 1999 and R 484, 23rd April 1999.

'DISLODGING STEREOTYPES' *ANC Today.* October 2004 4: 22–28. (President's answer to questions in Parliament on 21 October 2004)

ANC. *A National Health Plan for South Africa.* 1994.

BARRETT, K, HEYWOOD M, STRODE A. (EDS.) *'HIV/AIDS and The Law: A Resource Manual',* third edition, the AIDS Law Project. 2003.

DEPARTMENT OF HEALTH. *'Operational Plan for Comprehensive HIV and AIDS Care, Management and Treatment for South Africa'*. November 2003.

DEPARTMENT OF HEALTH. *'National HIV and Syphilis Ante-natal Sero prevalence survey in SA'*. 2003. Government Printer. Pretoria.

GOVERNMENT COMMUNICATION AND INFORMATION SERVICE (GCIS) ON BEHALF OF THE PRESIDENCY. *'Towards a Ten Year Review'* October 2003.

HEYWOOD M, RICHTER M. 'Is South Africa's HIV/AIDS Programme "the largest and most comprehensive in the world"?' *AIDS Analysis Africa*. June/July 2002; 13: 14–16

HEYWOOD M. 'Preventing Mother to Child HIV Transmission in SA: Background, Strategies and Outcomes of the TAC Campaign Against the Minister of Health', *South African Journal on Human Rights* 2003; 19: 278–315.

SHISANA O, BEZUIDENHOUT F, BROOKES HJ, CHAUVEAU J, COLVIN M, CONNOLLY C, DITLOPO P, KELLY K, MOATTI JP, LOUNDOU DA, PARKER W, RICHTER L, SCHWABE C, SIMBAYI LC, DAVID STOKER D, TOEFY Y, VAN ZYL J. *Nelson Mandela/HSRC Study on HIV/AIDS*. Human Sciences Research Council. Cape Town 2002.

JOCHELSON K, MOTHIBELI M, LEGER J-P. 'Human Immunodeficiency Virus and Migrant Labour in South Africa', *International Journal of Health Services*, 1991; 21: 157–173.

MINISTER OF HEALTH AND OTHERS V TREATMENT ACTION CAMPAIGN AND OTHERS. 2002 (5) SA 721 (CC).

MSIMANG S AND EKAMBARAM S. 'Moving Beyond the Public: The challenge of women's political organising in the time of AIDS', *Development Update*. 2004; 53: 53–76

MSOMI S. 'Mbeki's Extreme Makeover', *Sunday Times*. Johannesburg. April 11, 2004

PRESIDENTIAL AIDS ADVISORY PANEL, FINAL REPORT. March 2001 available at: www.info.gov.za/reports/2001/aidspanelpdf.pdf

REPRODUCTIVE HEALTH RESEARCH UNIT (RHRU). *'HIV and Sexual Behaviour Among Young South Africans: A National Survey of 15 to 24 years olds'*. 2004.

STATISTICS SOUTH AFRICA. Mid-Year Population Estimates 2004.

CHAPTER 25
The impact on ethics

Jerome Singh

HIV CLINICAL TRIALS IN the developing world are fraught with ethical dilemmas. However, an approach that is responsive to the social, political, economic and infrastructural milieu of the study population should be the realisable goal of researchers and sponsors and not remain just a hypothetical construct. This should be so even if the preferred course of action of the host country does not seem to resonate with that of the sponsoring country. Study populations must be protected from exploitation.

The health care needs of a population must dictate the study design. However, the shortcomings implicit in overprotecting research participants in the developing world must also be recognised. Blindly presuming that a first world standard of health care is inherently the gold standard to be applied universally can ultimately compromise the interests of those it is intended to help. Besides such a stance being paternalistic, it can potentially hamstring research in these settings when the gold standard cannot be attained on logistic, financial or physiological grounds. The grounding of such research because of such factors would run counter to the interests of the intended study population.

Under normal circumstances clinical practice is a fertile ground for dual loyalty dilemmas. HIV/AIDS merely compounds that problem. While the recommendations suggested here are by no means exhaustive, definitive or even necessarily always universally applicable, in the absence of a better solution they can help health professionals resolve difficult ethical dilemmas.

Concerns have been raised about exploitation, standards of care and the informed consent process in the conduct of research, and in some cases, clinical practice, in sub-Saharan Africa in the light of HIV/AIDS.

The ethical imperatives for research, however, are clear, as this region carries a disproportionate burden of HIV infection in developing countries and indeed in the world. This chapter explores some of the ethical issues that arise for researchers and clinicians dealing with HIV/AIDS and attempts to offer guidance on how they could approach these issues. Part 1 appraises standards of care in HIV clinical trials. Part 2 focuses on how dual loyalties and conflicts of interest arise in the HIV/AIDS clinical care landscape and how such dilemmas could be resolved.

Part 1

Standards of care in HIV clinical trials: Identifying the key ethical issues

Prior to its revision in 2002, the 'standard of care' provisions in the Declaration of Helsinki on Ethical Principles for Medical Research Involving Human Subjects read as follows :

> The potential benefits, hazards and discomfort of a new method should be weighed against the advantages of the *best proven* diagnostic and therapeutic method.
>
> In any study, every patient – including those of a control group, if any – should be assured of the *best proven* diagnostic and therapeutic method. (author's emphasis)

In the context of HIV research, standard of care debates have centred on two related concerns: first, the legitimacy of employing placebos in the control arm of a trial when an effective and proven intervention exists; and secondly, whether the 'best proven' therapeutic method should be seen in a local or global context. Building on earlier remarks by Robert Levine, Alex London summarises the debate as follows:

> When Helsinki calls for the 'best proven therapeutic method' does it mean (A) the best therapy anywhere in the world? Or does it mean (B) the standard that prevails in the country in which the trial is conducted?

Before we consider how this dilemma could be resolved, the debate needs to be reviewed more fully.

In 1994, the AIDS Clinical Trial Group (ACTG) 076 regimen of zidovudine (hereafter regimen 076) was shown to reduce maternal-infant HIV transmission rates by more than half. In September 1997, the use of placebo-control groups in clinical trials designed to test the efficacy of a short-course of zidovudine for the prevention of maternal-infant HIV infection in sixteen Southeast Asian, Caribbean and sub-Saharan African countries elicited damning indictments in *The Lancet* and *The New England Journal of Medicine*. Lurie and Wolf criticised such studies, arguing that all except one of the trials employed placebo-control groups despite the fact that zidovudine had by then clearly been shown to substantially cut the rate of vertical transmission and had been recommended in the United States for all HIV-infected pregnant women.

Another outspoken critic of the studies, Marcia Angell, argued that 'only when there is no known effective treatment is it ethical to compare a potential new treatment with a placebo'; only if there was genuine doubt about the benefit of prophylaxis would the use of a placebo group be ethically justifiable. When effective treatment does exist (as was the case with regimen 076 for maternal-infant HIV transmission) a placebo should not be used. In the light of the relevant provisions in the Declaration of Helsinki, Angell argued, such studies would be considered unacceptable in a developed country and as such, should be equally unacceptable in the developing world. To adopt a standard of care for developing countries that fell below that of developed nations was accordingly unethical. Angell took particular exception to the argument that prophylaxis can be withheld in a study if no prophylaxis is the local standard of care. She argued that unless there are specific indications to the contrary, the safest and most reasonable position is that people everywhere are likely to respond similarly to the same treatment.

Just prior to the debate erupting, the American sponsors of the studies – the Secretary of Health and Human Services, the directors of the National Institutes of Health (NIH), and the Centers for Disease Control and Prevention (CDC) – had defended the design of their studies in a Department of Health and Human Services report released in July 1997. They argued that the standard of care in the study sites was no prophylactic intervention at all and that the inclusion of placebo controls would result in the most rapid, accurate, and reliable answer about the value of the intervention being studied. In response to their critics, the directors of the NIH and CDC, Harold Varmus and David Satcher respectively, also argued in a separate commentary published in *The New England Journal of Medicine* that, as regimen 076 was unavailable in the countries involved in the studies, the standard of care that governed the citizens of those countries was no treatment at all. They argued that interventions that could be expected to be made available in countries like the United States might be well beyond the financial resources of a developing country or exceed the capacity of its health care infrastructure. They pointed out, for example, that in Malawi the cost of zidovudine in the 076 regimen for just one mother and child was, at the time, 600 times the annual per capita allocation for health care. They argued that in the absence of particular prophylaxis in a developing country, they would support a study of a new drug in that country if the burden of disease made such a study compelling and that even if there were risks associated with intervention, such a trial would pass the test of beneficence and should thus be permitted.

In the studies at issue, Varmus and Satcher argued that zidovudine is a powerful drug and its safety in the populations of developing countries – where the incidence of other diseases, anaemia and malnutrition are higher than in developed countries – was unknown. As such, they reasoned, even though regimen 076 was proven to be effective in some countries, it was unlikely that it could be successfully exported to other countries. They argued that besides the fact that placebo-controlled trials usually provide a faster answer with fewer side-effects, such studies also provided definitive answers about the safety and value of an intervention in a particular setting. Commentators such as Aaby et al and Halsey et al agreed. They criticised Lurie and Wolfe's paper, Angell's editorial, and *The Lancet* editorial as showing a lack of understanding of the realities of health care in developing countries.

Despite these rebuttals, in October 1997 investigators discontinued the use of placebos in an NIH-funded study of two short-course zidovudine regimens in Ethiopia. In February 1998 the CDC and the Thai government announced that their placebo-controlled study of a short-course zidovudine regimen in Thailand had shown a 51% reduction in perinatal HIV transmission rates, but with the CDC making it known at the same time that the use of placebos would cease in that study and another then underway in Côte d'Ivoire.

In 1998, developing world HIV scientists like Edward Mbidde and Salim Abdool Karim lent their support to defenders of the trials. While Abdool Karim agreed with Lurie and Wolfe that researchers and research agencies from developed countries should not conduct research in developing countries that would be considered unethical in their own countries, except under justifiable extenuating circumstances, he argued that the position in countries like South Africa was somewhat different. He pointed out that much of the research was sponsored by local agencies and the United Nations Program on Acquired Immunodeficiency Syndrome (UNAIDS) and involved local scientists. Using two large South African perinatal trials then underway as examples, he argued the reasons why the use of regimen 076 in a control arm for either study was inappropriate in the South African context. He noted, among other things: (a) that regimen 076 was then not affordable in South Africa; (b) the high home birth frequency (which made efficacious drug intake difficult to monitor); (c) the high frequency of late booking for antenatal care appointments (which made the widespread use of the perinatal component of the 076 regimen virtually impossible); and (d) that breastfeeding was common in rural areas (which meant that HIV-positive women participating in a 076 study would have to be discouraged from breastfeeding, a factor that necessitated the free or heavily subsidised provision of breast-milk substitutes, both of which have substantial cost implications).

Abdool Karim also noted that standard of care criteria differ across countries, and across the world. He stated that while regimen 076 was the standard of care in some countries it was not an international standard as established by the World Health Organisation. As such, its non-provision in the control arm of a study, in deference to high-quality routine care, could not be construed as causing undue risk or harm to study participants. Since no therapy that participants might otherwise have received was being withheld from them, such studies were, in his view, not unethical. Abdool Karim argued therefore that in these circumstances the provision even of a known beneficial agent (in this case regimen 076) in a study's control arm could not be justified. In the light of all these factors, Abdool Karim concluded that a placebo-control arm is ethically justifiable in such circumstances.

The case for less efficacious interventions in clinical trials in the developing world was further explored by Wilkinson, Abdool Karim and Coovadia in an editorial in the *British Medical Journal* in February 1999. They argued that the benefit levels from antiretroviral drugs in developed nations are unlikely to be matched in Africa. They noted that most African women have little choice but to breastfeed their young: if short-course antiretroviral drugs were available in Africa some children would be saved from HIV but many others would remain at risk of acquiring HIV from the breast-milk of their infected mothers. Nor would formula feeding necessarily be the solution as it might stigmatise HIV-infected women. They noted that even in relatively resource-rich South Africa, and allowing for a cut in the price of zidovudine, implementation of a short-course regimen would consume a substantial proportion of a region's health budget. Moreover, the rapid implementation of a costly, vertical programme might also draw financial and human resources away from other programmes. They pointed out that many of Africa's women – those who live in remote rural areas, urban slums, or war zones; those who will not or cannot access prenatal care; those who deliver outside a health setting; and those who deliver prematurely – have no hope of ever receiving antiretrovirals. In these circumstances, they argued, only by having a placebo for comparison could the efficacy of an intervention be truly judged. The equivalency design is inappropriate if the effect in the treatment arm is expected to be substantially weaker than that in the (antiretroviral drug) control arm. Nor did it make sense to insist that the control arm of a trial should consist of an intervention that is not, and is never likely to be, the standard of clinical care in the country where the study is done. Was this not, they asked, 'merely ethical imperialism [to insist] on such a control arm in a study clinic when a few kilometres up the road women continue to receive no intervention at all?'

International guidelines: Standards of care and the employment of placebo arms

By 1999, existing international ethical guidelines were being called into question by various critics and in September 2000 the South African Department of Health published its own guidelines on clinical trials – *Guidelines for Good Practice in the Conduct of Clinical Trials in Human Participants in South Africa* (Clinical Trials Guidelines or CTG). The use of placebos for trials in South Africa is addressed in Paragraph 9.3.2. This provision states that the use of placebos in a South African trial after an intervention has been shown to be effective is generally to be regarded as unethical. However, the CTG acknowledges that with increasing disparities in health care between wealthy and poor countries, therapy that has been shown to be effective is often unaffordable in resource-poor settings. It therefore concludes that it may be justifiable to use placebos in South Africa if: first, a community does not have access to interventions that are the standard of care in resource-rich settings; and secondly, the balance between potential harms and benefits are such that the potential benefits to the community would considerably outweigh the harm. It recognises that this issue is controversial and that there is no international consensus. It therefore advises that widespread consultation should take place prior to embarking on such studies.

In the same month Solly Benatar and Peter Singer, both prominent bioethicists involved in promoting developing-world health issues, challenged the conventional notion that the ethical nature of a trial could simply be deduced from a reading of the text of a declaration. They noted that the debate surrounding standard of care remained incomplete for three reasons: first, the failure to adequately define 'standard of care'; second, the incorrect assumption that standards set by developed countries can be considered the norm; and thirdly, inadequate concern on the part of commentators on research ethics with the injustice implicit in the fact that 90% of all medical research being undertaken was for diseases that cause just 10% of the global burden of disease.

For Benatar and Singer, declarations, like constitutions, need interpretation: 'Determining what is ethical goes beyond merely following prescriptions and requires moral reasoning'. Echoing the sentiments of Abdool Karim, they too note that little attention is paid to the fact that there are many differences between pregnant women in developing countries and those in countries where the 'best proven' treatment has been established. According to Benatar and Singer, whether a placebo arm is justified in a trial requires careful consideration of potential harms and benefits in specific contexts. The relevant standard of care to be adopted should take into account the context of the trial and must be sensitive to the social, economic and political milieu. They condemn placebo trials as unethical in instances when such trials are undertaken for the purpose of what they term self-serving 'me-too' marketing – showing that a new drug is more effective than placebo when existing and cheaper drugs are already on the market (making the pursuit of such research redundant and thus unethical). They feel that in situations where there are good reasons to conduct placebo-controlled trials these should be considered on their merit rather than be precluded by a bluntly-designed prohibitive clause in ethics declarations. Benatar and Singer call for an expanded standard of care understanding. They argue that the highest achievable standard of care should be the goal. They suggest that reasonable limits can be negotiated in specific contexts. The objective should be to ratchet the standard upwards rather than to set utopian ideals that cannot be met.

In October 2000 the 52nd World Medical Association (WMA) General Assembly adopted a revised version of the Declaration of Helsinki at its congress in Edinburgh, Scotland. On the issue of standards of care and the legitimacy of conducting placebo-controlled trials, paragraph 29 of the revised version of the declaration reads:

> The benefits, risks, burdens and effectiveness of a new method should be tested against those of the best current prophylactic, diagnostic and therapeutic methods. This does not exclude the use of placebo, or no treatment, in studies where no proven prophylactic, diagnostic or therapeutic method exists.

This revision did nothing to quell the debate surrounding what standard of care ought to apply to developing world clinical trials. Neither did it placate Benatar and Singer's concerns about providing guidance on how the 'standard of care' should be determined.

In April 2001 the US National Bioethics Advisory Commission (NBAC) published *Ethical and Policy Issues in International Research: Clinical Trials in Developing Countries*. The report explored the issue of whether and if so, under what circumstances, researchers and sponsors have an obligation to provide an established effective treatment to the control arm even if it is not available in the host country. The NBAC uses the phrase 'established effective treatment' to refer to a treatment that is established (it has achieved universal acceptance by the global medical profession) and effective (it is as successful as any

in treating the disease or condition). According to the NBAC, established effective treatments are not limited to what is routinely available
in the country in which the research is being conducted and the
NBAC does not intend this phrase to refer to a single best treatment,
since agreement may be lacking about what treatment is best.

According to the NBAC, if in a proposed clinical trial the control
group were to receive less care than would be available under ideal
circumstances, the burden on the investigator to justify the design
would be heavier. The NBAC recommended that representatives of the
host country, including scientists, public officials and persons with
the condition under study, should have a strong voice in determining
whether a proposed trial is appropriate. Recommendation 2.2 of the
report states:

> Researchers and sponsors should design clinical trials that
> provide members of any control group with an established
> effective treatment, whether or not such treatment is available
> in the host country. Any study that would not provide the
> control arm with an established effective treatment should
> include a justification for using an alternate design. Ethics
> committees must assess the justification provided, including
> the risks to participants, and the overall ethical acceptability of
> the research design.

In 2002 the ensuing debate about standards of care and the implications of guideline 29 of the Helsinki Declaration forced the WMA
General Assembly sitting in Washington, D.C. to issue a note of clarification about the provision:

> The WMA hereby reaffirms its position that extreme care must
> be taken in making use of a placebo-controlled trial and that in
> general this methodology should only be used in the absence
> of existing proven therapy. However, a placebo-controlled trial
> may be ethically acceptable, even if proven therapy is available,
> under the following circumstances:
> - Where for compelling and scientifically sound methodologi-
>   cal reasons its use is necessary to determine the efficacy or
>   safety of a prophylactic, diagnostic or therapeutic method;
>   or
> - where a prophylactic, diagnostic or therapeutic method is
>   being investigated for a minor condition and the patients
>   who receive placebo will not be subject to any additional
>   risk of serious or irreversible harm.

In November 2002 the Council of International Organizations of
Medical Sciences (CIOMS) issued its revised guidelines on biomedical
human research. Guideline 11 contains a formulation of the

well-established principle that patients should not be deprived of treatment when they participate in research. When an 'established effective intervention' exists, it states, research subjects in a control group of a clinical trial should receive this intervention. The guideline then proceeds to describe three circumstances that make it 'ethically acceptable' to use a placebo arm:

- when there is no established effective intervention;
- when withholding an established effective intervention would expose subjects to, at most, temporary discomfort or delay in relief of symptoms; and
- when use of an established effective intervention as comparator would not yield scientifically reliable results and use of placebo would not add any risk of serious or irreversible harm to the subjects.

The way forward

Despite the revisions to the Helsinki Declaration and CIOMS Guidelines outlined above, the world is no closer to agreeing upon an appropriate standard of care for clinical trials. Part of the solution to the impasse between the two opposing camps may lie in recognising that the beliefs of those who support placebo trials are actually underpinned by two related but different rationales. These may be articulated as follows:

Rationale 1: where there is genuine doubt about the *efficacy of a drug in a particular setting, placebo-control trials should be permitted.*

Rationale 2: where there is doubt about the realistic *implementation of a particular drug in a particular setting on logistic, financial or physiological grounds, placebo-control trials should be permitted.*

Rationale 1

It seems a reasonable presumption that commentators like Angell and her critics come from diametrically opposed viewpoints on the issue of placebo-controlled trials and appropriate standards of care. However, this might not be, nor does it necessarily have to be, the case. Both camps share a concern for the welfare of trial participants and the scientific integrity of the trial design. Earlier we noted Angell's contention that 'only when there is no effective treatment is it ethical to compare a potential new treatment with a placebo' and it is here that possible common ground may exist between the rival camps.

London has noted that Angell's claim can be interpreted in two different ways:

- Only when there is no known effective treatment for illness x anywhere in the world is it ethical to compare a potential new treatment with a placebo.

- Only when there is no known effective treatment anywhere in the world for illness x within a population p is it ethical to compare a potential new treatment with a placebo in population p.

Angell's position has traditionally been assigned the first interpretation. But there are at least two good reasons why the second interpretation is preferable. Not least, this position would resonate with that of some of her critics, thus bringing the opposing camps closer together to the benefit of research participants in the developing world. As some commentators point out, many differences exist between participants in developing countries and those in countries where the 'best proven' treatment has been established. These factors influence treatment efficacy. According to them, whether a placebo arm is justified in a trial requires careful consideration of potential harms and benefits in specific contexts. They have argued that treatment efficacy is not necessarily universal.

Looking at the second interpretation, if an intervention has been proven efficacious on a population elsewhere in the world but not on the proposed study population (and genuine doubt exists about whether the drug will be effective in the proposed study population) one can assume that no effective treatment exists anywhere in the world for the study population (at least, not until it is proven effective in the new study population). The use of a placebo arm in a study on such a population, despite the existence of effective treatment elsewhere in the world for another population, is then not necessarily unethical. Besides such an interpretation resonating with the concerns of some of the proponents of placebo-controlled trials, it would also address Angell's concern that genuine doubt must exist about the benefit of prophylaxis before the use of a placebo group can be deemed ethically justifiable. This interpretation provides the basis for a common ground between some of the proponents and critics of placebo-control trials. It can thus hopefully help move at least two camps involved in the standard of care debate beyond their current impasse.

There is also another reason why Angell's statement should be assigned the second interpretation. It was earlier noted that some commentators like London criticised Angell on the grounds that adopting the best known standard of care in the control arm would mean that clinical equipoise, the fundamental requirement of any clinical trial, would effectively be violated (as using a proven treatment in a control arm versus an unproven intervention in the study arm would mean that researchers would be knowingly favouring the participants of the control arm over the intervention arm – something considered untenable in research circles). This point is difficult to refute. Using the second interpretation, Angell et al escape this.

Rationale 2

Commentators such as Abdool Karim argue that when the known effective treatment for illness x cannot practically be implemented within a population p it is ethical to compare a new treatment with a placebo in population p.

Those in this camp would probably be of the view that the appropriate standard of care for a particular setting should be dictated by the maxim 'best available, best sustainable in the local public health sector context'. Procedurally, such a stance would see the proposed standard of care in a particular setting being deemed ethically sustainable if it is considered reasonable and justifiable in that setting. This determination would ideally be based on the consensus of the host country's regulatory bodies, research ethics committees, study community and proposed research subjects, and on the health needs and priorities of that country. In such a model the support of regulatory bodies and research ethics committees in the sponsoring country on the proposed standard of care of the host setting should be deemed preferable, but not a *sine qua non* for the research to continue. In the absence of consensus between relevant role-players in the host and sponsoring countries, the wishes of the host country should prevail. A failure to do so could result in charges of ethical imperialism being levelled at the sponsoring country.

Admittedly, such a system might not be suitable for a country that lacks a research regulatory environment and/or competent research ethics committees. However, in the absence of a formal protective framework the views of the local scientific community and the wider local community, especially those of the intended subjects of the study, must assume increased importance. Their engagement must be established through a careful and thoroughly informed consultative process. In the absence of consensus between the role-players in host and sponsoring country, notwithstanding the absence of a formal regulatory mechanism, the wishes of the host country should still prevail. Such an approach would respect the needs and hopefully further the interests, of the host population.

Dual loyalties and conflicts of interest in the HIV/AIDS clinical care landscape

Loyalty to the patient, the practitioner's duty of care, is one of the oldest paradigms in the ethics of healing, but health professionals today face mounting pressure to subordinate the interests of their patients to those of a third party, such as an employer, research sponsor, or the state. We shall explore here the loyalty conflicts that can arise in therapeutic settings in the context of the HIV/AIDS pandemic.

Dual loyalty and conflict of interest

Health professionals, both clinicians and researchers, often have obligations to third parties, such as employers, sponsors, insurance companies or governments that may conflict with undivided devotion to the patient or research participant. This can be called a dual loyalty. In 2003 the Dual Loyalty Working Group (DLWG), a multinational, multidisciplinary team of experts in law, bioethics, and human rights, proposed a comprehensive set of guidelines on conflicts of this nature: *Dual Loyalty & Human Rights in Health Professional Practice: Proposed Guidelines and Institutional Mechanisms.*

Convened by Physicians for Human Rights and the Health Sciences Faculty of the University of Cape Town, the DLWG defines a dual loyalty as a *clinical* role conflict between professional duties to a patient and obligations – express or implied, real or perceived – to the interests of a third party.

While the DLWG report does not explicitly deal with dual loyalty issues in medical research, the clear and traditional demarcation between research and therapeutic practice is becoming increasingly blurred. Although our main concern in the present discussion will be the dual loyalty dimensions of therapeutic practice, it is important not to lose sight of the ethical dimensions of the practice – research nexus. In this latter context particularly, 'conflict of interest' signifies a situation where a professional judgement about a primary interest becomes unduly influenced by a secondary interest. Discussions on conflicts of interest in research have traditionally centred on researchers receiving undue or improper financial incentives or industry kickbacks. In the HIV/AIDS pandemic, however, the more pressing concern is likely to be the conflicts of interest that can arise when the role of clinician and researcher merge. In the practice–research context this translates to the physician-researcher's primary interest (duty of care towards the patient-subject) being undermined by secondary factors (such as loyalty to the study/sponsor).

How dilemmas can arise

In the context of HIV/AIDS, dual loyalty dilemmas for clinical practice can arise in at least two ways: first, when physicians link their practice with research; and secondly, when state physicians encounter unreasonable or irrational state health polices. I will briefly explore the implications of both.

Practice linked with research

Clinical practice and research are normally regarded as separate domains but, increasingly, community-based physicians are drawn into research projects through the enrolment of their patients in clinical trials, while medical researchers in community-based studies take on therapeutic responsibility for their research participants. In both instances the juggling of clinician-researcher roles can create confusion for the research participant/patient and present conflict of interest dilemmas for the health professional. A well-known HIV observational study illustrates this point.

Case study

In 1997 a study by Quinn et al focusing on the relationship between viral load and heterosexual transmission of HIV-1 in couples who were serodiscordant at baseline drew sharp criticism from ethicists. The study was carried out in ten clusters of rural villages in Uganda. The primary purpose was to delineate the risk factors associated with heterosexual transmission of HIV. Villagers were surveyed on five occasions at ten-month intervals. Participants were asked questions about their sexual practices and medical histories. In addition, blood and other bodily fluids were drawn for testing for HIV-1 and other sexually transmitted infections (STIs). To determine whether STIs such as syphilis and gonorrhoea increased the risk of HIV transmission, the study gave residents in five of the ten sites intermittent antibiotic treatment to reduce the prevalence of STIs. In other words, researchers assumed a therapeutic clinical role. The study was strongly criticised by Marcia Angell in an editorial in *The New England Journal of Medicine*.

She pointed out, among other things, that the study meant that for up to thirty months several hundred people with HIV and other STIs were observed but not treated by researcher-clinicians. Moreover, in the case of HIV-discordant couples the decision to disclose HIV-positive status to the seronegative partner was left to the seropositive partner even though both were regularly seen by researcher-clinicians. Angell argued that the caregivers in question ought to have informed seronegative partners of their partner's risk profile so that they could have taken steps to guard against the harm of transmission. In this case the researcher-clinicians were faced with a conflict between serving the interests of science and the sponsor (which would necessitate their remaining silent about their knowledge and adhering to the role of passive observers despite the ethical implications thereof) or the interests of their patients (which would necessitate their taking measures to protect the interests of the patient-subject or other persons at risk).

A study such as this raises many difficult ethical questions. If researchers assume the role of clinicians, do they automatically assume, too, the ethical responsibilities of that role? Should they step into that role? Are there differences in the ethical duties owed by a researcher and clinician? Should there be? The recommendations that follow attempt to offer some guidance on these issues.

Recommendations

Research can be clearly distinguished from therapy. Research is subject to prospective third-party control while therapy is reviewed retrospectively. Similarly, the roles of research scientist and clinical practitioner are also very different. Morin et al describe the difference as follows:

> Investigators act to generate scientific knowledge that potentially will result in future therapeutic benefits. Practitioners are focused on present health and welfare of patients.

Goldern notes that in therapeutic encounters health workers are expected to attend almost entirely to the patient's welfare. On the other hand, in research encounters, patient-subjects are being used for scientific ends. He notes that investigators therefore have commitments both to present patient-participants and to abstract, future patients, thereby causing a conflict between competing primary interests. In such a situation, Goldner argues that an investigator must educate the potential research participant on the critical distinction between clinical practice and research. In addition, the investigator must correct the patient-participant's perception that an invitation to participate in research is a professional recommendation solely intended to serve the individual's treatment needs.

But the distinction between research and treatment may be far from clear to the patient-participant and since it is quite probable that subjects may misconceive the nature of a research project, particular attention must be paid when researchers offer some medical benefit that can be integrated into a course of treatment. Although trial patient-participants are offered a treatment of unproven efficacy, many may think they are receiving 'cutting edge' treatment guaranteed to improve their condition. Moreover, they may well believe that the purpose of a clinical trial is to benefit them rather than just gather data for the purposes of contributing to scientific knowledge, a mistaken state of mind that has been termed 'therapeutic misconception'. Morin et al note that this perception may be reinforced when subjects receive the experimental treatment from the same physician who has administered all their care in the past, rather than being referred to a clinical investigator located in an academic setting with a reputation for conducting research. In these instances the US National Bioethics Advisory Commission has advised that researchers make clear to research participants, in the initial consent process and throughout the study, which activities are elements of research and which are elements of clinical care. They should also indicate in their research protocols how they would minimise the likelihood that potential participants will mistakenly believe that the purpose of the research is solely to administer treatment rather than to contribute to scientific knowledge.

The informed consent process might also be compromised when the physician-investigator responsible for enrolling patients in a trial and obtaining their informed consent stands to gain financially from each participant enrolled. According to Morin et al, the physician-investigator may accordingly be less inclined to emphasise how the experimental treatment differs from the care that is ordinarily provided, the additional risks involved, or the lack of direct benefit to the participant. In such instances, they recommend that funding and financial incentives offered to the physician-researcher must be disclosed to the potential participant as part of the informed consent process. Moreover, the physician who has ongoing responsibility for treating a patient should not be the person responsible for obtaining that patient's informed consent to participate in a trial to be conducted by the physician himself or herself. In such instances patients may feel indebted to their physician or hesitate to challenge or reject his or her advice to participate in the research.

In the Quinn study, researchers had an ethical duty to inform the HIV-seronegative partners at risk. The need to breach confidentiality and warn an identifiable party at risk was established as a principle in the leading case of *Tarasoff* v. *Regents of the University of California*. Although this was an American case, its rationale has been endorsed by professional medical associations around the world. Moreover, researchers in the Quinn study had an ethical duty to treat their patients for the HIV-related and sexually transmitted conditions with which they had been diagnosed. The conclusion must be that researchers who commence a therapeutic relationship with their patient-subject cannot hide behind their researcher status to evade their ethical responsibilities.

The preamble of the 2002 CIOMS *International Ethical Guidelines for Biomedical Research Involving Human Subjects* states:

> Professionals whose roles combine investigation and treatment have a special obligation to protect the rights and welfare of the patient-subjects. An investigator who agrees to act as physician-investigator undertakes some or all of the legal and ethical responsibilities of the subject's primary-care physician. In such a case, if the subject withdraws from the research owing to complications related to the research or in the exercise of the right to withdraw without loss of benefit, the physician has an obligation to continue to provide medical care, or to see that the subject receives the necessary care in the health-care system, or to offer assistance in finding another physician.

Contending with irrational or unreasonable state health policies

When state policies set a state at odds with its own constitutional or other legal obligation to realise its citizens' right to the highest attainable standard of health, health professionals experience the consequences of such policies at first-hand and may well find themselves thrust into dual loyalty conflicts.

Let us presume, for example, that a state adopts a policy on HIV/AIDS that is widely recognised as irrational or unreasonable even though it has the capacity and infrastructure to address the malady and a legal obligation to do so. If state physicians recognise these factors they could experience a conflict of interest between performing the duty of care towards their patients (which would ideally require them to actively protect and promote the interests of their patients by protesting such policy to the relevant authorities) and between their duty to serve the interests of their state employer (which might arguably require the physician to remain silent about the irrationality or unreasonableness of the state's policy).

Conversely, a government's openly negative views about certain HIV/AIDS treatment options could influence loyal or misguided state physicians to voluntarily not *want* to provide objectively verifiable and reasonable care to, or protect the interests of, state patients. This could conceivably occur where the physician comes to believe in the state's rationale. This mindset could conflict with the physician's ethical duty to care for the patient according to recommended guidelines. There are at least two instances in South Africa where physicians involved in HIV/AIDS clinical care were faced with conflicts of this nature.

Case study

In 1999, unable to secure a budget or staff to improve his hospital's existing internal services, a hospital superintendent, Dr Thys von Mollendorff in Nelspruit, Mpumalanga province, authorised a local volunteer charity organisation, the Greater Nelspruit Rape Intervention Project (GRIP), to use an unused office in his hospital to provide free counselling, fresh clothes, legal advice, and free HIV antiretroviral treatment to rape survivors.

The strategy took its lead from existing government policy for other community-focused initiatives, under which 49 other charities such as Alcoholics Anonymous and Life-Line also worked in the hospital. According to Von Mollendorff, GRIP made a significant impact on the lives of rape survivors treated at the hospital. The rape survivors were treated immediately and received intensive private counselling, clean clothes and help with legal procedures. Most importantly, according to Von Mollendorff, the free antiretroviral drugs GRIP supplied within 72 hours of the rape saved at least 100 lives. At the time, the use of antiretrovirals was prohibited in state hospitals (despite it being available in the private sector). When Von Mollendorff ignored the provincial Health Minister's order to cease the practice, he was charged with insubordination. His view was that adhering to the government's policy meant denying medication to those in need, which, he believed, unjustifiably subordinated his obligation to affirm his patients' right to the highest attainable standard of care. Von Mollendorff was suspended from duty in November 2001. On February 15, 2002, he was found guilty of gross insubordination and on February 22, 2002 was dismissed from his post. In March 2003 Mollendorff successfully challenged his dismissal in an arbitration hearing before the Public Service Health Sectoral Bargaining Council. As a result, the Mpumalanga health department withdrew all charges and agreed to pay his legal costs. Mollendorff was also paid a year's salary and his lost pension benefits. His earlier finding of guilt on charges of insubordination was also declared null and void. Dr Mollendorff decided against reinstatement as Superintendent of Nelspruit Hospital.

In a related matter, despite growing national and international evidence for the effectiveness of antiretrovirals in preventing mother-to-child transmission (MTCT), together with the spiralling HIV epidemic among South Africa's black female population, the South African government throughout 2000 and 2001 persistently refused to provide antiretrovirals as part of a comprehensive MTCT prevention programme. As the DLWG notes, this treatment was not only affordable, but the government was under an obligation to provide it in terms of their constitutional requirement to realise citizens' rights to access to health care. Faced with spiralling HIV infection among his infant patients and the intransigence of the government on the issue, a state paediatrician, Dr Salojee, testified against the government in a Constitutional Court hearing. His supporting affidavit, and those of others, eventually moved the Constitutional Court to compel the South African government to develop a comprehensive MTCT programme.

As the DLWG notes:

> The clinicians in both the two cases faced inequitable policies that denied the right of access to health care to vulnerable and marginalised populations, and both chose to act in favour of the rights of their patients, the former by resisting state restrictions, the latter by actively joining arms with an advocacy nongovernmental organisation to challenge state policy.

Other clinicians might not be as decisive about how to respond to such dilemmas. The following will hopefully provide guidance on the issue.

Recommendations

In the face of dual loyalty obligations such as we have illustrated here, the DLWG Guidelines are designed: to help the health professional identify situations where subordination of patient interests to those of the state or other third party implicates human rights; to clarify the responsibilities of the health professional in these situations; and to enable the health professional to respond appropriately, especially where he or she faces personal or professional risks by adhering to obligations to the patient.

According to the guidelines, where the state has failed to take necessary steps to establish a health system that affords equitable access to health services, the health professional participating in that system has an obligation to press for alternative policies designed to end the violations. Article 3 of the Guidelines advises, moreover, that the health professional must place the protection of the patient's human rights and wellbeing first whenever there exists a conflict between the patient's human rights and the state's interests. This responsibility includes affirmatively resisting demands or requests by the state or third party to subordinate patient human rights. It would seem that the actions of Mollendorf and Salojee exemplify this principle. According to Article 6 of the Guidelines the health professional should recognise that passive participation, or acquiescence, in violation of a patient's human rights is a breach of loyalty to the patient.

Accordingly, passivity in the face of state requirements that violate patients' human rights is not excused.

Article 13 of the Guidelines recommends that the health professional should act individually and collectively to bring an end to policies and practices that prevent him or her from providing core health services to some or all patients in need. Such practices would include failure by the state to take appropriate steps to achieve the highest attainable standard of health for all; inequity in allocation of health resources or benefits; discrimination (or tolerance of discrimination) in health on grounds of sex, race, ethnicity, class, sexual orientation, refugee and immigrant status, religion, language, caste or class or disability; and denial of health information (such as information about reproductive health). The Guidelines explicitly state that its provisions also apply in private practice where the state's obligations extend to ending discrimination and assuring the highest attainable standard of health.

The DLWG takes the position that health professionals have a positive obligation to end practices that effectively lower the extent and quality of health services they provide to certain individuals. In this view, when the professional denies or limits appropriate care to an individual because of constraints caused by unfair or inequitable allocation of public resources, institutionalised discrimination, or state failure to address the needs of vulnerable groups, he or she becomes an instrument in the violation of protection against discrimination or the right to the highest attainable standard of health. Rather than adjust his or her practice to the constraints imposed by discrimination or state failure to develop a fair and equitable allocation of health resources, the health professional should act to remove those constraints.

The DLWG recognises that there are obvious limits to protecting a patient's human rights, especially where the violations are structural and pervasive. In these instances the DLWG suggests that the only means by which health professionals can protect, respect and fulfil the human rights of their patients is through collective action or through professional organisations working to bring about a fairer and less discriminatory system.

According to Article 14 of the Guidelines the health professional should support colleagues individually and collectively – through professional bodies – when the state acts to impede or threaten their ability to fulfil their duty of loyalty to patients. Mollendorf's case is an example of where strong collective action could yet be beneficial to discourage similar victimisation by the state. The DLWG position is that collective action is necessary to provide redress and that each individual health professional has the responsibility to support colleagues at risk of intimidation or reprisal for challenging unjust state policy.

Bibliography

AABY P, BABIKER A, DARBYSHIRE J, NUNN A, BARRETO S, ALONSO P ET AL. 'Ethics of HIV trials'. *Lancet* 1997; 350: 1546.

ABDOOL KARIM SS. 'Placebo-controls in HIV perinatal transmission trials: A South African viewpoint. *American Journal of Public Health* 1998; 88: 564–566.

ANGELL M. 'The ethics of clinical research in the third world'. *New England Journal of Medicine* 1997; 337: 847–849.

ANGELL M. 'Investigators' responsibilities for human subjects in developing countries'. *New England Journal of Medicine* 2000; 342: 967–8.

APPELBAUM PS ET AL. *'False hope and best data'.* Hastings Centre Report 1987, 17: 20–24.

ANONYMOUS. 'Another HIV-1 trial loses placebo-control'. *Lancet* 1997; 350:831.

BALETA A. 'South African Judge Reaffirms Judgment to Expand Access to AIDS Drug'. *Lancet* 2002; 359: 954.

BEAUCHAMP TL, CHILDRESS JF. 1994. *Principles of Biomedical Ethics.* 4th ed. New York. NY: Oxford University Press: 441.

BENATAR S, SINGER PA. 'A new look at international research ethics'. *British Medical Journal* 2000; 321: 824–826.

CENTERS FOR DISEASE CONTROL. *'Short-course regimen of AZT proven effective in reducing perinatal HIV transmission: Offers hope for reducing mother-to-child HIV transmission in developing world'.* February 24, 1998.

CONNON EM ET AL. 'Reduction of maternal-infant transmission of Human Immunodeficiency Virus Type I with Zidovudine treatment'. *New England Journal of Medicine* 1994; 331: 1173–1180.

EDITORIAL. 'The ethics industry'. *Lancet* 1997; 350: 897.

EICHENWALD K, KOLATA G. 'Drug trials hide conflicts for doctors'. *New York Times* May 16, 1999.

EICHENWALD K, KOLATA G. 'A doctor's drug trial turns into fraud'. *New York Times* May 17, 1999.

GOLDNER JA. 'Dealing with conflicts of interest in biomedical research: IRB oversight as the next best solution to the abolitionist approach'. *Journal of Law Medicine and Ethics* 2000; 28: 379–404.

HALSLEY ET AL. 'Ethics and international research'. *British Medical Journal* 1997; 315: 965–966.

KATZ J. 'Human experimentation and human rights'. *St Louis University Law Journal* 1993; 329: 573–576.

LONDON L. 'Human Rights and Public Health: Dichotomies or Synergies in Developing Countries? Examining the Case of HIV in South Africa'. *Journal of Law, Medicine and Ethics* 2002; 30: 677–691.

MINISTER OF HEALTH AND OTHERS v TREATMENT ACTION CAMPAIGN AND OTHERS (No 2) 2002 (5) SA 721 (CC).

LEMMENS T AND FREEDMAN B. 'Ethics review for sale? Conflict of interest and commercial research review boards'. *The Milbank Quarterly* 2000; 78: 547–584.

LEVINE RJ. 'The "best proven therapeutic method" standard in clinical trials in technologically developing countries'. *IRB: A Review of Human Subject Research* 1998; 20: 5–9.

LURIE P AND WOLFE SM. 'Unethical trials of interventions to prevent or reduce perinatal transmission of the human immunodeficiency virus in developing countries'. *New England Journal of Medicine* 1997; 337: 853–856.

MBIDDE EK. 'Ethics of placebo-controlled trials of zidovudine to prevent the perinatal transmission of HIV in the third world'. *New England Journal of Medicine* 1998; 338: 837.

MORIN K, RAKATANSKY H, RIDDICK FA JR, MORSE LJ, O'BANNON JM 3RD, GOLDRICH MS ET AL. 'Managing conflicts of interest in the conduct of clinical trials'. *Journal of the American Medical Association* 2002; 287: 385–391.

MSAMANGA GI, FAWZI WW. 'The double burden of HIV infection and tuberculosis in sub-Saharan Africa'. *New England Journal of Medicine* 1997; 337: 849–851.

NATIONAL BIOETHICS ADVISORY COMMISSION. *'Ethical and Policy Issues in International Research: Clinical Trials in Developing Countries, Report and Recommendations of the National Bioethics Advisory Commission.* Volume 1. Bethesda, Maryland. April 2001.

NICOLL A. *'Are existing guidelines good enough?'* Nuffield Council of Bioethics Workshop on the Ethical Issues of Clinical Research in Developing Countries, 21–23 February 1999, London.

PHYSICIANS FOR HUMAN RIGHTS AND UNIVERSITY OF CAPE TOWN HEALTH SCIENCES FACULTY. *'Dual loyalty and human rights in health professional practice: Proposed guide-lines and institutional standards'.* Boston: Physicians for Human Rights (http://www.phrusa.org/healthrights/dual_loyalty.html).

QUINN TC, WAWER MJ, SEWANKAMBO N, SERWADDA D, LI C, WABWIRE-MANGEN F ET AL. 'Viral load and heterosexual transmission of human immunodeficiency virus type 1'. *New England Journal of Medicine* 2000; 342: 921–9.

RURAL DOCTORS ASSOCIATION OF SOUTH AFRICA. *'Victory for Dr Thys von Mollendorf'.* March 2003. http://www.rudasa.org.za/papers/mollendorf.php

SALOOJEE H. *'Affidavit in Support of the Treatment Action Committee Against the Minister of Health and Nine Provincial MEC's for Health.'* Transvaal High Court. 2001. Available on-line at: www.tac.org.za

SOUTH AFRICA, DEPARTMENT OF HEALTH *'Guidelines for Good Practice in the Conduct of Clinical Trials in Human Participants in South Africa'.* 2000.

SPERLING RS, SHAPIRO DE, COOMBS RW, TODD JA, HERMAN SA, MCSHERRY GD ET AL. 'Maternal viral load, Zidovudine treatment, and the risk of Human Immunodeficiency Virus Type I from mother to child'. *New England Journal of Medicine* 1996; 335: 1621–1629.

STUDDERT DM, BRENNAN TA. 'Clinical trials in developing countries: Scientific and ethical issues'. *The Medical Journal of Australia* 1998; 169: 545–548.

TARASOFF V. REGENTS OF UNIVERSITY OF CALIFORNIA. 17 Cal. 3d 425, 551 P.2d 334, 131 Cal. Rptr. 14 (Cal. 1976).

THOMPSON DF. 'Understanding financial conflicts of interest'. *New England Journal of Medicine* 1993; 329: 573–576.

UNITED STATES DEPARTMENT OF HEALTH AND HUMAN SERVICES. *'The conduct of clinical trials of maternal-infant transmission of HIV supported by the United States Department of Health and Human Services in developing countries'.* Washington, D.C., July 1997.

VARMUS H, SATCHER D. 'Ethical complexities of conducting research in developing countries'. *New England Journal of Medicine* 1997; 337: 1003–1005.

WILKINSON D, ABDOOL KARIM SS, COOVADIA H. 'Short-course antiretroviral regimens to reduce maternal transmission of HIV'. *British Medical Journal* 1999; 318: 479–480

CHAPTER 26
The economic impact of AIDS

Alan Whiteside

AIDS WILL AFFECT THE economy; growth will slow and the structure will change. However, economics is also a driver of the epidemic in that economic hardship can change people's behaviour in a way that will make them more susceptible to infection.

South Africa is a middle income country but one in which the distribution of wealth is still very uneven. Per capita growth in South Africa has been low in the last decade although overall the economy has grown. However, there have been fundamental changes in the structure of the economy. The primary (agriculture, forestry and mining) and secondary (manufacturing, electricity, gas, water and construction) sectors are shrinking as contributors to gross domestic product (GDP), while the tertiary sector (all services – banking, insurance, trade and tourism) is growing. The result has been rising unemployment.

The macroeconomic impact of AIDS is determined by the demographics of those most affected, the young and economically active, and in the costs of combating the disease. It is likely that economic growth will be less than it would be without AIDS, although the exact reduction is hard to determine. What is certain is that rising prevalence of HIV/AIDS lowers worker efficiency, raises costs, and reduces individual savings and firms' profits.

At a microeconomic level it appears that the impact on households will be severe as already strained finances are stretched even further by illness and death.

Understanding economics

All South Africans have a stake in the economy of the country. Our share of the country's wealth, government spending, and changes in employment are directly affected by economic performance and economic policies.

Inevitably, AIDS will affect South African economics. Conventional wisdom is that the economy will grow more slowly and its structure will change, possibly by decreasing employment and health care spending. But, if people's deaths did not affect the functioning of the economy, at a macroeconomic level and in purely economic terms, the survivors could be better off. However, all the evidence points to the disease increasing poverty and misery at the household level.

Equally, economics itself influences the epidemic, as one of the drivers and determinants of the scope and scale of the epidemic. For example, poverty drives many women into sexual associations to provide for themselves and their children. It also leaves women powerless in relationships. At the same time, the resources allocated to the disease, often determined by economists, will at least in part determine the responses to it.

Economics is the study of the allocation of scarce resources, the distribution of the products of these resources, and the consequences of this allocation and distribution. All economic decisions are driven by choice, scarcity and uncertainty. Choice, because if we have only R1000 and use it for prevention then we can't use it for care; scarcity, as there are not enough resources, including money, staff and infrastructure; and uncertainty because we do not know what the results of our decisions will be. In the case of HIV prevention the simple question 'what works?' has not been answered.

Broadly economics is divided into two, often interlinking, areas:

- Macroeconomics is the study of the whole economy, including national economies, how they operate and change and embrace national output, trends in employment and income distribution, price increases and money supply.
- Microeconomics is concerned with individual behaviour, what determines the decisions individuals make and how these decisions interact.

South Africa is defined as a middle-income economy. TABLE 26.1 provides economic data for South Africa, the USA (very rich) and Mozambique (very poor). Kenya and Botswana provide comparisons with other African countries.

By African standards, South Africa has a large economy and is, at first glance, well off. However, development is about more than

Country	Gross National Product (US billion)	Population (million)	GNP per capita	Human Development Index (HDI)	Gini coefficient
United States	8351	273	30600	0.934	40.8
Botswana	5.1	2	3240	0.577	Na
Kenya	10.6	29	360	0.514	44.5
South Africa	133.2	42	3160	0.702	59.3
Mozambique	3.9	17	230	0.323	39.6

wealth; it is also about the distribution of that wealth, still very uneven in South Africa. The Gini coefficient (a measure of distribution) gives another picture. Perfect distribution is indicated by zero; 100 shows that one person has it all. The Human Development Index (HDI) was constructed by the United Nations Development Programme to look beyond simple economic measures and combines measures of income, longevity and education.

Since 1994 there has been little per capita growth in South Africa. Ten years ago per capita incomes stood at R13 786. In 1997 they were R14 249 but fell to R14 013 in 1999. However, economies may change without affecting the macroindicators, adding complexity to the discussion. In South Africa the economy has been relatively stagnant in terms of per capita output, although in real terms output has grown. However, this disguises fundamental changes in the structure of the economy. The primary (agriculture, forestry and mining) and secondary (manufacturing, electricity, gas, water and construction) sectors are shrinking as contributors to gross domestic product (GDP), while the tertiary sector (all services – banking, insurance, trade and tourism) is growing. This new structure of production has resulted in a real decline in the numbers in formal employment, from 5 576 000 in 1991 to 4 864 000 in 1999. The unskilled have been worst affected, at a time when the economically active population is growing.

'Factors of production' that influence wealth in all sectors of the economy include human and non-human resources. Labour is the obvious human resource and the total number of people available and their willingness to enter the labour market (quantity) and their quality in terms of health, productivity and skill will vary. The non-human resources are land and capital, the latter being anything other than money that contributes to production. However, invested money is obviously crucial for economic growth, both through local savings and foreign investment.

What will the economic impact of AIDS be? Current projections are that the disease may have serious, long-term and adverse consequences. However, the impact is more than just economic and we need to be aware of this.

TABLE 26.1 Comparative Economic Data from the 2000/2001 World Bank, World Development Report (1999 data) and 2001 United Nations Development Programme Human Development Report *Source: World Bank, World Development Report 2000/2001, Oxford University Press. Washington 2000 and UNDP, Human Development Report 2001, New York 2001*

Macroeconomic impact

Will AIDS cause national economies to grow more slowly? This prospect is an important argument when lobbying for government and international action. On a government level, slower economic growth means less money and consequently a population poorer than it would be in the absence of AIDS. At company level, labour costs will rise, productivity decrease and markets will be affected. Furthermore, if for example, Africa's per capita growth were to be 0.7% lower than it would be in the absence of AIDS, this would have far-reaching international effects.

Such potential slowing of growth was predicted as early as 1992. Mead Over of the World Bank looked at the effects of AIDS in 30 African countries, examining the labour force, capital accumulation and other factors. His model projected economic growth rates with and without AIDS from 1990 to 2025 and suggested that:

- There are two key parameters: the distribution of infection and hence illness and death across the labour force; and the degree to which the illness will be funded from savings and limit investment.
- Under all scenarios AIDS meant economic growth rates would be 0.56% to 1.47% lower.
- GDP per capita impact was less clear cut. If the costs of AIDS are not financed from savings and most illness is among lower skill levels then per capita income could rise by 0.17% across the 30 countries and 0.13% in the ten worst affected. If all the costs were met from savings and illness is concentrated among the highest skill levels, then per capita income would fall by 0.35% across the 30 countries and 0.60% in the ten worst affected.

This work was done over a decade ago but nonetheless most subsequent models have come up with similar figures. Rene Bonnell, another World Bank economist, suggested that AIDS had reduced Africa's economic growth by 0.8% in the 1990s. HIV/AIDS and malaria combined, resulted in a 1.2% decrease in per capita growth annually between 1990 and 1995.

In South Africa, the Centre for Health Policy at the University of Witwatersrand suggested that the major initial impact would be on the public health service. In the longer term, the epidemic was expected to pose a threat to ongoing economic growth, affecting some sectors more seriously than others. Generally, the conclusion was that the overall effect would be sustainable for the economy for the next 15 years, although broader society would still be seriously affected.

Most of the work on the macroeconomic impact of AIDS in the developing world comes from South African investment groups and think tanks, most notably ING Barings, The Bureau for Economic Research and Standard Bank. Using demographic data from models developed by the Actuarial Society of South Africa, ING Barings has predicted the impact of AIDS on GDP, household disposable income, and real consumption expenditure. They also looked at the impact on demand components of GDP, government finances, components of domestic savings, trade and the current account, and financial variables and employment. The headline finding is that AIDS will cause the economy to grow more slowly. GDP growth in 2001 will be 0.3% lower because of AIDS, and for the period 2006 to 2010 it will be 0.4% lower each year. Household income and expenditure will decrease, as will government revenue and domestic savings.

In 2001 the Bureau for Economic Research noted that the basis of the economic impact of HIV/AIDS lay 'first and foremost' in the demographic effects and secondly in the costs of combating the disease. AIDS could mean that between 2002 and 2015 GDP growth could be between 0.3% and 0.6% lower than it would have been in the absence of the disease. But the conclusion was that the negative impact on GDP is gradual and the economy could continue to grow by 3% average real GDP growth over the next 10 to 15 years. Inflation could still average around 7% which is in line with the past few years in South Africa, and real interest rates may be only marginally higher. The point is that the impact is in comparison with a situation in which AIDS did not affect the region, something which we will never be able to quantify.

This research was confirmed by other studies such as that of Arndt and Lewis who note that by 2010 the economy would be 17% smaller than it would have been in the absence of AIDS; and by 2010 GDP per capita 8% lower than it would have been. The main drivers would be a shift in government spending towards health, increasing the budget deficit and reducing total investment, resulting in slower growth in productivity.

Despite the uncertainties of macroeconomic studies there is growing interest in what the disease will mean for South Africa. The impact of the epidemic is now inescapable as the scale and speed of the epidemic is worse than expected. The number of people infected with HIV in 2003 is considerably above that predicted in 1990 and known demographic effects are now such that recognition of economic consequences is unavoidable. There is also evidence of impact at micro-levels, making calculations of macro-impacts credible. In addition, the complexity of the disease and the scope of its consequences is better understood. For example, loss of key government workers means work is not done efficiently, investment is reduced, and economic growth slows. As the development consequences of the disease become apparent it is obvious that there must be a macroeconomic impact.

Furthermore, AIDS is an issue on the agenda of all investors, partly as a result of the adverse publicity surrounding the confusing response to the epidemic by government. AIDS feeds into the questions around the investment climate. Jeffery Sachs, former Director of the Centre for International Development at Harvard University commented in 2001 that the government's handling of the crisis had undermined business confidence in South Africa by causing bewilderment among investors over the policy judgement of the ruling party.

The headline finding of a 2002 Standard Bank workshop on the economic implications of AIDS was that models are correct to indicate an adverse impact on the economy but that the assumptions are variable and the outcome difficult to quantify. This fits in with the innovative work of MacPherson and colleagues. Their argument is that conventional economics misses the complexity and full significance of the epidemic. When the epidemic was in its early stages projections based on scenarios computed 'with AIDS' and 'without AIDS' were reasonable, but such comparisons are no longer valid. The disease cannot be treated as an 'exogenous' influence that can be 'tacked on' to models derived on the presumption that the work force is HIV-free. HIV/AIDS is an 'endogenous' influence in most African countries.

The authors point out that rising prevalence of HIV/AIDS lowers worker efficiency, raises costs, and reduces individual savings and firms' profits. The problem with economic decline is that once it begins it is not easy to halt. AIDS has the potential to push economies into decline and then keep them there.

In 2000 the South African Budget Review noted that the effects of HIV/AIDS on future population growth and labour force participation are difficult to predict, as is the economic and social impact. However, it suggested that population growth may slow to close to 0% by 2010, with the growth of the working age population declining from over 2% in 2000 to under 0.5% by 2008. Although it appeared that the Department of Finance was starting to take the threat of AIDS seriously, there was no further coverage of the epidemic in 2001 and 2002 budget reviews.

Unpacking macroeconomics – what do we know?

We know that AIDS is causing and will cause many hundreds of thousands of South Africans to fall ill and die. We know that already there are probably 200 000 excess adult deaths annually and that numbers will rise. Already many South African children have been orphaned, and again we know the numbers will increase, putting pressure on already stretched families. The consequence for social cohesion and political stability are unknown. We do know that if antiretroviral therapy is made available then some of the increase in morbidity, mortality and its consequences will be postponed. However, this too will have a cost. Resources used for antiretrovirals, be they financial, staff or infrastructural, cannot be used for other things (although they may represent a saving on other expenditure).

We also know that labour will be affected in a number of ways:

- There will be increased illness and death and so fewer people of working age.
- There may be effects on the quality of labour – people are sick but keep working.
- The education and training system may suffer.
- Productivity may decline because of the points above but also because morale is lower.

Government revenue and expenditure will be altered. Government will experience increased demands for social, welfare and health services. This will happen at a time when revenues are already adversely affected because of the macro- and microeconomic impacts. The impact of AIDS on the budget is one area which needs further study. According to the Institute for Democracy (Idasa) AIDS may put off foreign investors. This is a real concern but there is no published work on the impact of AIDS in investment flows. Internal investment may also be affected through lower levels of economic activity, increased interest rates, lower corporate profits and savings and a smaller national savings pool.

AIDS has an adverse macroeconomic impact. The complexity and long-term interrelated nature of this is beginning to be appreciated. Government and policy makers are not, and need not be, passive in the face of the epidemic. Innovative policies mobilising additional resources are needed. For example, skill shortages probably cannot be met from local sources and additional education and training for nationals requires long-term investment. The answer may be imported labour, requiring policies to speed up processing of work and residence permits and anathema to most governments. Welfare spending may have to be increased and directed at people who would not normally receive it.

Private sector and government
South African production, divided into sectors, is illustrated in TABLE 26.2.

	R million	%
Primary Sector	**94101**	10.6
Agriculture, forestry and fishing	27293	3.1
Mining and quarrying	66808	7.5
Secondary Sector	**213333**	24
Manufacturing	163880	18.5
Electricity, gas and water	23915	2.7
Construction (contractors)	25538	2.9
Tertiary Sector	**579659**	65.3
Wholesale and retail trade, catering and accommodation	115756	13
Transport, storage and communication	88384	10
Financial intermediation, insurance, real estate and business services	182202	20.5
Community, social and personal services	**193317**	21.8
General government services	140804	15.9
Other services	25667	2.9
Other producers	26846	3
Gross value added at basic price	**887093**	

TABLE 26.2 Gross value added by type of economic activity 2001 (current prices) *Source: South African Reserve Bank September 2002, Quarterly Bulletin*

The measured wealth of the country is produced by individuals, companies and the government, which grow the crops, make the goods and provide the services. Productive activities also take place between the macro- and micro-levels. There is surprisingly little information available on the impact of AIDS at this level.

Firm level studies

These are the most influential studies and include those from the Centre for International Health (CIH) at Boston University's School of Public Health showing that AIDS is equivalent to an additional payroll cost, so increasing the cost of doing business. TABLE 26.3 shows the estimated cost of AIDS to businesses and the benefits of prevention and treatment using company-specific data on employees, costs and HIV prevalence for five large enterprises in South Africa and Botswana.

While it is possible to study the impact of AIDS on larger companies, this is more difficult for smaller companies, the informal sector and subsistence agriculture. What research there is (mainly outside South Africa) shows that AIDS will reduce production because of illness and death. The tragedy of the disease is that if a person is employed, it is the illness that most disrupts production; death is an event that can be planned for. This is especially true for the public sector.

Sector	Heavy manufacturing	Agribusiness	Mining	Mining	Retail
Workforce size (number of employees)	>25 000	5 000–10 000	<1 000	<1 000	<1 000
Est. HIV prevalence 2002 (%)	9.9	24.4	33.6	24.1	11.2
Cost per infection by job level (present value, 2001 USD)					
Unskilled/semi-skilled	32 393	4 439	10 732	9 474	4 518
Technician/artisan	50 075	6 772	17 972	14 097	11 422
Supervisor/manager	83 789	18 956	63 271	45 515	24 149
Average cost per infection (multiple of median salary)	4.3	1.1	5.1	2.9	0.9
Liability acquired in 2002 (future cost of incident infections) (% of payroll)	5.0	2.4	9.4	5.9	0.9
Undiscounted cost of prevalent infections in 2006 (% of payroll)		4.8	18.1	12.2	1.8

With regard to subsistence agriculture there are a number of studies, all outside South Africa. The findings are similar. One study carried out for the Zimbabwe Farmers Union in one communal and small farm area found that any adult death resulted in a 45% decline in marketed output of maize, but where the cause of death was identified as AIDS there was a 61% loss.

TABLE 26.3 Costs of AIDS in five companies in South African and Botswana

What about productivity more generally? The Centre for International Health, Boston, notes that the general reason for lack of research is that in most settings, neither the health nor the productivity of an individual worker can be directly observed. The exception is in the commercial agriculture sector where workers may be paid by the amount harvested each day, and may receive health care from on-site, company-owned medical facilities. In these cases the estates have data on both the daily output and the health of each worker.

The Boston team were the first to look at the impact of AIDS on productivity and reviewed records of health and output over a five year period on a tea plantation in Kericho district, Kenya. During their last three years of life, tea pluckers who died of AIDS were absent from work almost twice as often as other tea pluckers. Most (58%) of this difference was comprised of unpaid (and unauthorised) leave. Output began to fall as early as three years before death for those infected with HIV. Over their last three years of life people living with HIV averaged only 91% of 'full' productivity (of controls). During their last year of life, productivity fell sharply to 82% and to 77% in the last three months. This points to labour being both more expensive (unless you shift the costs) and at the same time, less productive.

There was speculation in the mining industry in South Africa that the impact on productivity would go beyond the ill individual. The suggestion was that if one person on a 15-man gang was to fall ill then his workmates would tend to cover for him, lowering the productivity of the entire team. Of great concern is the public sector, where job security is often seen as a substitute for salary. People accept lower pay and expect to get other benefits including substantial sick leave. In normal times this can be (and is) factored in. However, AIDS leads to abnormal conditions, and it is probable that governments will operate increasingly inefficiently, with all the attendant consequences for the business climate, competitiveness and output.

Of particular concern are public sector health, education and welfare provision. In South Africa most children have access to education, there is a health service, and the welfare system transfers resources to the elderly through a state pension and to children through a number of grants. AIDS is having an effect in all these areas. The demand for health care is rising at a time when capacity to provide it is under threat. Unfortunately health workers are falling ill and dying from AIDS (or leaving the state sector to work in the private sector or emigrate). The increase in adult mortality is creating large numbers of orphans, and they in turn need government support. The elderly are facing ever-larger demands on their pensions as they take in grandchildren. In the education sector the illness and death of teachers means the capacity of the school system is declining.

Effectively production in the private and state sector is imperilled and likely to decline. This will have a macroeconomic impact. But more than that, there will be long-term effects on growth prospects. An unhealthy and uneducated population is not conducive to economic growth. The 2001 report of the Commission on Macroeconomics and Health makes the compelling argument that investing in health will result in macroeconomic growth, suggesting that good health is necessary (but not sufficient) for economic growth. Historical evidence from Europe, the USA and other OECD countries suggests that economic takeoff was supported by breakthroughs in public health, disease control, and better nutrition.

The Commission argues that societies with a heavy burden of disease have many severe impediments to economic progress. Most striking is the statement that 'a typical statistical estimate suggests that each 10% improvement in life expectancy at birth (LEB) is associated with a rise in economic growth of at least 0.3 to 0.4% points per year, holding other growth factors constant'. In high-income countries life expectancy at birth is 75 years for men and 81 for women (and rising). In sub-Saharan Africa it is 49 years for men and 52 for women (and falling). Thus the difference in growth will be about 11.6% per year, and this will cumulate rapidly. 'In short, health status seems to explain an important part of the difference in economic growth rates, even after controlling for standard macroeconomic variables'.

The report identifies four key channels of influence of disease on economic development:

- Disease reduces the number of years of healthy life expectancy.
- There is an impact on parental investment in children. High levels of infant and child mortality result in families having more children, reducing the ability of a family to invest in the health and education of the children.
- Disease reduces the returns to business and infrastructure investment in a number of sectors.
- Epidemic and endemic diseases can undermine social cooperation and even political and macroeconomic stability.

For South Africa the implications are bleak. Nonetheless, no matter how bleak they are at the macro and intermediate level, they are worse at the micro level. The full impact of the epidemic will ultimately be borne by households. As people lose their access to private support they will turn to the government for assistance. For government, AIDS increases demand for services while reducing capacity. When the state fails, or there is no state, people have to turn to their own resources. This includes the household, extended family and community. It is here that the full impact of the disease is being felt.

Microeconomic impact

What do studies on microeconomic impact show? Essentially that there is a close relationship between a household being affected by HIV/AIDS and its subsequent impoverishment, with children being particularly vulnerable. The impact at household level is considerable.

However, there are problems with household economic impact assessments:

- They concentrate on rural households.
- As their titles indicate, these are mainly *economic* studies.
- The problem is usually researched as a *household* study. This excludes information about relations between households.
- Survey methods fail to capture the most seriously affected households; those that have disintegrated before the survey starts.
- Policy makers, politicians and agencies demand quantitative, survey-based studies because they have a form of evidential 'truth'

which coincides with the demands of referees who are often academics. Such forms of academic 'truth', although valid, are partial and do not tell of the underlying misery.

- Single or even multi-visit surveys, unsupported by ethnographic methods, tend to underestimate impact.
- Commonly used survey methods fail to capture the dynamics of household and intra-household allocation and relations that underlie household decision making.
- AIDS may be seen as the major problem by the researcher, who has written and submitted a research proposal or is responding to a 'terms of reference' or 'scope of work' document. Communities and households may not have the same perception of its importance.

Therefore, while still important, these household economic impact assessments tend to be flawed and incomplete. Furthermore, such studies seldom provide clear directions on how the impact of HIV/AIDS on households can be mitigated.

A survey of households affected by HIV/AIDS in South Africa released in 2002 gives a clear indication of the impoverishing nature of the epidemic. The study surveyed more than 700 households with at least one person already sick with AIDS. It covered four South African provinces: Gauteng, Mpumalanga, Free State and KwaZulu-Natal. Significantly the sample was drawn from households already in contact with non-governmental organisations. It is a snapshot of HIV/AIDS-affected families but is not a representative sample of all affected households in South Africa. If anything it will underestimate the impact of HIV/AIDS among all affected households in the country.

The key findings were:
- Two thirds of the households in the survey reported loss of income as a consequence of HIV/AIDS.
- Almost half reported not having enough food and that their children were going hungry.
- Almost a quarter of all children under age 15 in the sample had already lost at least one parent.
- In 12% of the households, children were sent away to live else-where; in 8%, children under 18 were the primary caregivers; and in 25% of households, caregivers were over 60.
- More than two-thirds of the AIDS-sick individuals in the survey were women and girls, with an average age of 33.
- Only about 50% of the respondents have acknowledged publicly that the sick person they were caring for had HIV/AIDS; one in 10 reported hostility and rejection.

- Fewer than 16% of households in the survey were receiving government grants of any kind, even though all qualified for some form of assistance.
- Some 55% of AIDS-affected households paid for a funeral in the last year and spent, on average, four times their total monthly income on this.

New paradigm for analysis

Economics is known as 'the dismal science' and the conclusion here is dismal. Economics does not and cannot show the impact of AIDS, indeed it may even give the wrong message. There are three challenges facing South Africa in the decades ahead. First and foremost is prevention. We have to stop new infections. Second, we need to provide care and treatment for those infected. Finally we need to mitigate the impact on families, households, the elderly and orphans.

Most economic analyses provide little information that will help inform responses to the epidemic. The word 'mitigation' is frequently used as a possible response, as if it were a specific recommendation. In fact policymakers have a choice of a wide variety of ways to mitigate the impact of HIV/AIDS. Mitigating the impact of HIV/AIDS on households, for example, might include the provision of food, counselling, orphan support, educational support, employment opportunities, revolving loans, etc. Yet the reality is that most economists have instead focused on the size of the impact, rather than the effectiveness of the responses. This may have been important at the early stages of the epidemic, when simple 'awareness raising' was critical, but it is now crucial to move further towards finding the most appropriate way to mitigate impact.

Bibliography

ARNDT C, LEWIS J. 'The HIV/AIDS pandemic in South Africa: Sectoral impacts and unemployment'. *Journal of International Development* 2001;13: 427–449.

BARNETT T, WHITESIDE A. 2002. *'AIDS in the twenty-first century: Disease and globalisation'.* Basingstoke: Palgrave.

BUREAU FOR ECONOMIC RESEARCH. 2001. *'The Macro-economic impact of HIV/AIDS in South Africa'.* Stellenbosch: University of Stellenbosch.

CENTER FOR INTERNATIONAL DEVELOPMENT. *'Policy and practice: Economic trends. South Africa – AIDS inaction concerns investors'.* September, 2001.

FOX M, ROSEN S, MACCLEOD, WASUNNA M ET AL. 'The impact of HIV/AIDS on labor productivity in Kenya'. *Tropical Medicine and International Health* 2004; 9: 318–324.

GOW J, DESMOND C. 2002. *'Impacts and interventions: The HIV/AIDS epidemic and the children of South Africa'.* Pietermaritzburg. Natal University Press.

GREENER R. 'AIDS and Macroeconomic Impact', in *State of the Art: AIDS and Economics*. Ed Steven Forsythe. Washington: The Policy Project, July (IAEN, State of the Art). 2002.

JOHNSON L, DORRINGTON R. *'The Impact of AIDS on orphanhood in South Africa: A quantitative analysis'*. Cape Town: Centre for Actuarial Research, University of Cape Town, October 2001 Care Monograph No. 4.

ROSEN SB, MACLEOD WB, VINCENT JR, FOX MP, THEA D, SIMON JL. *'Investing in the epidemic: The impact of AIDS on businesses in Southern Africa'.* [ThOrG1505], XIV International AIDS Conference, Barcelona, July 2002.

STEINBERG M, JOHNSON S, SCHIERHOUT G, NDEGWA D, HALL K, RUSSELL B, MORGAN J. *'Hitting home: How households cope with the impact of the HIV/AIDS epidemic: a survey of households affected by HIV/AIDS in South Africa'.* Health Systems Trust and The Kaiser Family Foundation, October 2002.

WHITESIDE A, SUNTER C. 2000. *'AIDS: The challenge for South Africa'.* Cape Town: Human and Rousseau Tafelberg.

WORLD HEALTH ORGANISATION. *'Macroeconomics and Health: Investing in health for economic development, Report of the Commission on Macroeconomics and Health'.* Geneva, WHO, 2001.

CHAPTER 27
AIDS-related mortality in South Africa

Debbie Bradshaw and Rob Dorrington

INFORMATION ON VITAL STATISTICS and mortality is important for planning resource allocation, identifying vulnerable households and communities and for town and regional planning. The rapid increase in young adult mortality in the late 1990s in South Africa, as estimated by the Medical Research Council's report on adult mortality, provides compelling evidence of the impact of the maturing HIV/AIDS epidemic, particularly among young women. This observation has been borne out from comparisons with data collected in two rural districts in South Africa. While there are anecdotal accounts of similar impacts in child mortality, the limited number of birth registrations makes the population register an unreliable tool for assessing trends in child mortality.

Models calibrated to available data have played an important role in estimating the cause of death profile. Estimates of the burden of disease show that by the year 2000, HIV/AIDS was already the biggest single cause of death. The Department of Health is in the process of rolling out a comprehensive treatment and care programme including antiretrovirals. Without better mortality data, and more timely production of statistics, it will be difficult, if not impossible, to monitor the impact of these programmes reliably. Urgent efforts are needed to improve the quality and timely production of statistics to monitor the effectiveness of these expensive and important programmes.

Definitions

Infant mortality rate (IMR) – the probability that an infant under one year of age dies. This is a key indicator of child health and also a measure of the health of the broader population. In the absence of highly active antiretroviral therapy and/or a prevention of mother-to-child-transmission (PMTCT) programme, the infant mortality rate is a sensitive marker of the prevalence of HIV among pregnant women in areas of high prevalence.

Under five mortality rate (u5MR) – the probability of a child dying before the age of five years. This is a preferred indicator of child health as it includes a measure of the vulnerability of toddlers that includes the impact of maternal and environmental health. Compared with the infant mortality rate, this indicator responds more slowly to changes in the HIV prevalence among pregnant women and will continue to increase over a longer period after the introduction of an antiretroviral programme and/or a PMTCT programme.

Adult mortality (45q15) – the probability of a 15-year-old dying before the age of 60 years. This indicator is affected by the increased mortality of young adults, including the ages when HIV is expected to have its greatest effect.

Life expectancy (e0) – the average age that an individual will live to from birth. As mortality rates increase, this summary measure decreases.

The lack of reliable vital statistics, including death statistics, in South Africa has made it difficult to monitor the impact of HIV on mortality. Indeed, mortality rates are key measures of the general state of development and health of a nation and are widely used for international comparisons. In developed countries, with well-established vital registration based on good quality medical certification of underlying causes, the rise in AIDS deaths prior to the introduction of HAART was clearly seen, with AIDS becoming the leading cause of death in certain age groups in the 1980s and continuing until the mid-1990s. Since the introduction of highly active antiretroviral therapy in industrialised countries, these trends have changed and the AIDS mortality rates have declined (FGURE 27.1).

Routine mortality statistics in South Africa are compiled by Statistics South Africa (Stats SA) from the vital registration system. The statistics are based on the medical certification of the cause of death, required by law, at the time of registration of the death with the Department of Home Affairs. However, the statistics are problematic, as death registration is known to be incomplete and to suffer from misclassification of cause of death. After 1994, the Government started extensive efforts to improve death registration and statistics. These involved the introduction of a new death certificate, dissemination of manuals on how to complete the death certificate and classify the cause of death and the establishment of a task team in each province to improve registration. This system improved the percentage of all deaths registered from a low of slightly more than 50% in

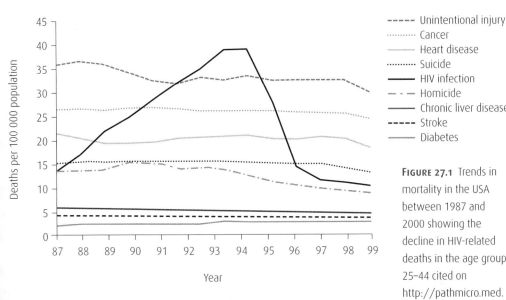

FIGURE 27.1 Trends in mortality in the USA between 1987 and 2000 showing the decline in HIV-related deaths in the age group 25–44 cited on http://pathmicro.med.sc.edu/lecture/hiv-usfigs.htm
Source: CDC

1990 to 78% in 1995 and over 80% in 1996. By 2000 about 90% of adult deaths were registered.

However, despite improved registration, delays continue to occur in the production of statistics with complete cause of death data. This makes it difficult to provide reliable information on AIDS mortality without careful interpretation and further analysis. There is still a degree of under-registration of deaths particularly in rural areas and there is mis-classification of causes of death. This problem is common to the interpretation of all causes of death. In the case of AIDS-related deaths in South Africa, it is often not specified because benefits such as pensions and life insurance pay outs may be withheld. In many instances the opportunistic infection present at the time of death is more likely to be reported as the cause of death. This problem is more pronounced in rural areas where death is often certified by a tradition-al leader who is not usually able to specify cause of death. Thus the statistics arising from the death certificates need careful considera-tion and interpretation with caveats.

Several attempts have been made to improve the recording of death statistics in rural areas. A study conducted in rural KwaZulu-Natal assessed the feasibility of using community health workers within the community to establish possible causes of deaths by conducting verbal autopsies with primary caregivers of the deceased. The com-munity health workers liaise closely with the traditional leaders and can provide more reliable data regarding causes of death. The use of verbal autopsies has been validated in other parts of South Africa, where they have shown to be reliable in assessing cause of death, even in rural areas. The use of a verbal autopsy instrument in rural districts has shown that death rates due to AIDS and pulmonary tuberculosis in the middle-aged and young are rising.

The impact of HIV/AIDS on mortality – empirical data

The South African Medical Research Council, in conjunction with the University of Cape Town, set up a system to monitor the changing pattern in mortality of the deaths recorded on the population register. This team released a report in 2001 that used reliable demographic

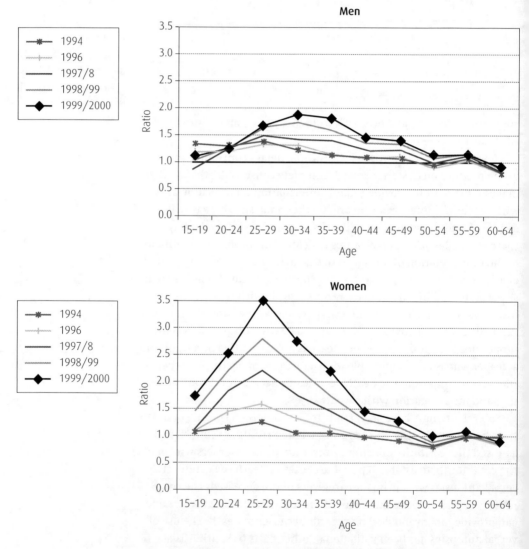

FIGURE 27.2 Estimated increase in adult death rates relative to the 1985 death rates
Source: Dorrington et al. 2001

techniques to adjust for the under-recording of deaths and demonstrated a steady increase in adult mortality during the late 1990s, irrespective of the cause. FIGURE 27.2 shows the relative increase in the estimated death rates for men and women. By the year 2000, it was estimated that the rates had increased 2.5 times for women aged 25 to 29 and 1.5 times for men aged 30 to 39. Having explored alternative explanations, it was concluded that HIV was the cause of this change. Based on the assumption that the increase could be attributed to HIV/AIDS, it was estimated that about 40% of mortality between the ages 15 to 49 years was due to HIV/AIDS and 25% of mortality across all ages. There is much more uncertainty about the extent of the impact of HIV/AIDS on child mortality than there is for adults as there are other very common causes of deaths in infants.

In response to this information, the South African Government set up an investigation into the reported causes of death. Stats SA processed a sample of death certificates for the years 1997 to 2001. The proportion of deaths attributed to HIV as the underlying cause rose from 5% of all deaths to 9%. However, the proportion of deaths due to external causes (which are likely to be more accurately recorded) decreased rapidly, indicating that natural causes had increased. Hence there was a concomitant increase in AIDS-indicator conditions such as TB (from 5% to 9%) and pneumonia (from 5% to 9%) confirming the rapid change in the cause of death profile arising from the maturing HIV epidemic.

The rise in the number of adult deaths in South Africa continues. Without adjusting for under-registration, the number of deaths on the population register increased in the last few years by nearly 70%. Part of this rise could be attributed to population growth (12%) and part to improved registration, both of persons on the population register and of deaths (less than 10% assuming that registration has not achieved full coverage), leaving a real increase of more than 40%. In the case of women aged 20 to 29 years, there has been an increase of 190% in the deaths registered which corresponds to a real increase in mortality of more than 150% once population growth and possible improvement in registration are taken into account. Thus far, the increase in adult mortality has continued unabated.

The impact of AIDS on adult mortality in rural South Africa

There are two externally funded district level population-based research sites in South Africa that include comprehensive demographic surveillance where deaths and their causes are carefully monitored. These are situated in the rural Bushbuckridge area of

Mpumalanga Province and part of the rural district of Umkhanyakude (Mtubatuba) in northern KwaZulu-Natal. Based on interviews
with the caregivers of the deceased, using relevant autopsy techniques, the causes of death have been identified by clinicians from
the disease history and the signs and symptoms prior to the death.

Both sites have found an increase in the young adult mortality
that can clearly be attributed to HIV/AIDS. The levels of mortality have
risen sharply, particularly in the late 1990s. For example, by the year
2000 the adult mortality rate (45q15) was 75% for men and 58% for
women in rural KwaZulu-Natal. The data from this district revealed
that AIDS, with or without TB, was the leading cause of adult death
accounting for 48% of the deaths of people aged 15 to 59 years.

Estimates of causes of death in South Africa

Given the limitations of the cause of death statistics, a national
burden of disease study was undertaken by the Medical Research
Council (MRC) to analyse all the available data in an attempt to derive
consistent and coherent estimates for the underlying causes of death
in South Africa. The Burden of Disease Research Unit of the MRC was
set up to collate and analyse data relating to health status and factors
affecting health. The ASSA2000 model was used by this MRC unit to
estimate the total number of deaths and the number of AIDS deaths.

The ASSA2000 model

The ASSA2000 model was developed by the Actuarial Society of South
Africa as a refinement of the ASSA600 AIDS and Demographic model.
These ASSA models are non-proprietary and allow users to alter
parameters to suit their needs. The original ASSA600 model models
the demographic impact of HIV/AIDS in the national population by
assuming that the population (those aged 15 to 29 at the start of the
epidemic and those turning 14 in each future year) can be split into
four risk-groups depending on the risk of transmitting/contracting
the virus. In the ASSA600 model these comprise the following:

- a small, high-risk group comprising sex workers and clients
- a much larger group, assumed to be at similar risk of transmitting/
  contracting the virus as people who regularly contract sexually
  transmitted infections (STIs)
- an even larger group who are at risk because of their sexual behaviour, but don't have STIs
- a similarly sized group who are assumed never to be at risk.

The ASSA2000 model incorporated new or updated information
about the population including 1988 to 2000 antenatal survey (ANC)

summary results, 1998 South African Demographic and Health Survey data and improved population estimates. There were also refinements such as allowing a better fit to the national ANC survey results and being able to model population groups and genders separately.

The national injury mortality surveillance system and the cause of death statistics processed by Stats SA were used to estimate the numbers of deaths due to other causes. The national injury mortality surveillance system was set up by the Medical Research Council at selected mortuaries to be able to track the causes of death in the case of injuries. Stats SA process the national death statistics – however, the injuries tend to have incomplete information about causes in this system – making it necessary to use both.

Careful analysis of several data sources was undertaken to assess the consistency of these estimates. The top causes of death thus identified are shown in TABLE 27.1, which shows that in 2000, the number of AIDS deaths was leading over other causes. These estimates also reflect the unique quadruple burden of disease experienced in South Africa with the co-existence of the pre-transition diseases related to under-development, the emerging chronic diseases, a high injury burden and recent impact of HIV/AIDS. FIGURE 27.3 shows the age distribution of the deaths in 2000 by broad cause group. The distinct age pattern of AIDS deaths among children and young adults is clearly apparent.

Mathematical model projections of AIDS mortality – ASSA

This increase in mortality was predicted by projections from mathematical models calibrated to the observed rapid increase in the prevalence of HIV. Projections based on the more recent version of the Actuarial Society of South Africa's ASSA2002 model include the impact of the roll-out of antiretroviral therapy (FIGURE 27.4). These show how the mortality is the third wave; following the incidence and the prevalence and that the prevalence reaches a plateau when the number of deaths matches the number of new cases.

Trends in key indicators of mortality suggest that infant mortality is expected to have peaked in about 2002 and started to decline with the under-five mortality rate following soon thereafter. Adult mortality rates are expected to increase until about 2006, with male mortality starting from a higher base and remaining higher than female mortality as shown by data from the ASSA2002 model. A further consequence of these increases will be an increase in the number of children who are orphaned (FIGURE 27.4).

Males				Females				Total			
Rank	Cause of death	Number	%	Rank	Cause of death	Number	%	Rank	Cause of death	Number	%
1	HIV/AIDS	80 089	26.4	1	HIV/AIDS	85 770	33.8	1	HIV/AIDS	165 859	29.8
2	Homicide/ violence	27 134	9.0	2	Stroke	18 184	7.2	2	Ischaemic heart disease	32 919	5.9
3	Tuberculosis	19 806	6.5	3	Ischaemic heart disease	14 539	5.7	3	Homicide/ violence	32 485	5.8
4	Ischaemic heart disease	18 380	6.1	4	Lower respiratory infections	10 430	4.1	4	Stroke	32 114	5.8
5	Stroke	13 930	4.6	5	Tuberculosis	9 748	3.8	5	Tuberculosis	29 553	5.3
6	Road traffic accidents	13 076	4.3	6	Hypertensive heart disease	9 458	3.7	6	Lower respira-tory infections	22 097	4.0
7	Lower respira-tory infections	11 667	3.8	7	Diabetes mellitus	8 081	3.2	7	Road traffic accidents	18 446	3.3
8	Diarrhoeal diseases	8 150	2.7	8	Diarrhoeal diseases	7 761	3.1	8	Diarrhoeal diseases	15 910	2.9
9	COPD	8 102	2.7	9	Low birth weight	5 427	2.1	9	Hypertensive heart disease	5 427	2.6
10	Low birth weight	6 449	2.1	10	Road traffic accidents	5 370	2.1	10	Diabetes mellitus	13157	2.4
11	Trachea/ bronchi/lung ca	5 085	1.7	11	Homicide/ violence	5 351	2.1	11	COPD	12 473	2.2
12	Diabetes mellitus	5 076	1.7	12	COPD	4 372	1.7	12	Low birth weight	11 876	2.1
13	Suicide	4 866	1.6	13	Nephritis/ nephrosis	3 505	1.4	13	Nephritis/ nephrosis	7 225	1.3
14	Hypertensive heart disease	4 774	1.6	14	Cervix ca	3 424	1.4	14	Trachea/ bronchi/ lung ca	7 173	1.3
15	Oesophageal ca	3 886	1.3	15	Asthma	3 227	1.3	15	Asthma	6 987	1.3
16	Asthma	3 760	1.2	16	Septicaemia	3 057	1.2	16	Suicide	6 370	1.1
17	Nephritis/ nephrosis	3 720	1.2	17	Breast ca	3 009	1.2	17	Septicaemia	6 047	1.1
18	Cirrhosis of liver	3 704	1.2	18	Inflammatory heart disease	2 559	1.0	18	Oesophageal ca	5 803	1.0
19	Protein-energy malnutrition	3 039	1.0	19	Protein-energy malnutrition	2 471	1.0	19	Cirrhosis of liver	5 672	1.0
20	Septicaemia	2 990	1.0	20	Trachea/ bronchi/lung ca	2 088	0.8	20	Protein-energy malnutrition	5 511	1.0
	All causes	303 081			All causes	253 504			All causes	556 585	

TABLE 27.1 Top twenty specific causes of death by sex, estimated for South Africa 2000
Source: Bradshaw et al. 2003

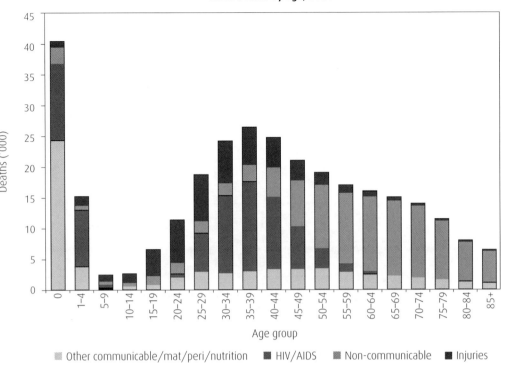

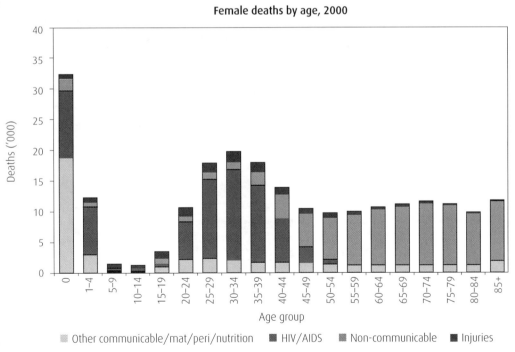

FIGURE 27.3 Age distribution of estimated deaths by group and sex, 2000 *Source: Bradshaw et al. 2003*

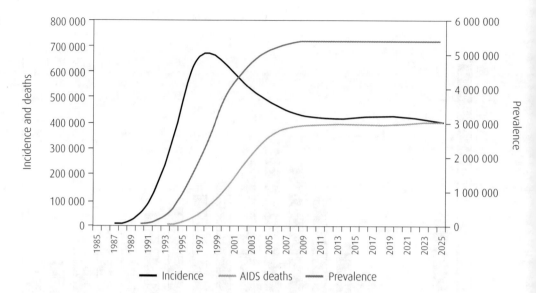

FIGURE 27.4 Projected number of incident and prevalence HIV cases and AIDS deaths based on ASSA2002 model. *Source: Authors*

Conclusion

The rapid increase in young adult mortality in the late 1990s in South Africa provides compelling evidence of the impact of the maturing HIV/AIDS epidemic, particularly among young women. However, the population register is unable to provide insight into the trends in child mortality as too high a proportion of children are not placed on the population register at birth. Models, calibrated to available data, estimate that, already by the year 2000, HIV/AIDS was the biggest single cause of death.

Bibliography

BAH S. 'A note on the quality of medical certification of deaths in South Africa , 1997–2001'. *South Arfican Medical Journal* 2003; 39; 239.

BRADSHAW D, GROENEWALD P, LAUBSCHER R, NANNAN N, NOJILANA B, NORMAN R, PIETERSE D, SCHNEIDER M. *'Initial Burden of Disease Estimates for South Africa, 2000'*. Cape Town: South African Medical Research Council. 2003. www.mrc.ac.za/bod/bod.htm

BRADSHAW D, LAUBSCHER R, DORRINGTON RE, BOURNE DE, TIMAEUS IM. 'Unabated rise in the number of adult deaths in South Africa.' *South African Medical Journal* 2004; 94; 278–279.

DORRINGTON RE, BOURNE D, BRADSHAW D, LAUBSCHER R, TIMAEUS IM. *'The impact of HIV/AIDS on adult mortality in South Africa'*. MRC Technical Report. MRC: Cape Town. ISBN 1-919809-14-7.

Dorrington RE, Bradshaw D, Budlender D. *'HIV/AIDS profile of the provinces of South Africa – indicators for 2002'* Centre for Actuarial Research, Medical Research Council and the Actuarial Society of South Africa. Accessed April 2003 at www.mrc.ac.za/bod/bod.htm

Groenewald P, Nannan N, Bourne D, Laubscher R, Bradshaw D. *'Identifying deaths from AIDS in South Africa'. AIDS* 2005; 19: 193–201.

Hosegood V, Vanneste AM, Timaeus IM. 'Levels and causes of adult mortality in rural South Africa: The impact of aids'. *AIDS* 2004; 18: 663–671.

Kahn K, Tollman SM, Garenne M, Gear JSS. 'Who dies from what? Determing cause of death in South Africa's rural north-east'. *Tropical Medicine and International Health* 1999; 4: 433–441.

Statistics South Africa. *'Advance release of recorded cause of deaths 1997–2001'.* Statistical Release P0309.2. Statistics South Africa, Pretoria. 2002.

Tollman SM, Kahn K, Garenne M, Gear JS. 'Reversal in mortality trends, evidence from the Agincourt field site, South Africa 1992–1995'. *AIDS 1999*; 13: 1091–1097.

SECTION 6
Treating HIV

CHAPTER 28
TB and HIV

Gavin Churchyard and Elizabeth Corbet

TB IS AN IMPORTANT GLOBAL public health threat and the burden of TB is increasing because of HIV infection. TB is the leading cause of death among HIV-infected Africans. South Africa not only has the highest number of HIV-infected individuals in the world, but has the 8th highest burden of TB worldwide.

In individuals with early HIV infection, the presentation of TB is similar to that in HIV-uninfected individuals and is usually pulmonary. But in those with severe immunosupression, presentation may be atypical.

TB is treated in the same way in HIV-infected and HIV-unifected individuals, but care must be taken when treating HIV and TB concomitantly because of interactions between anti-TB and antiretroviral drugs. Treatment with antiretrovirals can lead to immune reconstitution inflammatory syndrome in those coinfected with TB and HIV.

DOTS is reducing TB transmission in many countries, but is not enough to prevent the incidence of TB rising in areas of high HIV prevalence.

What is needed are efforts to reduce TB transmission through active case finding and preventing reactivation of latent TB through preventive therapy.

Tuberculosis (TB), a curable and preventable disease, remains an important public health threat globally. Approximately one third of the world's population is infected with *Mycobacterium tuberculosis* and the global burden of TB is increasing, in part because of the HIV epidemic, with a 0.4% per year increase globally, and a 6.4% per year increase in sub-Saharan Africa. An estimated 68% of all individuals who are co-infected with HIV and *M tuberculosis* (MTB/HIV co-infection) live in sub-Saharan Africa. East and southern Africa have been hit hardest by the HIV epidemic, and in this region even countries with well-run TB control programmes have reported more than four-fold increases in TB case-notification rates since 1990. The increasing burden of HIV-associated TB poses a growing threat to TB control in the wider community. Approximately one third of all TB cases in sub-Saharan Africa are directly attributed to HIV infection, and up to 75% of TB patients in some countries are HIV-infected. TB is the leading cause of death among HIV-infected Africans.

This chapter provides an overview of the epidemiology, pathogenesis, clinical presentation, treatment and control of HIV-associated TB, using South African examples where appropriate.

Epidemiology of TB and HIV in South Africa

South Africa has the highest number of HIV-infected and the 8th highest burden of incident TB of any country worldwide (TABLE 28.1). About two million South Africans are MTB/HIV co-infected, and the estimated incidence of all forms of TB was 509 per 100 000 population for 2002. Of these, 60% of adult cases are also HIV infected. Reported treatment outcomes for patients diagnosed in 2000 were disappointing because only 66% successfully completed treatment. The reported rate of death during treatment, 7%, is probably a considerable underestimate. This is because of under-notification of TB in patients who die without leaving hospital, misclassification of deaths as defaults from treatment, and failure to capture the high death rate among patients who transfer their care from urban to rural locations

Population, millions	43
Global rank (by estimated number of cases)	8
New cases of TB, all forms	
Number of cases, thousands	220
Incidence rate per 100 000 population	509
Change in incidence rate 1997–2000, %/year	8.7
HIV prevalence in new adult cases (15–49 years old), %	60
Adult cases attributable to HIV, %	50
Prevalent TB	
Smear positive TB, per 100 000 population	219
Smear positive, HIV-positive TB cases, %	21
Infection prevalence among adults	
Prevalence of MTB infection, %	42
Prevalence of MTB/HIV co-infection, %	8.3
Deaths from TB	
Deaths from TB, thousands	60
Deaths from TB, per 100 000 population	139
Adult AIDS deaths due to TB, %	18
TB deaths attributable to HIV, %	59

TABLE 28.1 TB-HIV estimates for South Africa for 2000 *Data extracted from Corbett et al. 2003*

because of terminal illness. The overall death rate from TB, including undiagnosed cases, was estimated as 139 per 100 000 population for 2000, giving a case fatality rate of 27%.

In sub-Saharan Africa TB incidence is strongly correlated with HIV prevalence: the higher the HIV prevalence estimates for the country, the higher the TB incidence. Although this is true for South Africa compared with other countries, and there is a relationship between HIV prevalence and TB case-notifications at the National level (FIGURE 28.1), the same relationship does not hold at provincial level (FIGURE 28.2).

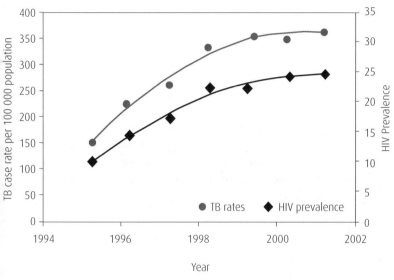

FIGURE 28.1 Trends in TB case notification rates and HIV prevalence among ante-natal clinic attenders in South Africa. Polynomial regression lines are displayed for TB case rates and HIV prevalence. Data based on the Department of Health's 2003 TB report

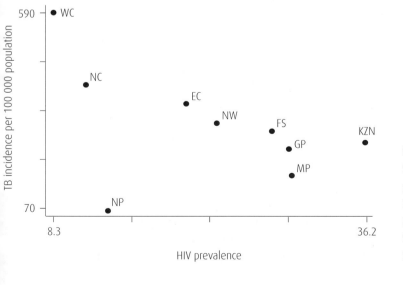

FIGURE 28.2 TB notification rates and HIV prevalence among ante-natal clinic attenders, by province (See Table 28.2 for abbreviations used for provinces)

This is because there is currently a strong gradient of diminishing HIV prevalence from East to West superimposed on an older pattern of increasing TB incidence from East to West that predates the HIV epidemic (FIGURE 28.2, TABLE 28.2).

TABLE 28.2 TB notification rates and HIV prevalence among ante-natal clinic attenders, by province *TB rates based on case notification rates for 2000 **HIV prevalence among ante-natal clinic attenders, 2000

Province	TB rates *	HIV prevalence **
	Per 100 000 population	
Eastern Cape (EC)	351	20.2
Free State (FS)	279	27.9
Gauteng (GP)	231	29.4
KwaZulu-Natal (KZN)	248	36.2
Mpumalanga (MP)	163	29.7
Northern Cape (NC)	400	11.2
Northern Province (NP)	70	13.2
North West (NW)	300	22.9
Western Cape (WC)	590	8.3
South Africa	**274**	**24.5**

In the Western Cape only a small fraction of TB cases can be attributed to HIV at present, whereas a high proportion are likely to be HIV-related in the Eastern Cape. Clearly these relationships will change if HIV prevalence becomes more homogenously distributed within South Africa. The attributable fraction estimates for all TB cases in South Africa, including adjustment for under-diagnosing and under-reporting, are that one-third of all TB cases in 2000 were directly attributable to HIV.

HIV and the risk of TB

TB incidence

HIV infection leads to an increased risk of active TB, either from reactivation of latent infection or from rapid progression to disease following recent infection. Strain-typing studies of African TB patients have found no association between HIV status and restriction fragment length polymorphism (RFLP) clustering, indicating that the proportion of disease due to recent transmission events is the same among HIV-positive as it is among HIV-negative TB patients.

HIV-uninfected individuals with TB infection have a ten to 20% lifetime risk of developing TB disease following MTB infection, whereas MTB/HIV-infected individuals have an annual risk of developing TB disease that can exceed 10%. TB incidence is greatest among those who are tuberculin skin test (TST)-positive, lowest among TST-negative individuals and variable among individuals unable to make any cutaneous response to other recall antigens such as mumps or candida (cutaneous anergy). Reported TB incidence rates for HIV-infected individuals who are TST-positive range from 3.4 to 16.2 per 100 person-years.

Estimates of relative risk

The WHO has estimated that HIV-infected individuals living in non-industrialised countries develop TB at six times the rate of HIV-uninfected individuals. This contrasts with an incidence rate ratio of 60 for HIV-infected individuals living in industrialised countries, where both MTB infection and HIV are relatively concentrated in a few minority groups.

In South Africa the only estimates of the relative risk of TB among HIV-infected individuals are from cohort studies of gold miners, which have shown that HIV-infected miners develop TB at 5.5 to six times the rate of HIV-negative miners. The susceptibility of gold miners to TB disease is increased further because of occupational exposure to silica dust, a strong risk factor for TB that interacts multiplicatively with the risk from HIV infection.

Immune status

Increased susceptibility to TB is evident from an early stage of HIV infection. Studies from Cape Town and among gold miners have documented that the risk of TB becomes more pronounced as the degree of immunosuppression increases, based on CD4 category or clinical stage.

Recurrent TB

As in other countries with endemic TB, recurrent disease accounts for a significant proportion of all TB in South Africa. HIV infection increases the risk of recurrence following successful treatment of TB. Risk factors for recurrence of HIV-associated TB are initial treatment regimens with less than six months of rifampicin, post-TB scarring, cavities, and low CD4 counts.

The role of ongoing exposure to high rates of TB transmission has been clearly shown in a prospective strain typing study in South African mining TB patients. HIV-infected miners had recurrent TB disease due to a new MTB strain (documented reinfection) at 18.7 times the rate in HIV-uninfected miners, but there was no increase in their risk of recurrent disease due to the original strain (documented recrudescence or late treatment failure). In settings of lower TB incidence, recurrent TB still occurs more frequently among HIV-infected patients, although the absolute difference is small. These observations suggest that that there is little to gain from intensifying the treatment regimens currently used in South Africa, but that it is important to consider secondary TB preventive therapy in high TB transmission settings.

HIV and TB transmission

Studies of household contacts have shown that HIV-infected TB patients may be less or equally, but not more, infectious than HIV-uninfected TB patients. In part this is because smear-positivity is strongly correlated with infectiousness. HIV-infected TB patients are less often smear-positive than HIV-uninfected TB patients. Even when smear-positive, MTB/HIV coinfected patients are still not strongly infectious. A second major factor tending to reduce average infectiousness is the relatively rapid course of HIV-associated TB disease. In South African miners, for example, the infectious interval between the onset of HIV-associated TB and diagnosis has been shown to be less than a third of that of HIV-negative TB patients.

Impact of TB on HIV progression

TB and HIV also have an interaction at the cellular level. TB disease leads to immune activation and increased viral replication and it has been postulated that this could result in an accelerated progression of HIV disease, or a period of increased HIV infectivity. If either possibility were true then preventing TB would be even more important.

The question of whether TB accelerates HIV progression has been studied extensively, but the clinical significance is still not clear. A number of observational studies have shown that HIV-infected patients who develop TB have a worse prognosis than HIV-infected patients who have been staged at a similar level of immunosuppression but remain free of TB disease. However, staging HIV is not very precise and it is difficult to reconcile this hypothesis with the lack of impact on survival reported by most TB preventive therapy trials. Prospective studies measuring viral load before and after an episode of TB support the view that intercurrent TB indicates profoundly impaired immunity rather than being the cause of it.

Clinical presentation and management of HIV-associated TB

Clinical presentation and diagnosis

TB can occur at any level of HIV-related immunosuppression, but the annual risk increases as immunosuppression becomes more pronounced. The extent of immunosuppression also modifies both the clinical and radiological features of TB. TB occurring early on in the course of HIV disease closely resembles HIV-negative TB: the most common presentation is with pulmonary disease involving the upper zones and cavities and smear-positive disease are common. By contrast, HIV-infected individuals with advanced immunosuppression are more likely to present with less classical radiological changes, such as hilar adenopathy with or without lower or mid-zone consolidation. Most highly immunosuppressed patients are smear-negative, and there is a high prevalence of extrapulmonary and disseminated TB.

A relatively high proportion of HIV-associated TB disease is extrapulmonary, and almost half of these patients have both extra-pulmonary and pulmonary sites of disease, a combination rarely seen in HIV-negative TB patients. The most commonly affected sites are lymph nodes, pleural cavities, pericardium, peritoneum, meninges, vertebral bodies and synovial tissue of other joints. Disseminated TB with mycobacteraemia is now a common cause of admission to hospital in areas of high HIV prevalence. Diagnosis is often delayed or missed, and mortality is high. About one third of all hospital deaths among HIV-infected Africans are from TB, and the diagnosis is made in life in only about half of the fatal cases. The presentation may be non-specific, although most patients report cough. Histologically there is multi-organ involvement including the lungs, liver, spleen and bone marrow, with a high bacilliary load and failure to mount a granulomatous response.

TB should be suspected in all patients presenting with cough for more than three weeks and in all patients with prolonged fever, night-sweats or unexplained weight loss. Diagnosis should be based on sputum smears whenever possible, and three sputum specimens should be collected from all TB suspects reporting a cough, even if extrapulmonary TB is suspected. Fine needle aspirate of asymmetri-cally enlarged lymphnodes has a high yield on microscopy and is a quick and easy investigation to carry out. Surgical biopsy of other sites is more invasive and the patient may be best served by empirical treatment. Radiological investigations may show characteristic find-ings that are strongly suggestive of TB, for example mediastinal or intra-abdominal lymphadenopathy with peripheral enhancement.

Establishing HIV status and giving broad-spectrum antibiotics early on in the work-up facilitates management of smear-negative TB suspects. Care needs to be taken in interpreting response to anti-biotics, however, since bacterial superinfection is a common compli-cation of HIV-associated pulmonary TB, and may result in a partial but transient response. TB cultures are helpful if positive in that they confirm the diagnosis and allow drug sensitivity patterns to be established. However, there is often a lengthy interval between taking specimens and receiving results and treatment should not be delayed if TB is suspected. WHO recommends that patients are started on full TB treatment, without withholding rifampicin. Treatment can be stopped and the patient denotified if there is no clinical response by one month.

Treatment outcomes, including mortality on treatment

HIV-infected TB patients are managed with the same treatment regimen as HIV-uninfected patients, as detailed in the South African National Guidelines. HIV infection does not alter the pharmacokinetic characteristics of standard anti-TB drugs, and sputum conversion and cure rates are similar to those of HIV-uninfected patients, provided that standard rifampicin-based regimens are used.

However, HIV-infected TB patients are at increased risk of dying during treatment and TB is now a leading cause of death in South Africa. During the first month the excess mortality is mainly due to TB itself and is concentrated in patients with severe forms of disease, such as meningitis, and those who have become moribund by the time of diagnosis. Mortality after the first month is mainly due to intercurrent opportunistic infections, such as bacterial infections, *Pneumocystis carinii* pneumonia (PCP) and cryptococcosis. Survival is highest in patients with early HIV disease.

Chemoprophylaxis with trimethoprim-sulfamethoxazole (TMP-SMX) reduces the risk of intercurrent opportunistic infection with a number of different pathogens, including *P carinii*, *Streptococcus pneumoniae*, enteropathogenic bacteria, *Plasmodium falciparum*, and *Toxoplasma gondii*. The survival of HIV-infected TB patients can be substantially improved by adding cotrimoxazole at a dose of 960 mg per day two to four weeks after TB treatment has been started. A slight delay is recommended to allow side-effects from cotrimoxazole to be distinguished from those of the anti-TB drugs. Lower doses may be ineffective because of increased metabolism in patients taking rifampicin. Cotrimoxazole should be continued after TB treatment is stopped. Antiretroviral therapy also has a substantial impact on survival of HIV-infected TB patients, and is discussed in more detail below.

Resistance to antituberculous drugs

Unlike in Europe, the USA and Thailand, HIV-infected TB patients in Africa are at no greater risk of having a drug-resistant strain than HIV-uninfected TB patients. Institutional outbreaks of primary multi-drug resistant TB (MDR-TB) affecting HIV-infected individuals have, however, been reported from many countries, including South Africa. An outbreak in Sizwe Tropical Disease Hospital, Johannesburg, occurred when HIV-infected in-patients receiving treatment for drug susceptible TB were exposed to a patient with chronic cavitary MDR-TB. Institutionally acquired MDR-TB has a high morbidity, with rapid progression to disease in HIV-infected patients and a very high mortality if not promptly diagnosed and treated with an appropriate MDR-TB regimen. Because of this, patients with known or suspected MDR-TB should be kept apart from HIV-infected patients as far as possible.

Diagnosis and treatment of latent TB infection

The most commonly used diagnostic test for identifying previous infection with MTB is the tuberculin skin test (TST). The TST reaction does not distinguish active tuberculosis disease from latent tuberculosis infection, and suffers from sub-optimal sensitivity and specificity. Specificity problems arise because the antigen preparation, purified protein derivative or PPD, is a crude extract that contains numerous antigens, many of which cross-react with environmental mycobacteria and BCG. Sensitivity is a particular concern in HIV-infected individuals, because the TST is an *in vivo* immunological test and is affected by immunosuppression. The prevalence of reactivity in HIV-infected African adults, typically about 25%, is only about half that found in HIV-uninfected African adults, even though a lower reaction size is used to define reactivity in HIV-infected individuals. Among HIV-infected individuals, the prevalence of TST positivity is lowest in those with low CD4 counts, many of whom demonstrate cutaneous anergy.

Despite the strong theoretical grounds for doubting the validity of the TST, it nonetheless remains a surprisingly good predictor of future TB risk and response to preventive therapy in HIV-infected individuals. When a low reaction size of 5 mm or more is used to define a positive response a number of different randomised clinical trials have demonstrated that TST-reactive individuals have considerable benefit from TB preventive therapy, whereas there is little or no benefit in TST negative or anergic individuals. Thus the TST allows preventive therapy to be effectively targeted to a relatively small minority of HIV-infected patients who will benefit from it. For this reason both the International Union Against Tuberculosis and Lung Disease and WHO recommend that TST reactivity be used to define latent TB infection and guide the need for preventive therapy as far as possible, once active TB disease has been excluded with a symptom screen and chest radiograph.

A number of different preventive therapy regimens have been used in HIV-infected individuals, including isoniazid alone, rifampicin plus pyrazinamide, rifampicin plus isoniazid, and rifampicin plus isoniazid plus pyrazinamide. Of these, isoniazid is the best established and cheapest option, with six to nine months of 300 mg daily being the standard course. Meta-analysis of all available trial data indicates a 76% reduction in TB incidence in TST-positive HIV-infected recipients, with most of the data being from trials in Africa (FIGURE 28.3). There is no significant benefit from treatment in TST negative HIV-infected individuals, however, and most clinical trials have found little or no effect on mortality (FIGURE 28.3), despite the major reduction in TB incidence.

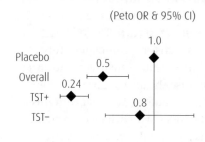

(Peto OR & 95% CI)

FIGURE 28.3 Efficacy of TB preventive therapy: Meta analysis. OR = odds ratio (diamond), CI = confidence interval (error bars), TST = tuberculin skin test, + = positive, − = negative. An OR<1 without overlapping confidence intervals suggests efficacy

Data extracted from Wilkinson 2002

The lack of survival benefit from preventive therapy seems paradoxical given that TB is the most common cause of death in HIV-positive Africans. This may reflect the relatively high standard of care and attention in diagnosing TB while patients are in clinical trials, and there is some evidence that there is indeed a pronounced survival benefit when isoniazid is used under operational conditions. However, there is also a suggestion that the effect of preventive therapy may wane with time, particularly where there is high TB transmission.

Isoniazid is well tolerated in most people. The most common side-effect is peripheral neuropathy, which can be prevented and treated with vitamin B12 (pyridoxine). Clinically significant hepatitis occurs in a small minority of patients, and fatalities can result if the drug is not stopped. Patients should be warned to stop treatment and report immediately if persistent nausea, vomiting or jaundice occur. The risk of fatal hepatitis is in the region of one in 10 000 persons treated, but increases with age, underlying chronic liver disease and high alcohol consumption. The Southern African HIV Clinicians Society guidelines recommend that patients with active alcohol abuse or liver disease should not be offered preventive therapy.

There is some evidence to suggest that the incidence of TB may increase with time after discontinuation of preventive therapy, and that the durability of rifampicin-containing regimens may be better than isoniazid alone. Rifampicin-containing regimens, where rifampicin is combined with pyrazinamide and/or isoniazid, only need to be administered for two to three months to achieve a comparable efficacy to that of isoniazid. However, they are less well tolerated and have not found wide acceptance in Africa, mainly because they are more expensive and because there is a strong emphasis on maintaining drug-sensitivity to rifampicin at all costs, within TB control programmes. The rifampicin-pyrazinamide combination has recently been withdrawn from routine use because of a high incidence of hepatitis in the United States, including some fatalities. In South Africa, the only strong indication for considering rifampicin-based preventive therapy is known exposure to drug-resistant TB, in which case at least two drugs to which the isolate is sensitive should be used.

Current international guidelines for TB preventive therapy among HIV-infected individuals are based on primary prevention in HIV-infected individuals with no previous history of TB. In the last few years, however, evidence has begun to accumulate that preventive therapy may also be effective in reducing TB recurrence rates in HIV-infected individuals who have already been treated for TB (secondary preventive therapy). The benefit may be particularly marked in areas of high TB transmission. Secondary isoniazid preventive therapy reduced the incidence of recurrent TB by 55% or more in three different studies (FIGURE 28.4), but with no major significant effect on mortality. Secondary preventive therapy may be easier to implement than primary preventive therapy and, in high TB prevalence areas, it seems reasonable to offer secondary preventive therapy in settings where primary preventive therapy is also being used. Only isoniazid 300 mg per day for one year or longer has been evaluated. The SA HIV Clinicians Society guidelines recommend secondary preventive therapy for HIV infected individuals who have had TB more than two years previously.

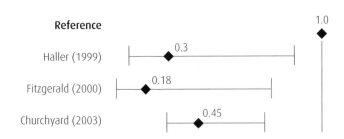

(Incidence Rate Ratios & 95% CI)

FIGURE 28.4 Efficacy of secondary TB preventive therapy. Incidence rate ratio of TB recurrence among HIV-infected individuals with a prior history of TB who received isoniazid compared with those who received placebo or with an historic cohort that did not receive isoniazid. Incidence rate ratios (indicated by diamond), CI = confidence interval (indicated by error bars) Incidence rate ratio less than 1 without confidence intervals overlapping suggest efficacy

Antiretroviral therapy

Antiretroviral therapy appears to be even more effective at reducing the incidence of TB disease among HIV-infected individuals than TB preventive therapy, although there have been no formal clinical trials. Antiretrovirals commenced during TB treatment reduces HIV viral load, the rate of AIDS-defining illnesses and has a pronounced effect on mortality. However, patients treated concomitantly for TB and HIV commonly experience adverse events, and both TB and HIV treatment can be compromised by drug interactions if care is not taken to choose compatible regimens.

The risk of TB, however, still remains high and is above that of HIV-uninfected individuals. The sparse data available from TB-endemic areas suggest that the greatest risk is in individuals in whom baseline CD4 counts were less than 200 cells/L when antiretroviral therapy was started (for example, this group had an incidence of TB of 3.4 per 100 person years in a study in South Africa). The continued high risk may be the result of a high prevalence of latent TB infection, or incomplete restoration of TB-specific immune responses with antiretrovirals.

Improvements in *in vitro* responsiveness to *M tuberculosis* following the start of antiretroviral treatment have been demonstrated in individuals previously treated for TB, those who had active TB when antiretroviral treatment was started, and those who have never had TB disease. However, despite successful control of viraemia, immune responses remain below those of HIV-uninfected controls and do not appear to recover completely. There is also *in vivo* evidence of immune restoration, in that the TST tends to increase in size with frequent conversion from negative to positive and immune reconstitution disorders are common in patients with diagnosed or undiagnosed active TB soon after antiretrovirals are started (see below).

Although at the individual level the benefit of antiretroviral therapy in reducing TB incidence seems clear, the impact at the population level is uncertain. Some authors have suggested that widespread uptake of antiretrovirals may be associated with a decline in TB incidence at a population level, particularly in industrialised countries, but other studies have not confirmed this. There is concern that widespread use of low potency antiretroviral regimens, or frequent short courses, may increase the absolute number of individuals with minimal or moderate immunosuppression who remain at risk of TB, which could actually increase TB incidence at a community level in settings with endemic TB.

Paradoxical reactions

HIV-infected and HIV-uninfected TB patients may experience new or worsening signs or symptoms of TB disease with TB treatment alone or with concomitant antiretrovirals. This phenomenon is referred to as a paradoxical reaction, or immune restoration inflammatory syndrome (IRIS). These reactions are thought to occur as a result of antiretroviral-mediated immune restoration with enhancement of the inflammatory response at sites containing *M tuberculosis* antigens. HIV-infected TB patients treated with antiretrovirals commonly experience paradoxical reactions when converting their TST from negative to positive, an event that usually occurs within a few weeks of staring antiretroviral treatment. The same phenomenon can occur among HIV-uninfected TB patients, in whom adult respiratory distress syndrome and other serious manifestations can result at the time of TST conversion, particularly in cases of miliary TB. Concomitant TB treatment and antiretrovirals is associated with a reported incidence of paradoxical reactions ranging from five to 36%, with extrapulmonary disease placing the patient at especially high risk.

The clinical manifestations are protean. Common symptoms and signs of paradoxical reactions include fever, lymphadenopathy and worsening of chest radiographic findings. However, virtually any site in the body can be involved, including the brain, pleural cavity and psoas muscles. There have been no reports of fatal reactions so far and most reactions are transient and self-limiting, although prolonged and severe reactions can occur. Recommendations for the management of paradoxical reactions include continuation of anti-TB treatment and antiretrovirals, use of nonsteroidal anti-inflammatories and corticosteroids when indicated. Indications for the use of corticosteroids include severe hypoxaemia, airways obstruction, neurological impairment and markedly enlarged painful lymph nodes. The ATS/CDC/IDSA guidelines recommend use of prednisone at 1 mg/kg with a gradual reduction after one to two weeks.

HIV-infected individuals living in communities with endemic TB have a high prevalence of undiagnosed active TB, which can be as high as 11% in severely immunosuppressed individuals. Initiation of antiretroviral treatment may unmask previously undiagnosed TB with an immune reconstitution disorder that can be very severe and may even be fatal. Current international and national guidelines make no recommendations about screening for TB prior to initiating antiretrovirals, but it seems prudent to do so using the same approach as for patients being considered for TB preventive therapy.

Concomitant antiretroviral and TB treatment

In South Africa most episodes of HIV-associated TB will occur among individuals who are unaware of their HIV status at the time of TB diagnosis: only a tiny minority will be patients already on antiretroviral therapy. Understanding the challenges of treating combined TB and HIV disease is important when introducing antiretrovirals into TB-endemic communities. The efficacy of both the TB and the HIV drug regimens can be compromised unless care is taken in the choice of antiretroviral regimen and the patient can also be exposed to an increased risk of drug toxicity.

Strategies to integrate TB and HIV treatment programmes need to be explored without compromising already overburdened TB control programmes. The most common approach used in the United States and Europe is to individualise both the TB and antiretroviral regimen. This type of approach is not ideal in endemic TB settings for a number of reasons: there is increased risk of TB treatment failure and generation of drug-resistant TB, and programmes could not cope with the large numbers of 'non-standard' TB patients that would result. Instead the WHO has proposed use of TB compatible regimens, and delayed start of antiretroviral treatment until the intensive phase of TB treatment is over where possible.

Drug interactions

Rifampicin is a critical component of all short-course TB regimens. Omission of this drug necessitates much longer treatment courses that have poor outcomes in HIV-infected patients. Unfortunately rifampicin is a potent inducer of the cytochrome P450-3A system and so affects the metabolism of many other drugs including most non-nucleotide reverse transcriptase inhibitors (NNRTIs) and protease inhibitors (PIs).

Rifampicin reduces the levels of most PIs by 75% apart from full-dose ritonivir or low-dose ritonivir in combination with saquinavir. Efavirenz levels are reduced by 20% when administered concomitantly with rifampicin, with a greater reduction occurring in patients weighing more than 50 kg. Metabolism of efavirenz may differ among individuals of different ethnic groups; white patients more affected than black Americans. Although rifampicin can be used together with efavirenz, some experts suggest increasing the dose of efavirenz from 600 to 800 mg to compensate for the slight decrease in efavirenz levels. Nevirapine and rifampicin can be used in combination, although nevirapine levels are reduced by about 30% and there may be an increased risk of hepatoxicity. Rifampicin also reduces the levels of zidovudine and abacavir. For this reason concern has been expressed about using the combination of these two drugs in a triple nucleocide regimen, such as trizivir.

An alternative to rifampicin, Rifabutin, has less effect on cytochrome P450-3A system and is often used as a substitute for rifampicin in affluent settings. However, it is extremely expensive and will not be available through the national TB programme.

When to treat

Deciding when to start antiretroviral treatment in a TB patient can be very difficult: delaying treatment in severely immunosuppressed individuals leaves them open to new complications of their HIV disease, some of which carry the risk of death or permanent disability, while starting antiretrovirals early has all of the problems discussed above.

The possible benefits and risks of starting antiretroviral therapy during TB treatment or delaying until TB treatment is completed are outlined in TABLE 28.3. These need to be determined on a case-by-case basis. The WHO and SA HIV Clinicians Society recommend that patients who are at high risk of AIDS-defining illnesses or death (CD4 count <200 cells/mm^3 or extrapulmonary TB) should be started on antiretrovirals during TB treatment. Patients with very advanced HIV disease (CD4 count <50 cells/mm^3) should start antiretroviral therapy as soon as TB treatment is tolerated. Antiretroviral treatment should be started in patients with CD4 counts between 50 and 200 cells/mm^3 after two months of TB treatment, as toxicities from TB drugs are greatest during this period. These recommendations, in the absence of clinical trial evidence, are based on clinical experience of the best time to start antiretrovirals in TB patients.

Antiretroviral regimens compatible with rifampicin-based TB regimens

The WHO recommend zidovudine (AZT) or stavudine (d4T) + lamivudine (3TC) + efavirenz (EFV) (600 or 800 mg/day) as a first-line regimen which is compatible with rifampicin-based TB regimens. Although saquinavir/ritonavir (SQV/RTV) (400/400MG bid), SQV/r (1600/200 mg qd in soft gel formulation) and lopinavir (LPV)/RTV (400/400 mg bid) are recommended by the WHO as alternatives to EFV, Roche and the US Food and Drug Administration have recommended that SQV/r *not* be used concomitantly with rifampicin, based on a recent Phase I study. The levels of other PIs are reduced to sub-therapeutic levels with rifampicin and are not recommended with rifampicin use. Abacavir (ABC) may also be substituted for EFV and has the advantage of reduced pill burden and requires no dose adjustment when given during TB treatment. The disadvantages include a significantly

ART during TB treatment	ART delayed until after TB treatment
Benefits	**Benefits**
• Less HIV-associated morbidity and mortality • Integrated HIV/TB care may lead to improved long-term ART adherence	• Reduced pill burden • No risk of drug interactions • Dose modifications not required • Reduced risk of paradoxical reactions • No need to alter ART regimen to accommodate TB treatment • Reduced adverse events from combined drug toxicities • Time for education and counselling in preparation for starting ART
Risks	**Risks**
• Increased pill burden that may lead to lower adherence to both TB and HIV treatment • ART dose modifications may be required • May need to alter ART regimen to accommodate TB treatment • More drug toxicities	• High risk of HIV-associated morbidity and mortality during TB treatment, particularly in individuals with advanced HIV disease

TABLE 28.3 Benefits and risks of starting ART during or following TB treatment

higher rate of virological failure compared to ZDV, 3TC and EFV and hypersensitivity reactions that may be difficult to distinguish from a paradoxical reaction. EFV is not recommended in woman of child-bearing age who may become pregnant. Nevirapine (NVP) is commonly substituted for EFV in these patients. There are limited data on the use of NVP with rifampicin. Although levels of NVP are reduced by rifampicin (TABLE 28.4), trough levels (which correlate best with virological response) remain in the therapeutic range. There may also be a greater risk of combined hepatotoxicity. WHO therefore recommend that NVP only be used when no other options are available. For women of childbearing age not on effective contraception, and pregnant women, SQV/r or ABC should be substituted for EFV.

The levels of other PIs are reduced to sub-therapeutic levels with rifampicin.

Once-daily antiretroviral regimens have acceptable potency, tolerability and safety. In a pilot study of 20 HIV-infected TB patients in KwaZulu-Natal, a directly observed once-daily antiretroviral regimen (didanosine (ddI), 3TC, EFV), co-administered with TB treatment was acceptable to patients and staff, safe and effective.

Antiretroviral therapy and isoniazid preventive therapy
It is recommended that prophylaxis of other opportunistic infections is continued until such time as sufficient immune reconstitution has

	Rifampicin	Rifabutin (daily)
NRTI	Caution when using triple nucleoside therapy	Normal dose
NNRTI		
Efavirenz	Efavirenz dose at 600–800 mg	Increase Rifabutin to 450–600 mg
Nevirapine	Nevirapine can possibly be used at normal dose in the absence of other options	Normal dose of each
Delaviridine	NR	NR
PI		
Amprenavir	NR	Decrease Rifabutin dose to 150 mg
Indinavir	NR	Decrease Rifabutin dose to 150 mg Increase indinavir to 1000 mg 8 hourly
Nelfinavir	NR	Decrease Rifabutin dose to 150 mg
Saquinavir	Can be used with low dose ritonavir	Normal Rifabutin dose
Ritonavir alone	Full dose ritonavir	NR
Lopinavir/ritonavir	NR	NR

TABLE 28.4 Dose adjustments between anti-retroviral therapy and rifamycins
NRTI = nucleoside reverse transcriptase inhibitors, NNRTIs = non-nucleoside reverse transcriptase inhibitors, PIs = protease inhibitors, NR = not recommended
Modified from Barnes et al. 2002

occurred. Although there are no data on which to base recommendations, isoniazid preventive therapy should probably be offered to TST-positive patients on antiretroviral treatment. TST-negative patients should have their TST checked again after a few months on antiretrovirals and should be offered isoniazid if it has converted to positive.

Controlling TB in the HIV era

DOTS

The current international and nationally recommended TB control strategy is DOTS (Directly Observed Therapy, Short course). DOTS aims to minimise TB transmission through prompt detection and cure of symptomatic infectious TB patients. The DOTS strategy has reduced TB prevalence, incidence and mortality in a number of countries with high burdens of endemic TB but low HIV prevalence rates. However, no country with a generalised HIV epidemic has managed to prevent TB incidence rates from rising, and it is clear that the DOTS strategy alone is inadequate in this case. There are some indications, however, that TB transmission rates can be kept at relatively stable levels by strong DOTS programmes, even when HIV prevalence and TB incidence rates are rising, and that favourable drug sensitivity patterns can also be maintained.

Beyond DOTS

Possible strategies for intensifying TB control include reducing TB transmission through enhanced or active case-finding and reducing reactivation of latent TB infection through use of preventive therapy.

Reducing TB transmission

Results of TB prevalence surveys suggest that there may be a significant burden of undiagnosed active TB in communities with endemic TB, including those with a high HIV prevalence. Community-wide TB active case-finding thus has the potential to reduce TB transmission. In endemic settings most TB episodes are the result of recent TB transmission events, so that a rapid fall in TB incidence could result from an effective intensified or active case-finding campaign.

The South African National TB Control Programme is actively exploring the possible options for enhancing case-finding, and some provinces have already started mobile TB clinics publicising the benefits of being tested for TB.

WHO recommend intensified case-finding for TB among known HIV-infected individuals, for example at voluntary counselling and testing centres and HIV care clinics. However, since HIV-uninfected TB makes a substantial contribution to TB transmission in the community and only a small fraction of HIV disease is diagnosed in South Africa, this approach has limited potential.

Reducing the risk of reactivation

TB preventive therapy as a strategy to improve TB control has limited potential when targeted to known HIV-infected individuals, because this will not affect the risk of disease and subsequent transmission from HIV-uninfected and undiagnosed HIV-infected patients. Similarly antiretroviral therapy may only have a modest impact on TB control, as it is too finely focused and would require widespread uptake by eligible individuals and excellent adherence to ensure that restored immunity is maintained.

A trial of community-wide preventive therapy in mineworkers, not targeted to known HIV-infected individuals, is being considered at present. This will provide data on the efficacy of an approach that has previously been successfully used to stop an epidemic of TB in native North Americans during the 1950s.

Integrating HIV and TB activities

A new strategic framework for reducing the burden of TB and HIV has been put forward by WHO, based on experience from the ProTEST initiative. Large-scale expansion of these programmes will be required if they are to have an impact on TB control at the community level.

Conclusions

Considerable progress has been made during the last decade towards the improvement of global TB control. DOTS, a clear strategy that is cost-effective, prevents drug resistance and reduces TB mortality and incidence in low HIV prevalence countries, has been developed and widely implemented. The drive to provide antiretroviral treatment to HIV-infected persons in the developing world has gained huge momentum and resulted in access to much cheaper drugs for Africans.

Despite these gains, there were still 8.5 million TB cases and 1.8 million deaths from TB in 2001, and the epidemic of HIV-associated TB continues to grow and drive global incidence rates upwards. Antiretroviral use is still very limited and we do not yet have a successful strategy for reducing TB incidence in high HIV-prevalence countries. The HIV epidemic has resulted in increasing TB case rates and mortality throughout sub-Saharan Africa, including South Africa.

Although HIV-associated TB may be more difficult to diagnose and carries a higher mortality than HIV-negative TB, the treatment outcomes among those who survive are good and it is possible to substantially reduce morbidity and mortality through the use of cotrimoxazole chemoprophylaxis and antiretroviral therapy. Integration and large-scale expansion of the HIV and TB control programmes, with universal access to HIV diagnosis, antiretrovirals and opportunistic infection prophylaxis has the potential to improve TB control and outcomes. The challenge for the coming decade is to successfully implement the interventions that we already know to be effective in reducing TB morbidity and mortality.

Bibliography

ANTONUCCI G, GIRARDI E, RAVIGLIONE MC, IPPOLITO G. 'Risk factors for tuberculosis in HIV-infected persons. A prospective cohort study. The Gruppo Italiano di Studio Tubercolosi e AIDS (GISTA)'. *Journal of the American Medical Association* 1995; 274: 143–148.

BADRI M, WILSON D, WOOD R. 'Effect of highly active antiretroviral therapy on incidence of tuberculosis in South Africa: A cohort study'. *Lancet* 2002; 359: 2059–2064.

BARNES PF, LAKEY DL, BURMAN WJ. 'Tuberculosis in patients with HIV infection'. *Infectious Disease Clinics of North America* 2002; 16: 107–126.

BRADSHAW D, SCHNEIDER M, DORRINGTON R, BOURNE DE, LAUBSCHER R. 'South African cause-of-death profile in transition – 1996 and future trends'. *South African Medical Journal* 2002; 92: 618–623.

CENTERS FOR DISEASE CONTROL AND PREVENTION. 'Updated guidelines for the use of rifabutin or rifampin for the treatment and prevention of tuberculosis among HIV-infected patients taking protease inhibitors or nonnucleoside reverse transcriptase inhibitors'. *Mobridity and Mortality Weekly Report* 2000; 49: 185–189.

CHURCHYARD GJ, FIELDING K, CHARALAMBOUS S, DAY JH, CORBETT EL, HAYES RJ ET AL. 'Efficacy of secondary isoniazid preventive therapy among HIV-infected Southern Africans: Time to change policy?' *AIDS* 2003; 17: 2063–2070.

CONRADIE FM, VAN DER HORST C, VENTER WDF, IVE PD, JENTSCH U, SANNE IM. *'Mycobacterium tuberculosis associated immune reconstitution syndrome and HAART in South Africa'.* [B10242] XIV International AIDS Conference, Barcelona. 2002.

CORBETT EL, CHURCHYARD GJ, CLAYTON TC, WILLIAMS BG, MULDER D, HAYES RJ ET AL. 'HIV infection and silicosis: The impact of two potent risk factors on the incidence of mycobacterial disease in South African miners'. *AIDS* 2000; 14: 2759–2768.

CORBETT EL, STEKETEE RW, TER KUILE FO, LATIF AS, KAMALI A, HAYES RJ. 'HIV-1/AIDS and the control of other infectious diseases in Africa'. *Lancet* 2002; 359: 2177–2187.

CORBETT EL, WATT CJ, WALKER N, MAHER D, WILLIAMS BG, RAVIGLIONE MC ET AL. 'The growing burden of tuberculosis: global trends and interactions with the HIV epidemic'. *Archives of Internal Medicine* 2003; 163: 1009–1021.

CRUCIANI M, MALENA M, BOSCO O, GATTI G, AND SERPELLONI G. 'The impact of human immunodeficiency virus type 1 on infectiousness of tuberculosis: a meta-analysis'. *Clinical Infectious.Diseases* 2001; 33: 1922–1930.

DEAN GL, EDWARDS SG, IVES NJ, MATTHEWS G, FOX EF, NAVARATNE L ET AL. 'Treatment of tuberculosis in HIV-infected persons in the era of highly active antiretroviral therapy'. *AIDS* 2002; 16: 75–83.

DEL AMO J, MALIN AS, POZNIAK A, DE COCK KM. 'Does tuberculosis accelerate the progression of HIV disease? Evidence from basic science and epidemiology'. *AIDS* 1999; 13: 1151–1158.

DYE C, WATT CJ, BLEED D. 'Low access to a highly effective therapy: A challenge for international tuberculosis control'. *Bulletin of the World Health Organisation* 2002; 80: 437–444.

GLYNN JR. 'Resurgence of tuberculosis and the impact of HIV infection'. *British Medical Bulletin* 1998; 54: 579–593.

GUIDELINES FOR TUBERCULOSIS PREVENTIVE THERAPY IN HIV INFECTION. 'Consensus guidelines from a workshop, 29–30 October 1999. HIV Clinicians Society of Southern Africa'. *South African Medical Journal* 2000; 90: 592–594.

HARRIES AD, HARGREAVES NJ, KEMP J, JINDANI A, ENARSON DA, MAHER D ET AL. 'Deaths from tuberculosis in sub-Saharan African countries with a high prevalence of HIV-1'. *Lancet* 2001; 357: 1519–1523.

JACK C, FRIEDLAND G, LALLOO U, EL-SADR W, CASSOL S, MURRMAN M ET AL. 'Integration of Antiretroviral Therapy into An Existing Tuberculosis Directly Observed Therapy Program in a Resource Constrained Setting (START Study)'. 10th Conference on Retroviruses and Opportunistic Infections 138. 2003.

KENYON TA, MWASEKAGA MJ, HUEBNER R, RUMISHA D, BINKIN N, MAGANU E. 'Low levels of drug resistance amidst rapidly increasing tuberculosis and human immunodeficiency virus co-epidemics in Botswana'. *International Journal of Tuberculosis and Lung Diseases* 1999; 3B: 4–1.

KORENROMP EL, SCANO F, WILLIAMS BG, DYE C, NUNN P. 'Effects of human immunodeficiency virus infection on recurrence of tuberculosis after rifampin-based treatment: An analytical review'. *Clinical Infectious Diseases* 2003; 37: 101–112.

MAHER D, FLOYD K, RAVIGLIONE MC. *'A strategic framework to decrease the Burden of TB/HIV'.* Stop TB Department, Department of HIV/AIDS, World Health Organization, WHO Report, WHO/CDS/TB/2002.296, WHO/HIV/2002.2. 2002.

MASUR H, KAPLAN JE, HOLMES KK. 'Guidelines for preventing opportunistic infections among HIV-infected persons – 2002. Recommendations of the U.S. Public Health Service and the Infectious Diseases Society of America'. *Annals of Internal Medicine* 2002; 137: 435–478.

MILLER S, ANDREWS S, COTTEN M, MAARTENS G, MARTEN D, WOOD R ET AL. 'Southern African HIV Clinicians Society Clinical Guidelines – Antiretroviral therapy in adults'. *Southern African Journal of HIV Medicine* 2002; 8: 22–29.

MUKADI YD, MAHER D, HARRIES A. 'Tuberculosis case fatality rates in high HIV prevalence populations in sub-Saharan Africa'. *AIDS* 2001; 15: 143–152.

POST FA, WOOD R, PILLAY GP. 'Pulmonary tuberculosis in HIV infection: Radiographic appearance is related to CD4++ T-lymphocyte count'. *Tuberculosis and Lung Disease* 1995; 76: 518–521.

SACKS LV, PENDLE S, ORLOVIC D, BLUMBERG L, CONSTANTINOU C. 'A comparison of outbreak- and nonoutbreak-related multidrug-resistant tuberculosis among human immuno-deficiency virus-infected patients in a South African hospital'. *Clinical Infectious Diseases* 1999; 29: 96–101.

SCOTT H, HAVLIR D, KLEMENT E, SCANO F, MALKIN J-L, DERFRAISSY J-F ET AL. Scaling up anti-retroviral therapy in resource-limited settings: Treatment guidlines for a public health approach. 2003 revision. World Health Organisation 2004. Geneva, Switzerland.

SHAFER RW, EDLIN BR. 'Tuberculosis in patients infected with human immunodeficiency virus: Perspective on the past decade'. *Clinical Infectious Diseases* 1996; 22: 683–704.

SONNENBERG P, MURRAY J, GLYNN JR, SHEARER S, KAMBASHI B, GODFREY-FAUSSETT P. 'HIV-1 and recurrence, relapse, and reinfection of tuberculosis after cure: A cohort study in South African mineworkers'. *Lancet* 2001; 358: 1687–1693.

WIKTOR SZ, SASSAN-MOROKRO M, GRANT AD, ABOUYA L, KARON JM, MAURICE C ET AL. 'Efficacy of trimethoprim-sulphamethoxazole prophylaxis to decrease morbidity and mortality in HIV-1-infected patients with tuberculosis in Abidjan, Cote d'Ivoire: a randomised controlled trial'. *Lancet* 1999; 353: 1469–1475.

WILKINSON D. *Drugs for preventing tuberculosis in HIV infected persons (Cochrane Review).* In: The Cochrane library. 2002.

WOLDAY D, HAILU B, GIRMA M, HAILU E, SANDERS E, FONTANET AL. 'Low CD4++ T-cell count and high HIV viral load precede the development of tuberculosis disease in a cohort of HIV-positive Ethiopians'. *International Journal of Tuberculosis and Lung Diseases* 2003; 7: 110–116.

WORLD HEALTH ORGANISATION. *'Global Tuberculosis Control: Surveillance, planning, financing.'* World Health Organisation. WHO Report 2003.WHO/TB/2003.316 2003.316. 2003. Geneva, Switzerland.

CHAPTER 29

Prevention of opportunistic infections in adults

Gary Maartens

MORBIDITY AND MORTALITY IN HIV is a consequence of opportunistic infections that occur with impaired immunity. Highly active antiretroviral therapy (HAART) is the best way to prevent opportunistic infections, but even when HAART is used, these infections may still occur.

Nearly all opportunistic infections are caused by infectious agents, or are malignancies associated with viruses. Many are preventable and critical questions must be asked before selecting a prevention strategy. For example, the incidence of the opportunistic infection, when in HIV infection it occurs, how effective and affordable the prevention is, and what risks are associated with its use.

Exposure to opportunistic infections should be prevented wherever possible by attention to safe water supplies, food hygiene, TB prevention and safe sex (chemoprophylaxis has a major role in late infection).

Immunisation is of limited benefit in the prevention of opportunistic infections, and active immunisations should be given early in HIV infection.

Almost all the morbidity and mortality associated with HIV infection is a consequence of opportunistic diseases that occur when immunity is impaired. The best way to prevent opportunistic diseases is to improve the level of immune function using highly active antiretroviral therapy (HAART). The use of HAART can reduce the incidence rate of opportunistic diseases by around 80%. However, even when HAART is used, opportunistic diseases continue to occur, as some patients will remain significantly immunesuppressed. This may occur if HAART is initiated with profound immunesuppression, if immune reconstitution is sub-optimal, or if immunity declines because resistance develops. Thus, even when HAART becomes widely available, the prevention of opportunistic disease remains an essential component of care for the HIV-infected person.

Almost all opportunistic diseases are infections, or are malignancies triggered by viral infections. Virulent organisms, such as *Mycobacterium tuberculosis*, are also regarded as opportunistic infections as they occur more frequently in the HIV infected and cause more severe disease. This chapter focuses on the prevention of opportunistic infections either by preventing exposure, immunisation or chemoprophylaxis.

Selecting prevention strategies

Many opportunistic infections associated with HIV infection are preventable. Critical questions need to be carefully answered before selecting a prevention strategy for a programme or an individual patient.

How common is the opportunistic infection?

Assessment of how commonly different opportunistic infections occur depends on good community-based prospective incidence studies. Most studies are unfortunately hospital-based and overestimate the incidence of certain severe opportunistic infections. TABLE 29.1 lists the potentially preventable opportunistic infections in southern Africa ranked according to how commonly they occur. The ranking is approximate and will vary from area to area – for instance malaria is geographically restricted and agents causing diarrhoea will be more common where there is no access to safe drinking water.

A further point is that opportunistic infections must not be considered in isolation, as some prevention strategies (notably trimethoprim-sulfamethoxazole, also known as cotrimoxazole) prevent several opportunistic infections that are common collectively, but uncommon individually.

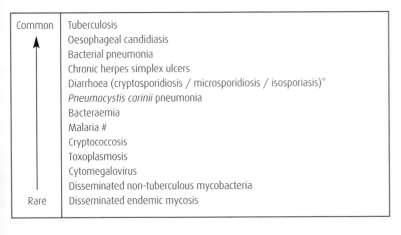

Common	Tuberculosis
↑	Oesophageal candidiasis
	Bacterial pneumonia
	Chronic herpes simplex ulcers
	Diarrhoea (cryptosporidiosis / microsporidiosis / isosporiasis)*
	Pneumocystis carinii pneumonia
	Bacteraemia
	Malaria #
	Cryptococcosis
	Toxoplasmosis
	Cytomegalovirus
	Disseminated non-tuberculous mycobacteria
Rare	Disseminated endemic mycosis

TABLE 29.1 Potentially preventable opportunistic infections approximately ranked by how commonly they occur in southern Africa
* Chronic diarrhoea is more common in areas without access to safe drinking water
# Incidence varies widely

At what stage does the infection occur?

There is no point in implementing a prevention strategy in early HIV disease if the risk of the opportunistic infection is restricted to late disease. However, immune responses to vaccination are poor in late disease and this prevention strategy should be used in early disease. Most of the major opportunistic infections occur when there is significant immunesuppression. The best marker of the degree of immunesuppression is the CD4 count. Infections caused by more virulent pathogens, such as *M tuberculosis* or *Streptococcus pneumoniae*, often occur with lesser degrees of immunesuppression. However, even the virulent pathogens occur more frequently as immunity declines. FIGURE 29.1 illustrates the approximate range of CD4+ T-lymphocyte counts for different opportunistic infections. As is evident from the figure, most opportunistic infections occur when the CD4 count is $<200 \times 10^6/\text{L}$. The least virulent pathogens occur when the CD4 count is $<50 \times 10^6/\text{L}$.

FIGURE 29.1 Timing of opportunistic infections according to CD4 counts (PCP = *Pneumocystis carinii* pneumonia, candida = candida oesophagitis, toxo = toxoplasmosis, MAC = *Mycobacterium avium* complex)

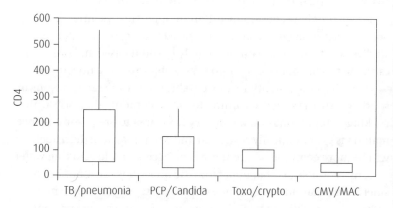

If CD4 counts are unavailable, then the total lymphocyte count can be used as a marker of immunesuppression. A total lymphocyte count of $<1.25 \times 10^9/\text{L}$ correlates with a CD4 count of $<200 \times 10^6/\text{L}$. Clinical evidence of immunesuppression also correlates with the risk of developing major opportunistic infections. Patients displaying clinical evidence of immune suppression (see TABLE 29.2) are at high risk of developing major opportunistic diseases and prevention strategies appropriate to patients with laboratory evidence of immunesuppression (CD4 count $<200 \times 10^6/\text{L}$) should be applied.

Oral candidiasis
Oral hairy leucoplakia
Unexplained weight loss
Chronic pathogen-negative diarrhoea

TABLE 29.2 Clinical features indicative of a high risk of developing major opportunistic diseases

How effective is the prevention strategy?

Ideally prevention strategies should be evidence-based. The strongest level of evidence, the randomised controlled trial, has only been conducted for a limited number of strategies. Even if a preventive strategy has been shown to be effective in a randomised controlled trial, the key question is, 'does it apply to the individual patient or population relevant to your practice?' There are major regional differences in the epidemiology and antimicrobial resistance patterns of opportunistic infections.

How affordable is the prevention strategy?

Affordability is related not only to the medication costs, but should also consider the number of patients needed to treat to prevent an infection and the infrastructure required to deliver the strategy.

What are the risks of the prevention strategy?

Clearly the benefits of the prevention strategy of chemoprophylaxis must outweigh the risks. Chemoprophylaxis carries the risk of adverse drug reactions. The risk of drug hypersensitivity is paradoxically increased in patients with severe immunesuppression; thus there is an increased risk of adverse drug reactions in advanced HIV disease.

A further risk of prophylaxis with antimicrobial agents is the development of resistance. This may be relevant for the individual (eg overgrowth of azole-resistant *Candida krusei* causing oesophagitis in patients on long-term fluconazole prophylaxis), or for the community (eg increased nasopharyngeal carriage of multiple antibiotic-resistant *S pneumoniae* in patients on cotrimoxazole prophylaxis with potential for spread to the community).

Preventing exposure

The best way to prevent opportunistic infections would be to prevent exposure to the infectious agent. However, this is only possible for a few opportunistic infections. The pathogenesis of several opportunistic infections is thought to be reactivation of latent/dormant infection after prior exposure – examples include tuberculosis, herpes simplex virus, cytomegalovirus and toxoplasmosis. Preventing exposure to these infections is obviously only an effective strategy before exposure has occurred. In developing countries exposure to cytomegalovirus is almost universal in childhood, thus there is no effective prevention strategy for cytomegalovirus in adults. Other opportunistic infections arise from overgrowth and invasion by normal flora, as occurs with mucosal candidiasis, and clearly exposure cannot be prevented. The most important and practical measure to prevent exposure is to ensure access to safe drinking water.

Safe water

Access to safe drinking water is very important, as many agents causing debilitating diarrhoea in HIV infection are waterborne. This is particularly true of the coccidian parasites, notably microsporidiosis. Microsporidiosis is the commonest cause of chronic diarrhoea in immunesuppressed patients in central Africa, where it is linked to drinking unsafe water. However, in South Africa over 80% of the population has access to safe water (2001 census) and microsporidiosis is uncommon – at least in urban areas.

Food hygiene

Food-borne illnesses are also important in HIV infection, notably *Salmonella* species, which cause bacteraemia and/or diarrhoea. Toxoplasma exposure is related to eating raw or undercooked meat. Serological surveys in South Africa show that about a third of the adult population has been exposed to *Toxoplasma gondii*. Approximately a third of patients with AIDS who are seropositive for *T gondii* will develop cerebral toxoplasmosis. People living with HIV infection need to be informed about food hygiene and the importance of adequately cooking meat.

Tuberculosis

Preventing exposure to tuberculosis is important in clinics where patients produce sputum specimens and in hospitals, especially tuberculosis hospitals. This topic is explored in more detail in CHAPTER 28.

Malaria vector control

Malaria is more severe in HIV infection and occurs more commonly with lower CD4 counts. Pregnant women in malarious areas are more at risk of severe malaria generally when they are primigravidae, but with HIV infection women of all gravidities are at risk. Thus HIV-infected individuals living in malarious areas should practise vector control. The simplest and most cost-effective way to achieve this is by using insecticide-impregnated bed nets. Other modalities of vector control that are of benefit to the community, such as reducing standing water, spraying with residual insecticides and larvicides, should also be implemented.

Safer sex

HIV-infected individuals should practise safer sex in order to reduce the transmission of HIV. Even if their partners are HIV infected, condoms should be used, as HIV mutants that are more virulent or have developed antiretroviral drug resistance can be transmitted. Safer sex will also lower the risk of acquiring herpes simplex virus and human herpes virus 8. The latter is an oncogenic virus strongly associated with the development of Kaposi's sarcoma.

Pets

Zoonotic infections acquired from pets are not common in people living with HIV infection in Africa. *T gondii* can be acquired from kittens or cat litter and people living with HIV infection should avoid handling either.

Chemoprophylaxis

Chemoprophylaxis refers to the use of antimicrobial agents to prevent opportunistic infections.

Primary and secondary prophylaxis

Primary prophylaxis is directed against preventing opportunistic infections that have not yet occurred. Secondary prophylaxis is used to prevent recurrence of opportunistic infections. This is necessary as many opportunistic infections recur after therapy. TABLE 29.3 lists secondary prophylactic regimens for common opportunistic infections in southern Africa. Recurrence rates are high in patients with chronic herpes simplex virus ulcers and oesophageal candidiasis, but they are not life-threatening and resistance can develop with prolonged use of prophylaxis. Resistant *C krusei* and herpes simplex virus infections are very difficult to treat. Thus secondary prophylaxis is not routinely recommended. Patients who experience frequent relapses can be given courses of therapy to initiate themselves as soon as symptoms start. Secondary prophylaxis may be indicated in highly

Infection	Secondary prophylaxis
Herpes simplex ulcers persisting >±4 weeks	Not usually recommended#
Tuberculosis	Not recommended
Candida oesophagitis	Not usually recommended#
Pneumocystis carinii pneumonia	Cotrimoxazole 960 mg daily OR Dapsone 100 mg daily
Toxoplasmosis	Cotrimoxazole 960 mg daily
Salmonella bacteraemia	Cotrimoxazole 960 mg daily *
Isosporiasis	Cotrimoxazole 960 mg daily
Cryptosporidiosis	No effective therapy
Bacterial pneumonia	Cotrimoxazole 960 mg daily *
Cryptococcal meningitis	Fluconazole 200 mg daily

TABLE 29.3 Secondary prophylaxis for opportunistic infections.
Recurrence rates are high with these infections, but they are not life-threatening and resistance can develop with prolonged use of prophylaxis
* High levels of resistance to cotrimoxazole exist in these bacteria in southern Africa, making cotrimoxazole prophylaxis less effective

selected patients – aciclovir 400 mg BD for chronic herpes simplex virus ulcers and fluconazole 100 mg daily for oesophageal candidiasis. Both secondary and primary prophylaxis can be discontinued when HAART results in immune reconstitution with CD4 counts increasing to >200 x 10⁶/L. It is prudent to wait until two CD4 counts are above this level before discontinuing prophylaxis.

Cotrimoxazole (trimethoprim-sulfamethoxazole)

Cotrimoxazole reduces the incidence of a number of opportunic infections (see TABLE 29.4). Randomised controlled trials have shown reductions in morbidity and, provided cotrimoxazole is not started in early disease, mortality. The efficacy of cotrimoxazole appears to be less marked in central and southern Africa as cotrimoxazole resistance in *Plasmodium falciparum* malaria, *S pneumoniae* and *Salmonella* species is common in this region. Nevertheless it is still effective and affordable.

The indications for initiating cotrimoxazole are either clinical evidence of immune suppression (WHO clinical stages 3 or 4 – including all forms of tuberculosis), or laboratory evidence of immune suppression (CD4 count <200 x 10⁶/L or, if this is unavailable, a total lymphocyte count of <1.25 x 10⁹/L).

Pneumocystis carinii pneumonia
Cerebral toxoplasmosis
Bacterial pneumonia
Bacteraemia
Isosporiasis

TABLE 29.4 Cotrimoxazole reduces the incidence of several opportunistic infections

Cotrimoxazole prophylaxis is well tolerated. The commonest side-effect is hypersensitivity causing a maculopapular rash. Many patients can continue receiving cotrimoxazole with the addition of anti-histamines unless there are systemic symptoms, extensive rash or mucosal involvement. If therapy is discontinued, desensitisation or rechallenge under antihistamine cover should be considered because cotrimoxazole reduces the incidence of many opportunistic infections. Both rechallenge or desensitisation appear safe, but should not be considered if the rash was accompanied by systemic symptoms or mucosal involvement. If cotrimoxazole cannot be tolerated then dapsone 100 mg daily should be substituted. Dapsone is equally effective at reducing the incidence of *P carinii* pneumonia, but has little or no effect on reducing the other opportunistic infections prevented by cotrimoxazole.

Tuberculosis

Preventive therapy for tuberculosis is indicated only for high-risk patients (e.g. tuberculin skin test positive or recent contacts). CD4 counts are not currently used to initiate tuberculosis preventive therapy. This topic is explored in more detail in CHAPTER 28.

Malaria

Malaria chemoprophylaxis should be offered to HIV-infected pregnant women in malarious areas, irrespective of their gravidity.

Chemoprophylaxis must be accompanied by vector control (see above). Resistance to sulfadoxine-pyrimethamine (Fansidar) has become widespread among *P falciparum* in southern Africa. Cotrimoxazole has the same mechanism of action as Fansidar and it is therefore no longer effective in most areas. Mefloquine is the agent of choice, but its safety in the first trimester is still unclear.

Immunisation

Prevention of infectious diseases by vaccination has been a highly effective public health tool. However, there are significant problems associated with vaccination in HIV infection. Vaccination with live organisms is contraindicated for patients with severe immunesuppression, irrespective of the cause. Furthermore, immune responses to vaccination are progressively impaired in HIV infection as the CD4 count falls. If the CD4 count is $<200 \times 10^6/\text{L}$ then immune responses to vaccination are very poor. The immune activation induced by vaccination leads to a transient rise in HIV RNA levels (viral load) – this does not appear to lead to more rapid HIV disease progression, but clinicians need to be aware of this phenomenon and avoid measuring viral load for a few weeks after vaccination.

Pneumococcal vaccination
Pneumococcal infections are a major cause of morbidity and mortality in HIV-infected individuals in sub-Saharan Africa. Thus pneumococcal vaccination has been advocated in HIV-infected adults. Unfortunately vaccination with the polysaccharide vaccine was not only ineffective in a large randomised controlled trial in Uganda, but vaccine recipients actually experienced more episodes of pneumonia. The newer, more immunogenic conjugated pneumococcal vaccines have shown benefit in HIV-infected children – trials in adults are awaited.

Hepatitis B vaccination
Hepatitis B is not generally regarded as an opportunistic infection, but both HIV and hepatitis B are sexually transmitted and HIV does alter the natural history of hepatitis B. Hepatitis B vaccination leads to reasonable immune responses provided the CD4 count is $> 200 \times 10^6/\text{L}$. There are no clinical trials to evaluate the efficacy of vaccination in HIV infection, but it should be offered in selected patients who are shown to be non-immune.

Influenza vaccination

Influenza vaccination appears to be beneficial in HIV-infected individuals in industrialised countries. It is unclear whether influenza causes significant morbidity in HIV-infected southern Africans and no trials of influenza vaccine in HIV infection have been conducted in developing countries.

Passive immunisation

Passive immunisation with specific antibodies is seldom indicated in HIV disease. It may be considered in patients with advanced disease who are exposed to chickenpox without prior immunity.

Bibliography

BADRI M, EHRLICH R, WOOD R, MAARTENS G. 'Initiating co-trimoxazole prophylaxis in adult HIV-infected patients in Africa: An evaluation of the provisional WHO/UNAIDS recommendations'. *AIDS* 2001; 15: 1143–8.

GRIMWADE K, SWINGLER G. 'Cotrimoxazole prophylaxis for opportunistic infections in adults with HIV infection'. *Cochrane Database Systematic Reviews* 2003; 3: CD003108.

GUMBO T, SARBAH S, GANGAIDZO IT ET AL. 'Intestinal parasites in patients with diarrhea and human immunodeficiency virus infection in Zimbabwe'. *AIDS* 1999; 13: 819–21.

LEOUNG GS, STANFORD JF, GIORDANO MF ET AL. 'Trimethoprim-sulfamethoxazole (TMP-SMZ) dose escalation versus direct rechallenge for *Pneumocystis carinii* pneumonia prophylaxis in Human Immunodeficiency Virus-infected patients with previous adverse reaction to TMP-SMZ'. *Journal of Infectious Diseases* 2001; 184: 992–997.

MAARTENS G (CORRESPONDING AUTHOR FOR THE SOUTHERN AFRICAN HIV CLINICIANS SOCIETY). 'The prevention and treatment of opportunistic infections in HIV-infected adults'. *South African Medical Journal* 2002; 92: 426–428.

VAN EIJK AM, AYISI JG, TER KUILE FO ET AL. 'HIV increases the risk of malaria in women of all gravidities in Kisumu, Kenya. *AIDS* 2003; 17: 595–603.

CHAPTER 30
Nutritional prophylaxis

Marianne Visser

THE CLINICAL OUTCOME OF HIV-infection and tuberculosis is adversely affected by malnutrition. At the household level, HIV infection is a major threat to food security in South Africa.

Weight loss of more than 10% predicts mortality in HIV-infected adults with advanced disease, independently of immune status and also leads to an increased incidence of opportunistic infections. Loss of lean mass is thought to be an independent predictor of survival.

Long-term use of highly active antiretroviral therapy is associated with changes in body fat distribution and can result in the lipodystrophy syndrome.

There is evidence that improved diet can improve the energy and nutrient intake of people living with HIV and AIDS. In industrialised countries, nutritional supplements are often used, but there is limited evidence of their effectiveness. This supplementation may be more beneficial in populations with poor baseline nutrition.

Asymptomatic micronutrient deficiences may occur among those living with HIV. There is evidence to suggest that low dietary intakes or blood levels of several vitamins and minerals may be associated with increased HIV disease progression and/or mortality. This may be due to the oxidative stress of HIV infection, as well as the role that micronutrients play in maintaining normal immune function. Adequate diet is the preferred method of correcting micronutrient deficiencies, but it is likely that daily micronutrient supplements will be needed in developing countries.

In South Africa, a national poverty eradication strategy is urgently needed to address the impact of HIV/AIDS on food security.

It has long been known that synergistic interactions exist between infection, nutritional status and immune function. Infectious diseases, no matter how mild, influence nutritional status. Conversely, almost any nutrient deficiency, if sufficiently severe, will impair resistance to infection. It is well recognised that the clinical outcomes of diseases such as HIV-infection and tuberculosis are worse when the host is malnourished.

The HIV epidemic is now the leading cause of death in sub-Saharan Africa and at a household level poses a major threat to food security as a result of diminished production, as well as the inability to purchase food. In a recent survey conducted among 728 AIDS-affected households in South Africa, weight loss was reported in 89% of households.

In this chapter, current data regarding the clinical significance of weight loss in HIV infection, the effect of antiretroviral therapy, as well as nutritional support, on body weight and body composition are reviewed. Furthermore, the role of micronutrient deficiencies in the pathogenesis of HIV infection and the effects of supplementation of various micronutrients on nutritional, immunological and clinical outcomes in HIV disease and the implications for clinical practice, are discussed.

Clinical significance of HIV-associated weight loss

A syndrome termed 'slim disease' was used in Uganda as early as 1985 to describe patients who presented with extreme wasting, accompanied by diarrhoea and fever. These features were subsequently incorporated into the World Health Organisation's clinical case definition used for AIDS surveillance in Africa. Furthermore, unintentional weight loss of less or more than 10%, is also included in current classification systems of HIV infection.

Weight loss (>10%) predicts mortality in HIV-infected adults with advanced disease independently of immune status. In addition, it has been shown that weight loss of 5 to 10% is related to an increased risk of opportunistic infections. However, it is important to remember that natural variations in body weight occur. A change in body weight of 5% has been described within a three month period among healthy adults. Weight loss typically falls into two categories in HIV-infected individuals. Patients who experience slow, progressive weight loss often suffer from gastrointestinal disease (<4 kg over four months), compared with those who experience acute intermittent episodes of weight loss (>4 kg within four months), usually associated with opportunistic infections. Among AIDS patients weight loss of 30% during a single episode has been documented. Weight recovery often occurs between such episodes and many patients remain weight-stable for prolonged periods.

Although the HIV-wasting syndrome was thought to be primarily an enteropathy, a post-mortem study from Côte d'Ivoire showed that 42% of patients with a clinical diagnosis of HIV-wasting syndrome, suffered from tuberculosis. Studies have confirmed that HIV-infected adults with tuberculosis are likely to suffer from more severe under-nutrition, as defined by a low Body Mass Index (BMI), than patients with HIV infection alone. In sub-Saharan Africa, HIV-infected patients are often unaware of their usual body weight and therefore weight loss is difficult to estimate. A recent study demonstrated that a BMI <20 kg/m^2 or <18.5 kg/m^2 in African HIV-infected men and women respectively, was associated with an increase in mortality. Among co-infected patients, a BMI <17.0 appears to be a strong predictor of mortality during the first four weeks of therapy.

Although weight loss in HIV infection features depletion of both lean and fat tissues, it is the lean compartment that is said to be an independent predictor of survival. Depletion of body cell mass (BCM), the metabolically active intracellular component of lean body mass, has been correlated with shortened survival, as well as impairment of strength and functional status of HIV-infected individuals. Limited evidence demonstrates that co-infection with tuberculosis results in greater declines in BCM than HIV infection alone. However, there do not appear to be large differences in body composition between co-infected adults and HIV-negative adults with tuberculosis.

Weight loss in HIV-infected women is characterised more by loss of body fat than by loss of lean body mass, a finding confirmed in studies in the USA and Africa. However, gender differences in body composition are minimised at end-stage illness. It may be that the relative degree of fat men and women tend to have available to provide energy is one cause for the disparity in body composition changes between genders. Changes in hormonal status, such as decreased testosterone in men and decreased oestrogen/progesterone in women may also be important.

The main causes of weight loss in HIV infection include a decreas-ed caloric intake, malabsorption and increased energy expenditure during systemic opportunistic infections (FIGURE 30.1). A number of metabolic abnormalities, such as increased protein turnover and increased *de novo* lipogenesis, may also contribute to the preferential wasting of lean tissue in patients with severe weight loss.

However, other studies imply a direct association between HIV infection and malnutrition. Depletion of BCM, as well as an increased resting energy expenditure (REE), have both been described in asymp-tomatic patients, suggesting that HIV infection *per se* may be a

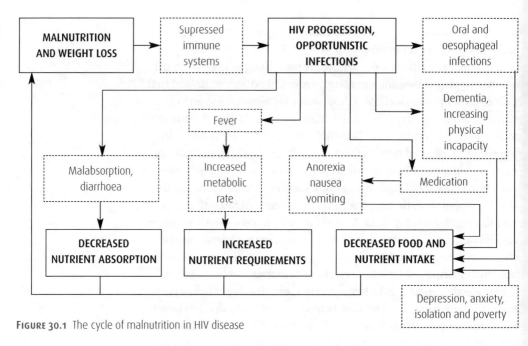

FIGURE 30.1 The cycle of malnutrition in HIV disease

contributing factor. Increasing plasma viral load has been associated with increases in REE in a cohort of HIV-infected men.

Effect of antiretroviral therapy on body weight/composition

Many patients report weight gain after the introduction of highly active antiretroviral therapy (HAART). However, the nature of the weight gain may vary. Some reports suggest the weight gain is mainly due to an increase in fat mass. Furthermore, a significant number of patients on HAART continue to suffer from weight loss.

Long-term use of HAART is associated with changes in body fat, as well as hyperlipidaemia and diabetes mellitus in some patients. Currently all these symptoms are classified as the lipodystrophy syndrome. Fat redistribution changes include loss of subcutaneous fat in peripheral limbs, face and buttocks (lipoatrophy) and/or visceral fat deposition (lipohypertrophy) in the abdomen, back and neck.

The complexity of body composition changes in the era of HAART is illustrated by the findings of a recent study in men with a clinical diagnosis of HIV-wasting syndrome, in whom increased truncal fat, as well as metabolic changes, was observed.

Other treatment options for the treatment of wasting have been explored in industrialised countries, including pharmacological agents such as recombinant human growth hormone. Growth hormone has been shown to increase weight and lean mass of patients with HIV-wasting and to decrease dorsocervical fat in HIV-infected persons. However, it should be noted that due to its lipolytic effects, it may potentiate further peripheral fat loss among patients with lipoatrophy.

Is nutritional intervention effective in the management of weight loss?

Limited evidence indicates that dietary counselling is an effective method to restore the energy and nutrient intake of people living with HIV/AIDS.

In industrialised countries high-energy, high-protein nutritional supplements often form part of the nutritional management of HIV-infected individuals. However, few studies have evaluated the effects of supplemental nutrition. An increase in body weight has been documented in some intervention studies. In some of these studies the increases in body weight were due to increased body fat and not lean body mass. Systemic infections may be one of the reasons for the failure to gain weight and/or accrue lean mass. The latter responds poorly to nutritional support, even if nutritional requirements are exceeded by the patient's intake. Thus, many authors concluded that simply providing nutrients to a malnourished patient is inadequate and suggest using anabolic agents such as recombinant growth hormone. The latter has been shown to promote the retention of lean tissue among those with secondary infections. On the other hand, specialised nutritional support containing medium-chain triglycerides has been shown to be of symptomatic benefit, particularly in the presence of chronic diarrhoea.

It is important to realise that nutritional care and support of people living with HIV/AIDS may be more beneficial in developing countries, because underlying factors contribute to poor baseline nutritional status. However, the extent to which nutritional therapy can reverse weight loss among HIV-infected individuals in Africa is largely unknown. Where resources are limited, food supplementation using maize-based supplements fortified with protein and micro-nutrients may be considered. As these type of supplements are energy dense, affordable and culturally acceptable, their efficacy needs to be urgently evaluated. Two recent nutrition intervention studies investigated the effects of such food-based supplements in HIV-infected individuals in South Africa. The first evaluated the effect of a soy/maize-based instant meal and though it proved acceptable to consumers, no significant effect on nutritional parameters or clinical outcome was shown, because of a small sample size. The results of a second study investigating the effects of a micronutrient, glutamine, pre- and probiotic enriched soy/maize-based liquid supplement are awaited. Supplementation of glutamine and arginine have been shown to prevent lean tissue loss or assist in the rehabilitation of patients with weight loss in the developed world.

Interventions that improve exercise capacity and functional performance may enhance the quality of life and reduce mortality of patients with AIDS wasting. Evidence suggests that aerobic exercise appears to be safe for HIV-infected individuals who are medically stable. Performing regular aerobic exercise results in an increased CD4 count, improved cardiopulmonary fitness and psychological wellbeing in this population. Further research is required to investigate the effects of aerobic exercise in people at varying stages of HIV disease, particularly those who are severely immunocompromised. The viability of these interventions has not yet been tested in Africa.

In conclusion, it appears that the impact of nutritional interventions on body composition will be most effective in the early rather than in the later stages of HIV infection. Early treatment for infections is probably one of the most effective ways of conserving the nutritional status of people living with HIV, as nutritional therapies without treatment of the underlying infection usually fail. Lean body mass changes measured by anthropometry are regarded by some as a valid tool for clinical practice. However, this would require trained nutritionists and the use of specialised equipment, such as skinfold calipers.

What is the role of micronutrient malnutrition?

Micronutrient deficiencies, the signs and symptoms of which are often lacking, may occur among HIV-infected patients. The relationship between micronutrients and HIV disease progression has been an area of great interest. Epidemiological evidence indicates that low dietary intakes or blood levels of several vitamins and minerals may be associated with increased HIV disease progression and/or mortality. As a result, the role of micronutrients in HIV/AIDS takes on special importance in populations with marginal intakes, which occurs in many communities in sub-Saharan Africa. In South Africa, low plasma levels of several micronutrients including vitamin A and zinc, have been described among stable HIV-infected adults and children. Those with more advanced disease were more likely to present with low plasma levels. Most studies investigating the micronutrient status of HIV-infected populations have used serum or plasma levels of micronutrients. However, it is important to bear in mind that serum concentrations of several micronutrients decline during the acute phase response. The serum micronutrient status of HIV-infected individuals with acute infections should therefore be interpreted with caution.

Semba and colleagues suggest the role of micronutrient deficiencies in the pathogenesis of HIV infection is based on two theories, the free radical theory and the nutritional immunological theory, as illustrated in FIGURE 30.2.

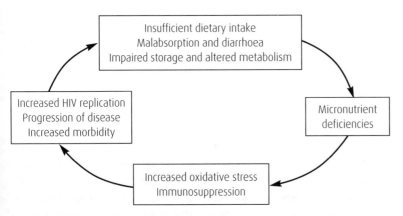

FIGURE 30.2 Cycle of micronutrient deficiencies and HIV pathogenesis

The role of oxidative stress

In HIV infection, oxidative stress may be caused by both overproduction of reactive oxygen intermediates (ROS) and a simultaneous deficiency of antioxidant defenses, such as glutathione and antioxidant nutrients such as vitamins E, C, β-carotene and selenium. One example of oxidative damage that may result from oxidative stress is lipid peroxidation, which could damage important cell membrane functions. Evidence suggests that chronic oxidative stress occurs in HIV infection and, in general, there is a decline in the status of several antioxidants that seems to correlate with disease severity. Several groups have demonstrated depleted cysteine or glutathione in the tissues of HIV-infected patients. A Canadian trial showed that supplementation of vitamin E (800 IU) and C (1000 mg) for a period of three months resulted in a significant reduction of oxidative stress parameters and plasma HIV-viral load. In contrast, β-carotene supplementation did not appear to offer any benefit to HIV-infected individuals who were already receiving a multivitamin supplement.

Glutathione (GSH) is a major intracellular thiol and is thought to inhibit nuclear factor kB, which is involved in the transcription of HIV. Selenium is an essential component of the antioxidant enzyme glutathione peroxidase (GSHPx), an important protective enzyme against oxidative stress. Decreases in serum selenium, plasma GSH and GSHPx activity have been shown to correlate with disease progression. Low serum selenium levels (<85 µg/L) have been shown to be independent predictors of mortality in both HIV-1-infected adults and children. Small selenium supplementation trials in HIV-infected individuals demonstrate increased glutathione status and GSHPX activity, but no effect on viral load. A recent clinical trial from the United States reported a significantly lower risk of hospitalisation among HIV-infected adults who were supplemented with 200 µg selenium per day.

Other treatment options include the supplementation of N-acetylcysteine (NAC), which may be associated with a slower decline in CD4 cell counts and a reduced mortality among HIV-infected individuals. Since whey protein is rich in cysteine, a recent trial investigated the effects of an oral supplement, enriched with whey protein, on plasma GSH levels in adults with advanced disease. Although significant increases in plasma GSH were observed, other clinical parameters remain unchanged.

The impact on micronutrient status of the the various drugs used in HAART needs to be considered. HAART regimes have been shown to improve glutathione status, and to increase levels of antioxidant vitamins. However, among intravenous drug users taking different HAART regimes, serum levels of vitamin E and carotenoids were significantly higher in those taking protease inhibitors (PIs). It is unclear whether these differences are due to differences in lifestyle or to a direct effect of PIs.

Maintaining host immunity

Many micronutrients play essential roles in maintaining normal immune function. Vitamin A plays a central role in the growth and function of T- and B-cells, antibody responses and maintenance of mucosal epithelia. Low blood levels of vitamin A are associated with accelerated disease progression and increased mortality in HIV-infected adults. In addition, low concentrations of vitamin A may be associated with increased mother-to-child transmission of HIV, higher infant mortality and child growth failure.

High-dose vitamin A supplementation has been shown to reduce diarrhoeal disease morbidity and AIDS-related mortality in HIV-infected children, and to improve the CD4 cell counts of children with AIDS. In contrast, two clinical trials have documented no beneficial effect of vitamin A supplementation in reducing mother-to-child transmission of HIV. Several studies have found no effect of vitamin A on HIV-viral load. However, there are potential biological mechanisms through which vitamin A supplementation may be beneficial in reducing morbidity and mortality in HIV disease.

Zinc is essential for the maturation and differentiation of T-lymphocytes and functioning of cells mediating non-specific immunity, such as neutrophils and NK cells. Several zinc-dependent enzymes play a role in antioxidant defence and hormones such as thymulin, which is essential for the formation of T-lymphocytes. Although low blood zinc concentrations have been associated with HIV disease progression and mortality, there may be problems with zinc supplementation. A single cohort study found that high dietary zinc intake was associated with increased disease progression. This is possibly because these individuals already had a high bio-availability of zinc, so did not require supplementation, and results of this study should not delay assessing the effect of zinc supplementation on the course of HIV infection in populations with marginal intakes. In a quasi-randomised trial study, the intake of 45 mg elemental zinc for one month in AIDS patients resulted in a reduction in opportunistic infections in the subsequent 24 months. However, in the absence of any zinc stores, it seems unlikely that zinc supplements have long-term effects. In Zambia, the supplementation of zinc, selenium, vitamins A, C and E to patients with persistent diarrhoea for a two week-period had no effect on morbidity or mortality. No significant increase in serum vitamin A concentrations was noted in the treatment group, suggesting severe malabsorption.

An Indonesian study investigated the combined effect of vitamin A and zinc supplementation to people with pulmonary tuberculosis and reported earlier sputum smear conversion times within two months of anti-tuberculous treatment. It has been suggested that zinc supplementation may be of great benefit for infections in which specific macrophage functions are central to resistance. Studies on the effect of zinc on mortality among African patients with pulmonary tuberculosis, of whom a large proportion are co-infected with HIV, are in progress. A trial investigating the role of zinc alone, or in conjunction with other micronutrients, on the morbidity and mortality of South African HIV-infected children is currently underway.

Severe iron deficiency results in anaemia, but may also contribute to decreased immune function. The pathogenesis of anaemia during HIV disease is likely to be multifactorial. Anaemia has been associated with increased mortality in studies conducted primarily in HIV-infected men. A study from Malawi showed that the prevalence of anaemia was 73% among HIV-infected pregnant women, the majority of whom suffered from iron-deficiency anaemia. Although it may be assumed that the reversal of iron-deficiency anaemia may prolong survival, concern has been raised that iron supplementation could prove to be harmful for HIV-infected individuals, as iron is a pro-oxidant and may promote viral replication. Retrospective studies have shown that a high iron status is associated with faster disease progression and higher mortality among HIV-infected adults. However, a recent study among pregnant Zimbabwean HIV-infected women concluded that the positive relationship between ferritin and viral load was not as a result of the acute phase response or iron accumulation due to advanced disease.

Low serum vitamin B12 has been associated with increased disease progression, while high dietary intakes of several B-vitamins have been linked with increased survival. In a retrospective survey, supplemental vitamin B was associated with slower disease progression among South African HIV-infected adults. High doses of B-vitamins, plus supplementation of vitamins C and E and iron resulted in increased CD4 cell counts among pregnant women and a reduction in the risk of adverse birth outcomes. Data from the same study show that children of infected mothers who took multivitamins while breastfeeding, were less likely to become infected and more likely to survive.

Micronutrient deficiencies may be involved in the pathogenesis of subclinical mastitis, illustrated by a study in which vitamin E-rich sunflower oil was found to reduce subclinical mastitis in Tanzanian women. Low plasma carotenoid levels have previously been identified as a risk factor for mastitis. Further research is needed.

Defining the role of micronutrient intervention

Although food sources are generally preferred, it is likely that daily micronutrient supplements will be required to reverse underlying deficiencies of HIV-infected populations, especially in developing countries. Few authors have attempted to formulate recommendations for the supplementation of micronutrients to HIV/AIDS patients. Some authors recommend the supplementation of vitamin A, along with anti-oxidants such as β-carotene, vitamins E, C and selenium, as well as annual biochemical monitoring. Others have concluded that the supplementation of twice the recommended daily allowance (RDA) for most micronutrients is likely to benefit the majority of HIV-infected individuals in Africa, since a range of micronutrient deficiencies usually co-exist. Clark *et al* concludes that the available data do not contraindicate the current practice of iron supplementation in developing countries where there is a high prevalence of HIV infection and iron deficiency. However, iron supplements should not be administered during opportunistic infections. For the management of HIV-infected children, the WHO guidelines for micronutrient supplementation in children with severe malnutrition may be used.

In addition, high dose vitamin A supplementation should be provided.

The role of other strategies to improve the micronutrient status of populations with a high HIV prevalence, such as dietary diversification or the fortification of foods, should not be overlooked. National nutritional guidelines by the Department of Health can be used as a basic guide to advise HIV-infected adults and children on dietary modification, with the aim of improving their intake not only of micronutrients, but also to ensure adequate energy and protein intake. Recently, the mandatory fortification of bread flour with several micronutrients was announced in South Africa, and is likely to contribute to an improvement of micronutrient status of all South Africans. Furthermore, a variety of fortified maize-based supplements are currently available, but research is needed on the effectiveness of these supplements on nutritional and clinical parameters of HIV-infected adults and children. Finally, there is a dire need in South Africa to develop a national poverty eradication strategy to address the impact of HIV/AIDS on household food security.

Bibliography

ALLARD JP. 'Oxidative Stress and Infections'. In: *Micronutrients & HIV Infection*. Friis H (Ed). CRC Press, Boca Raton, 2002.

AUKRUST P, MULLER F, SVARDAL AM, UELAND T, BERGE RK, FROLAND SS. 'Disturbed glutathione metabolism and decreased antioxidant levels in human immunodeficiency virus-infected patients during highly active antiretroviral therapy-potential immunomodulatory effects of antioxidants'. *Journal of Infectious Diseases* 2003; 188: 232–238.

BURBANO X, MIGUE-BURBANO MJ, McCOLLISTER K, ZHANG G, RODRIGUEZ A, RUIZ P ET AL. 'Impact of a selenium chemoprevention clinical trial on hospital admissions of HIV-infected participants'. *HIV Clinical Trials* 2002; 3: 483–491.

BUYS H, HUSSEY G. 'The role of micronutrients in the case management of HIV disease'. In: *Micronutrients & HIV Infection* . Friis H. (Ed). CRC Press, Boca Raton, 2002.

CARBONELL F, MASLO C, BEAUGERIE L. 'Effect of indinavir on HIV-related wasting'. *AIDS* 1998; 12: 1777–1784.

CASTETBON K, ANGLARET, TOURE S, CHENE G, OUASSA T, ATTIA A ET AL. 'Prognostic value of cross-sectional anthropometric indices on short-term risk of mortality in human immunodeficiency virus – infected adults in Abijan, Côte d'Ivoire'. *American Journal of Epidemiology* 001; 154: 75–84.

CHLEBOWSKI RT, BEALL G, GROSVENOR M, LILLINGTON L, WEINTRAUB N ET AL. 'Long-term effects of early nutritional support with new enterotrophic peptide-based formula vs. standard enteral formula in HIV-infected patients: Randomized Prospective trial'. *Nutrition* 1993; 9: 507–512.

CLARK RH, FELEKE G, DIN MD, YASMIN T, SINGH G, KHAN FA ET AL. 'Nutritional treatment for AIDS associated wasting using beta-hydroxy beta-methylbutyrate, glutamine, and arginine: A randomized, double blind placebo-controlled study'. *Journal of Parenteral and Enteral Nutritio*. 2000; 24: 133–139.

CLARK TD, SEMBA RD. 'Iron supplementation during human immunodeficiency virus infection: A double-edge sword?'. *Medical Hypotheses* 2001; 57: 476–479.

DEPARTMENT OF HEALTH, SOUTH AFRICA. 2001. 'The South African National Guidelines on Nutrition for People with TB, HIV/AIDS and Other Chronic Debilitating Conditions'. Department of Health, Pretoria.

DOWLING S, MULCAHY F, GIBNEY M. 'Nutrition in the management of HIV antibody positive patients: A longitudinal study of dietetic advice'. *European Journal of Clinical Nutrition* 1990; 44: 823–829.

ELEY BS, SIVE AA, ABELSE L, KOSSEW G, COOPER M, HUSSEY GD. 'Growth and micronutrient disturbances in stable, HIV-infected children in Cape Town'. *Annals of Tropical Paediatrics* 2002; 22: 19–23.

FAWZI W. 'Micronutrients and Human Immunodeficiency Virus Type 1 Disease Progression among Adults and Children'. *Clinical Infectious Diseases* 2003; 37(Suppl 2): S112–S116.

FILTEAU SM, LIETZ G, MULOKOZI G, BILOTTA S, HENRY CJ ET AL. 'Milk cytokines and sub-clinical breast inflammation in Tanzanian women: Effects of dietary red palm oil or sunflower oil supplementation'. *Immunology* 1999; 97: 595.

FRIIS H, GOMO E, MICHAELSEN KF. 'Micronutrient interventions and the HIV pandemic'. In: *Micronutrients & HIV Infection*. Friis H. (Ed). CRC Press, Boca Raton, 2002.

FRIIS H, GOMO E, NYAZEMA N, NDLOVU P, KRARUP H ET AL. 'Iron, haptoglobin phenotype, and HIV-1 viral load: A cross-sectional study among pregnant Zimbabwean women'. *Journal of Acquired Immune Deficiency Syndrome* 2003; 33: 74–81.

FRIIS H, SANDSTRÖM. 'Zinc and HIV infection'. In: *Micronutrients & HIV Infection*. Friis H. (Ed). CRC Press, Boca Raton, 2002.

GIBERT CL, WHEELER DA, COLLINS G, MADANS M, MUURAHAINEN N, RAGHAVAN SS ET AL. 'Randomized, Controlled Trial of Caloric Supplements in HIV Infection'. *Journal of Acquired Immune Deficiency Syndrome* 1999; 22: 253.

GRINSPOON S, CORCORAN, C, MILLER K. 'Body composition and endocrine function in women with acquired immunodeficiency syndrome wasting'. *Journal of Clinical Endocrinology and Metabolism* 1997; 82: 1332–1337.

HADIGAN C, CORCORAN C, STANLEY T, PIECUCH S, KLIBANSKI A, GRINSPOON S. 'Fasting hyper-insulinaemia in human immunodeficiency virus-infected men: Relationship to body composition,gonadal function, and protease inhibitor use'. *Journal of Clinical Endocrinology and Metabolism* 2000; 85: 35–41.

HOH R, PELFINI A, NEESE RA, CHAN M, CELLO JP ET AL. 'De novo lipogenesis predicts short-term body-composition response by bioelectrical impedance analysis to oral nutri-tional supplements in HIV-associated wasting'. *American Journal of Clinical Nutrition* 1998; 68: 154–163.

JAIN RG, FURFINE ES, PEDNEAULT L, WHITE AJ, LENHARD JM. 'Metabolic complications associated with antiretroviral therapy'. *Antiviral Research* 2001; 51: 151–177.

JOHNSON S, SCHIERHOUT G, STEINBERG M, RUSSELL B, HALL K, MORGAN J. 'AIDS in the Household'. Chapter 11 in: *South African Health Review*. Health Systems Trust, South Africa. 2002.

KANTER AS, SPENCER DC, STEINBERG M, SOLTYSIK R, YARNOLD PR ET AL. 'Supplemental vitamin B and progression to AIDS and death in black South African patients infected with HIV'. *Journal of Acquired Immune Deficiency Syndrome* 1999; 21:252.

KENNEDY CM, KUHN L, STEIN Z. 'Vitamin A and HIV Infection: Disease Progression, Mortality and Transmission. *Nutrition Reviews* 2000; 58: 291–303.

KENNEDY RD. '*Effects of a micronutrient, glutamine, pre- and probiotic enriched liquid supplement on nutritional status and immunity of adults with HIV/AIDS: a pilot study.*' Masters thesis. University Stellenbosch 2003.

Kotler DP, Tierney AR, Culpepper-Morgan JA, Wang J, Pierson RN. 'Effect of home total parenteral nutrition on body composition in patients with acquired immuno-deficiency syndrome'. *Journal of Parenteral and Enteral Nutrition* 1990; 14: 454–458.

Lucas SB, De Cock KM, Hounnou A, Peacock C, Diomande M, Honde M, Beaumel A, Kestens L, Kadio A. 'Contribution of tuberculosis to Slim disease in Africa'. *British Medical Journal* 1994, 308: 1531–1533.

Macallan DC, Noble C, Baldwin C, Foskett M, McManus T, Griffin GE. 'Prospective analysis of patterns of weight change in stage IV human immunodeficiency virus infection'. *American Journal of Clinical Nutrition* 1993; 58: 417–424.

Micke P, Beeh KM, Buhl R. 'Effects of long term supplementation with whey proteins on the glutathione levels of HIV-infected patients'. *European Journal of Clinical Nutrition* 2002; 41: 12–18.

Mulligan T, Tai VW, Schambelan M. 'Energy expenditure in human immunodeficiency virus infection'. *New England Journal of Medicine* 1997; 336: 70–71.

Nixon S, O'Brien K, Glazier RH, Wilkins AL. 'Aerobic exercise interventions for people with HIV/AIDS'. In: *The Cochrane Library* Issue 1, 2002.

Pichard C, Sundre P, Karsegard V et al. 'A randomized double-blind controlled study of 6 months of oral nutritional supplementation with arginine and omega-3 fatty acids in HIV-infected patients. Swiss HIV Cohort Study'. *AIDS* 1998; 12: 53–63.

Rabeneck L, Palmer A, Knowles JB et al. 'A randomized controlled trial evaluating nutrition counseling with or without oral supplementation in malnourished HIV-infected patients.' *Journal of American Dietician Association* 1998; 98: 434–438.

Rosenbaum K, Wang J, Pierson N, Kotler DP. 'Time-Dependent Variation in Weight and Body Composition in Healthy Adults'. *Journal of Parenteral and Enteral Nutrition* 2000; 24: 52–55.

Salomon J, De Truchis P, Melchior J-C. 'Nutrition and HIV infection'. *British Journal of Nutrition* 2002; 87(Suppl 1): S111–S119.

Salomon SB, Jung J, Voss T et al. 'An elemental diet containing medium-chain triglyc-erides and enzymatically hydrolyzed protein can improve gastrointestinal tolerance in people infected with HIV'. *Journal of the American Dietician Association* 1998; 98: 460–462.

Scrimshaw NS, San Giovanni JP. 'Synergism of nutrition, infection, and immunity: An overview'. *American Journal of Clinical Nutrition* 1997; 66: 464S.

Semba RD & Tang AM. 'Micronutrients and the pathogenesis of human immunode-fiency virus infection'. *British Journal of Nutrition* 1999; 81: 181–189.

Shabert JK, Winslow C, Lacey JM et al. 'Glutamine-antioxidant supplementation increases body cell mass in AIDS patients with weight loss: A randomized, double-blind controlled trial'. *Nutrition* 1999; 15: 860–864.

Shankar AH & Prasad AS. 'Zinc and immune function: The biological basis of altered resistance to infection'. *American Journal of Clinical Nutrition* 1998; 68(Suppl): 47S–63S.

Silva M, Skolnik PR, Gorbach SL, Spiegelman D, Wilson IB, Fernandez-DiFranco MG, Knox TA. 'The effect of protease inhibitors on weight and body composition in HIV-infected patients'. *AIDS* 1998, 12: 1645–1651.

Stack JA, Bell SJ, Burke PA, Forse A. 'High-energy, high protein, oral, liquid, nutrition supplementation in patients with HIV infection: Effect on weight status in relation to secondary infection'. *Journal of the American Dietician Association* 1996; 96: 337–341.

Steenkamp L, Dannhauser A. 'Nutritional Management of the HIV/AIDS patient – A practical approach'. *The South African Journal of HIV Medicine* December 2001, 31–36.

Suttman U, Ockenga J, Schneider H et al. 'Weight gain and increased concentration of receptor proteins for tumor necrosis factor after patients with asymptomatic HIV infection received fortified nutrition support'. *Journal of the American Dietetic Association* 1996; 96: 565–569.

Swenk A, Steuck H, Kremer G. 'Oral supplements as adjunctive treatment to nutrition counseling in malnourished HIV-infected patients: Randomized controlled trial'. *Clinical Nutrition* 1999; 18: 371–374.

Tang AM, Smit E, Semba RD et al. 'Improved Antioxidant Status Among HIV-Infected Injecting Drug Users on Potent Antiretroviral Therapy'. *Journal of Acquired Immune Deficiency Syndrome* 2000; 23: 321–326.

Thea DM, Kotler DP, Engelson ES et al. 'Comparison of HIV infection and other diseases upon the pattern of wasting in hospitalized African men and women'. *Journal of Investgative Medicine* 1995; 43: 350A.

Van Lettow M, Fawzi WW, Semba RD. 'Triple Trouble: The Role of Malnutrition in Tuberculosis and Human Immunodeficiency Virus Co-infection.' *Nutrition Reviews* 2003; 61: 81–90.

Venter CS, Jerling JC, Oosthuizen W, Hanson P, Mooko M, Bosman MJC, Scholtz SC. '*The effect of an instant soy-maize porridge on the well-being of young HIV+ volunteers*'. Nutrition Congress, Potchefstroom, South Africa, 2002.

Visser ME, Maartens G, Kossew G, Hussey GD. 'Plasma vitamin A and zinc levels in HIV-infected adults in Cape Town, South Africa'. *British Journal of Nutrition* 2003; 89: 475–483.

Wanke CA, Pleskow, D, Degiroiami PC et al. 'A medium chain triglyceride-based diet in patients with HIV and chronic diarrhoea reduces diarrhoea and malabsorption: A prospective, controlled trial'. *Nutrition* 1996; 12: 766–771.

Wheeler DA, Gibert CL, Launer CA et al. 'Weight loss as a predictor of survival and disease progression in HIV infection'. *Journal of Acquired Immune Deficiency Syndrome and Human Retrovirology* 1998; 18: 80–85.

Wilson D, Naidoo S, Bekker L, Cotton M, Maartens G (Eds). 2002. '*Handbook of HIV Medicine*'. Cape Town: Oxford University Press Southern Africa.

Woods MN. 'Dietary Recommendations for the HIV/AIDS patient'. In Miller TL and Gorbach SL. (Eds). *Nutritional Aspects of HIV Infection*. Arnold, London, 1999.

CHAPTER 31
Challenges in managing AIDS in South Africa

Douglas Wilson and Lara Fairall

SUITABLE INFRASTRUCTURE IS NEEDED to manage HIV-infected individuals at primary care level, but funding is not readily available and qualified health care personnel are in short supply.

Private health-care attracts most health care funding, but is accessed by less than 20% of South Africans. The standard of HIV care in the private sector is equivalent to that of the developed world.

The National Tuberculosis Control Programme's DOTS infrastructure may be a useful starting point for the development of a sustainable HIV service. Lessons learnt by the DOTS programme are relevant to HIV services.

Effective use of antiretroviral therapy requires meticulous adherence. Poverty, alternative disease constructs, stigma, gender and unpredictable drug supply are important factors influencing adherence. However, small studies in impoverished areas of South Africa have shown that excellent results can be achieved. Extensive community involvement and recruitment of lay counsellors is essential.

The management of TB and fungal infections in Africa is challenging because of limited facilities. Chronic diarrhoea and HIV-associated skin problems can be refractory to available treatments, and antibiotic resistance can develop as a result of the widespread and repeated use of antibiotics for serious bacterial infections.

Many HIV-infected individuals in South Africa will be unable to access antiretrovirals, and need palliative care, which can be therapeutically challenging and emotionally demanding. This needs to be acknowledged and proactively addressed.

South Africa is undergoing a period of profound socioeconomic development, and the HIV epidemic presents the medical system with extraordinary health care challenges. In 1994 the new democratically elected South African government inherited a divided and fragmented health system characterised by over-investment in hospital-based medicine in both the public and private sectors, with under-developed primary health care structures. Ten years later the health care system has undergone substantial changes, but remains ill-equipped to tackle the epidemic comprehensively. HIV affects every facet of South African society, characterised by wide discrepancies in income, with about 40% of households living in poverty. Evidence suggests, however, that survival among HIV-infected individuals is independent of racial group and socioeconomic status, provided there is equal access to health care. The success of the health sector in ameliorating the effects of the HIV epidemic will be measured by the extent to which human resources are mobilised and focused into coordinated and effective primary care programmes.

Funding is the most important issue driving the response to the HIV epidemic. In 1999, 56% of health care funding (R39 billion) was directed towards the private sector through the medical insurance industry and from household out-of-pocket payments. The public health services received the remaining 44% of health care funding (R31 billion) from government. What is worrying, however, is that less than 20% of the South African population access health care through the private sector. More than 80% of households therefore rely on the disproportionately under-funded public sector. Absolute increases to the public health sector budget have been under 1% annually since 1999 and although in 2003/4 there was an increase in funding for HIV/AIDS care, it was at the expense of other public sector projects. International donor agencies such as the Global Fund provide invaluable funding for the initiation of HIV treatment programmes, but do not provide a long-term solution to South Africa's funding needs.

The strengths and weaknesses of the current health care system in its ability to implement a sustainable programme for medical care for HIV-infected patients are summarised in TABLE 31.1.

The private sector

More than three quarters of the 5 400 doctors who were registered with the Southern African HIV Clinicians' Society in 2003 work within the private sector. Measurable outcomes in the private sector, when studied in the context of the country's largest managed care scheme, are comparable to the developed world (see FIGURE 31.1).

Experienced HIV clinicians are an invaluable national resource and public-private partnerships need to be developed. However, the private sector is by definition profit-driven, and HIV-infected patients may not be able to consistently access effective treatment (including

Strengths	Weaknesses
• Shift in government funding towards developing infrastructure in the primary care sector	• Ambiguous and conflicting messages from leaders in National Government
• Increasing government funding for HIV care	• The HIV epidemic being used for political point-scoring at the expense of rational and constructive debate
• Commitment to provide antiretrovirals in the public sector	• Severely limited human resources, especially nurses, pharmacists, doctors and clinical managers
• Increasing access to generic antiretrovirals	• Poor implementation of public health programmes with limited planning, training and follow through
• Experience acquired from implementing public health programmes such as the World Health Organisation's DOTS programme for tuberculosis treatment, the single nevirapine dose programme for the prevention of mother-to-child transmission, and termination of pregnancy in State facilities	• Inequity in primary care funding between provinces and districts
• A comprehensive National Treatment Programme for HIV/AIDS, which includes a role for traditional healers	• Inability of primary care facilities to meet current health care commitments
• Collaborative, multifaceted HIV research programmes with a substantial service component	• Insufficient space in primary care clinic buildings
• Increased regulation of the medical insurance industry, with a minimum benefits package	• Unpleasant working conditions
• HIV care (often with antiretroviral therapy) effectively delivered by private practitioners with the managed care component of the medical aid industry (for example the Aid for AIDS programme)	• Health care worker fatigue and burnout
• An increasing number of dedicated HIV clinicians in the public and private sector, with increasing access to training courses and educational material	• Excessive distances between rural clinics
• Comprehensive HIV care programmes instituted by large industries (such as the mining industry and automobile manufacturers)	• Poor lines of communication and referral between non-governmental organisations and provincial/municipal health care structures
• Highly committed non-governmental organisations (for example the Treatment Action Campaign)	• Lack of integration between governmental and non-governmental initiatives
• Government commitment to improve health care worker remuneration in the public sector.	• Inadequate information technology
	• Inadequate laboratory facilities outside of large urban areas
	• Lack of regulation of antiretroviral use in the private sector outside of the managed care industry.

antiretroviral therapy) in the private sector largely due to the high cost of care. This may result in patients being able to afford antiretrovirals only intermittently, with major implications for the development of resistance and treatment failure. Private practitioners may also provide ineffective antiretroviral treatment in the form of monotherapy or dual therapy, either because of cost constraints or misinformation. Patients may also not be informed that triple therapy can be purchased at discounted prices from large centralised pharmacies through SA HIV Clinicians Society initiatives. Currently there is no legislation to limit antiretroviral prescribing to suitably qualified practitioners, and the antiretroviral options of many patients may have been severely compromised by ineffective management. The National Treatment Plan has made no provision for patients'

TABLE 31.1 The ability of the South African healthcare system to meet the challenges imposed by the HIV/AIDS epidemic

FIGURE 31.1 24-month survival by CD4 count for patients on HAART, comparing a South African private sector HIV managed care scheme with two North American HIV care providers *Adapted from Hislop MS Maartens, G, Regensburg L. The influence of CD4 count at antiretroviral commencement on survival in HIV/AIDS patients in a managed care setting. South African AIDS Conference, Durban 2003.*

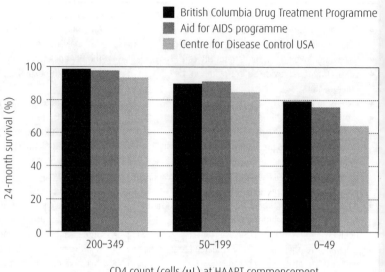

■ British Columbia Drug Treatment Programme
■ Aid for AIDS programme
■ Centre for Disease Control USA

CD4 count (cells/µL) at HAART commencement

self-funding of antiretrovirals from disability grants, from donations from their families, or from a small salary (in 2003 an individual earning R3000 a month needed to spend 25% of this income on antiretrovirals). It is anticipated that the price of antiretrovirals purchased by government after a tender selection process will be substantially less expensive, but the private sector is currently unable to access medications at tender prices. Local production of generic antiretrovirals, which should cost less than US$250 per year for triple therapy, will substantially reduce the cost of purchasing therapy in the private sector.

The public sector

The doctor-based private sector model is impractical if the majority of the five million South Africans living with HIV are to receive effective treatment and alternative models need to be explored. Most government-funded specialist HIV clinics are located in large regional and tertiary hospitals, making it difficult for patients to access care in these facilities, particularly as they are usually not located in high HIV prevalence communities. In contrast, most of the care given to symptomatic HIV-infected individuals is provided by community-based primary care clinics, which do not usually provide a dedicated HIV service. Outside the large urban centres primary care is usually provided by nurse practitioners who often function without support from an on-site doctor or who may not have a doctor available at all. At present primary care receives only 15% of state-derived funding, which must be increased if services targeting HIV-infected patients are to be developed. Inevitably there is competition for services between HIV-infected and uninfected users of the public health system: examples of health-related problems other than HIV with similar infrastructure and staffing requirements include chronic medical conditions such as diabetes, hypertension, cardiac failure, asthma, smoking-related lung disease, epilepsy and mental illness. Strong, ongoing political will is required to ensure that sufficient funding is obtained and allocated to HIV care at national, provincial and institutional level, without disrupting established acute and chronic care services. As the prevalence of HIV infection is likely to decline in the long term it is important to note, however, that infrastructure developed to treat HIV infection will be available to future generations of South Africans with other health problems.

The ideal community HIV clinic needs to provide: voluntary counselling and testing (VCT); referral to a conveniently located tuberculosis (TB) clinic; information on the benefits of safer sex, prophylaxis and antiretroviral treatment; a wellness programme (which offers isoniazid and cotrimoxazole prophylaxis); a drop-in clinic; and a well-managed antiretroviral programme. While specialist hospital-based HIV clinics may have a role in piloting a national antiretroviral treatment programme, in the longer term the burden will fall on nurse-based primary care services. Antiretroviral treatment programmes have been effectively implemented in a variety of resource-limited primary care settings both in South Africa and in other developing countries, with substantial involvement from nurse practitioners and lay counsellors (FIGURE 31.2). An often overlooked aspect of the antiretroviral rollout is that most South Africans will not need antiretroviral treatment for many years, but will require some form of psychological support and training in lifestyle modification. Lay counsellors who facilitate community-based support groups can effectively run wellness programmes that provide ongoing information, training and psychosocial care.

There are substantial management issues that need to be addressed, however, if antiretroviral therapy is to be made widely available in the public sector. It has been plausibly suggested that the management framework and infrastructure developed for tuberculosis control could be expanded to include HIV diagnosis and treatment. The performance of the National Tuberculosis Control Programme gives some insight into the challenges that may be encountered by a national antiretroviral therapy programme. The incidence of TB in South Africa (estimated in 2002 to exceed 520 cases per 100 000) is among the highest in the world, and about 60% of TB cases are also HIV infected. In 1997 the South African government adopted the World Health Organisation's DOTS initiative that aims to detect at

Baseline CD4 (cells/ul)	Duration on treatments in months								
At risk >=50	129	123	119	109	84	57	34	23	13
At risk <50	155	133	132	109	82	66	41	33	22
Deaths & loss to follow-up >=50		5	4	2	0	0	0	0	0
Deaths & loss to follow-up <50		23	2	2	1	0	0	0	0
Survival (%) 95% CI >=50		96.1 90.9-98.4	93.0 86.9-96.3	91.4 84.9-95.1	91.4 84.9-95.1	91.4 84.9-95.1	91.4 84.9-95.1	91.4 84.9-95.1	91.4
Survival (%) 95% CI <50		85.2 78.5-89.9	83.9 77.1-88.8	82.5 75.6-87.7	81.8 74.787.0	81.8 74.7-87.0	81.8 74.7-87.0	81.8 74.7-87.0	81.8 74.7-87.0

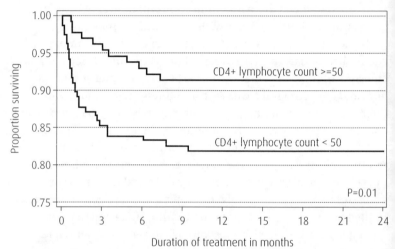

FIGURE 31.2 Survival of adults starting antiretroviral treatment, stratified by CD4 count, receiving treatment at the Médecins Sans Frontières Khayelitsha township clinic in Cape Town, South Africa *Adapted from: Coetzee D, Hildebrand K, Boulle A, Maartens G, Louis F, Labatala V, Reuter H, Ntwana N, Goemaere E. Outcomes after providing two years of antiretroviral therapy in Khayelitsha, South Africa. AIDS 2004; Apr 9;18(6): 887–95*

least 70% of new sputum smear-positive cases and successfully treat at least 85% of them with standardised six to nine month regimens. Sputum microscopy is an essential and inexpensive diagnostic tool for detecting smear-positive TB and should be uniformly available if the DOTS programme is fully implemented. In 2001 the availability of sputum microscopy ('bacteriological coverage') ranged from 90% in provinces such as Gauteng and the Free State, to 54% in KwaZulu-Natal. Nationally, 76% of smear-positive cases were successfully treated, ranging from 80% in the Western Cape to 67% in KwaZulu-Natal. Cure rates (documented conversion from smear-positive to smear-negative) were about 20% lower. Thirteen percent of smear-positive cases in the country interrupted treatment. The implications of these statistics for HIV care are significant. Laboratory investigations for monitoring HIV infection and treatment, such as the CD4 count and viral load used for monitoring HIV infection and treatment is much more expensive and sophisticated than sputum microscopy; and antiretroviral therapy, once initiated, should not be interrupted. The DOTS programme has proven difficult to implement, and it can be anticipated that an antiretroviral programme will be significantly more complex. Interestingly, some of the provincial programmes that performed relatively well were almost entirely based on care delivered by nurse practitioners.

In 1999 the WHO launched the ProTEST initiative that seeks to integrate effective TB diagnosis and treatment with voluntary counselling and testing for HIV infection, and improved prophylaxis and treatment for opportunistic infections. HIV and TB services are currently poorly integrated in South Africa, but by 2006 the Department of Health HIV/AIDS and TB Directorate plans to have implemented ProTEST in 174 districts. Currently, antiretroviral treatment is not included in the package of care, but the initiative has the potential to build the infrastructure necessary for the national antiretroviral programme.

An important strength of the South African DOTS programme is its ability to procure a sustainable supply of good quality antituberculous medications. Drug security is a crucial component of the antiretroviral rollout and the DOTS programme's experience is invaluable (see also CHAPTER 34). Many provinces rely on primary care nurse practitioners to perform most primary care-related clinical services. Given the scarcity and expense of primary care medical practitioners in the public service, nurse practitioners will also need to staff antiretroviral programmes. Carefully designed protocols for nurse practitioners on the safe and effective use of antiretrovirals need to be designed, tested and widely implemented. Again, the experience of the DOTS programme cannot be overlooked.

What is more debatable is whether, given sufficient funding, TB clinics should be also be functioning as HIV clinics. As a TB clinic's primary function is the detection of patients with sputum smear-positive TB, there is a very real risk of HIV-infected patients being repeatedly re-infected with *Mycobacterium tuberculosis* within the clinic building. It may be safer to situate HIV clinics in primary care facilities, in parallel with clinics used for the treatment of other chronic conditions such as diabetes, epilepsy and hypertension. The hypothesis that long-term antiretrovirals can be effectively delivered using directly observed therapy is being tested in several randomised controlled trials, the results of which will have a significant influence on the structuring of primary care antiretroviral programmes.

Excluding the cost of treatment, the most important barrier to the introduction of a national treatment programme is the limited capacity of the public health care system. While the last decade has seen health sector reform and a significant expansion in the number of primary care facilities (701 primary care clinics built in 10 years) this has not been matched by an increase in skilled health professionals. In contrast health professionals, discouraged by poor remuneration, lack of acknowledgement and poor working conditions have been lost to the private sector and abroad. This absolute shortage of skilled health professionals has been identified as the single biggest threat to the treatment programme. This shortage is worse in rural and under-resourced areas. In recent years community service medical officers, with limited experience and almost no support, have been sent to remote rural areas in an attempt to address this inequity. It is only now, with the announcement of a National Treatment Plan that the Rural Development Plan has been tabled. The Plan provides for pay incentives for health professionals who choose to work in rural areas.

The challenge of providing HIV- and antiretroviral-specific training is also considerable. At present HIV expertise in South Africa is limited largely to the private sector and to a small number of tertiary institutions in urban centres. Within these centres, antiretroviral therapy has largely been viewed as the task of the specialist, most of whom feel reluctant to delegate what is perceived to be complex clinical care to a lower level of expertise. But close on five million South Africans will qualify for treatment in the next decade. Realistically, even modest levels of access to care can only be achieved if nurses, not just doctors and certainly not just specialists, are equipped with the necessary skills. In order to be effective, such training programmes will need to be ongoing, with constant evaluation and support. Such training is not only costly but also of uncertain effectiveness given the difficulties of changing professional practice in health care. Commitment to the open-minded development and testing of training programmes and approaches is required if we are to identify those approaches which are effective and should be expanded with the treatment programme, while dropping those which are ineffective or potentially harmful.

Adherence and other barriers to effective care

Antiretroviral adherence and the spectre of resistance

When primary HIV care services have been developed, there still remain significant obstacles to the effective use of services and to the appropriate use of antiretrovirals, of which adherence is the most important. Inconsistent adherence allows HIV to acquire resistance to all known classes of antiretrovirals with notorious ease. Multi-drug resistant HIV is a significant problem in developed countries, and the sexual transmission of resistant virus is well established. The paucity of resources and the massive numbers of patients eligible for antiretrovirals in South Africa makes the development of widespread resistance a valid concern, which is best addressed by attempting to understand and address adherence and treatment issues (TABLE 31.2).

Patient Factors
Cost of antiretroviral treatment and care
Poverty
• unable to afford regular transport to point of care
• unable to afford food when appetite returns
Unstable domestic environments (forced migration to seek work)
Alternative constructs about the pathogenesis of HIV/AIDS
• traditional belief systems
• publicly endorsed dissident theories
Stigma (primarily a barrier to accessing services, but not for adherence)
Non-disclosure
Male gender
Affected but untreated family members/friends (drug spillage)
Antiretroviral Treatment Factors
Pill burden
Side-effects
Health System Factors
Absolute shortage of skilled staff (doctors, nurses, pharmacists)
Overburdened health facilities and staff
Poor HIV treatment knowledge and skills
Poorly integrated vertical services for people living with HIV/AIDS (eg TB and others)
Poor integration with private services
Unreliable drug supply systems
Lack of decentralised laboratories with HIV specific resources

The perception has been that people with little education and living in extreme poverty are not well positioned to follow complex treatment schedules. Increasingly, studies have shown this not be the case. See CHAPTER 32 for a complete discussion of antiretroviral therapy and viral resistance in South Africa.

TABLE 31.2 Barriers to the appropriate care of HIV/AIDS patients in South Africa

Adherence in Africa

Early studies from Uganda and Botswana reported adherence rates between 50 and 70%, comparable with those from the developed world. However, these studies report on data for patients enrolled in donor treatment programmes where patients were required to contribute a substantial portion of their monthly income to cover costs, at a time where triple therapy was still prohibitively expensive (US$400–800 for a month's supply). The cost of treatment was found to be the single most important barrier to adherence. These studies document forced treatment interruptions arising from financial restrictions. The Botswana study modelled the impact of various factors on adherence, and concluded that if cost restrictions were removed, adherence could be expected to increase from 54 to 71%. This is encouraging for the South African Treatment Programme where drugs will be provided free at point of care.

It is worth noting that, outside of forced treatment interruptions, adherence was excellent in a sizeable proportion of patients. This is consistent with studies from South Africa and Senegal that showed high rates of adherence among patients receiving treatment as part of clinical trials, where treatment was provided free of charge. Unpublished reports from the Botswana treatment programme, which has been providing free drugs since early 2002, are similarly impressive with adherence rates of up to 90% reported. In contrast with expectations, it would seem that adherence in Africa is comparable, if not better, than that in the developed world. This may be related to eligibility criteria since treatment has by and large been restricted to patients with symptomatic disease, and many have advanced AIDS at the time of starting therapy. Also, extremely limited access in the face of such a high burden of disease means that anti-retroviral treatment is regarded as a very high value commodity in Africa. Those who are fortunate enough to gain access to treatment are suitably adherent.

Nonetheless the impact of poverty on adherence remains a concern. Most studies from Africa are completed in treatment sites established in hospitals or large clinics in urban centres, with patients living in reasonably close proximity. Experience from the TB programme suggests that poverty may present a significant barrier to adherence in those living in poorly resourced rural areas. It is in these areas that adherence to short-course TB therapy has been limited by inability to pay for transport to TB clinics and uncertain home environments characterised by forced migration in search of work. TB is an impoverishing disease. Many patients lose their jobs after they fall ill, only to find themselves out-of-pocket and out-of-cupboard when their appetites improve on treatment. Complaints that TB treatment cures TB only to replace it with hunger are commonplace, and patients and health workers are left feeling unsure as how to deal with adherence, when even basic foodstuffs are unavailable. The same will be true of the South African antiretroviral programme. These deficiencies need to be anticipated and addressed to ensure an equitable chance of treatment success for those living in poor circumstances in rural South Africa.

Disease constructs in HIV: A potential barrier to adherence?

Another perceived challenge to treatment programmes in South Africa relates to concerns about how traditional constructs of disease play out at the level of adherence to western treatment regimens. Many Africans believe that witchcraft is a factor in the pathogenesis of HIV/AIDS. As a result, many seek care from traditional healers, and consume traditional medicines and remedies. The Botswana study reported that 47% of patients had sought care from traditional healers; this declined significantly after starting antiretrovirals. Patients did not consider seeking care from a traditional healer to be a barrier to adherence. This position is supported by many traditional healers who have indicated willingness to work alongside antiretroviral programmes in the management of patients with HIV/AIDS, referring patients to allopathic practitioners for treatment when necessary.

In South Africa, alternative constructs about the pathogenesis and treatment of HIV are not limited to traditional belief systems. Until quite recently the South African president and senior ministerial figures had adopted a widely publicised stance generally understood to mean that HIV does not cause AIDS. The treatment programme remains to be publicly and enthusiastically endorsed by the president, despite other leaders in the region playing a large and public role in the introduction of treatment programmes in their countries. The Minister of Health has promoted dissident alternative nutritional approaches such as immune boosters and encouraged ongoing research and development into traditional medicines in order to identify alternative treatments for AIDS. The extent to which this lack of endorsement of antiretroviral treatment will have an impact on South Africans' ability to access treatment and be adherent is not yet known.

In 2003 a well-known Gauteng radio personality went public with his HIV status and received much support and encouragement from his fans. Eight months after his diagnosis and public announcement he died from AIDS-related complications, without having attempted to effectively use antiretrovirals, despite having the financial means to do so. Initially he, like many South Africans, believed witchcraft had played a role in his illness and sought help from a traditional healer. He later embarked on a frantic search for help from dissident practitioners, among them the nutritionist who developed the much publicised alternative nutrition programme for HIV, which included the African potato, and who came with the national health minister's personal recommendation.

Stigma: A barrier to access but not adherence

Stigma is also known to present significant challenges to the provision of antiretrovirals in the public sector. Botswana's treatment programme MASA (Setswana for 'new dawn') started in January 2002 under the personal supervision of President Mogae, who chairs the National AIDS Co-ordinating Council (NACA). The programme aimed to deliver treatment to about 19 000 HIV-infected citizens in the first year, and expand to an additional 20 000 patients per year in following years. Disappointingly, by the end of 2002 only 3 200 people had enrolled in the programme. This was consistent with low recruitment rates reported by NGOs operating free prevention of mother-to-child transmission (PMTCT) programmes. Health care workers reported that stigma was playing a large role in preventing HIV-infected people from accessing services. Provision of formula milk as part of the PMTCT programmes identified women as being HIV positive, in a society where women lack status and are in no position to demand safer sex practices without the risk of being ostracised from their partners, in-laws and family.

Adherence studies from Botswana report similar findings; most patients on treatment withhold their status from their families and communities for fear of being stigmatised. Importantly, however, patients don't perceive stigma to be a barrier to adherence and only 15% report that stigma affects their ability to follow treatment schedules. Rather stigma would seem to be a barrier to accessing HIV/AIDS services, as people fear being identified as positive when seeking care in dedicated programme areas of clinics and hospitals. This poses a significant challenge to South Africa where it is likely that, at least initially, treatment programmes will be implemented in a vertical manner to ensure that a reasonable standard of care is delivered. Inadvertent waiting room disclosure places a major restriction on patients seeking care from these services. This is especially true of rural and disadvantaged areas where patients are frequently required to wait for long periods before they are seen by a nurse or doctor (in South Africa an average clinic visit consumes a full working day). This fact, combined with the absence of alternative infrastructure, has transformed clinic waiting rooms into hubs of social exchange where being identified as HIV positive can result in the rapid dissemination of one's status along community grapevines.

Introduction of prevention of mother-to-child transmission (PMTCT) and post-exposure prophylaxis (PEP) after rape has driven voluntary counselling and testing (VCT) in women, but where these services do not exist, VCT has been poorly utilised. This is a function of two elements of the HIV epidemic in South Africa – stigmatisation of the disease and, until now, the non-availability of effective treatment. Why know your status when the diagnosis offers little more than stigma? The Médecins Sans Frontières' experience in Cape Town has clearly documented this health-seeking behaviour and describes it as a new social contract: 'Break the fatality and we will break the silence'. It also describes the relationship between treatment and prevention. A 2002 study by the Centre for AIDS development documented high levels of condom use and willingness to practise safer sex – in part attributable to a more comprehensive approach to the disease.

The question of gender

HIV is stigmatised primarily because it is sexually transmitted. This brings into question the role of gender in managing the epidemic. The plight of African women has received much attention. In much of Africa, women are considered second-class citizens with limited ability to influence decisions about sexuality and accessing health care.

This holds true for many South African women. But when it comes to HIV in South Africa, gender discrimination has not been restricted to women. South African NGO treatment initiatives report a preponderance of women seeking treatment, in contrast with the rest of Africa where women and men have enrolled in treatment programmes in almost equal proportions. In part this is explained by HIV/AIDS programmes which to date have prioritised access to antiretrovirals for PMTCT and PEP. This has preferentially driven testing rates in women, while most men have remained untested. In addition men have been blamed for the spread of the disease, particularly as a result of migratory labour practices, when they are removed from their families and sexual partners for prolonged periods. Women often attend treatment programmes without disclosing this to their untested and untreated partners, while continuing to practise unprotected sex with them. The risk of re-infection and spread of resistant virus is considerable. Until this imbalance is addressed, and men distanced from blame for the spread of the disease, interventions to encourage safer sex practices can be expected to be of limited effectiveness.

Spillage: More than just a black market

International response to the long-awaited decision to provide free antiretrovirals to HIV-infected South Africans with AIDS has been tempered by concerns about the development of a global black market and the attendant potential for unregulated treatment and consequent rapid emergence of drug anarchy. South Africa has more HIV-infected citizens than North America and Europe combined. Its treatment programme will fast become the largest distributor of antiretrovirals in the world, with drugs provided free at point of care.

This brings with it the potential for system leakage of drugs and the development of crime syndicates operating in black market trade. Already reports from Kenya indicate that antiretrovirals are being sold at reduced prices on Kenyan markets. Strategies for increasing accountability of health care professionals, especially those working in the poorly supervised areas of the health system, and enhanced community participation are needed in order to ensure such leakage is kept to a minimum.

Concerns about spillage are not restricted to conventional black market theories. Discordant treatment status within relationships and families has potentially disastrous consequences for adherence. Once clinically well, patients on treatment may be tempted to share drugs with sick partners, friends and children who have not yet accessed services. This highlights the role of stigma in accessing services, and prioritises the development of treatment programmes which provide for relatively anonymous entry into care programmes by integrating this function into existing primary care services, while simultaneously setting up a dedicated service which operates once patients are on treatment and are more at ease with their status.

The question of mothers sharing drugs with their children is less easily resolved. Paediatric treatment is part of the National Treatment Programme, but is unlikely to be rolled out at a pace comparable with the adult programme given its relative complexity and care requirements (such as taking blood from infants, adjusting dosages at regular intervals, and educating caregivers on how best to give antiretrovirals to young children). The result will be that many women may find themselves feeling better on treatment while their children are dying. The instinct to share treatment will be compelling and difficult to overcome. Programmes that provide for simultaneous treatment of mothers and children provide a promising model to address this problem.

Issues in caring for individuals with AIDS in South Africa

There is a very substantial literature on the management of HIV infection in the developed world. Problems experienced by HIV-infected patients and their caregivers in the South Africa are much less well documented and ongoing, relevant research is essential. This section will broadly discuss important clinical issues affecting AIDS patients in South Africa.

Smear-negative tuberculosis

TB is the commonest opportunistic infection among HIV-infected adults, and is associated with substantial morbidity and a high mortality. The WHO places much emphasis on diagnosing highly contagious pulmonary TB that is sputum smear-positive for acid-fast bacilli (AFB). The HIV epidemic limited the relevance of this approach as between 40 to 60% of HIV-infected individuals have sputum smear-negative disease, and are consequently unable to easily access the effective antituberculous therapy offered by the tuberculosis programme. Sputum induction with hypertonic saline is a simple, inexpensive and under-utilised tool that improves the yield of AFB from patients with an non-productive cough. Mycobacterial culture, widely used in the developed world to diagnose smear-negative tuberculosis (SNTB), is relatively costly and often takes several weeks to provide a diagnosis. Outside of large urban centres in South Africa, TB culture is not readily available and clinicians caring for HIV-infected adults with suspected tuberculosis need to rely on clinical skill and experience to diagnose HIV-associated SNTB.

The WHO has provided guidelines for the diagnosis of SNTB: at least three sputum-negative specimens; there are radiographic abnormalities consistent with active pulmonary TB; and no response to a course of broad-spectrum antibiotics. Although useful, the sensitivity and specificity of these guidelines are compromised by a number of important factors including clinical difficulty in assessing response to antibiotics, and in distinguishing between tuberculosis and other sub-acute or chronic pulmonary conditions such as post-TB bronchiectasis, *Pneumocystis* pneumonia, nocardiosis, cryptococcosis, Kaposi's sarcoma, and lymphocytic interstitial pneumonitis. Up to 10% of patients with HIV and pulmonary TB will have a normal chest radiograph, and some will have subtle abnormalities that may be overlooked by clinicians who have not had training in pulmonary radiology. Recently the WHO also outlined criteria for the diagnosis of extra-pulmonary tuberculosis where the diagnosis is based on one culture-positive specimen, or histological or strong clinical evidence consistent with active extra-pulmonary TB, followed by a decision to treat with a full course of anti-tuberculous chemotherapy. Strikingly, in the absence of mycobacterial culture or histology these guidelines are entirely dependent on the clinical judgement of a doctor, a problem in South Africa where junior doctors or primary care nurses deliver much of the clinical care in the state sector. Most doctors working in high HIV/TB prevalence settings are unaware of the WHO's guidelines, and the TB control programme nurses have not had sufficient training in HIV-associated TB, and may be reluctant to continue antituberculous therapy where they feel that the client's TB has not been adequately diagnosed with sputum smears.

Simple case definitions for the diagnosis of SNTB need to be developed and validated. The utility of one set of case definitions for the diagnosis of SNTB is shown in TABLE 31.3.

Case definition	Number	TB diagnosis		Positive predictive value
		Confirmed	Response to therapy	
Pulmonary (a)	83	64	10	89%
Lymphadenitis (b)	118	102	9	94%
Serositis (c)	36	25	9	94%
Constitutional (d)	11	4	0	36%

TABLE 31.3 Positive predictive value of clinical case definitions for the diagnosis of pulmonary and extrapulmonary tuberculosis in HIV-infected patients with tuberculosis symptoms and negative sputum smears.
(a) Cough > 21 days; pulmonary opacification or nodular infiltrate on chest radiograph; PCP excluded; no resolution after treatment with a broad-spectrum antibiotic (except for patients with diffuse micronodular [miliary] infiltrate on chest radiograph who should be treated for TB immediately).
(b) Significant peripheral nodes (long axis e3 cm) plus fever e38 °C OR drenching sweats for >2 weeks; visceral nodes (mediastinal or abdominal nodes seen on imaging) plus fever e38 °C on 2 occasions OR drenching sweats for >2 weeks.
(c) Pleural effusion (lymphocytic exudate); pericardial effusion (effusion on ultrasound, plus fever e38 °C on 2 occasions OR drenching sweats for >2 weeks [aspiration reserved for patients with haemodynamic compromise]); ascites (lymphocytic exudate plus fever e38 °C on 2 occasions OR drenching sweats for >2 weeks).
(d) Wasting (body mass index of <18.5 or documented weight loss of 10% body weight in a month) with fever e38 °C on 2 occasions OR drenching sweats for >2 weeks.
Adapted from: Wilson D, Nachega J, Chaisson R, Maartens G. Validation of expanded case definitions smear-negative tuberculosis in HIV-infected South African adults. Abstract MoPeB3229 15th International AIDS Conference 2004

A number of small clinical studies have shown that patients with TB respond in a fairly predictable manner to antituberculous therapy, showing improvements in weight, haemoglobin, and Karnofsky score, and a fall in serum C-reactive protein.

A strategy that combines clinical recognition of SNTB case definitions with documenting objective response to antituberculous therapy may hold promise for diagnosing SNTB until new, inexpensive, effective and robust laboratory-based diagnostic techniques are developed. Responsibility falls on the WHO to provide leadership in the difficult area of TB diagnostics if the large numbers of patients with HIV-associated TB are to be effectively treated.

All professional and lay health care workers in South Africa need to have a very high index of suspicion for TB among HIV-infected patients. Weight loss, cough and drenching sweats are very suggestive symptoms and testing for sputum AFB is an essential first step in making the diagnosis. Interactions between TB and HIV are discussed in more detail in CHAPTER 28, as is the use of isoniazid prophylaxis.

Fungal infections

Three potentially fatal fungal infections occur commonly in HIV-infected individuals with advanced immune suppression (CD4 count <200 cells/μL). All present clinicians with diagnostic challenges in resource limited settings.

Pneumocystis pneumonia (PCP) caused by *Pneumocystis jiroveci*, commonly presents with a pulmonary syndrome that can be difficult to distinguish clinically from pulmonary TB and community acquired pneumonia. In developed countries the diagnosis of PCP is confirmed by demonstrating the fungal antigen (using a direct fluorescent antigen test) or fungal DNA (using the polymerase chain reaction) in bronchial fluid obtained after sputum induction or bronchoscopy. South African clinicians often do not have access to these sophisticated investigations. Clinical features such as increasing shortness of breath on exertion with non-productive cough developing over a period of days, hypoxia and bilateral pulmonary opacification (often with a 'ground-glass' alveolar pattern) are helpful pointers towards the diagnosis.

PCP responds to high-dose cotrimoxazole that is widely available in inexpensive generic formulations. The addition of high-dose prednisone improves the prognosis of patients with hypoxia. Secondary prophylaxis with cotrimoxazole prevents relapse. The use of cotrimoxazole as primary prophylaxis is discussed in CHAPTER 28. *Pneumocystis* resistance to cotrimoxazole has been described, but the clinical significance is unclear.

Cryptococcal meningitis (CM) is caused by infection with *Cryptococcus neoformans* and presents with a gradually developing headache suggestive of raised intracranial pressure, behavioural changes, reduced level of consciousness, cranial nerve palsies (usually the abducent nerve) and seizures. There may be a history of weight loss and sweats preceding the headache, and meningism is often absent. Abnormalities in the cerebrospinal fluid (CSF) are often minimal and a florid pleocytosis is unusual. The India ink stain demonstrating budding yeasts in the CSF is an inexpensive and very specific investigation, but the sensitivity is poor. The cryptococcal latex agglutination test performed on either serum or CSF is about 90% sensitive for culture positive CM and technically simple to perform. However, due to its relatively high cost it is often not available outside large urban

centres attached to academic institutions. This important investigation needs to be more widely available.

Oesophageal candidiasis (oc), caused by *Candida albicans* (or other
Candida species), presents with increasing pain on swallowing, proceeding to the point where afflicted patients are entirely unable to eat
or drink. Traditionally the diagnosis has been made on oesophago-
scopy, which shows extensive pseudomembranous plaques with
underlying erythema and contact bleeding. Fortunately, the finding
of oral candidiasis in a patient presenting with painful swallowing
correlates well with the presence of oc, and the diagnosis can be
made clinically without the use of expensive endoscopy. The diagnosis of oc is more difficult if oral candidiasis is not present, is present
in a form other than the easily recognised pseudomembranous type,
or has been treated with topical antifungals. The doctor will then
need to decide whether to attempt a trial of fluconazole therapy or
try to obtain a barium swallow or endoscopy to exclude other, more
unusual causes of dysphagia.

The Pfizer fluconazole donation programme, started in 2000,
revolutionised the management of both cryptococcal meningitis and
oesophageal candidiasis. Fluconazole is a highly effective antifungal
agent that can be taken orally, but until the donation programme, its
price put it out of the reach of most state patients. The programme is
an outstanding example of collaboration between the ethical pharmaceutical industry and government. oc responds to a two-week course
of fluconazole, but frequently relapses. cm requires lifelong secondary prophylaxis with fluconazole to suppress the infection after an
initial month of high-dose therapy. The development of fluconazole
resistance, especially among *Candida* species, is a concern.

Bacterial sepsis

Up to 70% of HIV-infected adults will experience at least one bacterial
respiratory tract infection requiring treatment with antibiotics. With
more than 10% of the South African population living with HIV, antibiotic usage for respiratory tract infection is going to increase dramatically, as is the use of cotrimoxazole for primary prophylaxis. This
has major implications for the development of bacterial antibiotic
resistance. It is not unusual to find penicillin-resistant *Streptococcus
pneumoniae*, methicillin-resistant *Staphyloccccus aureus*, and multidrug-
resistant *Klebsiella pneumoniae* in the sputum of patients with advanced
HIV disease and community acquired infections. Non-typhoid salmonella species causing bacteraemia and severe sepsis in patients with
advanced HIV infection are usually resistant to first-line antibiotics in
South Africa. Blood culture can only be accessed with difficulty,

usually due to the unavailability of culture bottles in public sector emergency units. Doctors caring for patients with severe bacterial sepsis are required to make a judgement call on the antibiotic resistance profile of the infecting organism. The tendency is to treat severe sepsis of unknown aetiology with a cephalosporin and aminoglycoside or quinolone. This strategy, while effective in managing individual patients, has significant cost implications and may accelerate the development of broad antibiotic resistance.

The widespread use of cotrimoxazole as primary prophylaxis may render this antibiotic ineffective for the treatment of bacterial infections. Ongoing research is needed to quantify the extent and magnitude of antibiotic resistance in HIV-infected patients, and to monitor trends over time in order to inform empiric antibiotic choices.

Chronic diarrhoea and the wasting syndrome

Ongoing profuse watery diarrhoea due to small bowel enteropathy is a common and troublesome feature of very advanced HIV infection. It has a significant negative impact on patients' quality of life: each episode exhausts the patient; periods of rest are disrupted; major electrolyte losses occur; and oral intake is voluntarily curtailed as eating tends to provoke episodes of cramping and diarrhoea. Infestation with coccidian parasites is the usual cause, although *Mycobacterium avium intracellularae* and *Mycobacterium tuberculosis* infection can present in this way. Special staining techniques are needed to demonstrate the coccidian parasites, and access to these investigations is usually restricted to larger centres. Patients with fever and drenching sweats should be investigated for TB. Those without constitutional symptoms can be managed symptomatically with antidiarrhoeals or opiates. If the diarrhoea is refractory to symptomatic treatment a case can be made for treating empirically with a two to four week course of cotrimoxazole to cover for infestation with *Isospora* and *Cyclospora*, and with metronidazole to treat possible giardiasis. Albendazole treats one species of microsporidia, but a four-week course is costly, and identifying the microsporidium species in a stool specimen requires sophisticated technology. The most effective treatment is antiretroviral therapy, which is the only effective treatment available for *Cryptosporidium* and *Microsporidium*.

Profound wasting in the absence of an obvious cause is usually attributed to a very high HIV viral load, which can be primarily responsible for fatigue, fever and sweats. Worryingly, however, up to one third of patients diagnosed with the wasting syndrome have been found to have occult TB. Further research in this area is essential.

Dermatological and oral problems

Skin rashes, while seldom life threatening, can make patients living with HIV feel anxious and miserable. Pruritic papular eruption (PPE) (also called prurigo) is due to an abnormal response to insect bites and is associated with significant immunesuppression. The intensely itchy inflamed papules are very visible (patients dress in long-sleeved shirts and trousers to hide the lesions) and fade to leave disfiguring pigmented macules. The rash responds to a potent topical corticos-teroid ointment, which is not routinely available in primary care. If the patient has scabies (which mimics PPE), this needs to be treated before steroids are used. Shingles (caused by the varicella zoster virus) is very common, occurring at all stages of HIV disease, and can cause extensive superficial skin loss and incapacitating neuralgia. The diag-nosis is easily made clinically, but should be made within 72 hours of the initial symptoms if the course of the infection is to be modified by treatment with high-dose aciclovir, again not routinely available in primary care. Ichthyosis (dry skin) is associated with advanced HIV infection and causes intense, diffuse itching that responds to liberal application of hydrating agents such as cetomacrogol and aqueous cream. Dermatophyte (fungal) infections can cause large 'ring-worm' rashes and disfiguring hair and nail loss. The infection responds to topical clotrimazole or oral griseofulvin. Itraconazole or terbinafine are ideal agents for the treatment of fungal skin and nail infections, but are prohibitively expensive. It is essential to treat facial rashes in order to preserve patients' self-esteem and to prevent social withdrawal and depression. Nodular acne responds to topical benzoyl peroxide and a one to three month course of oral doxycycline. Seborrhoeic dermatitis can be treated with a mild potency steroid cream.

Oral candidiasis and gingivitis responds to an antiseptic mouth-wash (such as chlorhexidine). Severe oral candidiasis can be treated with nystatin or amphotericin lozenges, and gingivitis with a course of metronidazole and amoxycillin.

Skin rashes occurring as a complication of treatment with the non-nucleoside reverse transcriptase inhibitors (NNRTI) is discussed in CHAPTER 32.

The importance of effectively managing skin and mouth conditions to preserve quality of life cannot be over-emphasised. Clinic managers and policy makers must ensure that appropriate medications in suffi-cient quantities are available at primary care level to treat the large numbers of patients who will develop these conditions.

Patients starting successful antiretroviral therapy may develop local-ised atypical inflammation in response to foreign antigens that the compromised immune system was previously unable to detect. This phenomenon has come to be called the immune reconstitution inflammatory syndrome (IRIS) or immune reconstitution disease and can cause significant morbidity during the first months of therapy. Previously occult infections can be unmasked or, more problemati-cally, infections that are already being treated can appear to flare, causing symptom exacerbation. The latter phenomenon is probably due to the immune system recognising antigen from non-viable organisms that had not been effectively cleared from the body. Pro-foundly immunosuppressed patients seem more likely to develop the condition. Comprehensive data on IRIS have yet to be published, especially from the developing world.

The commonest pathogen provoking IRIS in South Africa is proba-bly *M tuberculosis*. The presentation of IRIS-associated TB is atypical. Florid peripheral or central lymphadenopathy, pleural or pericardial effusions and atypical infiltrates seem to be commoner than cavi-tating pulmonary disease. Biopsy may show an exuberant granuloma-tous inflammatory response with few acid-fast bacilli. It is essential to screen patients for tuberculosis symptoms and to exclude active infection before starting antiretroviral therapy. Primary care practi-tioners are ideally positioned to exclude active disease with serial weight and symptom review. Treatment is with standard antitubercu-lous therapy according to the national protocol. The management of a tuberculosis-associated syndrome occurring in patients already on antituberculous therapy is controversial. A pragmatic approach is to treat the manifestations of the syndrome with oral prednisone (usually 60 mg daily), and to consider extending the course of the antituberculous therapy for a further three months. TB-associated IRIS should not be confused with the TB paradoxical reaction where TB lesions (such as pulmonary infiltrates, tuberculomas, adenitis and effusions) can increase in size when antituberculous therapy is commenced in both HIV-infected and uninfected individuals. Conceptually, the paradoxical reaction relates to massive antigen release due to mycobacterial lysis, whereas IRIS relates to immune recovery. Clinically it can be difficult to distinguish the two condi-tions when both antiretroviral and antituberculous therapy are started at about the same time.

Both PCP and CM can flare in patients receiving secondary prophy-laxis. As discussed above, diagnosis can be problematic. PCP should be treated with high-dose cotrimoxazole and prednisone, and CM with fluconazole and serial lumber punctures to relieve intracranial pressure. Fungal CSF culture is useful to distinguish between failed prophylaxis and IRIS.

Pruritic papular skin rashes occurring early in the course of anti-retroviral therapy are probably also a manifestation of IRIS. The rash can resemble PPE or facial acne that is slightly atypical as pruritis is often marked. Importantly, the rash needs to be distinguished from that due to NNRTI allergy. Topical corticosteriods are effective. Patients often worry that the manifestations of IRIS are due to anti-retroviral failure or treatment side-effects. Strong reassurance is needed, and patients need to be told that the development of IRIS means that the treatment is working and the immune system is beginning to function again.

Screening for serious adverse effects of antiretrovirals

Serious complications of antiretroviral therapy are unusual, but given the large numbers of patients taking these drugs health care workers will occasionally encounter life-threatening antiretroviral-related events. A comprehensive overview of antiretroviral side-effects is given in CHAPTER 32. Three of the most serious acute adverse effects are lactic acidosis, acute pancreatitis and drug-induced hepatitis, all of which present with abdominal symptoms. Patients should be counsel-led to come into their clinic if they experience severe abdominal pain or vomiting persisting for more than 24 hours, or become jaundiced. Health care workers should have rapid and easy access to the results of serum lactate, lipase, transaminases and bilirubin. Most skin rashes associated with the use of nevirapine are benign and can be treated symptomatically or by switching to efavirenz. A small percentage of patients taking nevirapine develop life-threatening skin necrosis (Stevens-Johnson syndrome) that may be associated with fever, hepatitis and eosinophilia as part of a hypersensitivity syndrome. Health care workers need to be aware of the possibility of severe nevirapine-induced rash.

The decision to discontinue antiretroviral therapy should not be made lightly and junior doctors need to be able to discuss clinical cases and laboratory results with experienced colleagues at any time. Ensuring that the necessary infrastructure and expertise are available is a major challenge to public sector antiretroviral programmes that needs to be innovatively addressed by public-private partnerships.

The curative to palliative care pendulum

The prognosis of very advanced HIV disease is poor. Most South Africans do not have the option of antiretroviral therapy in advanced disease. Health care workers, especially in primary care and in medical wards, need to become accustomed to working with terminally ill patients and with the aims and philosophy of palliative care. The WHO defines palliative care as the active total care of patients whose disease no longer responds to curative treatment. The key word in this definition is 'active'. Evaluation for, and treatment with palliative care should be pursued vigorously in both out-patient and in-patient settings.

Many patients with AIDS die from an opportunistic infection or bacterial sepsis that may be entirely treatable. The typical example is TB, which markedly exacerbates immunosuppression. Patients with TB can present in a moribund state, with other conditions such as oesophageal thrush, severe wasting and chronic diarrhoea. Treatment of the TB is associated with improved immune function, weight gain and marked improvement in quality of life. At the initial presentation it may have been entirely appropriate to initiate palliative care with the expectation of a poor outcome, focusing on attending to physical conditions such as pain, pruritis, dyspnoea and diarrhoea, and the patient's psychosocial and spiritual concerns. However, this process needs to proceed in parallel with evaluation for a treatable condition that may have precipitated the patient's decline. Ideally this should be done in hospital, but resource limitations often mean this happens in out-patients with support from the patient's family and friends who interact closely with the health care team. Should a treatable condition be identified, and the patient's condition improve, the focus of care shifts away from palliation. During the last one to two years of an individual's life, focus can shift a number of times between curative care and palliative care. Doctors should not avoid prescribing opiates, such as morphine, should the patient's symptoms prove refractory to other forms of treatment. Addiction does not occur when prescribed for a physical condition such as pain and treatment can be safely withdrawn should the patient's condition improve.

The greatest challenge around palliative care in the South African public health sector is that the same team seldom treats individual patients for any period of time. Many young patients present for the first time in an apparently terminal condition to the formal health care system. Primary care workers seldom have the time to discuss palliative care in the comprehensive, empathic manner required to explore end of life issues. Young doctors performing internship and community service (frequently under sub-optimal supervision) may not yet have the degree of life experience and emotional maturity required to meaningfully grapple with questions around palliation. Maartens and Bekker have published data suggesting that palliative care is the preferred option if a patient has no antiretroviral options, has laboratory evidence of severe immune suppression (CD4 count <50 cells/μL, or total lymphocyte count <0.75 x 10^6/L), and poor quality of life with no reversible illnesses.

The decision to implement palliative care, once made, can be difficult. Hospice beds are in short supply, and most patients need to be cared for at home. Access to palliative care medications, especially morphine, can be difficult as a valid prescription is required each month, and the patient's family needs to take time off work to queue to collect the treatment. Many primary care clinics do not have the facilities required to stock morphine.

Government has attempted to deal with some of the practical problems around palliation by establishing home-based care (HBC) programmes, where care is provided by non-governmental organisations, community structures and religious groups. These organisations lack clinical expertise and may find it difficult to obtain medical advice, and are vulnerable to misinformation on the benefits of nutritional and folk remedies in advanced HIV disease. Very problematically, while government provides infrastructure and disposable items, the HBC workers are often not paid for their work. The often unglamorous and repetitive nature of HBC can exhaust even the most dedicated volunteer, who may only commit to a given individual for a period of time. Nonetheless invaluable care is provided to large numbers of terminally ill patients living in impoverished conditions.

Resource allocation

One of clinical medicine's most taxing aspects is that of who to treat with a scarce and costly intervention such as admission to a regional hospital ward, mechanical ventilation in an intensive care unit, or haemodialysis. Again junior doctors are in the front line of the decision-making process. Decisions often need to be made after-hours on critically ill patients with minimal collateral information. Patients' HIV status may not be known at the time of presentation, and ideally should not affect the decision-making process. Essential information such as a previous CD4 count or total lymphocyte count may not be available, and family members may not give a full history of HIV-associated illness in order not to prejudice the patient's chances of getting optimal treatment. A judgement-call on the possibility of underlying immunosuppression and probability of successful treatment outcome frequently needs to be made based on the presence of severe wasting, severe oral candidiasis or oral hairy leucoplacia, or skin lesions such as Kaposi's sarcoma. As general rule HIV-infected patients who are not severely wasted, who have not had a prior AIDS-defining diagnosis (or who are known to have a CD4 count >200 cells/μL), or who have good antiretroviral options should be considered for aggressive medical therapy, including ventilation and dialysis.

There are similar issues of resource allocation around the use of antiretrovirals in the government's antiretroviral rollout. Not everyone wanting and needing antiretrovirals will be able to receive treatment immediately, and some form of screening may be needed, should the ability to effectively provide treatment be exceeded by the demand. Each clinic will need to arrive at a pragmatic selection process that is seen to be fair and equitable by the local community. Insisting that patients complete an antiretroviral treatment training and adherence programme may be one solution to the problem.

Recruiting health care workers to AIDS care

AIDS patients pose an extraordinary challenge to the people responsible for their care. Many are poor; few can access antiretrovirals, and most are subject to repeated debilitating illnesses that respond indifferently to the medications available on the primary care Essential Drug List. As the epidemic matures the numbers of patients with advanced HIV disease increase exponentially, threatening to overwhelm the country's frail public health system. Nurses, counsellors and doctors have to cope with daily exposure to suffering, hopelessness and death. Loss of job satisfaction, frustration and emotional burnout are almost inevitable, and health care workers at the frontline of AIDS care seldom have an opportunity to express feelings of despair and grief. Primary care nurses are especially at risk as they live in the communities they serve, and are responsible for breaking bad news not only to patients but also to friends and families in their community. Doctors working with impoverished patients in urban areas are relatively protected from the psychological impacts of providing care, but are still exposed to the repeated loss of established patients, and to therapeutic nihilism. The workplace ethos places a high premium on silence and coping, and many health care workers have little choice but to succumb to stress, or to leave when coping skills are exhausted. There is a need for empathetic counselling services for health care workers.

The extraordinary fact remains that many people choose to remain in the field of HIV/AIDS. Reasons for this are diverse. Simple nursing, counselling and medical interventions can dramatically improve patients' quality of life. Satisfaction in doing a task well, and patients' and families' appreciation, can enhance health care workers' feelings of self-worth and self-sufficiency. Communities reward health care workers who are personally involved in the epidemic by respecting and acknowledging their professional status and expertise. Dedicated HIV/AIDS workers should be encouraged and supported by management and given the autonomy to build 'winning teams'. Many provinces have developed simple and effective guidelines for the treatment of common HIV-related conditions that provide a clear framework within which to work. Ongoing professional development and training opportunities are essential, as is being given the opportunity to participate in research. Management should promote clinic leaders who network within the community, and respond innovatively to challenges.

The HIV epidemic in South Africa places unprecedented demands on the health care system. These demands can be used in positive and constructive ways to explore and build new ways in which to promote health and deliver effective care. Twenty-first century health care workers have an opportunity to practise holistic medicine, and to enjoy the existential rewards that accompany belonging to one of the caring professions.

Bibliography

BENATAR SR. 'Health care reform and the crisis of HIV and AIDS in South Africa.' *New England Journal of Medicine* 2002; 351: 81–92

DOHERTY J, THOMAS S, MUIRHEAD D, McINTYRE D. *Health Care Financing and Expenditure.* Health Systems Trust. 2003.

FARMER P, LÉANDRE F, MUKHERJEE JS, CLAUDE MS, NEVIL P, SMITH-FAWZI MC, KOENIG SP, CASTRO A, BECERRA M, SACHS J, ATTARAN A, KIM JY. 'Community-based approaches to HIV treatment in resource-poor settings'. *Lancet* 2001; 358: 404–409.

HARRIES AD, NYANGULU DS, HARGREAVES NJ, KALUWA O, SALANIPONI FM. Preventing antiretroviral anarchy in sub-Saharan Africa. *Lancet* 2001; 358: 410–414.

IJUMBA P. '*Voices of Primary Health Care Facility Workers*'. Health Systems Trust. 2003.

KIRONDE S, BAMFORD L. '*Tuberculosis*'. Health systems Trust. 2003.

KITAHATA MM, TEGGER MK, WAGNER EH, HOLMES KK. 'Comprehensive health care for people infected with HIV in developing countries'. *British Medical Journal* 2002; 325: 954–57.

LANIECE I, CISS M, DESCLAUX A, DIOP K, MBODJ F, NDIAYE B, SYLLA O, DELAPORTE E, NDOYE I. 'Adherence to HAART and its principal determinants in a cohort of Senegalese adults.' *AIDS* 2003; 17(suppl 3): S103–S108.

MÉDECINS SANS FRONTIÈRES SOUTH AFRICA, THE DEPARTMENT OF PUBLIC HEALTH AND THE UNIVERSITY OF CAPE TOWN, AND THE PROVINCIAL ADMINISTRATION OF THE WESTERN CAPE, SOUTH AFRICA. *Antiretroviral Therapy in Primary Health Care – Experience of the Khayelitsha Programme in South Africa.* World Health Organization 2003 available at http://www.who.int/hiv/en

ORRELL C, BANGSBERG D, BADRI M, WOOD R. 'Adherence is not a barrier to successful antiretroviral therapy in South Africa'. *AIDS* 2003; 1: 1369–1375.

WEIDLE P, MALAMBA S, MWEBAZE R, SOZI C, RUKUNDO G, DOWNING R ET AL. 'Assessment of a pilot antiretroviral drug therapy programme in Uganda: Patients' response, survival and drug resistance'. *Lancet* 2002; 360: 34–40.

WEISER S, WOLFE W, BANGSBERG D, THIOR I, GILBERT P, MAKHEMA J ET AL. 'Barriers to Antiretroviral Adherence for Patients Living with HIV Infection and AIDS in Botswana'. *Journal of Acquired Immune Deficiency Syndrome* 2003; 34: 281–288.

WENDO C. 'Africans advocate antiretroviral strategy similar to DOTS'. *Lancet* 2003; 362: 1210.

WORLD HEALTH ORGANISATION. *HIV/TB: A Clinical Manual.* WHO/HTM/TB2004.329 [http:www.who.int/tb]

CHAPTER 32
Antiretroviral therapy

Robin Wood

THE MAIN AIM OF antiretroviral therapy is to delay or prevent the progression to AIDS and death of HIV-infected patients. However, even successful therapy does not completely prevent clinical events, particularly when started in advanced disease. Furthermore, antiretroviral therapy is required for life, since it cannot eradicate latent HIV.

Commonly used drug categories include nucleoside reverse transcriptase inhibitors (NRTIs), non-nucleoside reverse transcriptase inhibitors (NNRTIs) and protease inhibitors (PIs).

Current guidelines on when to start antiretroviral therapy are based on US and international HIV treatment recommendations that use a combination of evidence from randomised clinical trials, observational cohorts and expert opinion. All the guidelines emphasise initiating antiretroviral therapy for patients with HIV-related symptoms.

Poor adherence is the major cause of failure to achieve viral suppression and remains a particular challenge in the developing world, although studies have shown that adherence is possible where patients are supported.

Indications for changing antiretrovirals include drug toxicity, drug intolerance and treatment failure.

Drug resistance is a problem in the face of a highly mutation-prone virus. This is exacerbated by drug pressure and measurement of drug resistance can be helpful in guiding treatment.

Scaling up of antiretroviral programmes in the public sector in South Africa will require standardisation and simplification of treatment regimens.

The antiretroviral treatment era started in 1987 with the approval of zidovudine (AZT), a thymidine nucleoside analogue that targets the reverse transcriptase enzyme, necessary for the replication of the human immunodeficiency virus (HIV). Clinical benefit of AZT was demonstrated in a placebo-controlled trial that showed significant short-term clinical and survival improvement in patients with advanced disease. During the late 1980s other nucleoside reverse transcriptase inhibitors (NRTIS) were developed. Subsequent studies of monotherapy with AZT or the other NRTIS failed to show significant survival benefits when therapy was initiated at earlier stages of HIV infection. As more antiretroviral drugs of different classes became available, triple combination therapy was shown to have greater and more durable benefits than either mono- or dual therapy. While clinical benefits of therapy were relatively easy to demonstrate in patients at late stages of HIV infection, when mortality and the rate of new AIDS-defining events are high, the low rate of clinical events in early HIV infection required studies to be both large and prolonged, in order to have sufficient statistical power to show superiority of different combinations of therapies. The development of surrogate markers of HIV disease progression allowed the benefits of antiretroviral therapy to be monitored during both late and the earlier asymptomatic phase of HIV infection. CD4 T-cell counts provided the first reliable marker of disease progression. In 1996 the highly active antiretroviral therapy (HAART) era began with the availability of protease inhibitors (PIS), a new class of antiretrovirals and a commercial polymerase chain-reaction-based assay, which allowed accurate monitoring of viral response to potent therapy. Improvements in the newer molecular quantitative viral assays have allowed circulating plasma HIV to be measured to a lower threshold of 50 copies of HIV RNA per ml. An increase in CD4 counts and percentage of patients achieving viral suppression below 50 copies/ml are now standard endpoints of HAART trials. It should, however, be remembered that surrogate markers do not precisely reflect clinical outcomes.

A third class of antiretrovirals, the non-nucleoside reverse transcriptase inhibitors (NNRTIS), was developed soon after the first protease inhibitors became available and combinations of drugs from these three classes of antiretrovials now constitute HAART, which represents the 'standard of care' for antiretroviral therapy. While dual NRTIS constitute the conventional backbone of HAART, dual nucleoside therapy alone is no longer recommended because viral suppression is sub-optimal and can result in increased development of drug resistance. Where HAART has been made available to HIV-infected populations there have been dramatic decreases in rates of mortality and morbidity, improved quality of life and changed perceptions of HIV infection from that of a death sentence to a manageable chronic illness.

Aims of treatment

The primary aim of antiretroviral treatment is to stop or delay the inexorable progression to AIDS and death of HIV-infected patients. Successful HAART does not totally prevent clinical events and when therapy is initiated in advanced HIV disease at CD4 counts <50 cells/ml, new AIDS diagnoses can still occur in 10 to 15% of individuals despite virological suppression. Clinical benefits of therapy are hard to demonstrate in early HIV disease. Favourable responses to therapy usually include a decline in plasma HIV-1 RNA and increase in CD4 counts. Reductions in plasma viraemia achieved by HAART account for much of the clinical benefit of therapy and a sustained suppression of plasma viral load has become the most important measurable goal of therapy. Continued viral suppression is usually associated with an increase in CD4 counts. However, individual responses are quite variable and the correlation between CD4 response and viral load in any individual is weak. CD4 counts can also increase with incomplete viral suppression. Long-term cohort studies and national death registers have confirmed the sustained benefits of HAART.

Limitations of therapy

HAART is effective in controlling viral replication but is unable to eradicate latent HIV-1, which persists in the host, integrated within the genome of metabolically inactive but long-lived memory CD4+ T-cells. This reservoir of latently infected cells allows resurgence of viraemia when therapy is discontinued and life-long therapy is therefore necessary. Effective antiretroviral therapy increases naïve and memory CD4+ T-cells with partial restoration of immunity to some opportunistic infections, however there is a failure to restore HIV-1 specific immune responses. The ability to restore immune responses is diminished when therapy is initiated late in the clinical course and the ability of the adult thymus to repopulate the immune repertoire also declines with age. The consequent desire to initiate HAART to halt disease progression before the occurrence of significant immunological deterioration led to the philosophy of 'hit early-hit hard', during the late 1990s.

Increasing awareness of adverse events associated with long-term drug use, including metabolic and mitochondrial toxicities, has subsequently led to a more conservative approach, which in turn has been reflected in the evolution of treatment guidelines. Metabolic abnormalities of lipid and glucose metabolism include hyperlipidaemia, insulin resistance and frank diabetes mellitus. As the life expectancy of patients on HAART has increased, so increasing temporal exposure to metabolic toxicity has resulted in increased risk of cardiovascular events. Changes in body habitus have also been increasingly recognised in patients on HAART, which is associated with changes in lipid and glucose metabolism. Both peripheral fat wasting of the face, limbs and buttocks and increased fat deposition in the abdomen and other subcutaneous areas including submental, retroauricular regions and the 'buffalo hump' constitute the lipodystrophy syndrome. These long-term metabolic complications of HAART were first thought to be limited to patients receiving PIs but have been shown to be associated with all currently licensed drug classes. Although NRTIs primarily target the reverse transcriptase enzyme of HIV they also have differing affinities for a related human mitochondial enzyme, DNA polymerase gamma, which encodes for mitochondrial structural sub-units necessary for the oxidative phosphorylation pathway. Mitochondrial dysfunction particularly results from the inhibition of this enzyme by the dideoxy-NRTI drugs such as ddC, d4T and ddI. Mitochondrial toxicity has protean manifestations including acute life-threatening lactic acidosis, asymptomatic lactic acidaemia, chronic myopathy or peripheral neuropathy. Lipodystrophy, mitochondrial toxicity and other chronic side-effects such as gastrointestinal intolerance impact negatively on quality of life and result in poor adherence to HAART. The recognition of the negative impact of these toxicities on tolerability has led to the development of new members of each drug class, which are better tolerated and have improved metabolic profiles.

Drug categories

Nucleoside Reverse Transcriptase Inhibitors (NRTIs)

NRTIS (TABLE 32.1) have closely related structures that are analogues of the nucleosides adenosine, thymidine, cytidine and guanosine, required for DNA synthesis. They differ from the natural nucleosides by the absence of a hydroxyl group at the 3'-position of the ribose ring. These nucleoside analogues are prodrugs, which require phosphorylation by intracellular kinases to become the pharmacologically active tri-phosphorylated form. Different human cell phenotypes phosphorylate nucleosides at differing rates. During the process of reverse transcription, these triphosphorylated nucleotide analogues bind with the viral reverse transcriptase enzyme, competing with naturally occurring nucleotides for incorporation into the DNA copy of HIV RNA. Once incorporated into the DNA, the absence of a 3'-hydroxyl group does not allow the development of a new 3',5'-phosphodiesterase bond with the next nucleotide, resulting in chain termination. Intracellular concentrations of the tri-phosphorylated forms of the NRTIs determine antiviral activity, rather than the serum concentrations of the prodrugs. The half-life of intracellular AZT-triphosphate is considerably longer than serum AZT half-life and recognition of this has allowed the dosing interval to be increased from the originally recommended four to 12 hourly. Resistance to NRTIs can arise by several mechanisms. Mutations in the *Pol* gene can alter the structure of reverse transcriptase, resulting in preferential binding of natural deoxy-nucleotide triphosphates or by selectively excluding NRTIs. Chain termination can also be reversed by removal of the 3' terminal nucleotide monophosphate by binding to free pyrophosphate or free nucleosides. NRTIs such as AZT require the step-wise acquisition of several mutations before the development of significant resistance. In contrast, a 1000-fold resistance to 3TC can result from a single mutation at codon 184 (M184V). The relationship between NRTI-resistant mutations is complex, with resultant changes in viral replicative capacity, cross-resistance to other specific NRTIs and even delay or reversal of resistance to other members of the class. Interpretation of genotypic resistance patterns should be made in conjunction with the patient's present and past history of antiretroviral exposure.

Generic name	Abbreviation	Trade name	Usual dosage	Common side-effects (comments)
Zidovudine	AZT, ZDV	Retrovir	300 mg b.i.d. (2 tabs daily)	Bone marrow suppression, GI disturbance, headache, myopathy
Didanosine	ddI	Videx	200 mg b.i.d. (125 mg b.i.d. if <60 kg) or 300–400 mg q.d. (4 tabs daily)	Peripheral neuropathy, pancreatitis, nausea, diarrhoea (take on empty stomach)
Zalcitabine	ddC	Hivid	0.75 mg t.i.d. (3 tabs daily)	Peripheral neuropathy, pancreatitis, oral ulcers
Stavudine	d4T	Zerit	40 mg b.i.d. (30 mg b.i.d. if <60 kg) (2 caps daily)	Peripheral neuropathy
Lamivudine	3TC	Epivir	150 mg b.i.d. (2 tabs daily)	Anaemia, GI disturbance, myalgia rarely
Abacavir	ABC	Ziagen	300 mg b.i.d (2 tabs daily)	GI disturbance, hypersensitivity reaction 5%

TABLE 32.1 Nucleoside reverse transcriptase inhibitors

Non-nucleoside Reverse Transcriptase Inhibitors (NNRTIs)

NNRTIS (TABLE 32.2) are relatively free of the long-term metabolic complications associated with PI use and in combination with two nucleosides have gained popularity as initial therapy. They have no activity against HIV-2. NNRTIs do not require chemical modification to become pharmacologically active and the different members of the class have diverse chemical structures. They are small molecules, which act by non-competitive binding to an active receptor site close to the polymerase domain of reverse transcriptase. Binding of NNRTIS to this catalytic receptor site results in a change in the three-dimensional structure of reverse transcriptase and subsequent impairment of polymerase activity. High-level resistance to these agents can develop rapidly if used as monotherapy, as a result of single-point mutations affecting the NNRTI catalytic binding site. Cross-resistance to all other first generation NNRTIs is very common. Class adverse effects include acute skin rash and hepatotoxicity, which is more frequent in the first three to four months of therapy.

Generic name	Abbreviation	Trade name	Usual dosage	Common side-effects (comments)
Nevirapine	NVP	Viramune	200 mg q.d. for 14 days then 200 mg b.i.d. (2 tabs daily)	Rash, elevated transaminases, hepatitis
Delavirdine	DLV	Rescriptor	400 mg t.i.d. (12 tabs daily)	Rash, headache
Efavirenz	EFV	Stocrin	600 mg QD (3 tabs daily)	Rash, central nervous system symptoms, elevated transaminases

Protease Inhibitors (PIs)

TABLE 32.2 Non nucleoside reverse transcriptase inhibitors

PIS (TABLE 32.3) are structurally diverse molecules, which do not require any chemical modification to become pharmacologically active. PIs are metabolised in the liver and gut by the P450 enzyme system (predominantly the CYP 3A4 isoenzyme) resulting in many pharmacological interactions with other hepatically metabolised drugs. The PI target is the HIV-encoded protease enzyme, which is necessary for the cleaving of the long HIV protein precursor transcript into Gag, Gag-Pol subunits prior to virion assembly and export of new infectious virus from the infected cell. They are small molecules, which bind to the central active cleavage site of the HIV protease heterodimer. Resistance mutations clustered around the active site alter the active binding site with resultant decreased drug binding. PIs have multiple overlapping patterns of resistance, with specific single mutations such as D30N associated with nelfinavir resistance, shared resistance profiles for indinavir and ritonavir, and distinctive patterns for saquinavir, amprenavir and lopinavir.

The variable pathways to resistance affecting single or groups of PIs allows for sequential use of members of this class following failure of a primary PI regimen. Class-related adverse events include acute gastrointestinal symptoms in the first few weeks of therapy and long-term metabolic complications such as insulin resistance, hyperlipidaemia, and morphological changes in fat distribution (lipodystrophy). Both peripheral fat wasting and central fat accumulation have been reported after prolonged PI use. Newer PIs such as atazanavir are thought to be relatively free of these metabolic side-effects, however, long-term experience with these agents is limited.

Generic name	Abbreviation	Trade name	Usual dosage	Common side-effects (comments)
Saquinavir	SQV	Invirase/ Fortovase	600 mg t.i.d. 1200 mg t.i.d. (9 caps daily)	GI disturbances (mild) (take with a fatty meal, or up to 2 h after meal), headache, elevated transaminases, hyperglycaemia
Indinavir	IDV	Crixivan	800 mg q 8 hr (6 caps daily)	Kidney stones, hyperbilirubinaemia (take on an empty stomach), GI disturbances, hyperglycaemia, headache.
Ritonavir	RTV	Norvir	600 mg b.i.d. (12 caps daily)	GI disturbance, circumoral and extremities paresthesias, diarrhoea, fatigue, hepatitis, taste perversion, hyperglycaemia
Nelfinavir	NFV	Viracept	750 mg t.i.d. or 1250 mg b.i.d. (9 caps daily)	Diarrhoea (take with food), hyperglycaemia
Amprenavir	AMP	Agenerase	1200 mg b.i.d. (16 tabs daily)	Rash, headache, GI disturbance

TABLE 32.3 Protease inhibitors

Boosted protein inhibitors

The P450 enzyme system is a family of isoenzymes, which are important in the metabolic degradation of PIs. Ritonavir is a potent inhibitor of the main CYP3A4 iso-enzyme present in both gut and hepatic tissue, which is important in the determination of plasma concentrations of PIs. Inhibition of CYP3A4 activity in the gut wall improves PI bioavailability by reducing local drug metabolism and subsequently increasing levels in the portal vein. Inhibition of hepatic CYP3A4 metabolism of PIs with relatively good bioavailability results in prolongation of plasma half-life, allowing for decreased frequency of drug dosing. The bioavailability of saquinavir is increased by co-administration of ritonavir resulting in an approximately 20-fold increase in peak plasma concentration (C_{max}). Co-administration of ritonavir and lopinavir results in an increase in C_{max}, prolongation of plasma half-life and increased trough levels (C_{min}). The combination of lopinavir and ritonavir increases lopinavir exposure (area under curve (AUC)) by 100-fold.

The addition of ritonavir to other PIs such as amprenavir, atazanavir, indinavir and nelfinavir prolongs plasma half-lives and increases C_{min} and AUC allowing less frequent dosing. Based on pharmacokinetic interaction studies, the use of ritonavir boosting has rapidly evolved from an investigational concept to widespread clinical practice, particularly for the management of antiretroviral-experienced patients. The long-term risks and toxicities of ritonavir boosted PI regimens have, however, not been clearly delineated.

New therapies

Tenofovir disoproxil fumarate (Viread) is an ester prodrug of the nucleotide analogue of adenosine 5'-monophosphate. It is generally well tolerated with some gastrointestinal adverse events and has increased bioavailability when administered with food (35%). The prolonged elimination half-life allows once-daily administration, with the major route of elimination being renal. The recommended dosage is one 300 mg tablet daily, if creatinine clearance is >60 ml/min. There is little interaction with PIs or NNRTIs. However, co-administration with didanosine results in didanosine levels that are significantly raised by 30–60%. Retrospective analysis of pooled data from placebo-controlled trials suggests that tolerability of didanosine in combination with tenofovir is similar to didanosine and placebo but it is recommended that the dose of didanosine is reduced from 400 mg to 250 mg per day. Efficacy has been shown to be similar to stavudine and resistance is associated with the K65R mutation, which occurs infrequently in patients receiving tenofovir. When combined with stable antiretroviral therapy, tenofovir has shown antiretroviral efficacy in both antiretroviral experienced and naïve patients. Adverse events associated with tenofovir include asthenia, headache and gastrointestinal disturbance. Nephrotoxicity, particularly tubular dysfunction, is less common than reported with use of the earlier nucleotide compound adefovir.

FTC (Emtricitabine) is a fluorinated cytidine analogue closely related to lamivudine but with a longer elimination half-life allowing once daily administration. Potency and resistance profile are similar to lamivudine. The prescribed dose of emtricitabine is a single 200 mg capsule once a day.

Videx EC is an enteric-coated formulation of ddI, which does not contain the antacid buffer component of standard formulation ddI. Videx EC is taken once daily on an empty stomach but the absence of antacid allows other medications to be taken at the same time with fewer gastrointestinal side-effects.

Capravirine is a second-generation non-nucleoside drug, which requires two or three key mutations to develop high-level resistance, in contrast to currently licensed non-nucleosides that have high-level resistance associated with a single mutation of the *Pol* gene. In patients previously failing NNRTI therapy, capravirine in combination with nelfinavir and two NRTIS was superior to placebo, nelfinavir and two NRTIS.

Atazanavir (Reyataz) is an azopeptide PI with freedom from the cholesterol and triglyceride abnormalities that are associated with other members of the protease inhibitor class. Oral bioavailability is variable but is improved when taken with food. There is a low pill burden and the recommended dosage is 400 mg (two tablets) taken once daily. The main side-effect is an increase in unconjugated bilirubin, which is related to serum drug level and patients' glucoronidation enzyme genotype (Gilbert's trait). Once daily dosing and a benign metabolic profile make this an attractive first line PI, particularly in those with increased cardiovascular risk factors. Atazanavir blood levels are boosted by co-administration with ritonavir but the role of this combination in salvage therapy has not been delineated.

Fosamprenavir is a phosphate salt of amprenavir. Fosamprenavir is a prodrug formulated into 476 mg tablets with a side-effect profile that is similar to the parent drug. The adult dosage of three to four tablets twice daily results in a considerably decreased pill burden compared with amprenavir (16 tablets). Once-a-day dosing is possible if fosamprenavir is combined with ritonavir.

T20 or enfuvirtide (Fuzeon) is a large polypeptide molecule, which inhibits HIV fusion with T-cells and thereby inhibits cellular infection. The molecule acts extracellularly at nanomolar concentrations by binding and preventing the conformational changes in viral gp41 necessary for membrane fusion. As gp41 binding and fusion is a time-dependent process, T20 may be synergistic with other fusion inhibitors which block and delay the binding process. Mutations in the binding area of gp41 can result in resistance to T20. However, there is no evidence of cross-resistance to other antiretrovirals including the newer fusion inhibitors under development. The usual dosage of T20 is 90 mg (1 ml) administered by subcutaneous injection twice daily and should be combined with other potent drugs. The formulation is a lyophilised powder, which should be dissolved in sterile water prior to use. The reconstituted solution should be refrigerated and used within 24 hours. Irritation at the injection site is the commonest adverse event and hypersensitivity reactions are rare (<1%). Manufacture of T20 is complex, requiring multiple steps, and is likely to remain costly.

Current US and international HIV treatment guidelines are based on a combination of evidence from randomised clinical trials, observational cohorts and expert opinion. Most of the randomised trials have been conducted in patients with advanced HIV disease, have been of limited duration and have utilised virological rather than clinical endpoints. As HIV disease has now become a chronic condition requiring management over decades, short-term trials with virological endpoints are insufficient to guide treatment.

Since the advent of HAART in 1996, United States Department of Health and Social Services (USDHSS) Guidelines have undergone a process of evolution, first towards more aggressive therapy and subsequently towards a more conservative approach. In 1996 the recommendations were to treat patients with less than 500 CD4 T-cells/ml and all those with viral load above 30 000 copies/ml. In 1997 the 'hit early-hit hard' strategy expanded treatment to include all with viral load >10 000 copies/ml, regardless of CD4 count. By 2000 treatment was restricted to those with <500 CD4+ T-cells/ml or those with viral loads >30 000 copies/ml, and in 2002 to those with CD4 T-cells <500 cell/ml or having a viral load >55 000 copies/ml. More recently emphasis has been on treating those with CD4 T-cells <350 and allowing clinical judgement to be exercised at earlier stages of disease. Internationally there has been a convergence of recommendations of all the major guidelines. The Southern African HIV Clinicians Society guidelines have evolved similarly, with the 2002 version being more conservative than before and now mirroring the recommendations of the British HIV Association (BHIVA). The WHO recommendations for expanded access in developing countries are influenced by the lack of medical and laboratory infrastructure in many countries which have a high burden of HIV and AIDS. The WHO guidelines do not include viral load criteria but emphasise treatment of significant symptomatic disease and those with <200 CD4 T-cell/ ml or total lymphocyte counts <1200 T-cell/ml. A comparison of guideline recommendations for initiation of HAART is given in TABLE 32.4.

All of the guidelines emphasise initiation of antiretrovirals or symptomatic patients with HIV-related symptoms (CDC B and C or WHO stages 3 and 4). The decision to initiate treatment of asymptomatic patients is more complex and is based on the patient's readiness to adhere to long-term therapy, together with an assessment of the level of existing immunodeficiency, the risk of disease progression and the risks and costs of therapy. In resource-poor settings, the threshold for entry into an antiretroviral treatment programme will also need to take cognisance of the resultant numbers to be treated,

Guideline	Criteria	WHO 4	WHO 3	WHO Stages 1 & 2			
	CD4 ranges			<200	200–350	350–500	>500
WHO	Clinical & CD4 or TLC*	Treat	Treat if CD4<200*	Treat	Defer	Defer	Defer
BHIVA & SAHIVCS	Clinical & CD4	Treat	Treat†	Treat	Treat if CD4 declining	Defer	Defer
European	Clinical,CD4 & viral load	Treat	Treat	Treat	Treat	Treat if viral load >50 000	Treat if viral load >100 000
USDHSS	Clinical, CD4 & viral load	Treat	Treat	Treat	Treat	Treat if viral load >55 000	Treat if viral load >55 000

TABLE 32.4 Comparison between World Health Organisation (WHO) British HIV Association (BHIVA), Southern African HIV Clinicians Society, European and United States Department of Health and Social Security (USDHSS) antiretroviral treatment guidelines

* WHO guidelines utilise a total lymphocyte count of <1200 cells/μL as a surrogate for CD4 T-cell count <200 cells/μL when CD4 T-cell counting technology is unavailable

† SAHIVCS guidelines exclude pulmonary tuberculosis from HIV-related clinical diagnostic indications for antiretroviral therapy

available financial and medical infrastructure and the resources necessary to identify treatment beneficiaries.

Adherence

Poor adherence is the major cause of failure to achieve viral suppression with existing antiretroviral regimens. At present antiretroviral therapy is not curative and once started the patient must be motivated to commit to life-long therapy and to maintain high levels of adherence to therapy over many years. Doctors have been shown to be poor at predicting their patient's adherence. Another more reliable subjective measure of adherence is the patient self-reported recall form of pill taking over the prior 72 hours. There are some objective measurements of adherence, including routine pill counting, random pill counts and electronic containers with incorporated memory chip. None of these is a perfect measure of pill-taking behaviour and each has its limitations. Viral RNA quantitation can be a good surrogate for adherence. Suppression of circulating viral load to less than 50 copies per ml is an indicator of good recent adherence. Viral failure following initial successful treatment may result from either poor adherence or interpersonal variations in metabolism or pharmacokinetic interactions resulting in inadequate inhibitory drug concentrations. Primary viral failure may result from poor adherence, initial infection with resistant virus or inadequate inhibitory drug concentrations. Local South African pilot sites have reported high levels of adherence comparable to those achieved in the developed world. Poverty and low socioeconomic status were not shown to be associated with poor adherence whereas frequent dosing intervals and communication in home language were associated with better adherence. Co-morbid depression or alcoholism and drug dependency negatively impact on adherence, whereas disclosure and social support may impact positively. The South African private medical-aid sector has over 10 000 individuals on antiretroviral therapy. No specific adherence data has been published to date. However, reported viral suppression of 1.0–1.5 log at 12 months in contrast to more usual 2.5–3.0 log decline would not suggest good adherence in this population. The challenge in the public sector antiretroviral treatment rollout programme is to reproduce the high levels of adherence achieved in pilot sites to a large proportion of the population.

Who to treat?

Patients are chosen for initiation therapy on the basis of either the presence of clinical symptoms and/or laboratory immunological parameters. The benefits of antiretroviral therapy are greatest in those who have symptomatic HIV disease and efforts to target therapy at this group will maximise impact on health parameters. Those with clinical HIV disease frequently interface with the health services in primary care clinics, TB services and secondary and tertiary hospitals. In order to increase the number of symptomatic individuals who can benefit from antiretrovirals, HIV counselling and testing services including knowledge and benefits of therapy, need to be incorporated into these health services. Women who may benefit from antiretrovirals may also be identified via maternal to child transmission programmes, which will require recognition of HIV symptoms and laboratory access to CD4 T-cell counts. Identification of asymptomatic individuals is more resource-intensive and produces less programme benefits, requiring increased population access to voluntary counselling and testing programmes, together with widespread access to laboratory monitoring of CD4 T-cell counts.

Choice of initial antiretroviral therapy in adults

Cohort studies in the developed world, where the dominant viral subtype is clade B, have shown marked decreases in HIV-associated morbidity and mortality following access to HAART. Although data are not available from similar large cohorts receiving HAART in Africa, there is no strong evidence of lesser benefit in individuals infected with non-B subtypes. The choice of first-line therapy is particularly important, as a sub-optimal regimen will predispose to the acquisition of resistance mutations which in turn will negatively impact on subsequent treatment options as a result of cross-resistance.

Developed world treatment guidelines stress the need to individualise therapy, taking into consideration aspects of the past medical history such as lipid abnormalities, glucose intolerance, co-infection with hepatitis B or C and also those regimen characteristics which impact on adherence, such as pill burden, dosing frequency and food restrictions. In contrast, the WHO has encouraged resource-poor countries to develop a public health approach, utilising standardised antiretroviral therapy regimens. To date, no single drug regimen has been shown to be superior to all others and this absence of proven superiority is reflected by lack of consensus and variable national guideline recommendations. The United States Health and Social Services 2002 (DHSS) guidelines recommend initiation of therapy with two NRTIs and either a PI (indinavir or nelfinavir) or boosted PI (saquinavir/ritonavir or indinavir/ritonavir), while the British HIV Association treatment guidelines of 2001 recommended initial therapy with two NRTIs and an NNRTI. There has been some recent convergence of recommendations in the 2003 versions of DHSS and BHIVA guidelines, which now recommend either NNRTI- or PI-based initial regimens. The 2003 European guidelines are less prescriptive and make no specific recommendations while the WHO recommends any of two NRTI and one NNRTI, three NRTIs (zidovudine/lamivudine/abacavir) or two NRTIs and one PI. The SA HIV Clinicians Society 2002 guidelines parallel the WHO guidelines while recommending avoidance of protease inhibitors initially because of the long-term metabolic complications. Both NNRTI- and PI-based regimens have their protagonists and there are increasing data that regimens based on either class of drug combined with two NRTIs are well tolerated and effective. The triple NRTI regimen, however, have been shown to be less efficacious especially in patients with high viral loads (>500 000 copies/ml).

Choices of antiretroviral therapy to be avoided

All single-drug regimens are contraindicated for treatment of chronic HIV infection because of a lack of sustained potency. A role for AZT and single-dose nevirapine still remains for the prevention of HIV transmission to children of those pregnant women who do not require HAART.

Dual NRTI regimens are inferior to triple therapy and are considered sub-optimal as they are less likely to achieve sustained viral suppression. In South Africa, the high cost of antiretroviral treatment resulted in many patients being prescribed dual therapy. The recent decreases in local antiretroviral prices have reduced the differential cost between dual and triple therapy and triple therapy should now be prescribed whenever possible.

The thymidine derivatives, zidovudine and stavudine, have shown *in vitro* antagonism and are therefore not to be used together. The NRTI *dideoxy* derivatives, stavudine (d4T), didanosine (ddI) and zalcitabine (ddC) have overlapping toxicity profiles and combinations of these drugs should be avoided. The combination of stavudine with didanosine has been associated with an increased incidence of hepatic steatosis and lactic acidosis. Zalcitabine coadministration with didanosine or stavudine has been associated with increased risk of peripheral neuropathy.

Choice of antiretroviral therapy in women of childbearing potential

The choice of antiretroviral therapy in women with the potential to become pregnant must consider the possibility of *in utero* drug exposure of the foetus, particularly during the early vulnerable period of organogenesis. Pregnant and breastfeeding women are frequently excluded from clinical studies, resulting in a paucity of clinical trial data on antiretroviral therapy in these patients. The safety of antiretrovirals in pregnancy can be partially inferred from the results of studies of carcinogenicity, fertility, and teratogenicity in animal models. These pre-clinical data are supplemented by a few clinical human studies and observational non-experimental data from the Antiretroviral Pregnancy Registry. This registry collates data reports from doctors caring for women and children exposed to antiretrovirals during pregnancy. The FDA pregnancy category quantifies the safety data from the above sources. Didanosine, saquinavir, ritonavir, nelfinavir and tenofovir are FDA category B drugs, indicating that animal reproductive studies have failed to demonstrate risk to the foetus but well-controlled studies have yet to be performed. Zidovudine, zalcitabine, stavudine, lamivudine, abacavir, indinavir, amprenavir, lopinavir, nevirapine, delaviridine and efavirenz are in category C, indicating that safety in pregnancy has not been determined, animal studies are either positive for foetal risk or have not been performed and that the drug should not be used unless the potential benefit outweighs the risk to the foetus.

The following drugs and combinations should be avoided during pregnancy: efavirenz because of risk of spinal cord anomalies developing early in organogenesis; the combination of stavudine plus didanosine because of increased risk to mother and foetus of lactic acidosis; and indinavir because of increased risk of hyperbilirubinae-mia in the newborn.

Treatment during pregnancy aims to maintain the health of the mother and prevent mother-to-child transmission. In all scenarios the risks and benefits of therapy to both the mother and foetus need to be considered. Pregnant women with advanced disease who meet the initiation criteria for HAART should receive therapy. If pregnancy occurs while on HAART, the regimen should be continued whenever feasible unless specifically contraindicated. If there is drug intolerance or other toxicity then temporary discontinuation during the first tri-mester may be considered. A treatment-naïve pregnant woman quali-fying for therapy may consider delaying initiation of HAART until after the first trimester if her clinical status allows this as a safe option.

Choice of antiretroviral therapy in HIV-2-infected individuals

HIV-2 infection is common in West Africa but relatively rare in South Africa and clinical data are less available. The virus is considered less pathogenic than HIV-1 and the natural history is characterised by a prolonged asymptomatic phase. Quantitation of HIV-2 viral load is not commercially available and therapy is initiated on the presence of symptoms, a CD4 T-cell count <200 cells/ml or a positive viral load. Currently registered NNRTIs do not inhibit HIV-2 reverse transcrip-tase. Amprenavir and nelfinavir are not active against HIV-2, and PIs in general may be less robust against the HIV-2. Treatment should be initiated with two NRTIs and two PIs or triple NRTIs.

Choice of antiretroviral therapy in Hepatitis B and C co-infected individuals

HIV-1, HBV and HCV share common routes of transmission and co-infec-tions are not infrequent. HIV-1 infection is associated with higher rates of chronic infection following exposure to either hepatitis virus. Chronic HBV and HCV co-infections with HIV-1 are characterised by increased levels of viraemia and abnormal liver transaminase levels and an associated increased risk of hepatotoxicity with use of nevirapine. Treatment for HBV is based on interferon alpha and lamivudine. Lamivudine should therefore be included in treatment regimens with the caveat that resistance will develop in 50% in two years. However, drug withdrawal may result in rebound HB viraemia with elevation of transaminases. Tenofovir has also been shown to have anti-HBV activity. Treatment of HCV is based on interferon-alpha and ribavirin. Ribavirin may potentially have additive toxicity when used in combination with NRTIS.

Choice of antiretroviral therapy in haemophilia

Use of PIs in haemophiliacs has been associated with episodes of spontaneous bleeding and increased requirement for factor VIII. The precise mechanism of this interaction has not been elucidated but risk of increased bleeding appears to be highest during the first month of PI therapy.

Choice of antiretroviral therapy in intravenous drug users

Intravenous drug use (IVDU) does not at present represent a significant risk behaviour for HIV infection in South Africa. However, patterns of recreational drug use are changing and IVDU is a major route of HIV infection in many other societies. Co-infection with HCV is increased with IVDU and needle sharing. Drug treatment programmes frequently use methadone for symptom control and this drug does have some pharmacokinetic interactions with antiretrovirals. NRTIs do not lower methadone levels but methadone does decrease the serum concentration of videx (ddI) by 40% and dose adjustment should be considered. The NNRTIs and several of the PIs significantly lower methadone levels, requiring upward dose titration to suppress drug withdrawal symptoms.

Initiation of antiretroviral therapy in patients with active opportunistic infections (OI) or malignant disease

Antiretrovirals may interact with OIs and their specific therapies in a variety of ways. Initiation of antiretroviral treatment may be associated with an improved response to specific therapy of an OI, there may be additive toxicity with specific therapeutic modalities or a worsening of the clinical manifestations of the OI itself. Antiretroviral therapy is the cornerstone of treatment for opportunistic diseases such as cryptosporidiosis, disseminated Kaposi's sarcoma and lymphoma when associated with profound immune suppression. Simultaneous initiation of antiretroviral and cytomegalovirus treatment, however, may lead to significant cytopaenias and therapy for CMV should be started before starting antiretrovirals. Clinical manifestations of TB, CMV retinitis and cryptococcal meningitis may be exacerbated by antiretrovirals and manifest as the immune restoration syndrome. In South Africa, because of the high frequency of co-infections, it is important to screen patients for these OIs and initiate specific treatment prior to the initiation of antiretroviral therapy.

Changing therapy

Indications for changing therapy include drug toxicity, drug intolerance and treatment failure. A decision to change treatment for drug toxicity should be based on the severity, potential risks and availability of suitable alternatives. Efforts should be made to restrict the need to change therapy for intolerance by preparing the patient for likely side-effects, prescription of symptomatic relief and reassurance that many of the initial troublesome symptoms may resolve with time. For both toxicity and intolerance it is appropriate to substitute the suspected offending drug with another of similar potency from the same class of agents. Examples of single-drug switches would be substitution of d4T for AZT-related haematotoxicity, substitution of abacavir or 3TC for ddI-related peripheral neuropathy, or substitution of nevirapine for efavirenz following neuropsychiatric events.

Treatment failure can be defined as ineffectiveness of a regimen to produce or maintain viral suppression. A progressive rise in viral load in a patient who initially had a good virological response to antiretroviral treatment is an ominous sign. Higher viral load increases the chance for development of viral resistance and will also allow ongoing damage to the immune system. Treatment failure should be confirmed with a repeat viral load estimation and should trigger a careful assessment of patient adherence to the drug regimen. It is believed that poor adherence is responsible for the majority of treatment failures. Unlike single-drug switches for intolerance or toxicity, failure should result in change of all components of the treatment regimen where possible. Resistance testing may allow recycling of components of a treatment regimen to which the virus is shown to be still sensitive.

Drug resistance

HIV, like all other life forms, adapts to its environment allowing it to replicate and transfer to new hosts to ensure ongoing survival. The reverse transcriptase enzyme necessary for the production of a DNA copy of the viral RNA, unlike other mammalian polymeraises, does not possess DNA 'proof reading' activity and is thus highly error-prone, resulting in frequent nucleotide substitutions, deletions and insertions. A high rate of viral replication together with the error-prone nature of the reverse transcriptase enzyme ensures that multiple mutations (quasi-species) exist at any time. Some of these genetic variants with mutations of the *Pol* gene result in changed structure and function of the reverse transcriptase (RT) and protease enzymes. These genetic variants generally have reduced fitness, putting them at a competitive disadvantage relative to 'wild type' virus and ensuring that they remain as minority subspecies in the untreated host. In the presence of drug pressure some of these minority subspecies may have increased replicative capacity relative to drug-sensitive 'wild type' virus and in the presence of continuing selective pressure can develop into the dominant sub-species. Selective pressure is increased when HIV is exposed to a drug regimen with low potency or inadequate drug levels as a result of sub-optimal drug adherence or pharmacokinetic factors.

Pharmacokinetic boosting of PIS using ritonavir as an inhibitor of the P450 enzymes present in the liver and gut can result in increased plasma drug levels, which exceed the inhibitory concentrations required to suppress both 'wild type' and partially resistant viruses. The rate of emergence of resistance-conferring mutations is also influenced by the genetic barrier of the component drugs within a regimen. The non-nucleoside reverse transcriptase inhibitors (NNRTIS) have a low genetic barrier and a single mutation in the RT gene can result in viral resistance to all currently registered members of this class of drugs. The genetic barriers posed by the NRTIS are variable with some members of the class such as lamivudine losing potency with a single mutation (eg M184V). However, other NRTIS require multiple sequential mutations before losing potency. Similarly the genetic barriers vary within the PI class, with only a single mutation of the protease gene (eg D30N) resulting in lowered sensitivity to nelfinavir while other members of the class require multiple primary and secondary mutations before loss of potency.

Measurement of drug resistance has been shown to be useful for guiding antiretroviral management. There are currently two types of assay available to quantify viral resistance: the genotype and the phenotype assays. Genotypic assays identify mutations in the viral RT and protease genes, which are associated with drug resistance. Identification of the relevant gene mutations can be achieved by polymerase chain reaction (PCR) amplification of the *Pol* gene and either subsequent sequencing of the entire RT and protease genes or by utilisation of DNA probes to detect the presence or absence of specific mutations.

Phenotypic assays assess the ability of HIV, isolated from patient plasma, to grow in various concentrations of antiretroviral drugs. Recombinant assays require the insertion of the viral *Pol* gene into laboratory cell lines. The ability of the resultant recombinant virus to replicate in the presence of differing concentrations of antiretrovirals is measured and reported as the concentration of drug required to inhibit 50% of viral replication (IC50). The ratio of IC50 of patient virus to the IC50 of test reference HIV allows calculation of FOLD-change in viral sensitivity.

Limitations of both phenotypic and genotypic assays include the lack of standardised methodology and quality assurance, high cost and loss of sensitivity at low copy number. Success of resistance determination is greatly decreased when viral copy numbers are less than 1000 copies per ml or if the resistant sub-species are present at a level of less than 20% of circulating virus. Resistance may also be missed following discontinuation of antiretroviral therapy, which will remove drug pressure allowing re-expansion of the 'wild type' drug-sensitive virus and consequently resistance assays should be performed while individuals are on therapy. Negative results of resistance determinations should be treated with caution as resistant sub-species may be present at low copy number and full interpretation requires knowledge of past antiretroviral exposure.

Choice of antiretroviral therapy in the South African public health setting

Scaling up of antiretroviral programmes in the public sector of South Africa will require standardisation and simplification of treatment regimens. Simplified regimens allow for a limited repertoire of drugs and side-effects with which medical staff can become familiar. The maintenance of a secure drug supply is easier when the number of drugs is limited. When the general population is receiving similar therapy then resistance can be monitored at a population rather than an individual level. Many factors impact on regimen selections including cost, tolerability, pill burden, safety, the potential for interaction with other commonly prescribed medications and the need to maintain future treatment options.

Tuberculosis (TB) is the commonest opportunistic infection in South Africa and standardised regimens must be carefully chosen to avoid adverse pharmacological interactions with TB drugs. Rifampicin is a potent CYP450 enzyme-inducer that results in lowered plasma levels of protease inhibitors and has an overlapping hepatic toxicity profile with nevirapine. There is considerable experience of rifampicin-containing TB treatment with co-administration of antiretroviral regimens including three NRTIS or two NRTIS with either efavirenz- or ritonavir-boosted saquinavir. However, a recent small Phase I study has resulted in Roche and the US Food and Drug Administration recommending that ritonavir-boosted saquinavir not be used concomitantly with rifampicin. There are early data indicating that co-administration of kaletra with additional ritonavir may be another option for patients receiving rifampicin.

As women of child-bearing potential constitute the majority of patients attending public sector HIV clinics, regimens must be available which are compatible with pregnancy. The need to have 'tuberculosis and pregnancy friendly' regimens and the constraints of a limited number of antiretrovirals currently registered in South Africa has resulted in convergence of regimens used in programmes. Many programmes are based on two standardised regimens, the first consisting of two NRTIs and one NNRTI and the second two NRTIs and a boosted PI. An example would be stavudine, lamivudine and efavirenz followed by zidovudine, didanosine and kaletra. Nevirapine should be substituted for efavirenz in women of child-bearing potential and boosted saquinavir for kaletra if tuberculosis therapy is required taking into account recent Phase I trial findings (see previous page).

Challenges in implementing HAART

Concerns have been raised that widespread use of antiretrovirals in developing countries, particularly in sub-Saharan Africa, will result in 'antiretroviral anarchy' and widespread viral resistance with subsequent population loss of therapeutic benefit. The need for high levels of adherence has led some to make parallels with the tuberculosis control programme and proposed use of directly observed treatment short course (DOTS). The logistics of delivery of lifelong DOTS to large numbers of people is likely to be very challenging. Until recently, high drug costs were a major constraint to widespread implementation, but now that drug costs have decreased, the lack of infrastructure may be a major constraint. The need to manage a programme within a limited national infrastructure has resulted in the exploration of several public sector delivery models. Models explored to date have included distribution of antiretrovirals at secondary hospitals, community clinics and tuberculosis services.

Bibliography

BRITISH HIV ASSOCIATION (BHIVA) 'Guidelines for the treatment of HIV-infected adults with antiretroviral therapy'. *HIV Medicine* 2001; 2: 276–313.

'*Department of Health and Human Services Guidelines for the use of antiretroviral agents in HIV-1-infected adults and adolescents*'. July 14th 2003; http://AIDSinfo.nih.gov

ORRELL C, BANGSBERG DR, BADRI M, WOOD R. 'Adherence is not a barrier to successful antiretroviral therapy in South Africa'. *AIDS* 2003; 17: 1369–1375.

SCALING UP ANTIRETROVIRAL THERAPY IN RESOURCE-LIMITED SETTINGS: '*Guidelines for a public health approach*'. World Health Organisation, Executive Summary April 2002, Geneva, Switzerland. 2002.

SOUTHERN AFRICAN HIV CLINICIANS SOCIETY 'Clinical guidelines for antiretroviral therapy in adults'. *SA Journal of HIV Medicine* July 2002; 8: 22–29.

THE EACS EUROGUIDELINES GROUP. 'European guidelines for the clinical management of HIV-infected adults in Europe.' *AIDS* 2003; 17 (supplement 2): S3–S26.

CHAPTER 33

The challenges of implementing anti-retroviral treatment in South Africa

Andrew Gray

THE MEDICINE MANAGEMENT CYCLE is an essential component when considering implementation of antiretroviral treatment in South Africa. This is traditionally portrayed as a cycle in which choosing medicines must be followed by procurement, distribution and use. These processes must be used to learn from each cycle and ensure its continuation.

The dichotomy between the public and private sector in South Africa continues to complicate all parts of this cycle.

Examining all aspects of the medicine management cycle is essential when considering the most effective way to implement antiretroviral treatment in South Africa.

As with any other highly contested terrain, debates around the provision of antiretroviral treatment in South Africa, and in particular in the public health sector, have been characterised by starkly stated and firmly held opinions. Such opinions have reduced the space for meaningful debate about the very real challenges of implementing antiretroviral treatment in the country. The debate has instead become a contest between notions of toxicity and/or infrastructural deficiencies on the one hand, and the moral and ethical imperative to take immediate action on the other. This chapter will try to clarify some of the challenges facing the health system as a whole. The framework for discussion will be the medicine management cycle. However, this should not be read in any way as detracting from the very real challenges in related areas, such as human resource management, laboratory services and clinical services. Instead, it will seek to show how these areas affect, and are affected by, the key policy decision to widely deploy antiretroviral therapy in South Africa.

The medicine management cycle

Medicine management is traditionally portrayed as cyclical (FIGURE 33.1). A choice of a medicine or group of medicines (selection) must be followed by processes to ensure its efficient purchase (procurement), then by actions that ensure accessibility at the point of care (distribution), followed by steps to ensure the necessary conditions for effective prescription, supply and ultimate consumption by the patient (use). The final step is to make sure that future selection decisions are informed by these steps, so continuing the cycle. The cycle is supported by various management functions (including the organisational design features and operation of the health system, its financing mechanisms, information technology resources and human resources), as well as by the policy and legal framework within which the system operates. There are challenges implicit in each of these steps and supporting mechanisms.

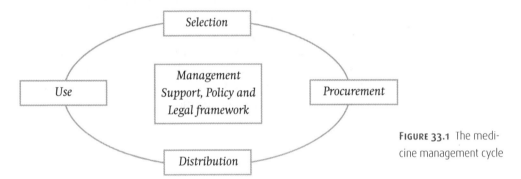

FIGURE 33.1 The medicine management cycle

Selection

The South African health care system has in the past used two opposing models of medicine selection. In the private sector, this has traditionally been left to the individual practitioner, particularly the doctor. In contrast, the public sector has used an essential medicines list since 1996. This list satisfies the health care demands of most cases, providing safe medicines, of known efficacy, which can be procured at a price the patient and the health care system can afford. This concept, first clarified by the WHO Director-General in 1975, has been considered a basic principle of the Primary Health Care approach since the 1978 Alma Ata conference. An initial South African Essential Medicines List, drawn from the Standard Treatment Guidelines (STGs) for Primary Health Care, was published in 1996. This was updated in 1998 and supplemented by guidelines and lists for the management of adult and paediatric patients in hospitals. However, the 1998 documents avoided making any selection of antiretrovirals, other than for post-exposure prophylaxis (PEP). Expensive drugs were specifically excluded, except possibly for limited use in academic and research situations. According to the document, a decision on widespread implementation of such treatment could only be made after direction from the DOH.

This directive has now been issued by Cabinet, and must be implemented by the Department of Health. One of the key challenges facing the health system is to integrate HIV and AIDS management into mainstream health services. In this way, additional resources mobilised to implement the Cabinet's political statement would strengthen the overall system, rather than divert resources and skills away from primary health care (PHC) and hospital-based care.

This is also true of medicines selection. Not only must official mainstream selection documents in the public sector reflect the Cabinet decision, but the structures responsible for such decisions must be allowed to complete their tasks without exception. A revised PHC set of STGs and an Essential Drugs List for PHC has been finalised. While it provides more guidance on the management of HIV-infected patients, it makes no mention of antiretroviral therapy. The selection of first- and second-line antiretrovirals for the state rollout plan was completed in late 2003, but without the direct involvement of either provincial pharmacy and therapeutics committees (PTCs) or the National Essential Drugs List Committee (NEDLC). Individual members of these committees did contribute to the process, but this lack of involvement reinforced the idea that HIV was somehow 'off limits'. A similar process was followed in deciding the post-rape PEP protocol (Policy Guideline for Management of Transmission of Human Immunodeficiency Virus (HIV) and Sexually Transmitted Infections in Sexual Assault). In this, azithromycin was suggested for prophylaxis of sexually transmitted infections, but was not available in public sector facilities. The challenge remains to urgently accelerate selection processes (as was the case with the cabinet-driven policy process), but to ensure that procurement, distribution and use can occur.

The initial choice of first- and second-line antiretrovirals for the state rollout also follows WHO guidelines to the management of HIV in resource-limited settings. However, the choice of antiretroviral treatment is far from simple and the following factors should be considered:

- evidence of efficacy in similar settings – almost entirely lacking, especially evidence of hard outcomes (survival) rather than intermediate outcomes (viral loads and CD4 counts at specific times). In addition the evidence of which first-line approach is most effective and durable is continually being updated

- evidence of the effect of regimen choice on the emergence of resistance – the concept of the 'durability' of regimens is receiving increased attention, but recommendations are as yet based on incomplete data
- the toxicity profile of the agents – in particular, the degree of laboratory monitoring necessary to ensure safe use and the impact of expected common adverse effects on patient adherence
- evidence of important drug interactions – this is especially important given the need to manage significant co-morbid conditions such as tuberculosis (TB)
- ease of administration – pill burdens, dose intervals and routes of administration
- cost and availability of suitable, reliable suppliers – while a significant barrier to access in the past, this is becoming less of an issue as generic entry and local production increase, but remains a major factor in terms of second-line and rescue regimen choices.

Patients in the private sector often appear to have been treated suboptimally, largely because of the costs involved and the difficulty of continuing to pay for antiretrovirals. Considerable improvements have been achieved by medical aids that contracted disease management programmes to develop treatment algorithms and to support individual doctors. These programmes have become an important repository of expertise and experience. The challenge in the private sector is to simplify and preferably standardise the selection of at least first-line antiretrovirals, while ensuring that this does not contribute to a greater emergence of resistant mutants than does their use in far greater numbers in the public sector. A common approach in both sectors will aid communication, simplify procurement and also allow for effective training of all health workers. One of the more significant recent shifts has been the relaxation of voluntary licence conditions by at least two multinational pharmaceutical manufacturers, which will allow local generic firms to sell into state and private markets. A continued mismatch between the state and private sector could result in the 'antiretroviral anarchy' feared by many in the industrialised world, particularly if single- or dual-drug regimens are used in the private sector. It is not yet known to what extent the state will intervene directly to make this less likely. At least one African country set the precedent of stopping private sector sale of antiretrovirals once state provision started. Similar action is not expected in South Africa, but this does not mean that greater contact between the public and private sectors should not be pursued.

Procurement

The prerequisites for access to antiretroviral treatment are rational selection, affordable prices, sustainable financing, and reliable health and supply systems. It is sustainable financing that is particularly vital for procurement, which involves many more processes when widespread access is planned.

In the private sector in South Africa, procurement has generally been left to individual patients, using traditional sources such as retail and distance-dispensing services (courier pharmacies). Online pharmacies have not been a feature of the local supply chain. Disease management programmes and the Southern African HIV Clinicians Society have engaged in negotiations to aid procurement by securing preferential pricing arrangements. For example, antiretrovirals are generally supplied at wholesale prices, with a R50 per prescription handling fee added (and VAT), rather than the usual 50% mark-up and then variable discount rate. It is important to make sure that these arrangements are not jeopardised by the new legislation on discounts, rebates or any form of incentive scheme in the sale of medicine that came into effect after 2 May 2004.

Public sector procurement is far more complex. It involves the purchase of medicines by the whole health system, subject to complex state procurement requirements. Needs are difficult to forecast accurately because past consumption records are not available. As a result only incomplete morbidity data can be used for these calculations. Predicting the off-take at any given time and place in the country will also be very difficult in the initial stages of the treatment rollout and quantification will have to depend on the following:

- estimates of overall population prevalence, as extrapolated from antenatal surveillance at sentinel sites and modified by population-based prevalence studies
- estimates of the proportion of HIV-infected persons needing antiretroviral treatment, based on expected progression to a set CD4 count and/or functional level
- estimates of the uptake of voluntary counselling and testing, then of acceptance of treatment (if warranted), and finally of adherence to the treatment programme
- estimates of the degree of penetration of the health care system, from initial pilot sites to full coverage over time.

The political outcome of poor quantification could be as dangerous as the economic consequences – too cautious an approach will be seen as a delaying tactic, while too optimistic estimates of off-take will not only result in the wastage of medicines and money but will also be interpreted as incompetence.

Choosing a procurement method is largely a matter of policy and practice, determined for the state as a whole. The tender system for medicines has been in place since the late 1980s, but it is not in a position to provide truly competitive prices when many medicines are under patent. The Medicines Act has been amended to allow for international tender, but still requires registration by the Medicines Control Council (MCC) of any products procured in this way. However, the time from application to registration is not likely to be less than 24 months. Delays caused by regulatory authority demands are both understandable and difficult to avoid as they ensure the safety, efficacy and quality of medicines entering the local market. However, this process needs to be streamlined. One option might be to establish formal reciprocity agreements, where registration by another country's regulatory body, which is accepted as stringent enough to substitute for MCC scrutiny, is accepted as sufficient to allow market entry. However, given the geographical position of South Africa and the relative strengths of surrounding regulatory authorities, this would appear to be a more useful mechanism for use by neighbouring states than for South Africa itself. A related issue is the extent to which South Africa will allow procurement to be guided by the WHO pre-qualification process, rather than by local registration or exemption from registration. The latter mechanism, using section 21 of the Medicines Act, is intended for small-scale and clinical trials access and not for large-scale access and is of limited use. However, WHO pre-qualification will, from the end of 2004, be entrenched as a pre-requisite for procurement using Global Fund monies, unless the local regulatory authority is considered stringent. Stringent in this case is defined by membership of the International Conference on Harmonisation (a closed group of the US, European and Japanese authorities) or the Pharmaceutical Inspection Co-operation Scheme (of which South Africa's MCC is as yet not a member). Current procurement by South African recipients with Global Fund grants is likely to result in a conflict between sovereign rights and multilaterally imposed conditions, which needs to be avoided.

Parallel importation is also possible, but is limited by the scarcity of markets from which reliable quantities of patented medicines can be procured at much lower prices than those offered locally or through preferential pricing mechanisms. Recently patent holders have agreed to offer voluntary licences to generic manufacturers, which promises to improve access to lower cost generic versions of a number of the antiretrovirals needed for the first- and second-line regimens currently favoured. However, some key agents are still not accessible by this route. This keeps the pressure on the government to either use (Agreement on Trade-related Intellectual Property Rights) TRIPS-compliant mechanisms, such as compulsory licensing or government use provisions, or to exert pressure by other means to ensure that voluntary licences or agreements not to pursue patent infringements are obtained from the patent holders. South Africa has a TRIPS-compliant Patents Act, and could, if it chose, simplify the process for obtaining a compulsory licence without offending its international obligations. However, it is likely that there will be demands to enshrine so-called TRIPS-plus provisions as part of free trade negotiations with major market partners such as the US. This will strengthen provisions that make it more, not less difficult to launch generic medicines, such as lengthened periods of data protection. The potential impact of this mechanism is difficult to measure. However, a clear challenge to the state will be to ensure sustainable local production, to supply not only the South African market but the region as a whole. Procurement choices made in the early stages of the rollout will set the scene for this market. However, delaying until local production of the entire first- and second-line regimen is achieved is not an option. Equally, setting prices over too long a period (two years is preferred in the normal tender process) is also not possible in this rapidly changing environment. Nevertheless, some stability in pricing is necessary to allow for sustainable budgeting over the medium term.

Part of the procurement process is ensuring the quality of products purchased, not only at tender adjudication, but throughout the supply cycle. In the past, the private sector has been able to rely on the fact that all medicines procured, whether made locally or imported, were locally registered and hence subject to MCC Good Manufacturing Practice inspections. However, this is not likely to be sufficient for the public sector if international tender is used as a procurement method. The current infrastructure for quality assurance in the provincially operated pharmaceutical depots is clearly insufficient. Most sites rely on visual inspection, with some rudimentary laboratory services at two or three depots. It has also been a problem to ensure that suppliers adhere to the terms of tender contracts in terms of lead times and expiry dates. Greater effectiveness and efficiency in logistics systems is therefore a major challenge, requiring an upgrade in the information technology used. There is some progress in creating a data warehouse and Pharmaceutical Management Information System (PharMIS), but this is still in development and requires continued support. As will be argued later, this lack is even more keenly felt throughout the supply chain from depot to hospital and clinic.

How can the artificial divide between the public and private sectors be bridged? While volumes (and hence economic power) are certainly going to be greater in the public sector, there are pockets of skill and capacity in the private sector which could be tapped. Out-sourced laboratory functions are an obvious option, as are out-sourced information technology functions (see later). It may well be that pooled procurement between the state and disease management programmes (servicing large medical aids or groups of medical aids, or particular industries) is an option.

Distribution

Some of the elements of the distribution cycle have already been discussed. As a cycle, this traditionally starts with procurement, then port clearing (where procurement is external), receipt and inspection, inventory management, storage, requisition of supplies, delivery and dispensing to patients. The cycle ends with consumption reporting, which allows future quantification and procurement.

In the private sector, in stark contrast to the public sector, information technology plays a large part in the management of the distribution cycle. While every community pharmacy in South Africa has online ordering and claims processing, and every private hospital has access to a sophisticated billings system, such IT resources are generally lacking in provincial hospitals and clinics. Provincial depots and those out-sourced to specialist logistics firms have basic inventory systems in place, but they cannot compare with the sophisticated systems found in most of the private sector wholesale and distribution pharmacies. The minimal capacity to enable the safe and effective distribution of antiretrovirals needs to be created in the public sector. However, this capacity must not be built in as a vertical programme, but must contribute to the overall improvement of the logistics capacity of the public health care system. The state has acknowledged that those depots that do not have access to strong security and inventory-tracking information management systems experience higher levels of theft and stock-outs. Unplanned and unpredictable medicine changes due to stock-outs will negatively impact on the durability of chosen antiretroviral regimens. The ready market for stolen antiretrovirals, both in South Africa and abroad, means that stock diversion will pose serious threats to the distribution system in the public and private sectors. The greater the price differential between the two, the greater the chance of diversion from the state to the private sector.

Beyond the depots, the private and public sectors are clearly differentiated by lack of access to electronic patient records in the state system. This has received considerable attention in the state's rollout plan, but is going to be very difficult to implement. There have been two attempts to address this. Over a number of years, there has been a concerted effort to rationalise and improve the collection, transmission and use of health management information at the district level. Studies at pilot sites have shown that it is feasible to implement paper-based data capture systems and computer-based district-level collation and transmission systems. However, getting this system to operate effectively over larger areas without the intensive support that characterises pilot projects has been difficult. Although data from the District Health Information System are becoming available for routine use, their quality varies widely, making interpretation difficult. The other example is the attempt by the Northern Province (now Limpopo) Department of Health and Welfare to introduce a hospital information system. External evaluations have described this as a 'how not to' model, clearly showing how the introduction of new technology can fail. However, the introduction of a sophisticated paperless hospital system at the Inkosi Albert Luthuli Central Hospital in Durban has shown that the public sector can use computer technology.

It is all too easy to point to public – private partnerships as the panacea for all state sector capacity problems. However, the history of previous attempts to service public sector patients via contracted private sector facilities has not always been a happy one. The district surgeon system, which in previous years used retail pharmacies to supply medicines to the elderly and those with chronic illnesses, was swiftly dismantled post-1994. Evidence of fraud, diversion and over-servicing was partly responsible for this. What it has left is a deep sense of disquiet about any proposals that entail the use of state stock by private practitioners. Re-building trust in such delivery mechanisms is a major challenge. The sheer scale of the implementation hurdles faced by the state rollout of antiretroviral therapy requires that this is overcome. Most pharmacists and doctors practise in the private sector, catering for those wealthy enough to pay directly and for those with medical aid cover, the latter being roughly 17% of the population. Where services are not provided by the state (such as antiretrovirals, prior to the Cabinet decision of 2003), or are thought to be inferior or are inconvenient to access, a proportion of those considered state-dependent have in the past used the private sector. In the event of an effective state-led antiretroviral rollout, mechanisms that will mobilise all available resources from all sectors will be needed. It would be inefficient not to use the approximately 2400 community pharmacies in the private sector, the extensive private wholesale and distribution networks and the private hospitals. Finding a way to harness these resources while still building capacity in the public sector and utilising a wide range of distribution channels, yet still

Use

The final stage in the medicines management process of antiretrovirals is perhaps the most challenging. It is the least easy to capture in simple, systematic, cyclical terms, and involves the greatest spread of organisational elements, health workers and patients, and general society. The traditional cycle of using medicines involves diagnosis, prescription, dispensing and adherence to medication by the patient. Continued care completes the cycle, through follow-up and reexamination of the diagnosis and prescription. Each of these deserves closer scrutiny to identify the challenges facing the South African health care system.

The diagnosis of AIDS, and the decision to start antiretrovirals, is not without controversy. Highly active antiretroviral treatment (HAART) has been developed over only eight years and so is relatively new to most health practitioners, and was certainly not covered during the undergraduate training of most prescribers and dispensers. The use of HAART, in terms of combinations of antiretrovirals, their doses and durations and the optimal timing of initiation, is evolving rapidly. A WHO expert conference in 1985 defined rational drug use as when 'patients receive medications appropriate to their clinical needs, in doses that meet their individual requirements, for an adequate period of time, and at the lowest cost to them and their community'. Answering the questions of who, what, when, for how long and at which cost, requires access to relevant and appropriate data and its application, both at the level of policy-making and in individual patient care. The policy level demands have already been described in the section under Selection. However, while enabling the appropriate selection structures (provincial PTCs and the national EDL Committee) to make these decisions is relatively easy, ensuring equitable access to such expertise across the whole health care system is not.

The first choice that has to be made for the public sector is the level at which such services are provided. Equitable access demands that the lowest effective level be chosen, which must imply that antiretroviral therapy is provided through clinics. This also suggests using nurse practitioners or training and deploying a new category of doctor assistants. To start with, medical officers must be trained to provide antiretroviral therapy in the public sector. However, lessons learned in the private sector must also be applied. Where a large number of inexperienced private practitioners were seen to be providing inadequate care and inappropriate medication, the solution was access to high-quality advice from a centralised point – the disease management programme. Choices were restricted by, for example, creating reimbursement rules rationalising the use of laboratory testing. The public sector already has the advantage of standardised treatment approaches and algorithms through an essential medicines list. But this needs to be supplemented with an operative system of both up- and down-referral, access to medicines information and clinical advice and the necessary information systems to allow effective quality assurance.

The public sector challenges of the first steps of use (diagnosis/ follow-up and prescribing) include:

- developing clear treatment algorithms that identify the patients eligible to receive antiretrovirals and show how to make choices of initial and subsequent therapy and monitoring, in a way that is compatible with available laboratory and clinical infrastructure yet still ensures safety and durability of the programme
- training, deploying and retaining sufficient and appropriate health practitioners to identify such patients, and to initiate and monitor treatment over time, but at a cost that is affordable to the health care system and using facilities that are convenient to most patients.

Safe prescribing and follow-up of patients receiving these antiretrovirals requires access to a minimal laboratory service for routine biochemical and haematological tests, mostly to exclude adverse events. It also requires access to sophisticated tests for monitoring the patient's immunological responses, particularly the CD4 count, the virological response, in terms of viral load, as another marker of the clinical effect of treatment and, at some stage, the resistance mutations developed by the virus in response to treatment. There are two main problems with these requirements. First, access to cheaper test materials is needed. This must also be coupled with access to sufficient trained personnel to perform these tests, and even more importantly (and particularly with resistance testing) the capacity to interpret the results.

The demands of establishing an efficient logistics system were mentioned in the section on Distribution. However, dispensing medicine is more than a logistics function. The 1996 National Drug Policy recognised the need to upgrade the capacity of pharmaceutical personnel to ensure the rational use of medicines, and also the need to involve and empower the patient. The use-cycle steps of dispensing and adherence are linked. Patients who are prescribed antiretrovirals must have access to an effective dispensing service that includes not only a check on the rationality of the prescription, but also an effective adherence support strategy through individual counselling and community-based information and education programmes. It could be argued that effective monitoring of adverse events also requires an effective pharmaceutical system. Clearly, if the system is to provide convenient access at clinic level, then access to a pharmacist at all points will not be possible. Suitable support personnel (pharmacist's assistants) are being trained but are not available in sufficient numbers at present. Greater reliance on nurses will be an ongoing feature of the public sector response, and will require closer coopera-tion between nursing and pharmacy services. Nurses will also have to perform many logistic management tasks. This demand for access to a suitable, comprehensive pharmaceutical service also provides ammunition for arguments that favour public – private cooperation and partnership, drawing on the resources of community and private hospital pharmacies, distance-dispensing services and wholesale/ distribution facilities. A fully operational pharmacovigilance system must ensure that information flows from all possible sources, both public and private. It must effectively interact with the overall medi-cines regulatory system and mobilise resources such as academic departments of pharmacology and pharmacy, private medicines information services and consumer movements. However, there are still improvements to be made in the rationality and quality of anti-retroviral use and monitoring in the private sector. Disease manage-ment programmes can only do so much, and must be supplemented by a clearer link between quality assurance efforts in the public sector and those in the private sector. These might include:

- accreditation of sites that provide antiretroviral services, in both sectors (but without this becoming a barrier to access)
- institutionalisation of ongoing quality improvement systems in both sectors, based on the routine collection, analysis and publica-tion of data regarding selected quality measures (be those process or outcome measures)
- effective application of measures, such as the certificate of need and dispensing licences, designed to improve the quality and distribution of services and to promote equitable access.

This chapter has so far paid more attention to challenges which lie within, rather than outside, the orthodox health care system. However, a comprehensive treatment of the topic demands that those outside at least be listed – including, for example:

- involvement by consumer and treatment access advocacy groups, particularly if education is to form part of the new contract between those taking antiretrovirals and the provider/state (the essence of the concept of concordance)

- some form of cooperation with, if not cooption of complementary and traditional health care delivery systems (beyond research into the long-term possibilities of finding effective antiviral agents and immune boosters among traditional medicines)
- attention to the marketing and sale of unregistered complementary medicines, food supplements and miracle cures for HIV and AIDS.

Conclusions

Looked at in their entirety, the challenges of providing antiretroviral treatment in South Africa are just a summary of the systems challenges that were left by apartheid. A system fractured into a well-resourced private sector for the affluent and an under-resourced public sector for an impoverished majority must find new common ground, a common approach to quality and delivery, and an equitable distribution of resources, skills and capacity. Experience and skill built up in the for-profit environment must be harnessed for the common good, but in ways that are commercially viable. A public sector that has managed with poor infrastructure and inadequate resources, both human and material, must ensure the safe deployment of a sophisticated intervention and also ensure its sustainability. A constitutional commitment to a human rights approach, to an entrenchment of social and economic rights, must find expression in a massive mobilisation of new resources. A well-intentioned policy stance of self-reliance and fiscal discipline must be replaced by one that finds ways of accommodating large-scale donor-funded interventions, that retains national sovereignty in areas such as medicine regulation and trade policy, and yet relies on and actively shapes multilateral responses and international trade practices. These challenges are by no means trivial, and involve every aspect of the South African response to the HIV and AIDS pandemic. Only a concerted, co-ordinated, multi-sectoral approach will suffice.

Bibliography

ATTAWELL K, MUNDY J. 'Provision of antiretroviral therapy in resource-limited settings: A review of experience up to August 2003'. WHO, UK Department for International Development, London, 2003.

BENNET S, VELÁSQUEZ G, QUICK J. 'Public-private roles in the pharmaceutical sector'. Health Economics and Drugs DAP. Series No. 5. World Health Organisation, Geneva, 1997.

CORREA CM. 'Implications of the Doha Declaration on the TRIPS Agreement and public health'. Health Economics and Drugs EDM Series No. 12. World Health Organisation, Geneva, 2002.

Fresle DA, Wolfheim C. 1997. *Public education in rational drug use: A global survey.* World Health Organisation, Geneva.

Grubb I, Perriëns J, Schwartländer B. 2003. *'A public health approach to antiretroviral treatment: Overcoming constraints'.* World Health Organisation, Geneva.

Myhr K, Ewen M, Creese A. 2003. *Medicine prices – a new approach to measurement.* World Health Organisation and Health Action International, Geneva.

Quick JD, Rankin JR, Laing RO, O'Connor RW, Hogerzeil HV, Dukes MNG, Garnett A. 1997. *Managing Drug Supply* (2nd Edition). Kumarian Press, West Hartford, CT.

Schneider H (Ed). *'Scaling up the use of anti-retrovirals in the public sector: What are the challenges?'* Seminar proceedings. School of Public Health & Perinatal HIV Research Unit, University of the Witwatersrand, 1 August 2003.

Velásquez G, Boulet P. 1997. 'Globalization and access to drugs. Implications of the WTO/TRIPS Agreement'. *Health Economics and Drugs DAP Series No. 7.* World Health Organisation, Geneva.

Velásquez G, Vidal J. 2003. 'IPR, innovation, human rights and access to drugs. An annotated bibliography'. *Health Economics and Drugs EDM Series No. 14.* World Health Organization, Geneva.

WHO *Scaling up antiretroviral therapy in resource-limited settings: Treatment guidelines for a public health approach (2003 Revision).* World Health Organisation, Geneva, 2003.

WHO/UNAIDS *Emergency scale-up of antiretroviral therapy in resource-limited settings: Technical and operational recommendations to achieve 3 by 5.* Report of the WHO/UNAIDS international consensus meeting on technical and operational recommendations for emergency scaling-up of antiretroviral therapy in resource-limited settings, 18. 21 November 2003, Lusaka, Zambia. 2003.

WHO *Working document on monitoring and evaluating of national ART programmes in the rapid scale-up to 3 by 5.* WHO work in progress, 2003.

WHO *Human capacity-building plan for scaling up HIV/AIDS treatment.* World Health Organization, Geneva, 2003.

WHO *'Interagency Guidelines. Guidelines for price discounts of single-source pharmaceuticals'.* WHO, UNAIDS, UNCF, UNFP, Geneva, 2003.

CHAPTER 34

The political history of AIDS treatment

Nawaal Deane

'Human beings are perhaps never more frightening than when they are convinced beyond doubt that they are right.' – Laurens van der Post

THE POLITICAL RESPONSE TO the treatment of AIDS in South Africa has been characterised by misunderstanding and controversy. In September 2003, the Cabinet of the South African government announced the adoption of the national antiretroviral rollout plan. This major accomplishment is the culmination of a long and checkered history littered with conflict and legal challenges in the face of dire need. While there has been government support for bogus 'AIDS cures' such as an industrial solvent, a coal-derivative and a nutritional cocktail of garlic and vegetables, there has been a corollary lack, until compelled, of government support for antiretroviral drugs for rape survivors, prevention of mother-to-child HIV transmission and treatment of AIDS.

However, at the time of writing, there does appear to be political will to continue with the planned rollout of antiretrovirals across all provinces. At the same time, differences in infrastructure and capacity between provinces present a major challenge to government, both national and provincial.

In September 2003, the South African Cabinet announced the free provision of antiretroviral drugs for the treatment of AIDS in the public health care service. This heralds one of the most significant milestones in the country's response to the AIDS epidemic as it has farreaching consequences for the effort to change the devastating course of the HIV/AIDS epidemic in South Africa.

Until this point, the HIV/AIDS epidemic in South Africa, and the government's unique response to it, has been marked by a series of controversies. No account of the South African HIV/AIDS epidemic would be complete without a description of some of the key controversies that have shaped perceptions of the South African approach to treating AIDS.

There were great expectations in 1994, a dawn of a new era. The new democratic government was faced with the huge challenge of building a new society and undertaking to deliver essential services. Its efforts were predicated on a constitution born of a human rights ethos. Upon assuming the mantle of authority, the new government started its efforts with good intentions and well-developed plans. However, this did not extend to the critical need to implement antiretroviral prophylaxis or treatment. This chapter explores the various controversies surrounding treatment for AIDS, including the South African 'AIDS cures' supported by government such as virodene, oxihumate-K and the nutritional cocktail of garlic and vegetables while there has been steadfast opposition to antiretroviral drugs developed by multinational drug companies for both prevention and treatment.

Virodene

Political drama around miracle AIDS cures, immune boosters, toxicity of antiretroviral drugs and the benefits of nutrition versus treatment have dominated media coverage. But first in the line was the Virodene scandal, which caused international embarrassment for the South African government in 1997.

Virodene, put forward as an anti-AIDS drug, was developed by three scientists from Pretoria. Virodene was backed by senior politicians including the Deputy President and the Health Minister in 1997 after a Cabinet presentation by the researchers, which included patient testimony of being miraculously cured of AIDS. This political endorsement of Virodene before scientific peer review made it easier for the cryogenics researcher, Olga Visser, and cardiothoracic surgeons, Dirk du Plessis and Kallie Landaure to ask for R3.7 million to research and promote Virodene.

The controversy broke after several South African researchers, as well as the international medical community, questioned the scientific validity of the Virodene research. This led to a subsequent joint enquiry by the University of Pretoria and the Gauteng Provincial Department of Health into the drug, which revealed that Virodene contained the highly toxic industrial solvent (dimethylformamide) which could cause serious liver damage and cancer.

Patients on Virodene reported burning sensations, shortness of breath, swelling of the throat, physical discomfort and irritation after using the drug. None of the three Virodene researchers were experts in HIV, virology, or microbiology and the explanation provided for the mechanisms for Virodene's claimed selective anti-HIV activity were unfounded. The Medicines Control Council (MCC) raised concerns over the methodology and ethics of the research. The MCC stood its ground despite political pressure to treat Virodene as a special trial. The MCC refused leading eventually to the Minister of Health appointing a new chairperson of the MCC.

The political scandal occurred after it was revealed that political office-bearers may have bought or received donated shares in Virodene. A British TV-channel broke the story that the ANC would have received a 6% share from projected annual profits of £100 million had the Virodene project gone through. The ruling party denied ever being aware of the offer. However, media coverage continued to uncover political connections to the backers of Virodene. Eventually, these concerns were laid to rest when President Mbeki wrote in an article entitled 'The War against Virodene', that 'Neither the ANC nor anyone in its leadership, whether working inside or outside government, has been or will be involved in any financial arrangement related to Virodene.'

Oxihumate-K

In 2001, an article in a South African newspaper, the *Mail & Guardian*, uncovered another AIDS 'snake oil' treatment funded by the government. Enerkom, a state-owned company, developed an anti-AIDS treatment based on oxihumate-k (made from burnt coal) and tested it on Tanzanian soldiers without the approval of the Tanzanian authorities. The trials took place at the same Tanzanian military hospital where Virodene was tested. Tanzania's National Institute for Medical Research, which rejected the Virodene experiments, had not given its approval to trials of oxihumate-k.

It was unclear how much South African government support there was for Enerkom's project. The Department of Health distanced itself from the trials, saying that the Minister of Health knew nothing about them. However, the Department of Minerals and Energy, which oversees Enerkom, had backed the trials.

In 2002, Enerkom and all its research and production facilities were auctioned off without a whisper of accountability for taxpayers' money that was wasted in the abortive immune booster.

Nutrition: Garlic, beetroot and lemons

The politicisation of the AIDS debate became polarised between nutrition versus antiretroviral treatment in the year 2003 when the

Minister, Manto Tshabalala-Msimang began to put emphasis on nutrition as the best treatment for people with HIV. After the controversy over dissident comments of the 'toxicity' of antiretroviral drugs, the health minister extolling the benefits of a Mediterranean concoction of lemon, ginger, olive oil, garlic and beetroot was met with ridicule by the media and AIDS activists. Although she defended her support for the herbal remedies her emphasis on nutrition rather than anti-retroviral treatment reinforced the perception that she still felt that antiretrovirals are not the best option.

The appointment of controversial dissident, Roberto Giraldo, as her nutritional advisor in March 2003 further reinforced the wide-spread idea that the health minister was still a denialist who sought to delay the national treatment plan.

Subsequently, it emerged from an investigative newspaper report that a self-proclaimed 'nutritionist', Tine van der Maas, had put a number of AIDS patients on the diet. She claimed that the 'immune system was strengthened' after taking combinations of lemon blended and grated, mixed with extra virgin olive oil and water, crushed garlic, ginger cut in small pieces, spinach, beetroot and a solution of extracts from the African potato. She said more than 800, 1500 and 42 patients had been given the foods at government provincial hospitals in Mpumalanga, Eastern Cape and Limpopo province respectively. Van der Maas claimed that her patients did not need antiretroviral drugs once they were on the diet.

These ambitious claims of therapeutic benefit for this nutritional combination came under scrutiny by Janicker Visser, a dietician from the University of Stellenbosch, who disputed this and argued that there was no scientific evidence to support the claim that these ingredients boost the immune system. A safety and efficacy study of the African potato was abandoned because some patients who had taken the extract had shown severe bone-marrow suppression. Visser said certain forms of garlic damaged stomach membranes and caused an increase in bleeding time in some people, while onions increased gastrointestinal discomfort. But despite this finding the health minister continued to defend the diet – saying she had seen people in Durban, crippled by AIDS-related complications, regain the ability to walk. She backed up her theory by saying that the World Food Programme has found that food is the first line of defence against HIV and AIDS.

Support for bogus AIDS treatments was unfortunately matched by the lack of support for the use of scientifically proven AIDS treatments developed outside South Africa, usually by multinational drug companies.

Antiretroviral prophylaxis for rape survivors

The explosion of the AIDS epidemic coupled with the high incidence of rape in the country meant that women and girls, without the provision of post-exposure prophylaxis (PEP), faced possible death sentences after sexual abuse. In April 2002 the government committed to providing free PEP to all rape survivors ensuring that within 72 hours the chances of contracting HIV would be minimised. The battle had been particularly difficult until that point especially for the Greater Nelspruit Rape Intervention Project, based in Mpumalanga. The organisation that provided PEP for rape survivors had been repeatedly evicted from hospitals by the Provincial Health Minister of Executive Committee (MEC), Sibongile Manana, who accused the Greater Nelspruit Rape Intervention Project (GRIP) of supplying medicines to, and endangering the lives of, poor black people.

Access to PEP by rape survivors is still patchy in much of the country with many women and children unaware of this service. According to Human Rights Watch, 'The South African government has taken a crucial step in recognising the importance of HIV prevention for rape survivors. But there is a deadly disconnect between the government's stated intention to provide drugs that can prevent HIV and the reality for rape survivors who can't get them.'

The 73-page report released on: 'Deadly Delay: South Africa's Efforts to Prevent HIV in Survivors of Sexual Violence', found that police and nurses who should have been helping rape survivors get anti-HIV drugs didn't do so, sometimes because they had no idea that the programme even existed. And some service providers may not have offered these drugs even when they knew about them, because they thought that doing so was against government policy.

Nevirapine for PMTCT

Nevirapine has been at the centre of political debate and several court battles. Nevirapine has been shown to reduce the chances of a child contracting HIV from its mother during birth by up to 50%.

In 1998, Minister of Health Dlamini-Zuma shocked the AIDS community by refusing to make nevirapine available to pregnant women on the basis that it was too expensive to administer in the public sector. The Department of Health then put on ice pilot programmes designed to test the feasibility and cost-effectiveness of the regimen on the basis that the money available would be utilised for broad-based AIDS awareness campaigns.

Her successor, Minister of Health Tshabalala-Msimang, continued this policy and did not make nevirapine freely available to HIV-positive pregnant women attending government hospitals despite the drug being provisionally registered for this use in 2001. Nevirapine had also been offered free by the drug's manufacturer, Boehringer Ingelheim, to the governments of developing countries for use in the public sector health service in 2000 but the South African Department of Health rejected the offer.

The situation was exacerbated by a comment by the late presidential spokesperson, Parks Mankahlana, in an interview with the American journal *Science*, who further undermined the move towards implementing a prevention of mother-to-child-transmission (PMTCT) programme. He said that the South African government was worried that providing nevirapine to curb vertical transmission of the virus would burden the state with caring for the surviving orphans.

The Treatment Action Campaign took their fight for nevirapine to the courts in August 2000. In a court statement, the TAC's secretary, Mark Heywood said: 'Since July 12th this year the South African government has known that a single 200 mg pill, given to a woman who has HIV and is about to go into labour, and another 6 mg pill, given to her child immediately after birth, can reduce the risk that she faces of transmitting HIV to her infant during delivery – and for a few months after – by nearly 50%. This drug is known as nevirapine (NVP).' Heywood's court statement continued with information that showed that this intervention, which could save at least 14 000 lives each year, would cost only R1.99 in additional taxes of each South African.

Government reasons for not implementing a PMTCT programme ranged from toxicity of the drug to the costs involved to the problems associated with breastfeeding. However, later in 2000, the government announced that it would dispense nevirapine in a total of 18 pilot sites around the country. This led to the TAC suspending its court action. But, when in 2001 the Department of Health referred the decision to use nevirapine back to the Cabinet, the TAC implemented legal action once more.

On December 14, 2001, the TAC won the lawsuit against Minister of Health Tshabalala-Msimang and nine provincial health ministers, compelling the government to provide nevirapine through the public health sector for PMTCT programmes. Five days later, the government announced that it would develop PMTCT programmes but at the same time appealed the judges' ruling.

At this time, doctors, non-governmental organisations, trade unions, religious leaders, and even some members of provincial and local governments opposed the stance of the national Ministry of Health. Some doctors continued to prescribe nevirapine to pregnant women in government hospitals in defiance of the official policy.

Two provincial health ministers defied the national government and announced that they would provide nevirapine for PMTCT within their provinces. In Mpumalanga province, however, the provincial Health Minister took disciplinary action against hospital doctors who prescribed nevirapine for PMTCT in defiance of official policy.

In March 2002 the Department of Health appealed the high court ruling to the Constitutional Court. The TAC won an interim order in the Constitutional Court that nevirapine should be provided by the state, where possible. The decision came as a victory for the TAC but was also significant for the newly formed democracy as it indicated the extent to which the courts will act on second-level rights and government policy.

The political 'turning point' came on April 17, 2002, when the Cabinet announced that it planned to have a universal PMTCT nevirapine programme in place by 2003 and it offered state-funded antiretroviral treatment to rape victims for the first time. The legal process culminated in July 2002, when the Constitutional Court ruled against the national Minister of Health and seven provincial Ministers, ordering the government to roll out PMTCT programmes using nevirapine across the country.

Antiretroviral drugs to treat AIDS

The confusion around President Mbeki's position on antiretroviral drugs for treating HIV/AIDS first began in 1999 when he told parliament that AZT (azidothymidine) is a toxic and failed drug and recommended that the Medicines Control Council (MCC) review the drug's status. After two reviews the MCC cleared the drug for use.

President Mbeki did not limit his doubts to a local audience. In April 2000, he wrote a controversial letter to world leaders where he defended the AIDS dissident's arguments: 'Toward the end of last year, speaking in our national parliament, I said that I had asked our Minister of Health to look into various controversies taking place among scientists on HIV-AIDS and the toxicity of a particular antiretroviral drug' in reference to the establishment of the Presidential AIDS panel, which included equal numbers of AIDS dissidents (such as Peter Duesberg and David Rasnick) and scientists who accept the conventional view that HIV causes AIDS. In an interview with *Time* magazine, President Mbeki said that he cannot accept that HIV is the sole cause of AIDS and he subsequently disputed the Medical Research Council's statistics that placed AIDS as South Africa's leading cause of death.

During this period, the Minister of Health supported the President's view that AZT is toxic. On March 16, 2000 she reinforced her scepticism about the drugs at an ANC youth league AIDS campaign where she denounced AZT and nevirapine as dangerous.

At the 14th International AIDS Conference in Barcelona in July 2002 in an interview with a *Newsday* journalist the Minister of Health said that antiretroviral drugs were 'poisons killing our people' but she later denied this.

Affordability of antiretroviral drugs was used as one reason for not implementing a national treatment plan. In December 2002, the Minister of Health told an international correspondent that the reason for not introducing antiretroviral drugs was because budgetary priorities meant her department could not provide drugs to the estimated 4.5-million South Africans with HIV. In the same month the Treatment Action Campaign launched their civil disobedience campaign to call for the rollout of antiretroviral drugs.

A joint treasury and health task team was appointed in 2002 to calculate the costs of antiretroviral treatment in public hospitals but the report was delayed for a year. In mid-2003, the Treatment Action Campaign embarked on a nationwide civil disobedience action to put pressure on government to not only release the report but adopt an antiretroviral treatment plan. The task team report was key to the cabinet giving the green light for the national antiretroviral rollout plan, but the constant delay to release it, eventually resulted in the TAC leaking a version to the media that found the government could afford a treatment plan. By August 2003 scientists, civil society and government gathered in Durban for the first National AIDS conference, where protest marchers disrupted the Health Minister's speech calling on all delegates to support the immediate implementation of a national treatment plan. Whether it was due to the protests, pressure at the conference or finally the cabinet recognising the urgency of the threat of AIDS – just days after the conference the Cabinet announced that it endorsed and supported the rollout of free antiretroviral drugs in the public sector. Celebrations and festivities erupted in all parts of the country, with AIDS activists expelling a collective sigh of relief and welcoming the decision. The health department was given a deadline of the end of September 2003 to come up with a draft plan that was anticipated as the largest ARV rollout plan in the world. A plan was released on November 19, 2003 that envisaged 'within a year' there would be at least one antiretroviral service point in each district and within five years 1.4 million people would be on treatment. Despite the years of waiting and protest, all AIDS activists and government officials knew that the most challenging part was still to come – implementation of the plan.

Conclusion

The political history of AIDS treatment in South Africa certainly appears to be 'a litany of controversies'. However, at the time of writing, the political will does appear to be there to roll out antiretroviral treatment at least where the infrastructure is present and provinces such as the Western Cape have already made major strides in this direction. Despite the optimism, many South Africans have been realistic about the challenges facing implementation. Major discrepancies in health care infrastructure and capacity between provinces meant that the rollout would not take place uniformly throughout the country. The wealthier provinces would forge ahead leaving behind poorer provinces with strained health care systems. The main concern for activists was for the treatment plan to be a catalyst that would strengthen the public health care system as opposed to weaken it. After the government rollout decision, one of the first things that the TAC did was pressure pharmaceutical giants, GlaxoSmithKline and Boehringer Ingleheim, to grant licences to generic companies to manufacture the drugs. But delays in the government tender process for procurement of the antiretroviral drugs has caused unnecessary delays in reaching targets set out in the plan.

A core challenge is to ensure that people are educated about the potential for resistance if the drugs are taken incorrectly. Treatment literacy is where the TAC has been playing a role in the rollout of the drugs. Human resources and the training of primary health care workers is seen as the backbone of the success of the rollout. With the brain drain, stress and poaching of nursing staff to the private health care sector, the government faces the huge task of providing the health care staff to deal with the extra work. But ten years of democracy was not nearly enough to improve health care systems in all provinces. The treatment plan is the greatest test of the South African Constitution to provide free health care to all South Africans.

Bibliography

BLOCK R. 'South Africa, Drug Firms Near Accord To Settle Court Case Over AIDS Drugs'. *Wall Street Journal.* New York. April 18, 2001

BRUMMER S. 'Virodene's unanswered questions'. *Mail & Guardian.* Johannesburg. March 1998

BRUMMER S, SOLE S. 'The ANC's Virodene backers'. *Mail & Guardian.* Johannesburg. July 2002.

CAMERON E. 'Lecture presented at the Harvard Law School's Human Rights Programme' *Mail & Guardian.* Johannesburg. April 2003.

DEANE N, SOGGOT M, MACFARLANE D. 'Coal-Fired AIDS Muti Tested On Soldiers'. *Mail & Guardian.* Johannesburg. September 28, 2001.

Deane N. 'South African Government Under Fire For Delaying Release of Global Funds' *Inter Press Service*. May 5, 2003.

Deane N, Haffajee F. 'What more must the minister do before she is removed'. *Mail & Guardian*. Johannesburg. April 2003.

Haffajee F. 'Aids and the ANC' *Financial Mail*. Johannesburg. March 2002.

Hennop J. 'AIDS: AIDS report in S Africa shows up divisions, draws criticism'. *Agence France Press*. April 5, 2001.

Kindra J. 'Aids drugs killed Parks, says ANC' *Mail & Guardian*. Johannesburg. March 2002.

Marais H. '*The Aids Review 2000 at the Centre for the Study of Aids'*. University of Pretoria April 2000.

McGreal C. 'Mbeki's AIDS experts split over link to HIV'. *The Guardian*. London. April 5, 2001

Malala J, Taitz L. 'Heath's damning Zuma dossier'. *The Sunday Times*. Johannesburg. 15 November 1998.

Sole S, Brummer S. 'Who's bankrolling Virodene?' *Mail & Guardian*. Johannesburg. 28 June 2002.

Swarns R. 'Study Says Aids Is Now Chief Cause of Death in South Africa' *New York Times*. New York. Oct. 16, 2001.

SECTION 7
What does the future hold?

CHAPTER 35
Models and trends

Brian Williams

'As far as the propositions of mathematics refer to reality, they are not certain; and as far as they are certain, they do not refer to reality'. Albert Einstein

OUR KNOWLEDGE OF HIV, of its mode of transmission, of the risk factors for and the consequences of infection, and of ways to reduce transmission, may be greater than for any other known pathogen as earlier chapters in this book testify. And yet, there is no convincing explanation for the dramatic regional variations in the prevalence of HIV infection. We do not know why the eight worst affected countries are all in southern Africa, the next six are in East and Central Africa, and the next fifteen are in West Africa if we exclude Haiti and Honduras. There is no convincing explanation for the fact that the median prevalence of infection among urban, low-risk groups, is about 30% in southern Africa, 17% in East Africa, 7% in West Africa and less than 1% in Brazil and India.

The problem is that we know a great deal about the immediate determinants of infection in individuals but little about the factors that determine the long term dynamics of infection and disease in populations.

In this chapter we use simple models to develop a conceptual framework within which we can pose and test key questions about overall disease dynamics. As we collect better and more extensive data we will need more complex models to explore more detailed questions that such data will raise.

There have been important successes in controlling the spread of HIV and managing the consequences of AIDS. In Thailand condom use has increased substantially while sexually transmitted infection (STI) and HIV rates have fallen dramatically, especially among sex workers; in Uganda increasing social stability and changes in behaviour have been associated with a 50% fall in the prevalence of HIV infection; in Brazil antiretroviral drugs have been made available to all who need them and AIDS deaths have declined dramatically. But there have also been failures. There is little evidence, for example, that public health interventions have had a significant impact on adult heterosexual transmission in southern Africa or indeed in most of sub-Saharan Africa.

If we are to control the epidemic of HIV and manage the personal, social and economic consequences of AIDS we need numbers. How many people are infected now? How many people will die in the next ten years? Would the number of future infections go down if we eliminated curable STIs? Would we reduce transmission rates significantly if sex workers used condoms routinely? What will the epidemic cost the country, the health services, communities and families? How many AIDS orphans will there be in twenty years from now? If we make highly active antiretroviral therapy freely available can the country afford it? How many lives will it save and for how long? With rates of tuberculosis infection in South Africa already among the highest in the world how will these rates change? Why are more women than men infected with HIV? Why are more people infected with HIV in KwaZulu-Natal than in the Western Cape?

These are empirical questions and depend primarily on the collection of good data. But data on their own are not enough. We need a conceptual framework within which we can formulate and test precise, quantitative questions. In order to do this we start with statistical analyses of the kind outlined in CHAPTER 3. If the prevalence of infection among women attending antenatal clinics (hereafter 'ANC women') is increasing can we estimate the rate of increase and how precisely? Is there evidence that the prevalence is reaching a plateau and if so at what level? Do infection rates vary significantly with age, sex, province, education and so on? Analyses such as these are an essential first step in deriving hard numbers from what is often soft data. However, epidemics of disease change over time, sometimes dramatically, as in the case of severe acute respiratory syndrome or SARS, sometimes more slowly, as in the case of HIV. But epidemics of disease are also non-linear and they often change in seemingly unpredictable ways. It may be for, example, that reducing transmission by 50% has little effect on the rates of infection while reducing it by a further 50% might eliminate the epidemic entirely. To understand the complex, often counter-intuitive patterns we observe in epidemics such as that of HIV/AIDS we need to develop dynamic, non-linear, mathematical models that we can fit to the data and use to make predictions about the future course of the epidemic and to explore the consequences of different interventions. But most importantly, models can help us to gain an understanding of the natural history of the epidemic, what drives it, where we might best seek to interrupt it and how we might finally eliminate it.

There are many ways to develop models and different people have different preferences. A typography of approaches to mathematical models might be as follows. The first question concerns the level of detail that should be included in a model; we may start from the simplest possible model adding complexity only as the data demand it or we may write down a 'complete' model that contains everything that we think is important for the problem at hand. The first approach helps us to focus on what is most important and tells us what each additional part of the model does, the second approach gives us more flexibility and power but cancelling errors can lead to false conclusions. If the purpose of the model is to help us understand the processes underlying the epidemic then we should adapt the former approach, but if it is to fit the data and provide scenarios for policy makers we might prefer the latter approach. The reliability and precision of predictions that models make are very important although here too a balance is required; a rather imprecise but very simple model will sometimes provide more insight than a very precise but rather complex model. It is often forgotten that a particular model structure necessarily imposes constraints on the possible outcomes and our forecasts may depend more on the structure of the model than on the precision of the data.

The second aspect of our typography of models relates to how we deal with uncertainty. Even if the model structure is adequate, there will be errors in the data to which we fit the model and these will be reflected in corresponding uncertainties in the fits and predictions. In general the best way to fit data to complex models is to use maximum likelihood methods, which are well developed and straightforward to implement. Once such estimates of the parameters have been made it is easy to obtain the covariance matrix of the parameters. Knowing the covariance of the parameters we can then explore the effects of variability in the data using Monte Carlo methods in which we generate random estimates of the parameters, chosen from the appropriate density functions, run the model many times and examine the variability in the outcomes. Very often estimates of the parameters that we use in our model are not available for the particular population that we are studying and we take them from other studies carried out at other times and in other places, which introduces further uncertainties. If we wish to account for both the prior uncertainty in the parameter estimates, derived from other studies, but simultaneously allow for the goodness-of-fit to the data through the likelihood function, we can use Bayesian techniques. These techniques combine prior estimates of the parameters with the likelihood function to obtain improved posterior estimates of the parameters. Bayesian techniques provide a powerful way of balancing our prior knowledge against the precision of the fit to the data, and Markov chain. Monte Carlo methods provide a particularly elegant way of implementing Bayesian fits, although they may be slow to converge.

The final aspect of our typography of models derives from the nature of the question that we are asking. If we wish to determine overall trends in incidence, prevalence and deaths, say, a conventional compartmental model, dealing with populations rather than individuals, will generally be sufficient. These are most easily constructed using Markov models but since their essential feature is that they carry no information about the history of the process being modelled and depend only on the present state of the system, it may be necessary to extend them in various ways. If we are concerned with the elimination of a disease, we may be concerned with chance processes among individuals and we would use a stochastic model, possibly even a micro-simulation model, in which we simulate individual people rather than populations of people. If we are trying to understand the importance of sexual networking we might wish to use network models which rely on graph and diffusion theory.

Most of the modelling work on HIV/AIDS in South Africa has used detailed compartmental models to fit the data for women attending antenatal clinics. The data have been supplemented by parameter estimates taken from the literature and related sets of data that may be less precise but constrain the range of model behaviour, such as national mortality figures. Unfortunately almost all data that we have in South Africa are for black and coloured people; data on white and Asian people are lacking and we focus our analysis on the former two population groups. Here we present the simplest possible model that is consistent with what we know about HIV/AIDS and will allow us to explore the consequences of various interventions.

The model is illustrated schematically in FIGURE 35.1. (An Excel spread sheet containing the model with details of the mathematical structure of the model, extensions to the Markov formulation, and how to run the model, is available on request.)

Taking estimates of the parameters from the literature and fitting the model to the data for women attending public antenatal clinics (see CHAPTER 3) gives the fit shown in FIGURE 35.2.

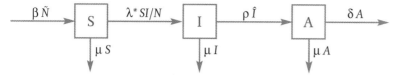

FIGURE 35.1 A simple model of HIV/AIDS in adults. N, the number of adults in the model, is equal to S, the number of susceptible adults, plus I, the number of infected adults and A, the number of adults with AIDS. People are born and enter into the population at a rate $\beta\tilde{N}$. Susceptible people become infected at a per capita rate λ/N, infected people develop AIDS at a per capita rate ρ, people with AIDS die at a per capita rate δ. Everyone dies at a background rate μ. The embellishments on the letters indicate extensions to the basic Markov formulation

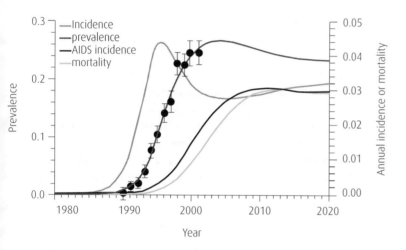

FIGURE 35.2 The model (Figure 35.1) fitted to the antenatal clinic data for South Africa. Details given in the text. Prevalence data show 95% confidence intervals. The prior parameter estimates used in the fit are $\beta = 0.023$ yr⁻¹, mean age of mothers, $g = 25.5$ yr, background mortality, $\mu = 0.0087$ yr⁻¹, Weibull median survival time, $\tau = 9$ yr, Weibull shape parameter, $w = 2.3$, median survival after AIDS, $\delta = 1$ yr. From the fit we are able to obtain estimates of the transmission parameter, $\lambda = 0.68 \pm 0.07$ months and the heterogeneity parameter, $\phi = 7.1 \pm 0.07$

From the fitted parameters we obtain an estimate of the initial doubling time, $d = 12.9 \pm 1.6$ months and an estimate of the asymptotic prevalence, equal to 27%. It is important to stress that these two parameters, together with a third, which determines the timing of the epidemic, are all that we can estimate directly from the ANC survey data. All other parameters that we estimate must be functions of these parameters and possibly also of other parameters derived from other studies.

The most important parameter in the epidemiology of any infection, which we can derive from our fitted value of the initial doubling time and our prior estimate of the survival distribution, is the case reproduction number, R_0, which gives the number of secondary cases for one primary case of infection. From the model fit our estimate of R_0 is 8.7 ± 0.9 so that to drive the epidemic to extinction we would have to reduce transmission by about nine times. The challenge presented by HIV/AIDS in South Africa is therefore substantial but not insurmountable.

FIGURE 35.2 also shows that if nothing changes then we would expect the prevalence to peak at about 27% and only decline slightly after that. The model suggests that the incidence peaked in 1995 at about 4.4%/year and will converge to about 3%/year over the next 20 years. The incidence of AIDS and AIDS-related deaths will rise to about 3%/year in about 2010. The model can also be used to show that the overall population of black and coloured people will stabilise over the next 20 years but will increase slowly after that.

All of these results apply to women attending public ante-natal clinics and we need to apply them to the whole population. It is generally assumed that the prevalence of infection among ANC women overestimates prevalence in young women and underestimates prevalence in older women so that the overall prevalence is about the same. In South Africa 54% of black and coloured women are between the ages of 15 and 49 years so that the prevalence among women of all ages is about 15% (excluding children infected vertically); we need to scale our estimate based on the fit to women attending ante-natal clinics accordingly. Strictly speaking we should standardise the infection rates for age but given the precision of the data and the level of detail included in the model, our estimate of 15% is probably good enough for our present discussion. Unfortunately there are very few data for men but a study in rural KwaZulu-Natal carried out in 1991 showed that the prevalence in men was 69% of the prevalence in women and in a mining town in 1998 the corresponding figure was 73%. Furthermore it is easy to show that if the rate of transmission per sex act from an infected man to an uninfected woman is, say, r times that from an infected woman to an uninfected man, then the prevalence of infection in women will be approximately equal to $\sqrt{r}$ times that in men. Since r is reckoned to be about three, the prevalence in men is expected to be 60% to 70% of the prevalence in women.

Drawing all of this together we note that in 2001 there were 20.6 million black and coloured women so that about three-million are infected with HIV; there were 18.8 million black and coloured men so that about two-million men are infected with HIV, giving a total of

5.0 ± 0.5 million. However, it is important to acknowledge the sources of uncertainty. If the prevalence in men was as high as in women then we would have to increase our estimate of the total number of people infected with HIV by about 780 000. If the prevalence of infection in white and Asian people was similar to that in black and coloured people then this would give a further 600 000 white and Asian people who are infected with HIV. Clearly much better and more extensive data on men and on white and Asian people are urgently needed.

Using the same logic and referring to the fit in FIGURE 35.2, about 3% of ANC women are currently being infected each year which translates into about 335 000 new infections each year in black and coloured women and 225 000 new infections each year in black and coloured men or a total of 560 000 per year. If the rates in men were similar to the rates in women this would increase the estimate by about 100 000 per year and if the rates in white and Asian people were similar to those in black and coloured women this would increase the estimate by a further 67 000 per year.

FIGURE 35.2 shows that AIDS-related mortality is likely to increase to about 3%/year among women attending antenatal clinics in 2010 so that in the population as a whole the crude death rate is likely to increase by about 1.6% per year, about twice the current crude death rate. But we must bear in mind that these deaths will be concentrated in young adults. If the epidemic reaches a steady state then the number of deaths will be close to the number of new infections each year so that after 2010 about 560 000 black and coloured people will die each year of AIDS and AIDS-related diseases. Again, depending on the actual rates in men and in other race groups, the true number could be as much as 30% higher.

More sophisticated models have been developed, but what this analysis shows is that there are still significant gaps in our knowledge of the basic data, especially relating to infection rates in men and in white and Asian people, so that however sophisticated we make our models the same limitations will apply.

What we can do with greater confidence, however, is to examine changes that are likely to occur as a result of interventions that may be implemented so that we are considering relative rather than absolute estimates. Let us first suppose that as the mortality rate increases, people are more likely to know someone who has died of AIDS and therefore to change their behaviour. To illustrate how we might go about estimating the impact of such behaviour change let us assume that for each person in someone's immediate family or close circle of friends who dies of AIDS each year, that person's risk of infection is cut by half. Then if they have, say, 50 such contacts, their risk of infection will fall by about 25% for each 1% increase in the adult mortality rate. With this assumption, and refitting the model to the data, we get the results shown in FIGURE 35.3.

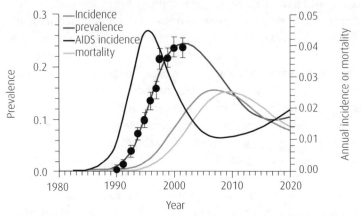

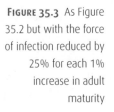

FIGURE 35.3 As Figure 35.2 but with the force of infection reduced by 25% for each 1% increase in adult maturity

As the AIDS-related mortality increases, risky behaviour decreases and incidence and then prevalence falls. But as AIDS-related mortality declines risk behaviour increases and we observe the oscillations shown in FIGURE 35.3. This rate of decline after the peak is not unlike the rate of decline observed in Uganda, where political leaders embraced the issue of AIDS and encouraged people to respond openly. This may partly explain the decline in Uganda. It has also been argued that in the United States rates of infection fell as death rates climbed but that the advent of antiretroviral therapies has led people to become less concerned about safe-sex and rates of infection may be increasing again.

As yet there is no evidence that such changes are occurring in South Africa perhaps because the level of denial concerning AIDS has remained high until very recently. But what then might be the impact of interventions aimed at reducing levels of transmission? Suppose that we were able to implement programmes involving behaviour change, increased condom use, effective reductions in the prevalence of STIs, and perhaps male circumcision. And suppose that the effect of these interventions was to reduce the risk of infection by 25% by 2010 and by 50% by 2015. The result would be as shown in FIGURE 35.4. Incidence and prevalence start to fall immediately, prevalence would start to fall soon and AIDS cases and deaths would peak at about the same rate in 2010 but would decline after that. By 2010 the prevalence, incidence and mortality would all be reduced by about 30%. This would improve the situation considerably and save many lives but greater reductions in transmission are needed to eliminate HIV.

Providing antiretroviral therapy to all those with AIDS is expected to extend their lives by a further ten years on average but with

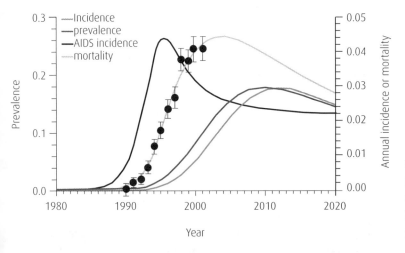

FIGURE 35.4 As Figure 35.2 but with the force of infection reduced by 25% by 2010 and by 50% by 2015

substantial variation about this expected value. Suppose that we start to implement an antiretroviral programme now and assume that by 2010 about 25% of those who need antiretrovirals are getting them and that by 2015 this proportion has increased to 50%. The impact of this programme is shown in FIGURE 35.5. As expected, it does little for prevalence or incidence but reduces AIDS deaths by about 50%.

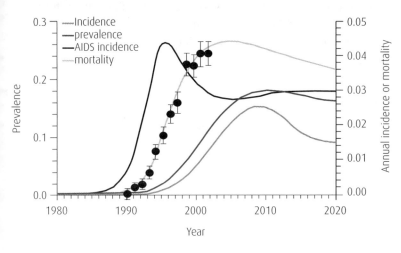

FIGURE 35.5 As Figure 35.2 but with 25% of people being given anti-retroviral therapy by 2010 and 50% by 2015

However, if we extend the data beyond 2020 the death rate begins to rise again as people on antiretrovirals begin to die. What is somewhat more problematical is that, as has been observed in Brazil, the number of people receiving antiretroviral therapy rises more or less linearly with time since people are kept alive each year and continue to need drugs while more people develop AIDS each year and add to the number already receiving antiretrovirals. At the current estimated incidence rate, about half-a-million people are being infected each year and about this number of additional people would need to be started on therapy each year so that by 2020 about eight-million people would be receiving drugs. While antiretroviral therapy will buy valuable time it will not in the end solve the problem, and prevention programmes will still be needed as urgently as ever.

These observations are made without explicitly including people's age. The influence of age on the outcome is particularly important in the case of sexually transmitted infections because the risk of infection increases dramatically at the age of sexual debut, which in South Africa is about 16 years, peaks around the age of 25 years in women and 30 years in men, and then declines slowly with age thereafter (See CHAPTER 3). It is perhaps interesting to note that among migrant workers the risk of infection appears to remain high until the age of 50 or more years. We can now use those results, from the model described in CHAPTER 3, to estimate the age-specific mortality by convoluting the age-specific incidence of infection (CHAPTER 3, FIGURE 3.7) with the mortality determined from the Weibull survivorship curve allowing for the change in prevalence over time. Clearly AIDS notification data will be very far from complete and in FIGURE 35.6 the data are normalised to have the same area under the curves. Comparing these model calculations with AIDS notification data from South Africa the good agreement between the shapes of the curves for men and for women is excellent giving us greater confidence in the underlying structure and therefore the reliability of our models.

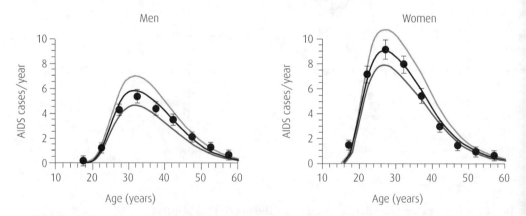

FIGURE 35.6 Age-specific notified cases of AIDS for men and women. Lines are obtained from incidence and survival estimates as described in the text. The points are AIDS case notification data for 1996 normalised (separately for men and for women) to have the same area under the curves

The discussion so far has been concerned with changes in the epidemic over time and with some of the effects of age. We have not asked questions about the spread of infection in space. The provinces of South Africa and some its neighbours are still bound by a system of oscillating migration which originated in the last century. The system was developed to ensure that the gold mines, in particular, had a secure supply of labour but also so that they would not be responsible for the health and social security of the men after they retired. At its peak, half-a-million men were brought to the gold mines each year from all over the southern African region, without their wives or families and were sent home each year to impoverished rural communities from where they would negotiate a new annual contract. The men were clearly placed at high risk of infection while away from their families; large numbers of sex workers gathered around the mines to earn money and wives were themselves at high risk living without the support of their husbands in rural areas. This system still persists with few changes.

In order to model the spatial spread of disease more complicated mathematical models are needed. The conceptual framework for spatial modelling involves a range of techniques from mapping and geographical information systems to more formal analysis. The latter includes reaction-diffusion equations with stochastic spatial effects and 'Small Worlds' theory which explores the way in which the properties of networks changes as their degree and pattern of connectivity changes. Although the details are complex and little work has so far been done in this area, we can illustrate the kinds of results that we expect to find quite easily. Suppose, for example, that every man in a certain town had sex with every woman who lived within one kilometres of his house. Clearly he would have relatively little sex with any particular woman but this would be a situation of extreme promiscuity. We have seen that the initial doubling time of the epidemic in South Africa is about one year so that on average he would infect one woman living within one kilometre in one year. If that woman had sex with every man living within one kilometre of her house it would take another year before she infected one man about one kilometre away. In other words the epidemic would spread at a rate of about one kilometre per year although the random nature of the process means that the actual rate is rather less. In 1937 R A Fisher considered the spread of mutant genes in natural populations and the beauty of mathematics is that we can now apply his results to the study of AIDS. In our hypothetical situation let us suppose that the mean-square-distance between a given person and their sexual partners is d kilometres. Let us also suppose that the number of infected people doubles every τ years and that each person lives for ε years. Then we can solve the Fisher equation to show that the epidemic front will spread out at
a speed, s, given by
$$s = d\sqrt{\frac{\ln(2)}{\tau\varepsilon}}$$

CHAPTER 35 MODELS AND TRENDS

so that if $d = 1$ km, $\tau = 1$ year and $\varepsilon = 10$ years, then the epidemic will spread at a rate of 260 metres per year and would take more than 2000 years to get from Johannesburg to Durban even if people were living densely packed all the way between the two cities and behaving in an extremely promiscuous fashion. It is clear that no amount of promiscuity, on its own, can explain the geographical spread of the epidemic. But if even a small number of people travel from Johannesburg to Durban and have sex in both places, the infection will spread rapidly from one city to the other.

We clearly need much more sophisticated models of geographical spread reflecting the actual population distribution (CHAPTER 3, FIGURE 3.5) and the patterns of migration which are themselves hard to define, measure and study. But it seems highly likely that much of the regional variation in HIV infection is a consequence of patterns of migration.

Finally, it has often been noted that if people only ever had sex with people who were born in the same year as themselves, HIV could not persist. If infections arose in certain age cohorts, the members of the cohort would grow older and die without spreading it to other age cohorts. The formal question then becomes: how wide does the average age range of people's sexual partners need to be in order for the epidemic to persist? Again we can solve a variant of the Fisher equation to show that if the standard deviation of the age range of people's sexual partners is α the infection spreads to younger (and of course older) ages at a rate of c years of age for each calendar year where

$$c \approx \frac{ln(2)\alpha}{\tau\sqrt{6}}$$

For an epidemic to persist, c must be greater than 1 or the age of infected people will increase more quickly than the infection spreads to younger people. In other words if the doubling time is one year then the age range of people's sexual partners must be at least ± 3.5 years. In a study in South Africa the age range of women's sexual partners was ± 5.4 years, sufficiently large to sustain the epidemic. However, if transmission were halved the age range needed to sustain the epidemic would be ± 6.2 years and the epidemic would only be marginally viable. But if a few girls have sex with much older men or a few boys with much lder women the infection will spread across the generations and persist.

Models can be used in many ways and for many ends. The detailed, demographic models developed by the Actuarial Society of South Africa (see CHAPTER 27) provide the best estimates of the numbers of infected people, the rate of new infections, the mortality rate, the number of AIDS orphans to be expected over the next ten to twenty years, and so on. Models such as these provide vital information for advocacy, planning, testing various scenarios and so on. The limitation of such models is that they take time to run and their complexity can make it difficult to know precisely which parts of the model are fitting which bits of the data. With simpler models it is easier to explore the natural history of the disease and in particular to put sensible bounds on our estimates using maximum likelihood methods, and to combine prior information of the parameter values with information from the likelihood functions to derive posterior bounds on the parameters and the trends in the measures of disease. Analytical models allow us to obtain algebraic expressions for the rate of spread of disease, for example, and are potentially much more powerful than any simulation model but require the use of sophisticated mathematical techniques and a high level of analytical skill. Even then such models can only be used to analyse particular, focused problems, although the price that is paid in extracting a small part of the system for analysis is often repaid many times over in terms of the understanding that it leads to.

With all the provisos, caveats and cautions noted above we can nevertheless make some statements with confidence. We know that the epidemic in South Africa is probably close to a steady state and is unlikely to increase much beyond its present levels. We know more or less how many people are infected, how many more people are being infected each year, how many people are going to die in the next ten years and how many children will be infected and will die. However, we also know that if nothing changes the current situation could persist indefinitely and the numbers are terrifying.

However, we also know that people are likely to change their behaviour as more and more people close to them die but that this will not happen unless we develop a supportive, open, well-informed attitude to HIV and AIDS. People's response to the perceived dangers could also be one of nihilism and despair in which case high-risk sexual behaviour could increase as the deaths become apparent. We know that if we can reduce transmission rates by about 50% we will have a substantial impact on the future course of the epidemic; to eliminate it completely we may have to reduce transmission by 80% or more but even that should not be impossible given time and commitment.

The modelling work described here is still in its infancy and if we truly wish to understand the course of the epidemic and how we might manage it, we need to bring together clinicians, molecular biologists, public health officials, epidemiologists, social scientists, economists, statisticians and mathematicians in a sustained effort to understand the dynamics of the epidemic, the risk factors, the effectiveness of various interventions, and the likely and possible future courses of the epidemic. These must feed directly into public health policy at the highest level. The world reacted rapidly and effectively to the epidemic of SARS by ensuring that people put aside their differences and personal ambitions and worked together to defeat the threat posed by this new infectious agent. There is no reason why we should not succeed in winning the battle against HIV/AIDS also.

This discussion also demonstrates the need for more and better data. We still rely heavily on the annual, national surveys of infection among women attending antenatal clinics. While these surveys enable us to estimate rates of infection in black and coloured women by province the sample size is insufficient to make statements at a finer than provincial scale and they provide little useful information about white and Asian women and no information about men. Our understanding of the epidemic could be greatly strengthened if the sample size were sufficient to examine geographical changes on a finer scale. We need also to establish routine surveillance among the other race groups and among men.

There are several alternatives to general population surveys which are expensive and difficult to carry out. One would be to use sputa from tuberculosis patients as a sentinel group for HIV. The epidemic of HIV is driving up rates of tuberculosis, especially in East and southern Africa. In Nairobi, for example, the annual notification rate has increased by ten times in ten years, from about 60 to 600 per 100 000 people almost entirely as a result of HIV infections and the links between HIV and tuberculosis are still being explored. While tuberculosis patients are biased in their own ways, the biases inherent there are no greater than those in other potential target groups and this would provide us with data from a wide cross-section of people, including men.

Another option is to set up sentinel sites where detailed studies are carried out not only of infection rates for HIV but also of other sexually transmitted diseases, such as syphilis, gonorrhoea and HSV-2 and AIDS-related opportunistic infections, such as tuberculosis. But these sites should also be used to monitor psychological and social markers of behaviour and to implement and run intervention programmes, including the provision of antiretroviral therapy. This would help us to develop a much more detailed and nuanced understanding of the epidemic. Work of this kind started eight years ago in the mining town of Carletonville and about ten years ago in the rural district of Hlabisa and the links between these two centres have been studied in some detail. A new study site of this kind is currently being established in the KwaZulu-Natal midlands. Similar studies are

needed in communities chosen to be representative of the different
social and economic conditions that are found in South Africa.

Here we have barely scratched the surface of the world of possibilities that modelling opens up to us. Models have been used to explore
the impact of HIV on TB, a particularly important matter in sub-
Saharan Africa, to investigate the likely impact of behavioural change
programmes and programmes to manage curable and treatable STIs,
to tell us how many people will die if we continue to do nothing and
how best to mount a serious response to the epidemic. Models
provide the broad framework within which we can pose sensible
questions and hopefully find meaningful answers that will help us to
manage and deal with the consequences of the epidemic of HIV.

Bibliography

ANDERSON RM, GUPTA S, NG W. 'The significance of sexual partner contact networks for
the transmission dynamics of HIV'. *Journal of Acquired Immune Deficiency
Syndromes* 1990; 3: 417–429.

AUVERT B, BUONAMICO G, LAGARDE E, WILLIAMS B. 'Sexual behavior, heterosexual
transmission, and the spread of HIV in sub-Saharan Africa: a simulation study'.
Computers and Biomedical Research 2000; 33: 84–96.

AUVERT B, BUVE A, FERRY B, CARAEL M, MORISON L, LAGARDE E ET AL. 'Ecological and
individual level analysis of risk factors for HIV infection in four urban populations in
sub-Saharan Africa with different levels of HIV infection'. *AIDS* 2001; 15 (Suppl 4):
S15–S30.

BEKKER LG, WOOD R. 'Antiretroviral therapy in South Africa – can we do it?' *South
African Medical Journal* 2002; 92: 191–193.

BRADSHAW D, SCHNEIDER M, DORRINGTON R, BOURNE DE, LAUBSCHER R. 'South African
cause-of-death profile in transition – 1996 and future trends'. *South African
Medical Journal* 2002; 92: 618–623.

BROOKMEYER R. 'AIDS, epidemics, and statistics'. *Biometrics*. 1996; 52: 781–796.

BUVE A, CARAEL M, HAYES RJ, AUVERT B, FERRY B, ROBINSON NJ ET AL. 'The multicentre
study on factors determining the differential spread of HIV in four African cities:
summary and conclusions'. *AIDS* 2001; 15(Suppl 4): S127–S131.

CHIN J, REMENYI MA, MORRISON F, BULATAO R. 'The global epidemiology of the HIV/AIDS
pandemic and its projected demographic impact in Africa. World Health Statistics
Quarterly'. *Rapport Trimestriel de Statistiques Sanitaires Mondiales* 1992;
45: 220–227.

CORBETT EL, WATT CJ, WALKER N, MAHER D, WILLIAMS BG, RAVIGLIONE MC ET AL. 'The
growing burden of tuberculosis: Global trends and interactions with the HIV
epidemic'. *Archives of Internal Medicine* 2003; 163: 1009–1021.

DORRINGTON RE, BRADSHAW D, BUDLENDER D. *'AIDS Profile in the Provinces of South
Africa: Indicators for 2002'.* Cape Town: University of Cape Town, Medical
Research Council, Actuarial Society of South Africa; 2002 November 2002.

DORRINGTON RE. 'How many people are currently infected with HIV in South Africa?'
South African Medical Journal 2002; 92: 196–197.

GILGEN D, WILLIAMS BG, MACPHAIL C, VAN DAM CJ, CAMPBELL C, BALLARD RC ET AL. 'The
natural history of HIV/AIDS in a major goldmining centre in South Africa: Results
of a biomedical and social survey'. *South African Journal of Science* 2001;
97: 387–392.

GILKS WR, RICHARDSON S, SPIEGELHALTER DJ. *'Markov Chain Monte Carlo in practice'*. London: Chapman & Hall; 1996.

GOUWS E, WILLIAMS BG. 'Science and HIV/AIDS in South Africa: A review of the literature'. *South African Journal of Science* 2000; 96: 274–276.

HARRISON A, SMIT JA, MYER L. 'Prevention of HIV/AIDS in South Africa: A review of behaviour change interventions, evidence and options for the future'. *South African Journal of Science* 2000; 96: 285–290.

KORENROMP EL, VAN VLIET C, GROSSKURTH H, GAVYOLE A, VAN DER PLOEG CP, FRANSEN L ET AL. 'Model-based evaluation of single-round mass treatment of sexually transmitted diseases for HIV control in a rural African population'. *AIDS* 2000; 14: 573–93.

MACPHAIL C, WILLIAMS BG, CAMPBELL C. 'Relative risk of HIV infection among young men and women in a South African township'. *International Journal of STD and AIDS* 2002; 13: 331–342.

MORRIS M, KRETZSCHMAR M. 'Concurrent partnerships and the spread of HIV'. *AIDS* 1997; 11: 641–648.

ROSEN S, SIMON J, THEA DM, VINCENT JH. 'Care and Treatment to Extend the Working Lives of HIV-Positive Employees: Calculating the Benefits to Business'. *South African Journal of Science* 2000; 96: 300–304.

ROSEN S, SIMON J, VINCENT JR, MACLEOD W, FOX M, THEA DM. 'AIDS is your business'. *Harvard Business Review* 2003; 81: 80–87, 125.

SCHALL R. 'On the maximum size of the AIDS epidemic among the heterosexual black population in South Africa'. *South African Medical Journal* 1990; 78: 507–510.

STOVER J, GARNETT GP, SEITZ S, FORSYTHE S. *'The Epidemiological Impact of an HIV/AIDS Vaccine in Developing Countries'*. The World Bank Development Group. Washington, DC. 2002.

STOVER J, WALKER N, GARNETT GP, SALOMON JA, STANECKI KA, GHYS PD ET AL. 'Can we reverse the HIV/AIDS pandemic with an expanded response?' *Lancet* 2002; 360: 73–77.

WILLIAMS B.G, TALJAARD D, CAMPBELL CM, GOUWS E, NDHLOVU L, VAN DAM J, CARAEL M, AUVERT B. 'Changing patterns of knowledge, reported behaviour and sexually transmitted infections in a South African gold mining community' *AIDS* 2003; 17: 2099–2017.

CHAPTER 36
The future of the HIV epidemic in South Africa

Salim Abdool Karim and Quarraisha Abdool Karim

THE HIV EPIDEMIC IN South Africa has evolved over the last 20 years and is now characterised by a levelling off of prevalence rates, amidst persistently high HIV incidence rates. The national incidence rate of HIV infection in antenatal clinic attendees is estimated to have peaked at 6.5% in 1997 and HIV transmission models have suggested that incidence has continued to hover at this level for the past five years. South Africa is now dealing with the full impact of the clinical burden of AIDS and the concomitant deaths that result. The introduction of free antiretroviral therapy in the public sector is a turning point that enables South Africa to purposefully and deliberately choose the future path of the HIV epidemic in this country. Choosing to implement treatment programmes without concomitant prevention interventions will result in an upward trend in the epidemic curve and an evergrowing unsustainable level of demand for antiretroviral therapy. However, South Africa has an opportunity to choose a better future; a future including the integration of HIV treatment and prevention programmes, which will result in a downward trend in the epidemic and our best hope for a bright future for South Africa.

It is well established in many industrialised countries that highly active antiretroviral therapy (HAART) can transform the natural course of HIV infection by reducing morbidity and mortality. HAART also symbolises hope for many communities. But access to these lifesaving drugs in resource-constrained settings, including South Africa, was severely restricted until the 2000 International AIDS Conference in Durban, South Africa. This conference paved the way for treatment access and changed the discourse on AIDS treatment in poor countries from 'if' to 'when'. Despite the change in discourse, most South Africans still did not have easy access to the life-saving drugs because of the lack of political will, availability of and prohibitive costs of the drugs.

Before 1994, the apartheid government's approach to dealing with AIDS was insufficient and lacked credibility. The Mandela government set about redressing this in 1994 by establishing AIDS as one of the 23 presidential lead projects and one of the 12 reconstruction and development programmes. This initial period of hope was, however, short-lived. Controversies followed at regular intervals and the trust and partnership between government and civil society broke down. The biggest setback came when President Mbeki (who took office in 1999) expressed doubt about whether HIV causes AIDS and questioned the safety of antiretrovirals. Subsequently, a presidential AIDS panel was created with equal numbers of AIDS denialists and orthodox AIDS scientists, but it predictably produced little of consequence. Several months later, the Constitutional Court's ruling against the government to provide nevirapine to reduce mother-to-child HIV transmission was a landmark decision and put further pressure on the government to provide antiretroviral treatment for AIDS.

The momentous decision of the South African government on 8 August 2003, to make antiretroviral therapy available in the public sector was a defining moment in the country's response to the challenges posed by the HIV/AIDS epidemic. It marked a turning point and signaled the end of past obtuseness.

Since the announcement that South Africans in need would be provided with antiretroviral drugs, the government's plan has got off to a slower than expected start. The Western Cape province was the first to provide AIDS treatment free of charge in selected government hospitals, building on experience from the Médecins Sans Frontières initiated and run treatment project in Khayelitsha, a poor community near Cape Town. The current number of people now on ARV treatment at public facilities nationally stands at 18 527 (TABLE 36.1)

TABLE 36.1 Patients receiving ARV treatment in public health facilities nationally. Summary compiled by the AIDS Law Project (late 2004). [Accuracy unsure]

Province	Operational Plan March 2004 target (Revised for 2005)	Approximate numbers on treatment (Adults and children)
Gauteng (19 sites)	10 000	5 588
North West (6 sites)	1 808	1 124
Northern Cape (5 sites)	790	[1 251]
Eastern Cape (10 sites)	2 750	1 525
Western Cape (28 sites)	2 728	5 137
KwaZulu-Natal (22 sites)	24 902	[2 500]
Limpopo (4 sites)	6 965	[300]
Mpumalanga (8 sites)	1 934	[500]
Free State (5 sites)	2 127	602
Total	54 004 (53 000)	18 527

yet the government's plan projected that 53 000 would be put onto treatment in 2003/4.

Efforts to overcome operational constraints to national coverage of AIDS treatment include: urgent procurement of medicines; speedy accreditation of treatment sites; resource allocation to underdeveloped sites to build capacity for site accreditation and treatment roll-out; clear, accurate and appropriate advice on testing, treatment, nutrition; and prevention, and training and support of health care personnel.

If the targets set out in the national AIDS treatment plan are to be met, South Africa will have to create one of the largest AIDS treatment programmes in the world – a feat that will need a concerted approach with assistance from all sectors of South African society as well as international support to achieve success (FIGURE 36.1)

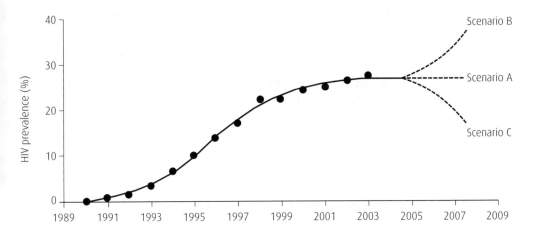

FIGURE 36.1 National HIV infection in antenatal clinic attendees in South Africa. The dots indicate actual HIV prevalence rates while the lines are projection scenarios

Besides the slower than expected scale up and the enormity of the tasks that lie ahead, if the provision of antiretroviral drugs in South Africa only utilises standard medical treatment models of AIDS care, it will fail to grasp the opportunity to have an impact on HIV/AIDS in South Africa. In addition to the need to develop simple and sustainable strategies for initiation and delivery of HIV care and therapy to large numbers of patients in the context of the existing underdeveloped health care delivery systems, the scale of the growing morbidity coupled with ongoing high HIV incidence rates demand an approach that addresses both treatment and prevention in an integrated manner.

To date, substantial resources and effort have been put into the prevention of HIV infection in South Africa (see CHAPTERS 9–15 for more details). This has included extensive condom distribution, public education, advertising campaigns, community-based programmes, and improved treatment of sexually transmitted diseases. Public health sector distribution of male condoms rose from 8 million in 1994 to 97 million in 1995, and 267 million in 2001. Unfortunately, HIV incidence rates remain unacceptably high and the burden of sexually transmitted infections has not abated, despite these prevention programmes (See CHAPTER 12).

Stigma, and concomitant discrimination, is one of the most critical reasons for the failure of prevention programmes as it is a major barrier to accessing HIV prevention, care and support services. Despite the widespread availability of HIV voluntary counselling and testing (VCT) services, it is estimated that less than a quarter of HIV-infected people are aware of their HIV status, and less than 1% know their CD4 count. People living with HIV and AIDS are afraid to speak openly about their HIV status. This, in turn, perpetuates secrecy and denial of personal risk as well as the presence and scale of the HIV epidemic. Not only does this have an impact on prevention, it also presents a major challenge to the provision of antiretroviral therapy.

Transforming AIDS into a treatable condition has the potential to change community perceptions of people living with AIDS. To realise this potential, the individual patient paradigm that currently exists for treating most medical conditions is inadequate as a modality for treating AIDS. Instead a public health model which integrates both prevention and care for HIV/AIDS is required. South Africa is reaching the peak of the epidemic curve, ie prevalence of HIV is leveling off because HIV incidence is currently similar to HIV mortality (FIGURE 36.1, SCENARIO A). The introduction of antiretroviral therapy without concomitant improvements in prevention is likely to lead to an upward turn in the epidemic curve (FIGURE 36.1, SCENARIO B) since new infections will continue to increase while deaths decrease. Indeed some studies have shown that initiation of HAART is associated with a subsequent resumption of sexual and drug use risk behaviors, particularly among groups of men who have sex with men. It is therefore essential for treatment to be accompanied by improved prevention so that both AIDS deaths and new HIV infections decrease leading to scenario C in FIGURE 36.1.

VCT is central to both prevention and treatment. The availability of antiretroviral drugs could be a catalyst to encourage the widespread uptake of VCT as a mechanism to counter the stigma and discrimination. Linking community outreach for VCT with programmes providing AIDS treatment and antiretroviral drugs for the prevention of mother-to-child transmission is one practical manifestation of the proposed approach. Further, linking condom promotion and STI identification and treatment to AIDS treatment and VCT programmes could reduce the number of high-risk discordant sexual acts by

Milestones in access to treatment for HIV in South Africa	
April, 2000:	Médecins sans Frontières and TAC start HAART provision at three government primary health care clinics in Khayalitsha.
July, 2000:	13th International AIDS Conference march for treatment access.
March, 2001:	Pharmaceutical industry withdraw court case against the state on parallel importation and generic drug procurement.
April, 2002:	Global Fund donate US$72 million to KwaZulu-Natal. Constitutional court rejects government appeal of the Pretoria High Court decision and orders government to provide drugs for the prevention of mother-to-child transmission of HIV at all public health care facilities in South Africa.
November, 2002:	Nelson Mandela Foundation sponsors workshop in Durban on treatment access.
August, 2003:	First South African AIDS conference, Durban.
September, 2003:	Government supports national treatment plan for AIDS treatment options in the public sector.
October, 2003:	Competition Commission rule that GlaxoSmithKline and Boehringer Ingelheim abused their dominant positions in antiretrovirals market.
January, 2004:	Western Cape government expands HAART rollout, and by the end of March, 2004, 2000 patients start treatment through an emergency drug procurement mechanism.
February, 2004:	Government accepts money from Global Fund March 2004: Boehringer Ingelheim threatens to disinvest from South Africa because of dissatisfaction about draft medicine pricing regulations of the Department of Health. TAC threatens to take legal action against the government if it fails to implement HAART programme.
April 1, 2004:	Announcement of AIDS treatment rollout in 27 pilot sites in four of nine provinces.

FIGURE 36.2 Milestones in access to treatment for HIV in South Africa *Abdool Karim Q. HIV treatment in South Africa: Overcoming impediments to get started.* Lancet 2004; 363:1394.

involving both HIV negative and HIV positive individuals in HIV prevention.

The increasing availability of antiretroviral therapy through resources from, among others, the President's Emergency Plan for AIDS Relief (PEPFAR) and the Global Fund against AIDS, tuberculosis and malaria is a major step forward in the global effort against AIDS. Recent World Trade Organisation agreements allowing developing countries under certain circumstances to acquire low-cost generic antiretroviral medication removes the biggest obstacle to affordable AIDS treatment. The provision of antiretroviral therapy can save lives and relieve the widespread suffering due to AIDS – it can also serve as an impetus for overcoming stigma and enhancing prevention through a public health model for integration of AIDS treatment and prevention.

Providing treatment for AIDS patients is only one piece of the puzzle in changing the course of the epidemic in South Africa. Indeed, a major challenge such as the AIDS epidemic will require much more to secure its defeat. AIDS affects almost every aspect of life. The response to the AIDS epidemic has to be commensurate, involving all sectors of society bound together by a common vision. This kind of social movement needs strong leadership at national level – it needs genuine partnerships between civil society, government, the military, the business sector and those infected and affected by HIV/AIDS. This is no small task at the best of times but is particularly so for an issue which shows up the schisms in society so sharply. But it can be achieved – indeed it *has* been achieved in several countries including Uganda. For South Africa, a country which is in the midst of reconstructing a nation from the devastation of apartheid, rising to this challenge has proved elusive. There have been too many other high priorities and distractions in the country and the nation has yet to be singularly focused and concerted in taking up the challenge of mitigating and overcoming this epidemic.

The government's critically important decision to provide antiretroviral treatment creates the opportunity to rebuild bridges and to make one more attempt at turning the tide of this epidemic. Treatment of AIDS in conjunction with a host of prevention strategies such as behaviour change, voluntary counselling and testing, STI diagnosis and treatment, widespread access to male and female condoms, and antiretroviral post-exposure prophylaxis provide the technical tools to control the HIV/AIDS epidemic. On their own, these tools could make a difference to the epidemic but if used in concert with political and national will as part of a broad-based social movement, they can change the course of the HIV/AIDS epidemic in South Africa. For now, these remain great hopes and expectations.

Bibliography

ABDOOL KARIM SS, ABDOOL KARIM Q, BAXTER C. 'Antiretroviral therapy: Challenges and options for South Africa'. *Lancet* 2003; 362: 1499.

ABDOOL KARIM SS, ABDOOL KARIM Q. 'Breaking the silence, one year later: Reflections on the Durban conference'. *AIDS Clinical Care* 2001; 70: 63–65.

CELENTANO DD. 'Sexual and drug risk-related behaviours after initiating highly active antiretroviral therapy among injection drug users'. *AIDS* 2001; 15: 2311–2316.

KASPER T, COETZEE D, LOUIS F, BOULLE A, HILDERBRAND K. 'Demystifying antiretroviral therapy in resource-poor settings'. *Essential Drugs Monitoring* 2003; 32: 20–21.

OSTROW DE, FOX KJ, CHMIEL JS, SILVESTRE A, VISSCHER BR, VANABLE PA, JACOBSON LP, STRATHDEE SA. 'Attitudes towards highly active antiretroviral therapy are associated with sexual risk taking among HIV-infected and uninfected homosexual men'. *AIDS* 2002; 16: 775–780.

Index

A

abacavir (ABC), 446–8, 508 & tab.
abstinence (from sexual acts), 251
aciclovir, 460, 496
acne, nodular, 496
acquired immune response, 120
Acquired ImmunoDeficiency Syndrome (AIDS)
    see AIDS
Acts
    Domestic Violence Act, 159, 161
    Medical Schemes Act (1988), 346
    Medicines Act, 529
    National Health Act (2004), 203, 204
adolescence, 263–4
    lack of access to health services, 276
    sexual decision-making process, 274–5
    see also young men; young women; youth
adoption, 363
adult mortality (45q15), 420
    see also deaths, AIDS-associated; mortality,
        AIDS-related
aerobic exercise, 468
African National Congress (ANC)
    50th Congress (1997) resolution on AIDS, 377
    HIV policy (pre-1994), 373–4
    A National Plan for Health, 374
    Reconstruction and Development Programme, 374
Agreement on Trade-Related Intellectual Property
    Rights (TRIPS), 530
AID for AIDS (AfA), 346
    HAART patients survival, US/SA comparison,
        480 fig.
AIDS
    deaths (see also deaths, AIDS-associated;
    mortality, AIDS-related)
        'disenfranchised' grief of survivors, 357–8
        projected incidence/prevalence/deaths,
            428 fig., 558–9 & fig.
    early cases (1981), 32
    economic impact, 405
    estimated costs to SA businesses, 413 tab.
    geographic spread in South Africa, 34 fig.

losses of skilled workers, 409–10
macroeconomic impact, 408–11
microeconomic impact, 415–17
mitigating measures for households, 417
mortality rates, 337, 420–1 & fig., 422 fig.,
    423–4
'notifiable disease' conflict, 376
    see also HIV infection; HIV/AIDS
AIDS Clinical Trial Group (ACTG)
    076 regimen of zidovine, 187, 385–9
AIDS consortium, 375
AIDS Law Project, 375
AIDS memorial quilts, 352, 367–8
AIDS Programme of the National Progressive
    Primary Health Care Network (NPPHCN), 35
AIDS Training, Information and Counselling
    Centres (ATICCS), 35, 170
AIDSVAX B/B trial results, 231
albendazole, 495
alcohol consumption
    effect on adherence to HAART, 515
    sex workers, 287–8 & tab., 290
Alexandra AIDS Orphan Project
    'Go-go grannies' initiative, 361
Alma Ata conference (1978), 525
amoxycillin, 496
amphetamines, 218
amprenavir (AMP), 510 tab.
anaemia, 471
anal sex, 249, 257, 277, 287 tab., 289, 290, 293
    & tab.
Angell, Marcia, 386, 392–4, 396
antenatal clinic surveys
    HIV prevalence/ages, 60 tab., 266–7 & tab.
    Hlabisa health district, Kwa-Zulu-Natal, 53,
        57 tab.
    mathematical model of adult HIV/AIDS,
        554–5 & fig.
    MTB notification rates/HIV prevalence, 435
        & fig., 436 & tab.
    national, annual, anonymous, 52, 61 fig.
    prevalence, 56 tab.

574

Western Cape district-wide, 52
anthropometry, 468
antibiotic resistance, 495
antibodies, 229
antigen presentation, 125–6, 127 & fig.
antigen processing cells (APC), 132
antigens, 125, 126 & fig.
antioxidants, 469
antiretroviral therapy, 45, 79, 82, 226, 481
    access, 380, 411, 501, 568 tab.
    adherence, 484, 504, 514–15
      in Africa, 485–6
    adverse side-effects, 498, 506–7
    changing therapy, 520
    choice of therapy, 515–16
    choices of therapy to be avoided, 516–17
    'drug anarchy', 489–90, 527
    drug resistance mutations, 116–17, 489, 504
    effect on body weight/composition, 466–7
    eligibility for treatment, 515
    generic drugs, 527, 529–30, 546
    government decision to provide
      (8 August 2003), 380, 526, 545, 568
    HIV-1 mutating ability, 111
    HIV-2 infection, 518
    immune reconstitution inflammatory
      syndrome (IRIS), 497–8
    impact estimates of mathematical models,
      557–60 & fig.
    integration of treatment/prevention of
      HIV, 237
    mining industry provision, 309
    mother-to-child HIV transmission prevention,
      187–90 & tab., 191, 400–1
    for MTB/HIV co-infection, 444–5
    national programme, 481–4
    versus nutrition therapy, 540–1
    pregnancy-compatible regimens, 517, 522–3
    as prevention strategy, 237
    primary aim, 506
    procurement problems/delays, 528–9
    resistance, 191
    spillage of drugs, 489–90, 531
    supplied by GRIP to rape survivors, 400
    and TB treatment, 448 tab.
    treatment failure, 520
    'tuberculosis/pregnancy friendly' regimens,
      523

    see also drug resistance; highly active antiretro-
      viral therapy (HAART)
apartheid system, 194
    migrant labour, 300 & fig., 310, 373.
    pervasive poverty legacy, 380–1
    race/gender burden of African women, 255
arginine supplementation, 468
asymptomatic infections, 199, 248
    and HIV transmission, 195
atazanavir (Reyataz), 512
azidothymidine, 544
azithromycin, 526
AZT
    see zidovudine (AZT)

B
bacterial pneumonia, 459 tab.
bacterial sepsis, 494–5
bacterial vaginosis, 195–6, 197 & fig., 198
Barre-Sinoussi, F, 32
bDNA (branched DNA, Bayer), 102, 103–4
Benatar, S, 389
β-carotene, 469
biological mechanisms of HIV transmission, 249,
    250 tab.
blood circulation/lymphatic circulation, 122 fig.
blood donors
    education/exclusion policy, 206
    informed consent, 215
    self-exclusion questionnaire, 206 tab., 209, 211
Blood Safety Policy (1999), 33
    outcome, 208 & fig.–209 & fig., 210 & tab., 212,
      213 & tab.
blood supply, 41
    ALARP (as low as reasonably possible) principle,
      211
    routine screening, 206, 211–12
    safe blood supply, 203, 205
    screening by Enzyme ImmunoAssay (EIA) test
      systems, 33
    screening for HIV-antibodies, 33
    window period of infectivity, 205 & fig., 212
blood transfusion
    legal aspects, 213–15
    recipients infection with AIDS, 33
    risk factor for patients, 211
Body Mass Index (BMI), 465

Boehringer Ingleheim
    generic manufacture licences, 546 (*see also*
    antiretroviral therapy, generic drugs)
boosted protein inhibitors, 510–11
border posts
    condom distribution/education, 310
Boston University School of Public Health Centre
    for International Health (CIH)
    cost of AIDS to businesses, 412–13 *tab.*
Botswana
    MASA stigma problem, 487–8
Brazil
    antiretroviral therapy, 552, 559
breastfeeding
    HIV-1 transmission, 185–7 & *tab.*
    stigma of milk formula provision, 487–8
British HIV Association (BHIVA)
    HIV treatment guidelines, 513, 516
Buffer Gel (microbicide), 234 & *tab.*–235 & *tab.*
Bushbuckridge district, Mpumalanga
    adult mortality rate, 424

C

caesarean section, 187–8, 190
Cameron, Justice E, 375
Candida albicans, 494
Candida krusei, 457, 459 & *tab.*
Candida oesophagitis (OC), 459 *tab.*, 460, 494
candidiasis, 197 & *fig.*, 198
    associated with HIV infection, 237, 339, 457,
        459 & *tab.*, 501
Cape Town
    heroin use, 219–21, 222 & *tab.*
capravirine, 512
Carletonville, Gauteng
    age/gender differences, 61, 62 *fig.*
    age-specific estimates of HIV incidence/
        prevalence, 73 & *tab.*, 74 & *fig.*, 560 & *fig.*
    HIV incidence rates, 67
    HIV infection prevalence, 291, 308
    HIV prevalence/ages of women, 60 *tab.*
    HIV/STI prevalence reduction, 161–3
    migrant labour, 289, 306
    peer education programme, 295
    sentinel site for data collection, 564
    sex workers, 287–8 & *tab.*, 289, 291, 310
    STI prevalence, 196 *tab.*
    see also Mothusimpilo project, Carletonville

Carraguard (microbicide), 234
Cavidi Tech ExaVir LOAD reverse transcriptase
    assay, 105
CCR5 co-receptor, 83
CD3+ T-cells, 124
CD4, 81, 82 *fig.*, 83–5, 87, 456
CD4+ count, 102–3, 129
CD4+ T-cells, 121, 122 *fig.*, 123 & *fig.*, 124 & *fig.*,
    134, 506
CD8+ CTL cells, 130
CD8+ T-cells, 121, 122 *fig.*, 123 & *fig.*, 124 & *fig.*,
    137, 228
    measuring response, 137
cellular immunity, 136
Centers for Disease Control and Prevention (CDC),
    Atlanta, 32, 386–7
Centre for Applied Legal Studies, 375
cerebral toxoplasmosis, 458
cerebrospinal fluid (CSF), 493, 497
cervical carcinoma, screening for, 237
chancroid, 195, 197
'Charter of Rights on HIV', 375
chemoprophylaxis, 440, 451, 454
    development of resistance risk, 457
child prostitiution, 354
child-headed households, 352, 361
children
    AIDS-associated deaths of family members,
        357–8
    as caregivers, 416
    'disenfranchised' grieving, 357–8
    HIV infection/deaths, 184, 340
    HIV positive diseases, 341
    'opportunistic infections', 342
    orphanages/residential care, 361
    peer integration, 359
    recreational facilities, 359
    see also orphans
chimpanzees, 114
chlamydia, 195, 196 *tab.*, 197 & *fig.*, 198, 292 & *tab.*
circulating recombinant forms (CRFs), 110
circumcision, male, 85, 226, 227, 239
clinical trials
    patient-participants' perceptions, 398
    placebo groups, ethics of, 385, 389–92
    researcher/clinician roles, 396–9
    standards of care, 391–2
clonal expansion, 123 & *fig.*, 127, 129

576

commercial polymerase chain-reaction-based assay, 505
Commission on Macroeconomics and Health (2001)
  health investment results in growth, 414
communication
  in sexual decision-making, 274–5, 279–80, 294
communities
  development interventions, 359
  home-based care by communities, 368
  preserving memories, 351–2, 367–8
  provision of essential services interventions, 363–4
community organisation model, 151–2
community organisations
  care/support for HIV/AIDS issues, 358, 368, 570
  child care committees, 362–3
  HIV prevention interventions, 276
community workers/social services, 359, 363–4
condoms, 40
  accessibility, 176–7, 281–2, 572
  barriers to use, 40, 175–6
  contraceptive efficacy, 169
  distribution to migrants, 309, 310
  efficacy, 167–8
  female, 169, 171 & fig., 172, 251
  history/construction, 167
  male, 168–9, 170–1 & fig., 251
  public sector distribution, 170–2 & fig.
  social marketing, 173–4
  targeted distribution, 177–8
  technological improvements, 178–80
  Thailand policy, 156–7, 252, 295
  use, 85, 145 & tab., 166, 197, 251, 263, 269 tab., 271 tab., 272, 295, 570
    linked to clinics' attitudes/availability, 148, 176
    prevalence, 174–5
    and self-esteem of youth, 147
Congress of South African Trade Unions (COSATU)
  HIV policy (pre-1994), 373
Constitution
  children's rights, 360
  social assistance guarantees, 363–4
  women's rights, 255
Constitutional Court
  rights of people with HIV, 375
  ruling to provide nevaripine to reduce MTCT, 380, 544, 568

consumer/treatment advocacy groups, 535
contraception
  practised by young women, 267–8
  use, 272–3
co-receptors, 83–4
cotrimoxazole (trimethoprim-sulfamethoxazole), 440, 451, 455, 460, 493–5, 497
  resistance, 457, 459 tab., 461, 493, 495
Council of International Organizations of Medical Sciences (CIOMS)
  International Ethical Guidelines for Biomedical Research Involving Human Subjects (2002), 391–2, 399
counselling
  voluntary, interactive, 155
  see also voluntary counselling and testing (VCT)
crack cocaine, 218, 288
CRF01_AE, 110
CRF04_cpx, 110
cross-presentation, 126, 127 & fig.
Cryptococcal meningitis (CM), 459 tab., 493, 497, 519
cryptococcosis, 440, 491
Cryptosporidiosis, 459 tab., 495, 519
cultural norms
  see sociocultural norms and values
cutaneous anergy, 436–7
CXCR4 co-receptor, 83
Cyclospora, 495
cysteine, 469
cytokines, 124, 125 & fig.
cytomegalovirus (CMV) pneumonia, 342, 457, 519
cytotoxic T-lymphocytes (CTL), 85, 124 & fig., 133, 228
  measuring activity, 137
  significance in vaccine design, 138
  see also CD8

D

dagga (marijuana), 290
dapsone, 460
de Klerk, FW
  action plan on AIDS, 375
deaths, AIDS-associated
  certification by traditional leaders, 421
  communities' attitudes, 357–8
  grief 'disenfranchisement', 357–8
  statistics interpretation, 421, 556–7 & fig.
  verbal autopsies, 421
  see also mortality

Declaration of Helsinki on Ethical Principles for
    Medical Research Involving Human Subjects,
    385, 390
delaviridine (DLV), 509 *tab.*
Demographic and Health Survey of 1998 (SADHS),
    144–5, 174, 256, 258, 269, 272, 425
dendritic cells (DC), 122, 123 & *fig.*, 126
depression
    effect on adherence to HAART, 515
detection of immunological response to HIV, 92
developing countries
    clinical trial ethics, 387–8
    nutritional interventions for HIV infected, 467
    'standards of care' debate, 390–1
diabetes type 1, 128
diagnostic technology, 92–5
diarrhoea, 342, 458, 495
didactic prevention messages, 155
didanosine, 508 *tab.*, 511, 517
Diffusion of Innovations theory, 156
discrimination phenomenon
    community awareness, 356
    'invisibility' of HIV epidemic (pre-1999), 376
    see also stigma phenomenon
District Health Information System, 532
doctors, junior
    lack of experience/maturity, 499–500
Domestic Violence Act, 159, 161
donovanosis, 197
DOTS (Directly Observed Therapy, Short course),
    449, 451, 477, 481–3
    in HAART implementation, 523
doxycycline, 496
DramAidE programme, 156, 281, 367
dried blood spots (DBS), 96
drug leakage/spillage ('anarchy'), 490, 527
drug resistance, 116–17, 191, 457, 459 *tab.*, 461,
    484–5, 489, 494, 508–10, 520–2
Dual Loyalty Working Group (DLWG)
    *Dual Loyalty & Human Rights in Health
    Professional Practice: Proposed
    Guidelines and Institutional Mechanisms*
    (2003), 395, 401–2
    on MTCT antiretrovirals provision by state, 401
dual technology platform (DTP), 103

E

economic development
    influence of disease, 44, 415
economic marginalisation, 254
economics, 44, 406–7
    comparative data, 407 *tab.*
education
    and HIV prevention interventions, 283
education system
    impact of HIV/AIDS, 414
efavirenz (EFV), 446, 447, 448, 449 *tab.*, 498, 509
    tab., 517, 522
ELISA screening test, 89–90, 93–4, 96, 97, 99, 379
    IgG capture assay, 100
Elispot assay, 137, 229
enfuvirtide (Fuzeon), 512
entry inhibitors, 84 & *fig.*
enzyme-dependent assays, 105
epidemics of disease, changing, 552, 564
epitopes, 125, 126 & *fig.*
Essential Drug List (public health sector), 501,
    525–6, 533
exposed seronegatives
    see highly exposed persistently seronegative
        individuals (HEPS)

F

family structures
    extended family care initiatives, 363–4
    food security, 463–4
    impact of AIDS, 43, 351
    integrated support for families/children, 366 *fig.*
    legal assistance and education, 365
    see also child-headed households; single-parent
        households
Fas-FasL (ligand) interaction, 124
femininity, 253, 259
flow cytometry/intracellular cytokine staining,
    137–8
fluconazole, 457, 460, 494, 497
    resistance, 494
follicular dendritic cells, 130
food hygiene, 454, 458
food-based supplements
    bread flour fortification, 473
    soy/maize-based, 467–8, 473
fosamprenavir, 512
foster care, 362, 365

578   Freire, Paolo, 152

FTC (Emtricitabine) (fluorinated cytidine), 511

funeral costs, 417

fungal infections, 493–4, 496

G

Gallo, R
    isolation of HIV, 32

gamma-interferon enzyme linked immunospot
    (Elispot) assay
    see Elispot assay

gastrointestinal intolerance, 507

Gauteng
    heroin use, 219–21, 222 & tab.
    mother-to-child (PMTCT) transmission
        studies, 53

gender inequality, 41–3, 147, 148, 194, 245, 283,
    313
    access to health services, 248
    determinants of HIV risk/vulnerability, 259,
        489
    Gupta model, 259, 260
    imbalance in power, 246
    sexual decision-making process, 274–5
    young women, 262, 265
    see also men; women

generic drugs
    see antiretroviral therapy, generic drugs

genital ulcer disease (GUD), 195, 197
    and HIV infection, 194–5, 238

genital warts, 195

genotype assays, 521

Ghana
    migration and HIV infection, 305 & tab.

giardiasis, 495

Gilbert's trait, 512

gingivitis, 496

Gini coefficient, 407 tab.

GlaxoSmithKline
    generic manufacture licences, 546

Global Fund against AIDS, tuberculosis and
    malaria, 478, 529, 571

glutamine supplementation, 468

glutathione (GSH), 469

glutathione peroxidase (GSHPX), 469

glycoprotein viral envelope, 79–80

gonorrhoea, 195, 196 tab., 197 & fig., 198, 292 tab.

grandparents
    care of orphans, 351–2, 361
    as primary caregivers, 416

Greater Nelspruit Rape Intervention Project (GRIP)
    free antiretroviral drugs, 400, 542

grief
    'disenfranchisement', 357–8
    traditional practices/customs, 358

Gupta model for reducing HIV risk, 259

H

haemophiliacs
    choice of antiretroviral therapy, 519
    infection with HIV, 33, 203

Hani, Chris, 369, 375

health behaviour theories, 150–1

health care system
    see primary health care facilities; private
        health care sector; public health care
        system

health care workers
    empathetic counselling services, 501–2
    HIV infection due to sexual behaviour, 348
    HIV infection risks, 347–8
    HIV prevalence, 337–8 & tab., 414
    job satisfaction/recognition, 501–2
    needlestick injuries, 347
    shortage of skilled professionals, 484

hepatitis B, 197, 203–4, 442
    choice of antiretroviral therapy, 518
    vaccination, 461

hepatitis C, 203–4
    choice of antiretroviral therapy, 518

heroin, 217–18, 219 & fig., 221, 222 & tab.
    trafficking/sales, 220–1

herpes simplex virus type 2 (HSV-2), 195, 197–8,
    226, 238, 292 tab., 457–9 & tab.
    increased risk of HIV infection, 238, 292 tab.
    seroprevalence, 197
    viral shedding, 195

heterosexual HIV transmission
    gender/age factor, 244, 245 & fig.

highly active antiretroviral therapy (HAART), 45,
    101, 237, 420, 454, 460, 505, 533, 567
    effect on body weight/composition, 466–7
    guideline recommendations for initiation of
        treatment, comparison, 513–14 & tab.
    impact on micronutrient status, 470

implementation challenges, 523
lipodystrophy syndrome, 466–7
resumption of sexual/drug use risk behaviours,
570
see also antiretroviral therapy
highly exposed persistently seronegative (HEPS)
individuals, 130, 133–4, 230
Hillbrow, Johannesburg
brothel-based STI treatment, cost-effectiveness,
296
sex workers, 289
HIV
'ABC' approach to prevention, 250–1
alternative constructs about pathogenesis/
treatment (eg politicians), 487
circulating recombinant forms (CRFs), 110
classification, 109, 110 & *fig.*
diagnosis, 92–4, 533
discrimination based on status, 282
diversification mechanisms, 40, 111–13, 112
fig., 113 *fig.*
drug resistance mutations, 116–17, 489
effect on incidence of STIs, 195
envelope proteins, 79–80
groups/clades, 110–11
immune-driven viral diversity, 40, 131–2
immunodominance, 132
interventions (*see* interventions)
'invisibility' (pre-1999), 376
and migration, in rural areas, 308
mutating ability, 39, 79, 111, 229
origin, 114
political activism, 380
political responses to developing epidemic, 373
recombination, 113 & *fig.*
seroprevalence surveys (1980s), 372–3
spread to/in South Africa, 38, 115–16
STIs as co-factor for transmission, 194–5
subtype distribution in Africa, 114, 115 *tab.*
TB impact on progression, 438
TB susceptibility, 437
traditional constructs of disease
(e.g. witchcraft), 486–7
transmission
biological mechanisms, 249, 250 *tab.*
by blood transfusion, 203–4
risk factor of migration, 298
see also AIDS; HIV infection; HIV/AIDS;
tuberculosis/HIV co-infection (MTB/HIV)

HIV clinical trials
dual loyalties/conflicts of interest, 395–6
ethical dilemmas, 385
use of placebo control groups, 385–92
HIV epidemic
early stage, urban/rural spread, 298
mature stage, rural local spread, 298, 307
HIV infection
age/gender differences, 41, 61, 62 & *fig.*,
63 *fig.*, 560 & *fig.*, 562
anal sex, 287 *tab.*, 289, 290, 293 & *tab.*
antibiotic resistance, 495
bacterial sepsis, 494–5
barriers to appropriate care, 485 *tab.*
cellular immune response, 228–9
chronic diarrhoea, 495
data sources
antenatal clinic surveys, 52–3
mother-to-child transmission (PMTCT)
studies, 53
national workplace survey, 54
population-based surveys, 53–4
sex workers/clients research, 54
dermatological problems, 496
detection of recent infection, 98–100
development pattern, 85, 86 & *fig.*
early primary HIV infection (PHI), 99–100
fungal infections, 493–4, 496
geographical distribution, 34 & *fig.*, 57–8 & *fig.*
HLA influence, 134–5
home-based community care, 359, 500
immune response factor, 139
immunisation, 461–2
immunosuppression, 129, 342, 456
impact on families, 347, 352–4
impact on health services, 336–9 (*see also*
individual health sectors (e.g. public,
private))
malnutrition, 464–6 & *fig.* (see also micronutrients; nutrition as therapy)
monitoring disease progression/antiretroviral
therapy responses, 102–5
natural resistance, alternative mechanisms,
135–6
neutralising antibodies, 86 & *fig.*, 87–8
opportunistic infections, prevention, 454
(*see also* opportunistic infections)
oral problems, 496
oxidative stress, 469–70

580

palliative care, 499–500
per-contact risk estimates, 250 *tab.*
persistence/antigen overload, 131
population dynamics model, 49 *& fig.*
prevalence, 246 *tab.*, 559 *& fig.*
prevention measures, 154–5, 167–70, 174–80,
    238, 250
prime boost strategy (combination approach),
    231
quality of life, 496
role of HIV viral load in prognosis, 86 *& fig.*
safer sex practice, 458–9
staging, 90–1
supplementation to maintain immunity,
    470–2
surrogate markers of progression, 505
TB preventive therapy, 450
transfusion-associated, 211
transmission risks, 85
viral structure, 80, 81 *& fig.*
wasting syndrome, 464–6, 495, 501
see also HIV/AIDS; tuberculosis/HIV co-infection
    (MTB/HIV)
HIV infection prevention interventions, 41, 252,
    569–71 *& fig.*
accurate, factual information, 279
communication/negotiation skills, 279–80
informed choices, 279
peer education, 280
Targeted AIDS Intervention (boys/young men),
    314–17
targeted at structural causes, 281, 310
HIV myths
among school-going youth, 268
among youth, 272, 279
'virgin cleansing', 149, 258
HIV testing, 39, 90–2
interpretation of results, 97
monitoring quality of testing, 106
technology, 92–5
test type/setting choices, 95
see also individual tests (e.g. ELISA, Western blot)
HIV vaccines, 227
cellular immune responses, 228–9
classes and types, 228 *tab.*
CTL/HLA significance in vaccine design, 138–9
development approaches, 88
envelope vaccine design, 230

humoral immune responses, 229–30
and immunogenicity, 136–7
implications of HIV diversity, 116–17
mucosal immune responses, 230
studies of HEPS sex workers, 133–4
trials, 97–8
and viral load, 136
HIV-1 M group, 109
diversity, 112 *fig.*
HIV-1 subtype B, 104
HIV-1 subtype C, 39, 48, 100
vaccine research, 231–2
HIV-1 subtype E, 99–100
HIV-1 type
antiretroviral drugs and, 111
co-receptors for entry, 83
entry inhibitors, 84 *& fig.*
genetic flow, 80 *& fig.*
immune responses and, 39, 111, 139
sequential interactions of gp120/host cell
    membrane, 84 *& fig.*
T-cell response, 130–1
viral replication, 81, 82 *& fig.*
viral structure, 80, 81 *& fig.*
viral targets, 82
HIV-2 type, 109, 110 *& fig.*
choice of antiretroviral therapy, 518
HIV/AIDS
Department of Health concerns (1994–1999),
    377
integrating gender into programmes, 259
mathematical model, 554–6 *& fig.*
personal account of LB Mboyi, 321–35
political issue (1999–2004), 377
state physicians/irrational state health policies
    conflict, 399–401
stigma/discrimination in community, 356
see also AIDS; HIV infection
HIV/HBV/HVC co-infection, 518
HIVNET 012, 188–9 & tab.
HIV/TB co-infection
see tuberculosis/HIV co-infection (MTB/HIV)
Hlabisa district, KwaZulu-Natal
age-specific estimates of HIV incidence, 73 *& fig.*
antenatal clinic surveys, 53, 57 *tab.*
demographic profile, 300 *& fig.*
HIV infection incidence of antenatal clinic
    attendees, 67, 338

HIV infection prevalence/incidence estimates, 71 & fig., 72 & tab.

HIV prevalence/ages of women, 59 & fig.

hospital admissions increase due to HIV and TB, 338 & tab.–339 & tab.

impact of increased hospital admissions, 344

sentinel site for data collection, 564

STI prevalence, 196 tab.

TB caseload/antenatal HIV infection, 64 & fig.

home-based care (HBC) programmes, 359, 500

homosexuals

diagnosed with AIDS, 33, 115

household economic impact assessments, 415–16

impoverishment due to AIDS, 416

HSV-2

see herpes simplex virus type 2 (HSV-2)

Human Development Index (UN), 407 tab.

human leukocyte antigen (HLA) system, 128, 134–5

peptide-binding, 139

significance in vaccine design, 138–9

human papillomavirus, 197

human T-lymphotropic virus type III (HTLV-III), 32

humoral immunity, 136, 229–30

hypoxia, 493

I

ICC assay, 229

icthyosis (dry skin), 496

identification of virus, 92

IFN(ELISPOT assay), 137, 229

immune reconstitution inflammatory syndrome (IRIS), 433, 444–5, 497–8, 519

patient reassurance, 498

immune responses, 119–20, 128–9

cellular, 228–9

humeral, 229–30

and micronutrients, 470

mucosal, 230

prime-boost strategy, 231

immune system anatomy, 121, 122 & fig.–125 & fig.

HIV-1 infection, 129–30

immunodominance, 132

incidence rates of infection, 51 & fig., 67

cohort studies, 68

estimates for antenatal clinic attendees, 70 & tab.

laboratory techniques, 68–9

mathematical/statistical estimating methods, 68, 558–9 & fig.

versus prevalence of infection, 74

indinavir (IDV), 510 tab., 517

infant mortality rate (IMR), 419

influenza vaccination, 462

ING Barings

impact of AIDS prediction, 409

Inkatha Freedom Party (IFP), 381

innate immune response, 120

insect bites, 496

Institute for Democracy (Idasa), 411

International AIDS Conference, Barcelona (XIV, 2002), 545

International AIDS Conference, Durban (XIIIth, 2000), 567

President Mbeki's speech, 379

interventions

design, 278 tab., 280

versus programmes, 278

intracytoplasmic cytokine (ICC) assay

see ICC assay

intravenous drug use (IVDU), 41

choice of antiretroviral therapy, 519

effect on adherence to HAART, 515

global report (2004), 244 & fig.

HAART/protease inhibitors (PIS), 470

heroin, 221–2

HIV/hepatitis transmission, 222

needle exchange programmes, 218, 222–3

needle sharing, 217–18, 249

investments

impact of AIDS, 410, 411

loss of confidence in government HIV/AIDS policies, 410

iron deficiency, 471–2

isoniazid, 441–2

Isosporiasis, 459 tab., 495

J

Jochelson, K, 373

K

kaletra, 522

Kaposi's sarcoma, 458–9, 491, 501, 519

screening for, 237

Karim, Salim Abdool, 394

clinical trials in developing countries, 387–9

582

Kericho district tea plantation, Kenya
   productivity study, 413
Klebsiella pneumoniae, 494
KwaZulu-Natal
   age/gender differences, 61, 62 *fig.*
   antenatal clinic surveys, 53
   antenatal women HIV infected, 267
   community-level intervention, 156
   HIV seroprevalence, 305 *tab.*, 306
   mother-to-child (PMTCT) transmission
      studies, 53
   population-based surveys, 53
   promotion of virginity testing, 258
   rural women's rights and customs, 254
   SAFA districts, 316 *fig.*
   sex workers anal sex practice, 257
   sex workers incidence rates, 67
   sex workers/clients, 54
   'Shosholoza Project' (1998), 315

L
lamivudine, 189 *tab.*, 447, 508 & *tab.*
life expectancy (e0), 420
lipid peroxidation, 469
lipodystrophy syndrome, 466–7, 507
London, Alex, 385, 392–4
long-term non-progressors (LTNP), 135
lopinavir (LPV)/ritonavir (RTV), 447, 449 *tab.*, 510–11
LoveLife intervention, 280, 282
lymph nodes, 121, 122 *fig.*, 130
lymphadenopathy-associated virus (LAV), 32, 339
lymphocyte count, 456
lymphocytic interstitial pneumonitis, 491
lymphogranuloma venereum, 197
lymphoma, 519

M
macroeconomics
   impact of AIDS, 408–11
macrophages, 126
major histocompatibility complex (MHC), 128
malaria
   chemoprophylaxis for HIV-infected pregnant
      women, 460–1
   cotrimoxazole resistance, 460
   vector control, 458, 461
Malawi
   health costs, 386

malignant disease
   choice of antiretroviral therapy, 519
malnutrition, 464–5, 466 *fig.*
   role of micronutrients, 468–9 & *fig.*
Mandela Foundation/HSRC population-based
   survey (2002), 53–4
Mandela, Nelson
   HIV prevention resources, 376
Mandrax (methaqualone), 219–20, 288
Masaka study (1994–2000), Uganda, 199
masculinity, 253, 259, 314, 316–17
mastitis, subclinical
   micronutrient deficiencies, 472
mathematical models, 46, 553
   Bayesian techniques, 554
   detailed compartmental models, 554
   Fisher equation, 561
   Markov models, 554
   Monte Carlo methods, 553
mathematical/statistical estimating methods, 68,
   199–200, 212, 237, 256, 257, 310, 428, 553
Mbeki, Thabo, President
   on AIDS and antiretroval therapy, 544–5
   on AIDS and mortality, 379, 544
   on poverty, 381
   presidential AIDS panel, 568
Mboyi, Lilian Benita
   autobiographical account, 43, 321–35
Médecins Sans Frontières, 488, 568
media advocacy theory, 153–4
medical aid industry, 43
   HIV and related diseases benefits, 346–7, 527
   see also private health care sector, managed
      health care programmes
Medical Research Council. Burden of Disease
   Research Unit
   ASSA2000 model, 424
Medical Schemes Act (1988), 346
medicine management cycle, 525 & *fig.*
Medicines Act, 529
Medicines Control Council (MCC)
   registration of medicines delays, 529
   virodene dispute, 376, 539–40
mefloquine, 461
Memory Box Project, 352, 367
   ameliorates 'disenfranchisement of grief', 367
men
   attitude to sexual partners, 314–15

balance of power factor, 246
blame for HIV infection spread, 489
constructive engagement in HIV prevention/
    intervention programmes, 42, 313–15
economic status and migration, 247
expectation of invulnerability, 254
involvement in HIV prevention, 42, 65, 260,
    313
mortality rates/causes, 426 tab., 427 fig.
partner violence, 147–8
social roles/sexual health context, 265–6
variety of sexual partners as cultural norm,
    253, 314–15
who have sex with men (MSM), 133 (see also
    homosexuals)
see also masculinity
Men as Partners intervention, 281
metabolic toxicity, 506–7
methadone programmes, 222, 519
metronidazole, 495, 496
microbicides, 84, 226, 233
    acceptability, 236
    clinical development, 235 & tab.
    mechanism of action, 234 & tab.
    obstacles to development, 235–6
micronutrients, 45
    malabsorption, 471
    and normal immune function, 470
    role in malnutrition, 468–9 & fig.
    role of intervention, 472–3
    supplements to maintain immunity, 470–2
microsporidiosis, 458, 495
migrants/migrant labour system, 42, 63, 149,
    194, 247, 300
    changing patterns, 301
    circular migration and HIV infection, 42, 247,
        299, 307–9, 561
    commercial sex market created, 306
    demographic data, 300 & fig., 561–2
    HIV spread from urban-rural areas, 296, 298,
        299 & fig.
    and HIV/STI incidence/prevalence, 304, 305 tab.,
        306 & tab., 307, 373
    HIV/STI risk of rural partners, 308
    and infectious diseases relationship, 299, 373
    interventions to limit HIV/STI infection
        spread, 309
    mining industry, 302–3

remittances to rural households, 302
    types, 303 & fig., 304
mining industry
    AIDS impact on productivity, 414
    interventions to prevent HIV/STI spread, 309
    TB susceptibility of HIV-positive miners, 437
mitochondrial toxicities, 506–7
mobile populations
    HIV information/education spread, 296
    spread of HIV virus, 296, 298
molecular quantitative viral assays, 505
monkeys, 130
monogamy, 251
Montagnier, L
    isolation of HIV, 32
morphine, 499
mortality
    AIDS-related, 44, 64
        impact on behaviour of survivors, 557–8
            & fig.
        infants (IMR), 419
        mathematical model projections of AIDS
            mortality, 425, 426 tab., 427 fig.–428
            fig., 556–7 & fig., 560 & fig.
    rates, 340 & tab., 419–20
mother-to-child transmission (PMTCT) of HIV-1,
    prevention of, 40, 183, 488, 570
    antiretroviral nevirapine course, 379–80,
        542–4
    antiretroviral treatment choices, 517
    children's morbidity/mortality rates, 340 & tab.
    diagnosis of infection in infant/mother, 101
    early cases (1981), 32
    HAART treatment eligibility, 515
    prevention, 187–90 & tab., 380
    responsibilities of women, 253
    risk factors, 185–7 & tab.
    routes, 184–5 & tab.
    state provision of antiretroviral therapy, 401
    studies, 53, 56, 57 tab.
    UN programme, 191
    see also antenatal clinic surveys; breastfeeding;
        nevirapine
Mothusimpilo project, Carletonville, 143, 152,
    157, 161–3
mouthwash, antiseptic (chlorhexadine), 496
Mpondombili Project, KwaZulu-Natal, 281

MTB/HIV co-infection
    see tuberculosis/HIV co-infection (MTB/HIV)
mucosal immune responses, 230
multi-drug resistance
    HIV, 484–5, 489
    TB (MDR-TB), 440
Mwanza study (1991-1994), Tanzania, 198, 308
Mycobacterium avium intracellularae, 495
Mycobacterium tuberculosis, 433, 455, 456, 495, 497
    danger of re-infecting HIV-infected patients,
        483
    see also tuberculosis (TB); tuberculosis/HIV
        co-infection (MTB/HIV)

N
N-acetylcysteine (NAC), 470
NAMES Project Foundation (1989), 367
National AIDS Conference, Durban (1st, 2003),
    545
National AIDS Convention of South Africa
    (NACOSA), 374, 375
National Essential Drugs Committee (NEDLC),
    526, 533
National Health Act (2004), 203, 204
National Institutes of Health (NIH), 386–7
National Medical and Dental Association
    (NAMDA), 374
National Network on Violence Against Women
    (NNVAW), 159, 161
national poverty eradication strategy, 463, 473
National Progressive Primary Health Care
    Network, 375
National Tuberculosis Control Programme
    DOTS infrastructure, 477, 481–4
needle exchange programmes, 222–3
    state intervention issue, 224
needlestick injuries, 347
negotiation in sexual decision-making, 274–5,
    279–80, 294
nelfinavir (NFV), 510 tab.
Nelson Mandela Human Sciences Research
    Council Survey of 2000 (HSRC survey), 144–5,
    273
    health care workers HIV prevalence, 348
Nelspruit, Mpumalanga
    volunteer charity organisation (GRIP) in
        hospital office, 400

nevirapine (NVP), 82, 446, 449 tab.
    for MTCT, 101, 188–9 & tab., 516, 542–4
    resistance, 191
    side effects, 498, 509 tab.
    women of child-bearing age, 448, 522
Nigerian drug traffickers, 220–1
non-nucleoside reverse transcriptase inhibitors
    (NNRTIS), 82, 446, 496, 504–5, 509 & tab., 521
nonoxynol-9 (n-9) vaginal gel, 234 & tab.
nucleic acid amplification technologies (NAT), 90,
    93, 98, 101
nucleoside reverse transcriptase inhibitors
    (NRTIS), 82, 504, 505, 507–8 & tab., 521
NucliSens HIV-1 QT (Organon Technica), 102–3
nutrition as HIV infection therapy, 540–1

O
opportunistic infections (OI), 45, 454–5 & tab.
    affordability of prevention strategy, 457
    chemoprophylaxis, 459–61
        risks, 457
    choice of antiretroviral therapy, 519, 522–3
    impact of malnutrition, 464–6 & fig.
    prevention strategies, 456–7
        by vaccination, 461–2
    regional differences in epidemiology/
        antimicrobial resistance patterns, 457
    as sentinel sites for data collection, 564
    timing according to CD4 counts, 456 fig.
oral candidiasis, 494, 496, 501
orphans, 40, 65
    adoption, 363
    care and support interventions, 360
    child care committees, 362–3
    cluster foster care, 362
    exploitation, 354
    extended family care, 361
    foster care, 362
    impact of AIDS-related deaths, 351, 353
    importance of peer integration, 359
    orphanages/residential care, 361
    surrogate parents, 362
    see also child-headed households
out-of-school youth, 278, 282
oxihumate-k trials, 540

P

p24 antigen test, 90, 91, 92, 102, 105

P450 enzyme system, 510

Paediatric AIDS Clinical Trials Group
(PACTG)(1994), US
protocol to decrease MTCT (regimen 076), 187,
385

paediatric health care services
estimated costs of HIV/AIDS epidemic, 343,
344 fig.
HIV-prevalence studies, 340–1 & tab.
hospital admission policies, 344, 345 fig.
simultaneous mother/children treatment, 490
see also mother-to-child transmission (PMTCT) of
HIV-1, prevention of

palliative care, 45, 499–500

paradoxical reactions to therapy, 445, 497

passive immunisation, 462

patients
blood transfusion consent, 214–15
human rights, 401–2
informed consent process, 398
perceptions of clinical trials, 396–8

peer education, 280, 309
men/boys, 314, 316

peptide-binding, 139

perforin, 124

peripheral blood mononuclear (PBMNC) cultures,
101

persons living with HIV and AIDS (PLHA) support
group, 359
memory boxes/books, 352, 367

PETRA trial, 188–9 & tab.

pets, 459

Pharmaceutical Management Information
System (PharMIS), 530

phenotype assays, 521

placebo-control groups
use in clinical trials, 385, 389–92

Planned Parenthood Association of South Africa
(PPASA), 170, 172

Plasmodium falciparum malaria, 460
resistance to Fansidar and cotrimoxazole, 461

pneumococcal vaccination, 461

Pneumocystis carinii pneumonia (PCP), 32, 342, 440,
459 tab., 491, 493

Pneumocystis jiroveci
see Pneumocystis carinii pneumonia (PCP)

political disturbances/violence, 194

population serosurveillance, 96–7

population-based surveys
Carletonville/urban population, 54, 62 fig.
Hlabisa district, KwaZulu-Natal, 53
Mandela Foundation/HSRC, 53–4

post-exposure prophylaxis (PEP) programme, 380,
488, 542, 572

poverty
and HIV prevention, 283, 380–2
influence on sexual behaviour, 149–50, 247,
406
and sex work, 247

prednisone, 493, 497

Presidential AIDS Panel (2000), 378–9, 544

President's Emergency Plan for AIDS Relief
(PEPFAR), 571

prevalence of HIV infection, 50 & fig., 51
age/gender differences, 61, 62 & fig., 63 fig.
geographical, 58 & tab.
racial differences, 63 tab.

prevention projects, 151–4, 560
community-level change, 156–7
implementing/evaluating problems, 157–8
personal/interpersonal level change, 154–5

primary caregivers
community support, 358 (see also home-based
care (HBC) programmes)

primary health care facilities
antiretroviral therapy for HIV-infected
patients, 483
availability of condoms, 148
impact of HIV-positive patients, 337, 338
& tab., 345, 348, 478–9 & tab., 480–1
judgemental attitudes of staff, 248
medical staff stress, 501–2
shortage of skilled professionals, 483–4, 498
wellness programmes, 481
youth-friendly services, 276, 282
see also paediatric health care services; private
health care sector; public health care
system

private health care sector, 345
communication with public health care
sector, 531
cost restraints of antiretrovirals, 478–9, 527
HAART treatment adherernce, 515
HIV policies, 346

586

ineffective management of HIV patients, 479
IT resources, 531
managed health care programmes, 346, 527, 531, 535
quality assurance, 535
private sector
impact of AIDS on productivity, 412–14 & tab.
measures to reduce AIDS economic burden, 346–7
PRO 2000, 234 & tab.–235 & tab.
productivity
AIDS impact, 413
programmes
versus interventions, 278
Project RESPECT (USA), 154–5
property rights
widows/orphans, 359
protease enzyme, 520
protease inhibitors (PIS), 446, 504–5, 509–10 & tab.
intravenous drug users on HAART, 470
protease virus, 79
provincial pharmaceutical and therapeutics committees (PTCS), 526, 533
proviral DNA, 81, 92, 101, 113 fig.
pruritic papular eruption (PPE), 496, 497
public health care system, 43
access to antiretroviral therapy, 533–4, 568 tab.
choice of antiretroviral therapy, 522–3, 526–7
communication with private health care sector, 531
Essential Drug List, 501, 525–6
high theft/stock-out levels, 531
hospital admissions policies, 344, 345 fig., 500–1
IT resources lacking, 531–2
laboratory service requirements, 534
national antiretroviral therapy programme, 481–4
nursing personnel upgrade, 535–5
pharmaceutical depots, quality assurance infrastructure, 530
pharmaceutical personnel upgrade, 535–5
procurement of antiretroviral drugs, 528–31
public-private partnerships, 532, 535
quality assurance, 535
secure drug supply, 522–3, 526
skilled professionals requirements/education, 534, 546

Standard Treatment Guidlines (STGs) for Primary Health Care (1996 rev. 1998), 525
see also primary health care facilities; private health care sector

Q

quality assessment, 106
quality assurance, 106
IFN(ELISPOT assay, 137, 229
quality control, 106
quality of life, 496

R

radioactive 51Cr release assay, 137
Rakai study (1994–1998), Uganda, 198, 308
rape survivors
GRIP counselling and assistance, Nelspruit, 400
post-exposure prophylaxis (PEP) programme, 380, 488, 542
rapid HIV test kits, 94–5
reactive oxygen intermediates (ROS), 469–70
recombinant growth hormone, 467
recombination, 113 & fig.
recreational substance use
sex workers, 287–8 & tab.
refugees, 304
regimen 076
see AIDS Clinical Trial Group (ACTG)
Reproductive Health Research Unit
brothel-based STI treatment, cost-effectiveness, 296
reproductive tract infections
and HIV, 194–5
research and development
clinical trials in developing countries: ethical issues, 44, 385–92
conflicts of interest in HIV/AIDS context, 395–6
investment required, 235–6
patient-participants' perceptions, 397–9
role of researcher versus clinician, 396–9
standards of care for clinical trials, 392
respiratory syncitial virus infection, 131
resting energy expenditure (REE), 465
restriction fragment length polymorphism (RFLP) clustering, 436
Retroviridae family
primate infecting lentiviruses, 109
reverse transcriptase (RT) enzyme, 520

reverse transcriptase virus, 79, 113 *fig.*, 505
    assay, 105
rhesus macaque monkeys, 117, 131, 133, 230
rheumatoid arthritis, 128
Rifabutin, 447
rifampicin, 437, 439, 440, 442–3, 446, 449 *tab.*
    compatible antiretroviral regimens, 447–8, 522
ritonavir (RTV), 447, 449 *tab.*, 510 & *tab.*, 511, 522
RNA assays, 81, 91, 92, 93, 99, 101, 102, 103–4
RT-PCR (Roche), 102, 103–4

S

Salmonella bacteraemia, 459 *tab.*
    cotrimoxazole, 460
Salojee, Dr, 401
saquinavir/ritonavir (SQV/RTV), 447, 449 *tab.*, 510
    tab., 522
scabies, 496
schools, 254
    dropouts, orphans as, 354
    and improved sexual health outcomes, 276–7
    institutional climate's effect on risk behaviour,
        148
    keeping youth in school, 282
    Life Skills programme, 280–1
    public sector condom provision, 178
secondary prophylaxis, 459 *tab.*, 460
selenium, 469–70
'self/non-self' concept in immunology, 120
Senegal
    HIV and seasonal migrants, 305 & *tab.*
seroprevalence surveys, 51
serosurveillance, 96–7
severe acute respiratory syndrome (SARS)
    epidemic, 552, 564
Sex Worker Education and Advocacy Taskforce
    (SWEAT), 172, 295
sex workers, 42
    anal sex practice, 257
    condom use, 290
    disempowerment, 294
    and drug trafficking, 220–1
    'dry sex' practice, 291
    HIV risk determinants, 286
    HIV-positive with bacterial STIs, 293 & *tab.*
    HIV/STI prevalence, 287 *tab.*
    illegal status/decriminalisation, 285, 288
    intravenous drug use/HIV infection, 217

mining industry, 285
periodic presumptive treatment of STIs, 199
racial subdivisions, 286–8
recreational drug/alcohol use, 288
STI infection prevalence, 291–2 & *tab.*
at truck stops, 54, 285, 287 *tab.*, 289
    HIV incidence rates, 67
    HIV prevalence/ages, 60 *tab.*
sexual behaviour, 268
    abstinence strategy, 273
    age differences of partners, 256
    age of debut/HIV and STI infection relationship,
        255, 268–70, 271 *tab.*
    coercion of girls, 258, 275, 282
    gender constructs, 245–6, 252–5, 265–6,
        313–14
    initiation before age 15, 274 *tab.*
    safer sex, 458–9, 558 (*see also* sexual risk
        behaviour)
    'secondary abstinence', 273
    self-reporting reliability, 157–8
    violence, 257, 275, 282
    see also young men; young women; youth
sexual power
    unequal distribution between men/women,
        148
sexual risk behaviour, 40, 255–8
    addressing personal/interpersonal influences,
        154–5
    death rate/safe-sex relationship, 558
    effect of institutional climate of schools, 148
    HIV prevention interventions, 154–7
    influencing factors
        distal context, 148–50, 156–7
        personal, 146–7, 154–5
        proximal context, 147–8, 156
    prevalence, 144–6 & *tab.*
sexually transmitted infections (STIs), 41, 63, 85,
    155, 167–70, 570, 572
    HIV transmission enhanced, 41, 193–4, 248
        & *fig.*, 291–2 & *tab.*
    prevalence, 196–8 & *tab.*, 560
    prevention treatment for sex workers, 295–6
    treatment/effect on HIV incidence, 198–200
    see also individual STIs (e.g. bacterial vaginitis,
        gonorrhoea, syphilis)
shingles, 496

588

simian immunodeficiency viruses (SIV), 110, 112
  fig., 230
Simple/Rapid Assays, 89–90
Singer, P, 389
single-parent households
  headed by grandparent, 351–2
  headed by women, 352
  'skipped generation' households, 352–3
single-platform technologies (SPT), 103
skin rashes, 498
smear-negative tuberculosis (SNTB) diagnosis,
  491–2 & *tab.*
social capital theory, 152–3
social grants, 365
social marginalisation, 254
  influence on sexual behaviour, 149
Society for Family Health, 172
  social marketing of condoms, 173
sociocultural norms and values, 148, 277
  about sexual expression, 265
  interventions to address stigma/discrimination,
    356–7
  men precluded from reproductive
    responsibilities, 316
  orphans, 353
  virginity, 277
  widows, 353
  women, 253, 254
  youth, 277, 283
socioeconomic conditions and STIs, 194
Soul City Institute for Health and Development
  Communication
  evidence of positive influence, 160–1
  project to reduce sexual risk behaviour, 143,
    154, 157, 158–61
South Africa
  AIDS policy (1981–1994), 34–5, 46, 373–5
  AIDS policy (1994–1999), 46, 375–6, 539
  AIDS policy (1999–2004), 35, 44, 170, 377–9,
    538, 540–6
  HIV infection statistics, 54, 55 & *fig.*, 56 & *tab.*,
    57 & *tab.*
  Patents Act, TRIPS compliant, 530
  production sectors/economic activity (2001),
    412 *tab.*
South Africa. Department of Health
  Annual Report (2004), 380

Essential Drug List (public health sector), 501,
  525–6
*Guidelines for Good Practice in the Conduct of
  Clinical Trials in Human Participants in South
  Africa (Clinical Trials Guidelines/*CTG), 389
national antiretroviral rollout plan, 545
National Drug Policy (1996), 534
national nutritional guidelines, 473
National Treatment Plan, 484
National Treatment Programme for HIV/AIDS,
  479 & *fig.*
*Policy Guideline for Management of Transmission of
  Human Immuno deficiency Virus (*HIV) *and
  Sexually Transmitted Infections in Sexual
  Assault,* 526
*Policy to Protect the Safety of the Blood Supply
  against the* HIV/AIDS *Pandemic (2000),* 204,
  213
*Policy with regard to Blood Transfusion in South
  Africa (1998),* 204, 213
Regulations regarding Blood and Blood Products, 213
Rural Development Plan, 484
'Sarafina 2' controversy, 376
Standard Treatment Guidlines (STGs) for
  Primary Health Care (1996, rev. 1998), 525
*Standards for the Practice of Blood Transfusion in
  South Africa,* 204, 213
see also state health policies
South Africa. Department of Social Development
  Community Driven Model, 366 *fig.*
  grants available, 365
  social services to HIV/AIDS affected people,
    363–4
South Africa. Government Communication and
  Information Services (GCIS)
  Towards a 10-Year Review (2003), 372, 380
South Africa. Government of National Unity (GNU)
  (1994–1999), 375
South African AIDS Vaccine Initiative (SAAVI),
  231–2
South African Budget Review (2000)
  HIV/AIDS epidemic coverage, 410
South African Health Workers Congress
  (SAHWCO), 374
South African Intrapartum Nevirapine Trial
  (SAINT), 188–9 & *tab.*
South African Medical Journal
  first AIDS report, (1983), 33

South African National Blood Transfusion Service (SANBS), 204–5
  Blood Safety Policy, 207–10 & fig.
  Clinical Guidelines on the appropriate Use of Blood, 215
  quality management system, 212
South African National Guidelines
  TB treatment regimen, 440
South African National TB Control Programme, 450
South African youth
  see youth
Southern African HIV Clinicians Society
  guidelines, 442–3, 478–9 & tab., 513, 516
  preferential pricing arrangements, 479, 528
specificity (in immunity), 125, 126 & fig.
spillage (of antiretroviral drugs)
  drug black market, 489–90
spondalysing ankylosis, 128
SQV/r, 447–8
Standard Bank workshop on economic implications of AIDS (2002), 410
Standard Treatment Guidlines (TGSs) for Primary Health Care (1996, rev. 1998), 525
standardised algorithm for recent HIV seroconversion (STARHS or 'detuned' ELISA), 68–9, 99
Staphylococcus aureus, 494
state health policies
  health professional's responsibilities, 401–2
  irrational/unreasonable health policies, 399–400
  procurement of antiretroviral drugs, 528–31
stavudine, 447, 508 tab., 517
Stepping Stones programme, 281
Stevens-Johnson syndrome, 498
stigma phenomenon, 354–5, 366, 570
  attached to milk formula provision, 487–8
  community awareness, 356
  and drug 'leakage', 490
  'invisibility' of HIV epidemic (pre-1999), 376
  preventing HIV infected from accessing services, 487–8
street children, 354
Streptococcus pneumoniae, 456, 494
  cotrimoxazole resistance, 460
  multiple antibiotic-resistance, 457
structural interventions
  rural development/job creation, 310

single-sex housing/family-friendly environments, 310
subsistence farming
  impact of HIV/AIDS on production, 413
  impact of HIV/AIDS on rural women, 353
sulfadoxine-pyrimethamine (Fansidar), 461
supplements
  see food-based supplements; micronutrients
syndromic management, 197, 198
syphilis, 195, 196 tab., 197 & fig., 198, 292 tab.
syringe exchange programmes
  see needle exchange programmes

T
T20 or enfuvirtide (Fuzeon), 512
Targeted AIDS Intervention (TAI)
  'Inkunzi Isematholeni' project, 315
  intervention with boys, 314–17
  'Shosholoza Project' (1998), 315
T-cell receptor (TCR), 127
T-cells, 121, 122 fig., 123 & fig., 124 & fig.
Teaching Men to Care intervention, 281
teenage pregnancy, 256–7, 263
tenofovir disoproxil fumarate (Viread), 511
Thailand
  100% Condom Programme, 156–7
  sex worker condom policy, 252, 295, 552
thymus gland, 121, 506
Toxoplasma gondii, 458, 459
toxoplasmosis, 457, 459 tab.
traditional healers
  death certification, 421
  HIV infected patients, 487
  HIV prevention interventions, 178
  traditional medicine research, 536
Treatment Action Campaign (TAC), 377
  nevirapine for MTCT, legal action, 543–4
  political activism around HIV, 380, 545
pressure to allow manufacture of generics, 546
treatment literacy, 546
treatment advocacy groups, 535
treatment failure, 520
Triangle Project, 172
trichomoniasis, 195–6, 197 & fig., 198, 292 & tab.
triglycerides, medium-chain, 467
trimethoprim-sulfamethoxazole
  see cotrimoxazole
triple combination therapy, 505, 517, 523

590 trizivir, 447

truck stops, KwaZulu-Natal
Du Cohort, 289–90
sex workers, 285, 287 tab., 289
STI/HIV infection incidence, 291–2 & tab.
truck drivers, prevalence of HIV infection, 293
& tab.

Tshabalala-Msimang, Manto
antiretroviral therapy controversy, 545
nevarapine therapy for MTCT debate, 542–4
nutrition therapy controversy, 540–1

tuberculin skin test (TST), 436, 441

tuberculosis (TB), 64 & fig., 481
adherence to treatment, problems, 486
ART/TB treatment benefits, 448 tab.
associated with HIV infection, 237, 336, 339,
433, 460, 552, 564
DOTS (Directly Observed Therapy, Short course),
449, 481–3
hospital admissions in Hlabisa district, 338
mortality rates, 422, 434
multi-drug resistant TB (MDR-TB), 440–1
prevention, 454, 458, 460
recurrent, 437
reducing reactivation risk, 450, 457
reducing transmission, 450
as sentinel sites for data collection, 564
vitamin supplementation, 471–2
see also MTB/HIV co-infection

tuberculosis/HIV co-infection (MTB/HIV), 45
antiretroviral therapy, 444–9 & tab., 451, 522–3
chemoprophylaxis, 440, 451, 454
clinical presentation/diagnosis, 438–9
immune reconstitution inflammatory
syndrome (IRIS), 433, 444–5
impact of malnutrition, 463
incidence, 434 & tab.
infectiousness, 438
integrating treatment programmes, 446
mortality, 440
paradoxical reactions to therapy, 445, 497
as sentinel sites for data collection, 564
smear-negative (SNTB), 491
TB preventive therapy, 441–3 & fig.
weight loss/BMI, 465

U

Uganda
first sex age/HIV infection decline relationship,
273
heterosexual transmission of HIV study (1997),
396–7
HIV infection in migrants, 305 & tab.
HIV prevalence, 50 & fig., 552, 572
range of HIV interventions, 252

Ukraine
HIV infections, 217

ultrasensitive p24 antigen assay (UPTA), 102

Umkhanyakude (Mtubatuba), KwaZulu-Natal
adult mortality rate, 424

UNAIDS Col-1492 Phase III microbicide trial
cohort of sex workers, 67, 68, 69 & tab.

under five mortality rate (U5MR), 420

United Democratic Front (UDC)
HIV policy (pre-1994), 373

United Nations Program on Acquired
Immunodeficiency Syndrome (UNAIDS)
2004 report on global HIV/AIDS: transmission
modes, 244 & fig.
global heterosexual component of HIV
infection (2003), 243
stigma/discrimination interventions, 356
youth behaviour change interventions, 278–9

United States (US)
policy to decrease MTCT (076 regimen), 191
sponsor of studies to reduce MTCT, 386–7

United States (US). Department of Health and
Social Services (USDHSS)
HIV treatment guidelines, 513, 516

United States (US). National Bioethics Advisory
Commission (NABC)
clinical trial patient-participants, 398
Ethical and Policy Issues in International Research:
Clinical Trials in Developing Countries (2001),
390

University of Cape Town
HIV vaccine research, 232

University of Pretoria
virodene dispute, 376

University of Stellenbosch
HIV vaccine research, 232

University of Stellenbosch. Bureau for Economic
Research
economic impact of AIDS, 409

University of Witwatersrand. Centre for Health Policy, 408
urethritis, 195

V

vaginal diaphragms
    HIV prevention, 180
vaginal microbicides, 236
valcyclovir, and HSV-2 transmission, 238
varicella zoster virus, 496
VaxGen trial results, 231
VCT Efficacy Study (Tanzania, Kenya, Trinidad), 155
VEE (Alphavax) adeno-associated virus, 232
Venezuelan Equine Encephalitis, 227, 232
verbal autopsies, 421
Videx EC, 511
violence, 257, 275, 282
viral diversity, immune-driven, 131–2
viral load assays, 102
virginity
    sociocultural norms, 277
    testing, 258, 277
Virodene dispute, 376, 539–40
vitamin A, 470
vitamin B12, 472
vitamin C, 469
vitamin E, 469
voluntary counselling and testing (VCT), 155, 237, 282, 355, 481, 488, 570, 572
    for HIV symptomatic individuals, 515
von Mollendorff, Dr Thys, 400

W

water supplies, safe, 454, 457–8
weight loss (wasting syndrome), 45, 464–6, 495
    effect of nutritional intervention, 467–8
welfare provision, impacts of AIDS, 414
Welkom, Free State
    sex worker STI prevention intervention, 309–10
Wellconal (dipipanone) 'pinks', 218–19
wellness programmes, 481
West Africa
    AZT/nevirapine trials, 189–90 & tab.
Western Blot (WB) confirmatory test, 90, 91, 92
Western Cape
    antenatal clinic surveys, 52
    antiretroviral therapy availability, 546, 568
    condom distribution, 172–3

HIV incidence rates, 67
Western Province Blood Transfusion Service, 204
wills
    education for AIDS affected, 365
women
    anal sex, 249, 277
    childbearing age
        antiretroviral therapy choice, 517, 522–3
        MTB/HIV co-infection therapy, 448
    economic status and HIV infection risk, 247
    empowering through life skills, 274–5, 279–80, 294
    empowering through microbicide use, 233, 236
    fear of violence and HIV infection risk, 258
    gender inequality, 42, 489
    HIV infection prevalence, 246 tab.
    HIV/AIDS burden, 313
    migrants, 304
    mortality rates/causes, 426 tab., 427 fig.
    partner violence and HIV infection, 147–8
    risk of acquisition of HIV infection, 245, 259–60
    sexual ignorance as cultural norm, 253
    social milieu for blacks, 254
    see also femininity; mother-to-child transmission (PMTCT); young women
workplace-based surveys, 54
World Health Organisation (WHO)
    Commission on Macroeconomics and Health (2001), 381
    criteria for diagnosis of extra-pulmonary TB, 491
    DOTS initiative, 481–2
    guidelines for children's micronutrient supplementation, 472–3
    guidelines for diagnosis of SNTB, 491
        guidelines for HIV treatment, 513
    pre-qualification process (antiretroviral drugs), 529
    PROTEST initiative to integrate HIV and TB services, 483
    'rational drug use', 533
    strategic framework for reducing MTB/HIV, 450
World Medical Association (WMA). General Assembly
    Declaration of Helsinki, 390, 391

Y

young men, 42
    gender expectations, 316–17
    HIV incidence, 245 & *fig.*
    multiple partners, 263, 270
    sociocultural factors, 265–6, 316
    TAI interventions, 315
    see also masculinity
young women, 42
    abstinence strategy, 273
    age of sexual debut/HIV infection relationship,
        268–70, 271 *tab.*, 560
    contraceptive practices, 267–8
    gender expectations, 316–17
    HIV incidence, 245 & *fig.*, 246, 266–7 & *tab.*
    mortality, 419
    older partners, 263, 266, 270, 275, 562
    sexual coercion, 263, 275, 282
    sexual risks, 267
    vulnerability to HIV infection, 265
    see also femininity; mother-to-child
        transmission (PMTCT) of HIV-1, prevention
        of; women

youth, 42, 263
    access to condoms, 281–2
    HIV prevention interventions, 278–9 & *tab.*
        (*see also* HIV infection prevention
        interventions)
    life skills interventions, 262, 277, 279–80
    out-of-school group, 278, 282
    palliative care, 499–500
    self-esteem, 147
    sexual risk, 264

Z

zalcitabine, 508 *tab.*
zidovudine (AZT), 82, 505, 507–8 & *tab.*, 516
    076 regimen, 187, 385–9
    for MTCT, 101, 189–90 and rifampicin, 446–7
    for TB patients, 447
Zimbabwe
    factory peer-education programmes, 156
    HIV prevalence, 50 & *fig.*
    male factory workers and HIV infection, 305 &
        tab.
    population-based seroprevalence survey, 256
zinc, 471
zoonotic infections, 459